Approxima...

m	ft and in		
1.22	4'0"		
1.23	4'½"		
1.24	4'1"		
1.26	4'1½"	...	5'8"
1.27	4'2"	1.74	5'8½"
1.28	4'2½"	1.75	5'9"
1.29	4'3"	1.76	5'9½"
1.31	4'3½"	1.78	5'10"
1.32	4'4"	1.79	5'10½"
1.33	4'4½"	1.8	5'11"
1.35	4'5"	1.82	5'11½"
1.36	4'5½"		
1.37	4'6"	1.83	6'0"
1.38	4'6½"	1.84	6'½"
1.4	4'7"	1.85	6'1"
1.41	4'7½"	1.87	6'1½"
1.42	4'8"	1.88	6'2"
1.43	4'8½"	1.89	6'2½"
1.45	4'9"	1.9	6'3"
1.46	4'9½"	1.92	6'3½"
1.47	4'10"	1.93	6'4"
1.49	4'10½"	1.94	6'4½"
1.5	4'11"	1.96	6'5"
1.51	4'11½"	1.97	6'5½"
		1.98	6'6"
1.52	5'0"	1.99	6'6½"
1.54	5'½"	2.01	6'7"
1.55	5'1"	2.02	6'7½"
1.56	5'1½"	2.03	6'8"
1.57	5'2"	2.04	6'8½"
1.59	5'2½"	2.06	6'9"
1.6	5'3"	2.07	6'9½"
1.61	5'3½"	2.08	6'10"
1.63	5'4"	2.10	6'10½"
1.64	5'4½"	2.11	6'11"
1.65	5'5"	2.12	6'11½"
1.66	5'5½"	2.13	7'0"
1.68	5'6"		

Adapted with permission from Webster-Gandy J, Madden A, and Holdsworth M (2006). Oxford Handbook of Nutrition. Oxford University Press: Oxford.

OXFORD MEDICAL PUBLICATIONS

Oxford Handbook of
Endocrinology and Diabetes

Published and forthcoming Oxford Handbooks

Oxford Handbook for the Foundation Programme 3e
Oxford Handbook of Acute Medicine 3e
Oxford Handbook of Anaesthesia 3e
Oxford Handbook of Applied Dental Sciences
Oxford Handbook of Cardiology 2e
Oxford Handbook of Clinical and Laboratory Investigation 3e
Oxford Handbook of Clinical Dentistry 5e
Oxford Handbook of Clinical Diagnosis 2e
Oxford Handbook of Clinical Examination and Practical Skills
Oxford Handbook of Clinical Haematology 3e
Oxford Handbook of Clinical Immunology and Allergy 3e
Oxford Handbook of Clinical Medicine – Mini Edition 8e
Oxford Handbook of Clinical Medicine 9e
Oxford Handbook of Clinical Pathology
Oxford Handbook of Clinical Pharmacy 2e
Oxford Handbook of Clinical Rehabilitation 2e
Oxford Handbook of Clinical Specialties 9e
Oxford Handbook of Clinical Surgery 4e
Oxford Handbook of Complementary Medicine
Oxford Handbook of Critical Care 3e
Oxford Handbook of Dental Patient Care
Oxford Handbook of Dialysis 3e
Oxford Handbook of Emergency Medicine 4e
Oxford Handbook of Endocrinology and Diabetes 3e
Oxford Handbook of ENT and Head and Neck Surgery 2e
Oxford Handbook of Epidemiology for Clinicians
Oxford Handbook of Expedition and Wilderness Medicine
Oxford Handbook of Forensic Medicine
Oxford Handbook of Gastroenterology & Hepatology 2e
Oxford Handbook of General Practice 4e
Oxford Handbook of Genetics
Oxford Handbook of Genitourinary Medicine, HIV and AIDS 2e
Oxford Handbook of Geriatric Medicine 2e
Oxford Handbook of Infectious Diseases and Microbiology
Oxford Handbook of Key Clinical Evidence
Oxford Handbook of Medical Dermatology
Oxford Handbook of Medical Imaging
Oxford Handbook of Medical Sciences 2e
Oxford Handbook of Medical Statistics
Oxford Handbook of Neonatology
Oxford Handbook of Nephrology and Hypertension 2e
Oxford Handbook of Neurology 2e
Oxford Handbook of Nutrition and Dietetics 2e
Oxford Handbook of Obstetrics and Gynaecology 3e
Oxford Handbook of Occupational Health 2e
Oxford Handbook of Oncology 3e
Oxford Handbook of Ophthalmology 2e
Oxford Handbook of Oral and Maxillofacial Surgery
Oxford Handbook of Orthopaedics and Trauma
Oxford Handbook of Paediatrics 2e
Oxford Handbook of Pain Management
Oxford Handbook of Palliative Care 2e
Oxford Handbook of Practical Drug Therapy 2e
Oxford Handbook of Pre-Hospital Care
Oxford Handbook of Psychiatry 3e
Oxford Handbook of Public Health Practice 3e
Oxford Handbook of Reproductive Medicine & Family Planning 2e
Oxford Handbook of Respiratory Medicine 2e
Oxford Handbook of Rheumatology 3e
Oxford Handbook of Sport and Exercise Medicine 2e
Handbook of Surgical Consent
Oxford Handbook of Tropical Medicine 4e
Oxford Handbook of Urology 3e

Oxford Handbook of
Endocrinology and Diabetes

Third edition

Edited by

John Wass

Professor of Endocrinology,
Oxford Centre for Diabetes,
Endocrinology and Metabolism (OCDEM),
Oxford, UK

Katharine Owen

Senior Clinical Researcher and Honorary Consultant,
Oxford Centre for Diabetes, Endocrinology and
Metabolism (OCDEM), Oxford, UK

Advisory editor
Helen Turner

Consultant in Endocrinology
Oxford Centre for Diabetes, Endocrinology and
Metabolism (OCDEM), Oxford, UK

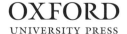

OXFORD
UNIVERSITY PRESS

OXFORD
UNIVERSITY PRESS

Great Clarendon Street, Oxford, OX2 6DP,
United Kingdom

Oxford University Press is a department of the University of Oxford.
It furthers the University's objective of excellence in research, scholarship,
and education by publishing worldwide. Oxford is a registered trade mark of
Oxford University Press in the UK and in certain other countries

First edition published 2002
Second edition published 2009
Third edition published 2014
Reprinted 2015, 2016, 2017, 2018, 2019

Impression: 6

Published in the United States of America by Oxford University Press
198 Madison Avenue, New York, NY 10016, United States of America

British Library Cataloguing in Publication Data
Data available

Library of Congress Control Number: 2013945298

ISBN 978–0–19–964443–8

Printed in China by
C&C Offset Printing Co. Ltd.

Foreword

Introduction to the Handbook of Endocrinology and Diabetes

It is clear that endocrinology is progressing fast and moving far from its original borders. Originally described as the study of the physiology and diseases of the endocrine glands, classical endocrinology encompassed the study of thyroid, hypothalamus, pituitary, adrenals, pancreas, parathyroids and the reproductive glands. Increasingly diabetes and metabolism are recognised as overwhelming issues, which are responsible for world epidemics with an enormous human and financial cost. Thus, lately it has become obvious that the initial definition is too narrow and does not encompass the breadth of the specialty—it needs to be redefined.

The speciality 'endocrinology' should be applied to every area in which hormones act, extending to brain neurohormones, cognition, oncology, and also bone diseases, the cardiovascular system and obesity … where hormones and growth factors interact closely. This new science is closer to the Hormonology that Starling described, than to Endocrinology as defined by Laguesse at the end of the 19th century.

This immense amount of knowledge is well summarised in the third edition of the Oxford Handbook of Endocrinology and Diabetes. Few of us have the talent of John Wass and Katharine Owen, and Helen Turner contributed to earlier editions. They have summarised with their colleagues, in an extensive though concise manner, our incredible specialty. This specialty develops every day and continues to rule our behaviours and diseases.

This Handbook of Endocrinology and Diabetes is a must for all physicians interested in hormones and related diseases, and in medicine in general.

Philippe Bouchard
President, European Society of Endocrinology
Member of the National Academy of Medicine

Preface to the second edition

The first edition of this handbook was well received and sold many copies. We were told by a number of specialist registrars in training and consultants that it was essential to have it in outpatients. We hope that the same will be true of the second edition.

Endocrinology remains the most exciting of specialties—enormously varied in presentation and management and with the ability to affect hugely and beneficially the quality of life over a long period of time. Our aims with this second edition remain the same, mainly to have a pocket handbook which can be easily transported in which all the pieces of information one so often needs are there as a reminder. We hope it will enable trainees to enhance their knowledge but also the older and so-called 'trained' will continue to have recourse to its pages when memory lapses occur. We regard it too as a companion to the *Oxford Textbook of Endocrinology and Diabetes*.

We are enormously indebted to our contributors who once again have provided timely texts full of practical detail. We are also hugely grateful to our external referees who have looked at all the chapters with great care and attention. Both have ensured that the text is as up-to-date as possible. As always we welcome comments for future editions and we hope this one proves as useful as the first one.

John A.H. Wass
Helen E. Turner
2009

Preface

We remain happy that this handbook has been well received both in its first and second editions. It has been translated into Chinese, and there is also an American version which has sold well. We want it to remain essential for specialist registrars in training and consultants who may have the occasional memory lapse.

Our subject remains one of the most exciting of the specialties; our aims with this third edition remain the same—to have, within a small volume, all the essential information that one needs to look after patients with endocrine problems and diabetes.

It is also an accompaniment to the Oxford Textbook of Endocrinology and Diabetes which has recently been published in its second edition (2011).

For this edition, we have completely revamped the diabetes section, and we hope and think that this has been made more readily accessible and assimilable.

We are enormously indebted to our contributors who have provided expertise and willing collaboration with our project. As always, we welcome comments which may enhance the next edition.

John Wass and Katharine Owen
2013

Contents

Contributors

Ramzi Ajjan
Senior Lecturer and Consultant
in Diabetes and Endocrinology,
Division of Cardiovascular and
Diabetes Research, The LIGHT
Laboratories, University of
Leeds, UK

Asif Ali
Consultant Physician (Diabetes
and Endocrinology), Department
of Medicine, Milton Keynes
Hospital, UK

Wiebke Arlt
Professor of Medicine and Head
of the Centre for Endocrinology,
Diabetes and Metabolism,
University of Birmingham, UK

Rudy Bilous
Professor of Clinical Medicine,
Academic Centre, James
Cook University Hospital,
Middlesbrough, UK

Pratik Choudhary
Senior Lecturer/Consultant,
Department of Diabetes and
Nutritional Sciences, The School
of Medicine, Kings College
London, UK

Peter Clayton
Professor of Child Health &
Paediatric Endocrinology;
Director, NIHR Greater
Manchester, Lancashire & South
Cumbria Medicines for Children
Research Network, University of
Manchester, UK

Gerard Conway
Clinical Lead in Endocrinology
and Diabetes, Department of
Endocrinology, University College
London Hospitals, UK

Ketan Dhatariya
Consultant in Diabetes,
Endocrinology and General
Medicine, Elsie Bertram Diabetes
Centre, Norfolk and Norwich
University Hospitals NHS
Foundation Trust, Norwich, UK

Julie Edge
Consultant in Paediatric Diabetes,
Oxford Children's Hospital, John
Radcliffe Hospital, Oxford, UK

Nick Finer
Consultant Metabolic Physician,
Centre for Weight Loss, Metabolic
and Endocrine Surgery, University
College London Hospitals, UK

Neil Gittoes
Consultant Endocrinologist and
Associate Medical Director,
Queen Elizabeth Hospital,
Birmingham, UK

Steve Gough
Professor of Diabetes
and Consultant Physician,
Oxford Centre for Diabetes,
Endocrinology and Metabolism
(OCDEM), Churchill Hospital,
Oxford, UK

Maggie Hammersley
Consultant Physician and Senior
Clinical Lecturer, John Radcliffe
Hospital, Oxford, UK

Niki Karavitaki
Consultant Endocrinologist,
Oxford Centre for Diabetes,
Endocrinology and Metabolism
(OCDEM), Churchill Hospital,
Oxford, UK

Fredrik Karpe
Professor of Metabolic Medicine,
Honorary Consultant Physician,
Oxford Centre for Diabetes,
Endocrinology and Metabolism
(OCDEM), Churchill Hospital,
Oxford, UK

Kim Lambert
Specialist Registrar, Wessex
Deanery, Winchester, UK

Alistair Lumb
Locum Consultant Physician,
Buckinghamshire Healthcare NHS
Trust, Aylesbury, Bucks, UK

Niki Meston
Consultant Chemical Pathologist,
Epsom and St Helier University
Hospitals NHS Trust, Surrey, UK

Helen Murphy
Senior Research Associate
Honorary Consultant, Department
of Clinical Biochemistry,
Addenbrooke's Hospital,
Cambridge, UK

Catherine Nelson-Piercy
Consultant Obstetric Physician,
Department of Obstetrics,
Guys and St Thomas' Hospitals,
London, UK

Sankalpa Neupane
Wolfson Diabetes and Endocrine
Clinic, Institute of Metabolic
Science, Addenbrooke's Hospital,
Cambridge, UK

Shwe Zin Chit Pan
Wolfson Diabetes and Endocrine
Clinic, Institute of Metabolic
Science, Addenbrooke's Hospital,
Cambridge, UK

Peter Scanlon
Consultant Ophthalmologist,
Gloucestershire and Oxford
Eye Units; Medical Tutor and
Senior Research Fellow, Harris
Manchester College, University
of Oxford; Visiting Professor
of Medical Ophthalmology,
University of Bedfordshire, and
Hertfordshire Postgraduate
Medical School, UK

Gary Tan
Consultant Diabetologist,
Oxford Centre for Diabetes,
Endocrinology & Metabolism
(OCDEM), Churchill Hospital, UK

Solomon Tesfaye
Professor of Diabetic Medicine,
Royal Hallamshire Hospital,
Sheffield, UK

Gaya Thanabalasingham
Specialist Registrar, Oxford
Centre for Diabetes,
Endocrinology and Metabolism
(OCDEM), Churchill Hospital,
Oxford, UK

Mark Vanderpump
Consultant Physician and
Honorary Senior Lecturer in
Diabetes and Endocrinology,
Royal Free Hampstead NHS
Trust, UK

Contributors to the second edition

Julian Barth
Consultant in Chemical Pathology and Metabolic Medicine, Leeds General Infirmary, Leeds, UK

Karin Bradley
Consultant Physician and Endocrinologist, Bristol Royal Infirmary and Honorary Senior Clinical Lecturer, University of Bristol, Bristol, UK

Emma Duncan
Consultant Endocrinologist, Princess Alexandra Hospital Senior Lecturer, University of Queensland, Austalia; Postdoctoral Research Fellow, UQ Diamantina Institute for Cancer, Immunology and Metabolic Medicine, Australia

Pam Dyson
Research Dietician, Oxford University, Oxford, UK

Mohgah Elsheikh
Consultant Endocrinologist, Royal Berkshire Hospital, Reading, UK

Stephen Gardner
Consultant Physician, Buckinghamshire Hospitals NHS Trust, UK

John Newell-Price
Senior Lecturer and Consultant Endocrinologist, University of Sheffield, Royal Hallamshire Hospital, Sheffield, UK

Peter Selby
Consultant Physician and Senior Lecturer in Medicine, Manchester Royal Infirmary, Manchester, UK

Kevin Shotliff
Consultant Physician and Diabetologist, Beta Cell Diabetes Centre, Chelsea and Westminster Hospital, London, UK

Sara Suliman
Specialist Registrar in Diabetes, Endocrinology and Metabolism, and Diabetes UK; Clinical Research Fellow, Oxford Centre for Diabetes, Endocrinology and Metabolism (OCDEM), Churchill Hospital, Oxford, UK

Janet Sumner
Lead Diabetes Specialist Nurse, Churchill Hospital, Oxford, UK

Vivien Thornton-Jones
Lead Endocrine Specialist Nurse, Churchill Hospital, Oxford, UK

Helen E. Turner
Consultant Endocrinologist, Department of Endocrinology, Churchill Hospital, Oxford, UK

John Wong
Consultant Chemical Pathologist, Kingston Hospital, Surrey, UK

Symbols and Abbreviations

📖	cross-reference
~	approximately
↑	increased
↓	decreased
1°	primary
2°	secondary
α	alpha
β	beta
γ	gamma
%	per cent
♀	female
♂	male
+ve	positive
−ve	negative
=	equal to
≡	equivalent to
<	less than
>	more than
≤	less than or equal to
≥	greater than or equal to
°C	degree Celsius
£	pound Sterling
®	registered trademark
►	important
►►	don't dawdle
ACA	adrenocortical adenoma
ACC	adrenocortical carcinoma
ACE	angiotensin-converting enzyme
ACEI	angiotensin-converting enzyme inhibitor
ACR	albumin:creatinine ratio
ACTH	adrenocorticotrophic hormone
AD	autosomal dominant
ADA	American Diabetes Association
ADH	antidiuretic hormone
ADHH	autosomal dominant hypocalcaemic hypercalciuria

aFP	alpha fetoprotein
AGE	advanced glycation end-product
AGHDA	adult growth hormone deficiency assessment
AHC	adrenal hypoplasia congenita
AI	adrenal insufficiency
AIDS	acquired immunodeficiency syndrome
AIH	amiodarone-induced hypothyroidism
AIMAH	ACTH-independent macronodular adrenal hyperplasia
AIT	amiodarone-induced thyrotoxicosis
AITD	autoimmune thyroid disease
alk phos	alkaline phosphatase
ALL	acute lymphoblastic leukaemia
ALP	alkaline phosphatase
ALT	alanine transaminase
a.m.	*ante meridiem* (before noon)
AME	apparent mineralocorticoid excess
AMH	anti-Müllerian hormone
AMN	adrenomyeloneuropathy
AMP	adenosine monophosphate
AN	autonomic neuropathy
ANCA	anti-neutrophil cytoplasmic antibody
APS	autoimmune polyglandular syndrome
AR	autosomal recessive
ARB	angiotensin II receptor blocker
ART	assisted reproductive technique
AST	aspartate transaminase
ATD	antithyroid drug
ATP	adenosine triphosphate
AVP	arginine vasopressin
AVS	adrenal vein sampling
bd	*bis in die* (twice daily)
BMD	bone mineral density
BMI	body mass index
BP	blood pressure
bpm	beat per minute
Ca	calcium
CAH	congenital adrenal hyperplasia
CBG	cortisol-binding globulin
CCF	congestive cardiac failure
CEA	carcinoembryonic antigen

CF	cystic fibrosis
CFRD	CF-related diabetes
CGM	continuous glucose monitoring
cGMP	cyclic guanyl monophosphate
cGy	centigray
CHD	coronary heart disease
CHO	carbohydrate
CK	creatine kinase
CKD	chronic kidney disease
CLAH	congenital lipoid adrenal hyperplasia
cm	centimetre
CMV	cytomegalovirus
CNS	central nervous system
COCP	combined oral contraceptive pill
COPD	chronic obstructive pulmonary disease
CPA	cyproterone acetate
CPK	creatine phosphokinase
Cr	creatinine
CRF	chronic renal failure
CRH	corticotrophin-releasing hormone
CRP	C-reactive protein
CSF	cerebrospinal fluid
CSII	continuous subcutaneous insulin infusion
CSMO	'clinically significant' diabetic macular oedema
CSW	cerebral salt wasting
CT	computed tomography
CTLA4	cytotoxic T lymphocyte antigen 4
cv	coefficient of variation
CV	cardiovascular
CVA	cerebrovascular accident
CVD	cardiovascular disease
CVP	central venous pressure
CXR	chest X-ray
DCCT	Diabetes Control and Complications Trial
DCT	distal convoluted tubule
DD	disc diameter
DEXA	dual-energy X-ray absorptiometry
DHEA	dehydroepiandrostenedione
DHEAS	dehydroepiandrostenedione sulphate
DHT	dihydrotestosterone

DI	diabetes insipidus
DIT	diiodotyrosine
DKA	diabetic ketoacidosis
DKD	diabetic kidney disease
dL	decilitre
DM	diabetes mellitus
DME	diabetic macular (o)edema
DN	diabetic neuropathy
DNA	deoxyribonucleic acid
DOC	deoxycorticosterone
DR	diabetic retinopathy
DRIP/TRAP	vitamin D receptor interacting protein/TR-associated protein
DRS	Diabetic Retinopathy Study
DSN	diabetes specialist nurse
DSD	disorders of sexual differentiation; disorders of sex development
DTC	differentiated thyroid cancer
DVA	Driver and Vehicle Agency
DVLA	Driver and Vehicle Licensing Agency
DVT	deep vein thrombosis
DXA	dual-energy absorptiometry
EBRT	external beam radiation therapy
ECF	extracellular fluid
ECG	electrocardiogram
EEG	electroencephalogram
eFPGL	extra-adrenal functional paraganglioma
e.g.	*exempli gratia* (for example)
eGFR	estimated glomerular filtration rate
EM	electron microscopy
EMA	European Medicines Agency
ENaC	epithelial sodium channel
ENETS	European Neuroendocrine Tumour Society
ENSAT	European Network for the Study of Adrenal Tumours
ENT	ear, nose, and throat
EOSS	Edmonton Obesity Staging System
ER	(o)estrogen receptor
ERT	(o)estrogen replacement therapy
ESR	erythrocyte sedimentation rate
ESRD	end-stage renal disease
ESRF	end-stage renal failure

ETDRS	Early Treatment of Diabetic Retinopathy Study
EUA	examination under anaesthesia
FAI	free androgen index
FAZ	foveal avascular zone
FBC	full blood count
FCHL	familial combined hyperlipidaemia
FDA	Food and Drug Administration
FDG	fluorodeoxyglucose
$FeSO_4$	ferrous sulfate
FGD	familial glucocorticoid deficiency
FGFR1	fibroblast growth factor receptor 1
FH	familial hypercholesterolaemia
FHH	familial hypocalciuric hypercalcaemia
FIHP	familial isolated hyperparathyroidism
FMTC	familial medullary thyroid carcinoma
FNA	fine needle aspiration
FNAC	fine needle aspiration cytology
FRIII	fixed-rate intravenous insulin infusion
FSH	follicle-stimulating hormone
FT_3	free tri-iodothyronine
FT_4	free thyroxine
FTC	follicular thyroid carcinoma
5FU	5-fluorouracil
g	gram
GAD	glutamic acid decarboxylase
GAG	glycosaminoglycan
GBM	glomerular basement membrane
GBq	giga becquerel
GC	glucocorticoid
GCK	glucokinase
GCS	Glasgow coma score
GDM	gestational diabetes mellitus
GDP	guanosine diphosphate
GEP	gastroenteropancreatic
GFR	glomerular filtration rate
GGT	gamma glutamyl transferase
GH	growth hormone
GHD	growth hormone deficiency
GHDC	growth hormone day curve
GHRH	growth hormone-releasing hormone

GI	gastrointestinal; glycaemic index
GIFT	gamete intrafallopian transfer
GIP	gastric intestinal polypeptide
GK	glycerol kinase
GLP-1	glucagon-like peptide-1
GnRH	gonadotrophin-releasing hormone
GO	Graves's orbitopathy
GO-QOL	Graves's Ophthalmopathy Quality of Life
GP	general practitioner
GRA	glucocorticoid-remediable aldosteronism
GRTH	generalized resistance to thyroid hormone
GTF	glucose tolerance factor
GTN	glyceryl trinitrate
GTP	guanyl triphosphate
GTT	glucose tolerance test
GWAS	genome-wide association studies
Gy	Gray
h	hour
HA	hypothalamic amenorrhoea
HAART	highly active antiretroviral therapy
Hb	haemoglobin
HbA1c	glycosylated haemoglobin
hCG	human chorionic gonadotrophin
HCO_3^-	bicarbonate ion
HDL-C	high-density lipoprotein cholesterol
HDU	high dependency unit
HFEA	Human Fertilisation and Embryology Act
hGH	human growth hormone
HH	hypogonadotrophic hypogonadism
HHS	hyperglycaemic hyperosmolar state
HIV	human immunodeficiency virus
HLA	human leukocyte antigen
hMG	human menopausal gonadotrophin
HMG CoA	3-hydroxy-3-methylglutaryl coenzyme A
HNF	hepatocyte nuclear factor
HNPGL	head and neck paraganglioma
HP	hypothalamus/pituitary
HPT	hypothalamo–pituitary–thyroid
HPT-JT	hyperparathyroidism-jaw tumour (syndrome)
HPV	human papillomavirus

HRT	hormone replacement therapy
HSD	11B-hydroxysteroid dehydrogenase
HSG	hysterosalpingography
5-HT2B	5-hydroxytryptamine 2B
HTLV-1	human T lymphotropic virus type 1
HU	Hounsfield unit
HyCoSy	hysterosalpingo-contrast-sonography
Hz	hertz
IADPSG	International Association of the Diabetes and Pregnancy Study Groups
ICA	islet cell antibodies
ICF	intracellular fluid
ICSI	intracytoplasmic sperm injection
IDDM	insulin-dependent diabetes mellitus
IDL	intermediate density lipoprotein
i.e.	*id est* (that is)
IFG	impaired fasting glycaemia
Ig	immunoglobulin
IGF	insulin growth factor
IGT	impaired glucose tolerance
IHD	ischaemic heart disease
IHH	idiopathic hypogonadotropic hypogonadism
IM	intramuscular
IPSS	inferior petrosal sinus sampling
IQ	intelligence quotient
IRMA	intraretinal microvascular abnormalities
ITT	insulin tolerance test
ITU	intensive treatment unit
IU	international unit
IUD	intrauterine contraceptive device
IUGR	intrauterine growth restriction
IUI	intrauterine insemination
IV	intravenous
IVC	inferior vena cava
IVF	*in vitro* fertilization
IVII	intravenous insulin infusion
K^+	potassium ion
kcal	kilocalorie
KCl	potassium chloride
kDa	kilodalton

kg	kilogram
KPD	ketosis-prone diabetes
L	litre
LADA	latent autoimmune diabetes of adulthood
LCAT	lecithin:cholesterol acyltransferase
LDL	low-density lipoprotein
LDL-C	LDL cholesterol
LFT	liver function test
LH	luteinizing hormone
LOH	loss of heterozygosity
Lpa	lipoprotein a
LPL	lipoprotein lipase
LVH	left ventricular hypertrophy
m	metre
MAI	*Mycobacterium avium intracellulare*
MAOI	monoamine oxidase inhibitor
MAPK	mitogen-activated protein kinase
MBq	mega becquerel
MC	mineralocorticoid
MCR1	melanocortin 1 receptor
MDI	multiple dose injection
MDT	multidisciplinary team
MEN	multiple endocrine neoplasia
mg	milligram
Mg	magnesium
MGMT	O-6-methylguanine DNA methyltransferase
mGy	milligray
MHC	major histocompatibility complex
MI	myocardial infarction
MIBG	metaiodobenzylguanidine
min	minute
MIS	Müllerian inhibitory substance
MIT	monoiodotyrosine
mIU	milli international unit
MJ	megajoule
mm	millimetre
mmHg	millimetre of mercury
MMI	methimazole
mmol	millimole
MODY	maturity onset diabetes of the young

mOsm	milliosmole
MPH	mid-parental height
MRI	magnetic resonance imaging
mRNA	messenger ribonucleic acid
MRSA	meticillin-resistant *Staphylococcus aureus*
MSH	melanocyte-stimulating hormone
MSU	midstream urine
mSv	microsievert
MTC	medullary thyroid carcinoma
mTOR	mammalian target of rapamycin
mU	milliunit
Na	sodium
NaCl	sodium chloride
NAFLD	non-alcoholic fatty liver disease
NASH	non-alcoholic steatohepatitis
NaU	urinary sodium
NB	*nota bene* (take note)
NDST	National Diabetes Support Team
NEC	neuroendocrine carcinoma
NEN	neuroendocrine neoplasia
NET	neuroendocrine tumour
NF	neurofibromatosis
NFA	non-functioning pituitary adenoma
ng	nanogram
NG	nasogastric
NHS	National Health Service
NICE	National Institute for Health and Care Excellence
NIDDM	non-insulin-dependent diabetes mellitus
NIS	sodium/iodide symporter
nmol	nanomole
NOGG	National Osteoporosis Guideline Group
NR	normal range
NSAID	non-steroidal anti-inflammatory drug
NSC	National Screening Committee
NSF	National Service Framework
NVD	new vessels on disc
NVE	new vessels elsewhere
O_2	oxygen
OA	osteoarthritis
OCP	oral contraceptive pill

od	*omne in die* (once daily)
OD	overdose
OGTT	oral glucose tolerance test
OHA	oral hypoglycaemic agent
OHSS	ovarian hyperstimulation syndrome
OR	odds ratio
PAI	plasminogen activator inhibitor
PAK	pancreas after kidney
PAL	physical activity level
PAR-Q	physical activity readiness questionnaire
PBC	primary biliary cirrhosis
PCOS	polycystic ovary syndrome
PDE	phosphodiesterase
PDR	proliferative diabetic retinopathy
PE	pulmonary embolism
PEG	polyethylene glycol
PET	positron emission tomography
pg	picogram
PHP	primary hyperparathyroidism
PI	protease inhibitor
PID	pelvic inflammatory disease
PIH	pregnancy-induced hypertension
PKA	protein kinase A
p.m.	*post meridiem* (after noon)
PMC	papillary microcarcinoma
pmol	picomole
PNDM	permanent neonatal diabetes mellitus
PNMT	phenylethanolamine-N-methyltransferase
PO	*per os* (orally)
PO_4	phosphate
POF	premature ovarian failure
POI	premature ovarian insufficiency
POMC	pro-opiomelanocortin
POP	progesterone-only pill
PPI	proton pump inhibitor
PPNAD	primary pigmented nodular adrenal disease
PRA	plasma renin activity
PRH	postprandial reactive hypoglycaemia
PRL	prolactin
PRRT	peptide receptor radioligand therapy

PRTH	pituitary resistance to thyroid hormone
PSA	prostate-specific antigen
PTA	pancreas transplant alone
PTH	parathyroid hormone
PTHrP	parathyroid hormone-related peptide
PTTG	pituitary tumour transforming gene
PTU	propylthiouracil
PUD	peptic ulcer disease
PVD	peripheral vascular disease
QCT	quantitative computed tomography
qds	*quater die sumendus* (four times daily)
QoL	quality of life
RAA	renin–angiotensin–aldosterone
RAI	radioactive iodine
RCAD	renal cysts and diabetes (syndrome)
rhGH	recombinant human growth hormone
rhTSH	recombinant human thyroid-stimulating hormone
RNA	ribonucleic acid
RR	relative risk
RRT	renal replacement therapy
rT3	reverse T3
RTH	resistance to thyroid hormone
s	second
SC	subcutaneous
SD	standard deviation
SDH	succinate dehydrogenase
SERM	selective (o)estrogen receptor modulator
SGA	small for gestational age
SH	severe hypoglycaemia
SHBG	sex hormone-binding globulin
SIADH	syndrome of inappropriate ADH
SLE	systemic lupus erythematosus
SNP	single nucleotide polymorphism
SNRI	serotonin noradrenaline reuptake inhibitor
SPK	simultaneous pancreas kidney
SSA	somatostatin analogue
SSRI	selective serotonin reuptake inhibitor
SST	short Synacthen® test
SSTR	somatostatin receptor
STED	sight-threatening diabetic eye disease

SU	sulphonylurea
T_3	tri-iodothyronine
T_4	thyroxine
TART	testicular adrenal rest tissue
TB	tuberculosis
TBG	thyroid-binding globulin
TBI	traumatic brain injury
TBPA	T_4-binding prealbumin
TC	total cholesterol
TCA	tricyclic antidepressant
TDD	total daily dose
T1DM	type 1 diabetes mellitus
T2DM	type 2 diabetes mellitus
tds	*ter die sumendus* (three times daily)
TENS	transcutaneous electrical nerve stimulation
TFT	thyroid function test
Tg	thyroglobulin
TG	triglyceride
TGF	transforming growth factor
TgAb	thyroglobulin antibody
TK	tyrosine kinase
TKI	tyrosine kinase inhibitor
TNDM	transient neonatal diabetes mellitus
TNF	tumour necrosis factor
TPO	thyroid peroxidase
TR	thyroid hormone receptor
TRE	thyroid hormone response element
TRH	thyrotropin-releasing hormone
TSA	transsphenoidal approach
TSAb	TSH-stimulating antibody
TSG	tumour suppressor gene
TSH	thyroid-stimulating hormone
TSH-RAB	thyroid-stimulating hormone receptor antibodies
TTR	transthyretin
U	unit
U&E	urea and electrolytes
UFC	urinary free cortisol
UK	United Kingdom
UKPDS	United Kingdom Prospective Diabetes Study

US	ultrasound
USA	United States of America
V	volts
VA	visual acuity
VEGF	vascular endothelial growth factor
VEGFR	vascular endothelial growth factor receptor
VHL	von Hippel–Lindau
VIP	vasoactive intestinal polypeptide
VLCFA	very long chain fatty acid
VLDL	very low density lipoprotein
VMA	vanillylmandelic acid
VRIII	variable-rate intravenous insulin infusion
vs	versus
VTE	venous thromboembolism
WBS	whole body scan
WDHA	watery diarrhoea, hypokalaemia, acidosis
WHI	Women's Health Initiative
WHO	World Health Organization
w/v	weight by volume
ZE	Zollinger–Ellison (syndrome)

Chapter 1

Thyroid

Anatomy

The thyroid gland comprises:
- A midline isthmus lying horizontally just below the cricoid cartilage.
- Two lateral lobes that extend upward over the lower half of the thyroid cartilage.

The gland lies deep to the strap muscles of the neck, enclosed in the pre-tracheal fascia, which anchors it to the trachea, so that the thyroid moves up on swallowing.

Histology
- Fibrous septa divide the gland into pseudolobules.
- Pseudolobules are composed of vesicles called follicles or acini, surrounded by a capillary network.
- The follicle walls are lined by cuboidal epithelium.
- The lumen is filled with a proteinaceous colloid, which contains the unique protein thyroglobulin. The peptide sequences of T_4 and T_3 are synthesized and stored as a component of thyroglobulin.

Development
- Develops from the endoderm of the floor of the pharynx with some contribution from the lateral pharyngeal pouches.
- Descent of the midline thyroid precursor gives rise to the thyroglossal duct, which extends from the foramen caecum near the base of the tongue to the isthmus of the thyroid.
- During development, the posterior aspect of the thyroid becomes associated with the parathyroid glands and the parafollicular C cells, derived from the ultimo-branchial body (fourth pharyngeal pouch), which become incorporated into its substance.
- The C cells are the source of calcitonin and give rise to medullary thyroid carcinoma when they undergo malignant transformation.
- The fetal thyroid begins to concentrate and organify iodine at about 10–12 weeks' gestation.
- Maternal TRH readily crosses the placenta; maternal TSH and T_4 do not.
- T_4 from the fetal thyroid is the major thyroid hormone available to the fetus. The fetal pituitary-thyroid axis is a functional unit, distinct from that of the mother—active at 18–20 weeks.

Thyroid examination
Inspection
- Look at the neck from the front. If a goitre (enlarged thyroid gland of whatever cause) is present, the patient should be asked to swallow a mouthful of water. The thyroid moves up with swallowing.
- Assess for scars, asymmetry, or masses.
- Watch for the appearance of any nodule not visible before swallowing; beware that, in an elderly patient with kyphosis, the thyroid may be partially retrosternal.

Palpation (usually from behind)
- Is the thyroid gland tender to touch?
- With the index and middle fingers, feel below the thyroid cartilage where the isthmus of the thyroid gland lies over the trachea.
- Palpate the two lobes of the thyroid, which extend laterally behind the sternomastoid muscle.
- Ask the patient to swallow again while you continue to palpate the thyroid.
- Assess *size*, whether it is *soft, firm or hard,* whether it is *nodular* or *diffusely* enlarged, and whether it *moves* readily on swallowing.
- Palpate along the medial edge of the sternomastoid muscle on either side to look for a pyramidal lobe.
- Palpate for lymph nodes in the neck.

Percussion
Percuss the upper mediastinum for retrosternal goitre.

Auscultation
- Auscultate to identify bruits, consistent with Graves's disease (treated or untreated).
- Occasionally, inspiratory stridor can be heard, with a large or retrosternal goitre causing tracheal compression (📕 see Pemberton's sign, p. 64).

Assess thyroid status
- Observe for signs of thyroid disease—exophthalmos, proptosis, thyroid acropachy, pretibial myxoedema, hyperactivity, restlessness, or whether immobile.
- Take pulse; note the presence or absence of tachycardia, bradycardia, or atrial fibrillation.
- Feel palms—whether warm and sweaty or cold.
- Look for tremor in outstretched hands.
- Examine eyes: exophthalmos (forward protrusion of the eyes—proptosis); lid retraction (sclera visible above cornea); lid lag; conjunctival injection or oedema (chemosis); periorbital oedema; loss of full-range movement.

Physiology

- Biosynthesis of thyroid hormones requires iodine as substrate. Iodine is actively transported via sodium/iodide symporters (NIS) into follicular thyrocytes where it is organified onto tyrosyl residues in thyroglobulin first to produce monoiodotyrosine (MIT) and then diiodotyrosine (DIT). Thyroid peroxidase (TPO) then links two DITs to form the two-ringed structure T_4, and MIT and DIT to form small amounts of T_3 and reverse T_3 (rT_3).
- The thyroid is the only source of T_4.
- The thyroid secretes 20% of circulating T_3; the remainder is generated in extraglandular tissues by the conversion of T_4 to T_3 by deiodinases (largely in the liver and kidneys).

Synthesis of the thyroid hormones can be inhibited by a variety of agents termed *goitrogens*.

- Perchlorate and thiocyanate inhibit iodide transport.
- Thioureas (e.g. carbimazole and propylthiouracil) and mercaptoimidazole inhibit the initial oxidation of iodide and coupling of iodothyronines.
- In large doses, iodine itself blocks organic binding and coupling reactions.
- Lithium has several inhibitory effects on intrathyroidal iodine metabolism.

In the blood, T_4 and T_3 are almost entirely bound to plasma proteins. T_4 is bound in ↓ order of affinity to thyroid-binding globulin (TBG), transthyretin (TTR), and albumin. T_3 is bound 10–20 times less avidly by TBG and not significantly by TTR. Only the free or unbound hormone is available to tissues. The metabolic state correlates more closely with the free than the total hormone concentration in the plasma. The relatively weak binding of T_3 accounts for its more rapid onset and offset of action. Table 1.1 summarizes those states associated with 1° alterations in the concentration of TBG. When there is primarily an alteration in the concentration of thyroid hormones, the concentration of TBG changes little (Table 1.2).

The concentration of free hormones does not necessarily vary directly with that of the total hormones, e.g. while the total T_4 level rises in pregnancy, the free T_4 level remains normal (📖 Endocrinology in pregnancy, p. 426).

The levels of thyroid hormone in the blood are tightly controlled by feedback mechanisms involved in the hypothalamo–pituitary–thyroid (HPT) axis (see Fig. 1.1).

- TSH secreted by the pituitary stimulates the thyroid to secrete principally T_4 and also T_3. TRH stimulates the synthesis and secretion of TSH.
- T_4 and T_3 are bound to TBG, TTR, and albumin. The remaining free hormones inhibit the synthesis and release of TRH and TSH.
- T_4 is converted peripherally to the metabolically active T_3 or the inactive rT_3.
- T_4 and T_3 are metabolized in the liver by conjugation with glucuronate and sulphate. Enzyme inducers, such as phenobarbital, carbamazepine, and phenytoin, increase the metabolic clearance of the hormones without ↓ the proportion of free hormone in the blood.

Table 1.1 Disordered thyroid hormone–protein interactions

	Serum total T_4 and T_3	Free T_4 and T_3
Primary abnormality in TBG		
↑ Concentration	↑	Normal
↓ Concentration	↓	Normal
Primary disorder of thyroid function		
Hyperthyroidism	↑	↑
Hypothyroidism	↓	↓

Table 1.2 Circumstances associated with altered concentration of TBG

↑ TBG	↓ TBG
Pregnancy	Androgens
Newborn state	Large doses of glucocorticoids; Cushing's syndrome
OCP and other sources of oestrogens	Chronic liver disease
Tamoxifen	Severe systemic illness
Hepatitis A; chronic active hepatitis	Active acromegaly
Biliary cirrhosis	Nephrotic syndrome
Acute intermittent porphyria	Genetically determined
Genetically determined	Drugs, e.g. phenytoin (see also Table 1.4, p. 11)

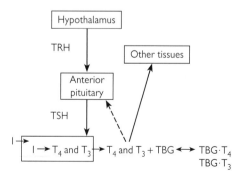

Fig. 1.1 Regulation of thyroid function. Solid arrows indicate stimulation; broken arrow indicates inhibitory influence. TRH, thyrotropin-releasing hormone; TSH, thyroid-stimulating hormone; T_4, thyroxine; T_3, tri-iodothyronine; I, iodine; TBG, thyroid-binding globulin.

Molecular action of thyroid hormone

- T_3 is the active form of thyroid hormone and binds to thyroid hormone receptors (TRs) in target cell nuclei to initiate a range of physiological effects, including cellular differentiation, post-natal development, and metabolic homeostasis. The actions of thyroid hormone are mediated by two genes (TRα, TRβ), which encode three nuclear receptor subtypes with differing tissue expression (TRα1: central nervous system, cardiac and skeletal muscle; TRβ1: liver and kidney; TRβ2: pituitary and hypothalamus).
- Both T_4 and T_3 enter the cell via active transport mediated by monocarboxylate transporter-8 and other proteins. Three iodothyronine deiodinases (D1–3) regulate T_3 availability to target cells. The D1 enzyme in kidney and liver is generally considered to be responsible for the production of the majority of circulating T_3. Although serum T_3 concentrations are maintained constant by the negative feedback actions of the HPT axis, intracellular thyroid status may vary as a result of differential action of deiodinases. In the hypothalamus and pituitary, 5'-deiodination of T_4 by D2 results in the generation of T_3, whereas 5'-deiodination by the D3 enzyme irreversibly inactivates T_4 and T_3, resulting in the production of the metabolites rT_3 and T_2. Thus, the relative activities of D2 and D3 enzymes in T_3 target cells regulate the availability of the active hormone T_3 to the nucleus and ultimately determine the saturation of the nuclear TR.
- TRs belong to the nuclear hormone receptor superfamily and function as ligand-inducible transcription factors. They are expressed in virtually all tissues and involved in many physiological processes in response to T_3 binding. TRα and TRβ receptors bind to specific DNA thyroid hormone response elements (TREs) located in the promoter regions of T_3-responsive target genes and mediate the actions of T_3.
- Unliganded TR (unoccupied TR, ApoTR) inhibits basal transcription of T_3 target genes by interacting preferentially with co-repressor proteins, leading to repression of gene transcription. Upon T_3 binding, the liganded TR undergoes conformational change and reverses the histone deacetylation associated with basal repression. Subsequent recruitment of a large transcription factor complex known as vitamin D receptor interacting protein/TR-associated protein (DRIP/TRAP) leads to binding and stabilization of RNA polymerase II and hormone-dependent activation of transcription.
- The roles of TRα and TRβ have been shown to be tissue-specific. For example, TRα mediates important T_3 actions during heart, bone, and intestinal development and controls basal heart rate and thermoregulation in adults, whilst TRβ mediates T_3 action in the liver and is responsible for the regulation of the HPT axis.

Abnormalities of development

- Remnants of the thyroglossal duct may be found in any position along the course of the tract of its descent:
  - In the tongue, it is referred to as '*lingual thyroid*'.
  - *Thyroglossal cysts* may be visible as midline swellings in the neck.
  - *Thyroglossal fistula* develops as an opening in the middle of the neck.
  - As thyroglossal nodules *or*
  - The '*pyramidal lobe*', a structure contiguous with the thyroid isthmus which extends upwards.
- The gland can descend too far down to reach the anterior mediastinum.
- Congenital hypothyroidism may result from failure of the thyroid to develop (agenesis). More commonly, however, congenital hypothyroidism reflects enzyme defects impairing hormone synthesis.

Further reading

Williams GR, Bassett JH (2011). Deiodinases: the balance of thyroid hormone: local control of thyroid hormone action: role of type 2 deiodinase. *J Endocrinol* **209**, 261–72.

Tests of hormone concentration

- Highly specific and sensitive chemiluminescent and radioimmunoassays are used to measure serum T_4 and T_3 concentrations. Free hormone concentrations usually correlate better with the metabolic state than do total hormone concentrations because they are unaffected by changes in binding protein concentration or affinity.
- See UK guidelines for the use of thyroid function tests. Association for Clinical Biochemistry, British Thyroid Association, British Thyroid Foundation (⅏ http://www.british-thyroid-association.org/info-for-patients/Docs/TFT_guideline_final_version_July_2006.pdf).

Tests of homeostatic control

(See Table 1.3.)

- Serum TSH concentration is used as first line in the diagnosis of 1°
  hypothyroidism and hyperthyroidism. The test is misleading in patients
  with 2° thyroid dysfunction due to hypothalamic/pituitary disease
  (📖 p. 127).
- The TRH stimulation test, which can be used to assess the functional
  state of the TSH secretory mechanism, is now rarely used to diagnose
  1° thyroid disease since it has been superseded by sensitive TSH
  assays. It is of limited use; its main use is in the differential diagnosis
  of elevated TSH in the setting of elevated thyroid hormone levels and
  in the differential diagnosis of resistance to thyroid hormone and a
  TSH-secreting pituitary adenoma (see Box 1.1).

In interpreting results of TFTs, the effects of drugs that the patient might
be on should be borne in mind. Table 1.4 lists the influence of drugs on
TFTs. Table 1.5 sets out some examples of atypical thyroid function tests.

**Box 1.1 Thyroid hormone resistance (RTH) (📖 see also
p. 50)**

- Rare syndrome characterized by reduced responsiveness to elevated
  circulating levels of free T_4 and free T_3, non-suppressed serum TSH,
  and intact TSH responsiveness to TRH.
- Clinical features, apart from goitre, are usually absent but may
  include short stature, hyperactivity, attention deficits, learning
  disability, and goitre.
- Associated with THβ gene defects, and identification by gene
  sequencing can confirm diagnosis in 85%.
- Differential diagnosis includes TSH-secreting pituitary tumour
  (📖 p. 180).
- Most cases require no treatment. If needed, it is usually β-adrenergic
  blockers to ameliorate some of the tissue effects of raised thyroid
  hormone levels.

Table 1.3 Thyroid hormone concentrations in various thyroid abnormalities

Condition	TSH	Free T$_4$	Free T$_3$
1° hyperthyroidism	Undetectable	⬆⬆	⬆
T$_3$ toxicosis	Undetectable	Normal	⬆⬆
Subclinical hyperthyroidism	⬇	Normal	Normal
2° hyperthyroidism (TSHoma)	⬆ or normal	⬆	⬆
Thyroid hormone resistance	⬆ or normal	⬆	⬆
1° hypothyroidism	⬆	⬇	⬇ or normal
Subclinical hypothyroidism	⬆	Normal	Normal
2° hypothyroidism	⬇ or normal	⬇	⬇ or normal

Table 1.4 Influence of drugs on thyroid function tests

Metabolic process	⬆	⬇
TSH secretion	Amiodarone (transiently; becomes normal after 2–3 months) Sertraline St John's wort (Hypericum)	Glucocorticoids, dopamine agonists, phenytoin, dopamine, octreotide, paroxetine
T$_4$ synthesis/release	Iodide, amiodarone, interferon α, lithium	Iodide, amiodarone, interferon alfa, lithium, sunitinib
Binding proteins	Oestrogen, clofibrate, heroin	Glucocorticoids, androgens, phenytoin, carbamazepine
T$_4$ metabolism	Anticonvulsants, rifampicin	
T$_4$/T$_3$ binding in serum	Heparin	Salicylates, furosemide, mefenamic acid

Table 1.5 Atypical thyroid function tests[1]

Test	Possible cause
Suppressed TSH and normal free T_4	T_3 toxicosis (approximately 5% of thyrotoxicosis)
Suppressed TSH and normal free T_4 and free T_3	Subclinical hyperthyroidism Recovery from thyrotoxicosis Excess thyroxine replacement Non-thyroidal illness
Detectable TSH and elevated free T_4 and free T_3	TSH-secreting pituitary tumour Thyroid hormone resistance Heterophile antibodies, leading to spurious measurements of free T_4 and free T_3 Thyroxine replacement therapy (including poor compliance)
Elevated free T_4 and low normal free T_3, normal TSH	Amiodarone
Suppressed or normal TSH and low normal free T_4 and free T_3	Non-thyroidal illness Central hypothyroidism Isolated TSH deficiency

Reference

1. Gurnell M, Halsall DJ, Chatterjee VK (2011). What should be done when thyroid function tests do not make sense? *Clin Endocrinol (Oxf)* **74**, 673–8.

Rare genetic disorders of thyroid hormone metabolism[1]

- An X-linked disorder of childhood onset with psychomotor retardation, including speech and developmental delay and spastic quadriplegia, caused by defects in the MCT8 gene encoding a membrane transporter. Male patients have elevated FT_3, low FT_4, and normal TSH levels.
- The deiodinase enzymes are part of a larger family of 25 human proteins containing selenocysteine. A multisystem selenoprotein deficiency disorder has been identified, manifested by growth retardation in childhood and male infertility, skeletal myopathy, photosensitivity, and hearing loss in adults. Thyroid function tests show raised FT_4, normal/low FT_3, and normal TSH levels due to functional D2 deficiency.

---

[1]Reviewed by Refetoff and Dumitrescu (2007) Syndromes of reduced sensitivity to thyroid hormone: genetic defects in hormone receptors, cell transporters and deiodination. *Best Pract Res Clin Endocrinol Metab* **21**, 277–305.

Antibody screen

High titres of antithyroid peroxidase (anti-TPO) antibodies and/or antithyroglobulin antibodies are found in patients with autoimmune thyroid disease (Hashimoto's thyroiditis, Graves's disease, and sometimes euthyroid individuals). See Table 1.6.

Screening for thyroid disease[1]

The following categories of patients should be screened for thyroid disease:

- Patients with atrial fibrillation or hyperlipidaemia.
- Periodic (6-monthly) assessments in patients receiving amiodarone and lithium.
- Annual check of thyroid function in the annual review of diabetic patients.
- ♀ with type 1 diabetes in the first trimester of pregnancy and post-delivery (because of the 3-fold increase in incidence of post-partum thyroid dysfunction in such patients) (🕮 p. 432).
- ♀ with past history of post-partum thyroiditis.
- Annual check of thyroid function in people with Down's syndrome, Turner's syndrome, and autoimmune Addison's disease, in view of the high prevalence of hypothyroidism in such patients.
- ♀ with thyroid autoantibodies—8× risk of developing hypothyroidism over 20 years compared to antibody −ve controls.
- ♀ with thyroid autoantibodies and isolated elevated TSH—38× risk of developing hypothyroidism, with 4% annual risk of overt hypothyroidism.
- Maternal thyroid antibodies are associated with miscarriage and preterm birth[2].

Table 1.6 Antithyroid antibodies and thyroid disease

Condition	Anti-TPO	Antithyroglobulin	TSH receptor antibody
Graves's disease	70–80%	30–50%	70–100% (stimulating)
Autoimmune hypothyroidism	95%	60%	10–20% (blocking)

NB TSH receptor antibodies may be stimulatory or inhibitory. Heterophile antibodies present in patient sera may cause abnormal interference, causing abnormally low or high values of free T_4 and free T_3, and can be removed with absorption tubes.

Reference

1. Tunbridge WM, Vanderpump MP (2000). Population screening for autoimmune thyroid disease. *Endocrinol Metab Clin N Am* **29**, 239–53.
2. Thangaratinam S, et al. (2011). Association between thyroid autoantibodies and miscarriage and preterm birth: meta-analysis of evidence. *BMJ* **342**, 1065.

Scintiscanning

Permits localization of sites of accumulation of radioiodine or sodium pertechnetate (^{99m}Tc), which gives information about the activity of the iodine trap (see Table 1.7). This is useful:

- To define areas of ↑ or ↓ function within the thyroid (see Table 1.8) which occasionally helps in cases of uncertainty as to the cause of the thyrotoxicosis.
- To distinguish between Graves's disease and a thyroiditis (autoimmune or viral—de Quervain's thyroiditis).
- To detect retrosternal goitre.
- To detect ectopic thyroid tissue.

The scan may be altered by:

- Agents which influence thyroid uptake, including intake of high-iodine foods and supplements, such as kelp (seaweed).
- Drugs containing iodine, such as amiodarone.
- Recent use of radiographic contrast dyes can potentially interfere with the interpretation of the scan.

Table 1.7 Radioisotope scans

	^{123}Iodine	^{99}Technetium pertechnetate
Half-life	Short	Short
Advantage	Low emission of radiation Has higher energy photons. Hence useful for imaging a toxic goitre with a substernal component	Maximum thyroid uptake within 30min of administration. Can be used in breastfeeding women (discontinue feeding for 24h)
Disadvantage		Technetium is only trapped by the thyroid without being organified
Use	Functional assessment of the thyroid	Rapid scanning

Table 1.8 Radionuclide scanning (scintigram) in thyroid disease

Condition	Scan appearance
Graves's hyperthyroidism	Enlarged gland Homogeneous radionucleotide uptake
Thyroiditis (e.g. de Quervain's)	Low or absent uptake
Toxic nodule	A solitary area of high uptake
Thyrotoxicosis factitia	Depressed thyroid uptake
Thyroid cancer	Successful ^{131}I uptake by tumour tissue requires an adequate level of TSH, achieved by giving recombinant TSH injection or stopping T_3 replacement 10 days before scanning

Ultrasound (US) scanning

Provides an accurate indication of thyroid size and is useful for differentiating cystic nodules from solid ones but cannot be used to distinguish between benign and malignant disease. There are several ultrasonographic findings that are suspicious for thyroid cancer (hypoechoic, microcalcifications, irregular margins, central vascularity, incomplete halo). The predictive value of these characteristics varies widely, and they can be used to select nodules for fine needle aspiration (FNA) biopsy.

* Microcalcification within nodules favours the diagnosis of malignancy; microcalcifications <2mm in diameter are observed in ~60% of malignant nodules but in <2% of benign lesions.
* Calcification is a prominent feature of medullary carcinoma of the thyroid.
* It can detect whether a nodule is solitary or part of a multinodular process.
* Sequential scanning can be employed to assess changes in size of thyroid over time.

NB Neither scintigraphy nor US is routinely indicated in a patient with goitre.

Fine needle aspiration cytology (FNAC)

- FNAC is now considered the most accurate test for the diagnosis of thyroid nodules. It is performed in an outpatient setting. One to two aspirations are carried out at different sites for each nodule. Cytologic findings are *satisfactory* or *diagnostic* in approximately 85% of specimens and *non-diagnostic* in the remainder.
- In experienced hands, FNAC is an excellent diagnostic technique, as shown in Table 1.9.
- Non-palpable nodules (discovered incidentally during other imaging procedures) have the same risk of malignancy as palpable nodules of similar size. US-guided FNAC can be performed for non-palpable nodules and for nodules that are technically difficult to aspirate using palpation methods alone, such as predominantly cystic or posteriorly located nodules. In patients with large nodules (>4cm), US-guided FNAC directed at several areas within the nodule may reduce the risk of a false –ve biopsy.
- Repeat FNAC after 3–6 months further reduces the proportion of false –ves.
- It is impossible to differentiate between benign and malignant follicular neoplasm using FNAC. Therefore, surgical excision of a follicular neoplasm is always indicated (📖 p. 99).
- See Table 1.10 for diagnostic categories from FNAC.

Table 1.9 Diagnostic features of FNAC

Feature	Range (%)	Mean value (%)
Accuracy	85–100	95
Specificity	72–100	92
Sensitivity	65–98	83
False –ve	1–11	5

Table 1.10 Diagnostic categories from FNAC

Category		Action
Thy 1	Non-diagnostic. Inadequate	Repeat sampling, using US if necessary
Thy 2	Non-neoplastic	Two samples, 3–6 months apart, showing benign appearances are indicated to exclude neoplasia. If rapid growth/pressure effects/high risk, diagnostic lobectomy may be indicated
Thy 3	(i) Follicular lesions	Lobectomy, with completion thyroidectomy if malignant (up to 20% risk of malignancy)
	(ii) Other suspicious findings	Discussion at thyroid cancer MDT
Thy 4	Suspicious of malignancy, e.g. papillary, medullary, or anaplastic carcinoma/lymphoma	Surgical excision for differentiated tumour (80% risk of malignancy)
Thy 5	Diagnosis of malignancy	Surgical excision for differentiated thyroid cancer (>95% risk of malignancy). Radiotherapy/chemotherapy for anaplastic thyroid cancer, lymphoma/metastases

Computed tomography (CT)

- CT is useful in the evaluation of retrosternal and retrotracheal extension of an enlarged thyroid.
- Compression of the trachea and displacement of the major vessels can be identified with CT of the superior mediastinum.
- It can demonstrate the extent of intrathoracic extension of thyroid malignancy and infiltration of adjacent structures, such as the carotid artery, internal jugular vein, trachea, oesophagus, and regional lymph nodes.

Positron emission tomography (PET)

- Up to 20% of thyroid incidentalomas found on PET scans may be malignant and thus require US-guided FNAC.
- Recurrent thyroid cancer that is fluorodeoxyglucose (FDG) avid positive on FDG PET scanning is unlikely to respond to even high-dose radioiodine therapy.

Additional laboratory investigations

Haematological tests

- Long-standing thyrotoxicosis may be associated with *normochromic anaemia* and, occasionally, *mild neutropenia* and *lymphocytosis* and, rarely, *thrombocytopenia*.
- In hypothyroidism, a macrocytosis is typical, although concurrent vitamin B12 deficiency should be considered.
- There may also be a *microcytic anaemia* due to menorrhagia and impaired iron utilization.

Biochemical tests

- *Alkaline phosphatase* may be elevated in thyrotoxicosis.
- Mild *hypercalcaemia* occasionally occurs in thyrotoxicosis and reflects ↑ bone resorption. *Hypercalciuria* is more common.
- In a hypothyroid patient, *hyponatraemia* may be due to reduced renal tubular water loss or, less commonly, due to coexisting cortisol deficiency.
- In hypothyroidism, *creatinine* kinase is often raised and the lipid profile altered with ↑ LDL cholesterol.

Endocrine tests

- In untreated hypothyroidism, there may be inadequate responses to provocative testing of the hypothalamo–pituitary–adrenal (HPA) axis.
- In hypothyroidism, serum prolactin may be elevated because ↑ TRH leads to ↑ prolactin secretion (may be partly responsible for ↓ fertility in young women with hypothyroidism).
- In thyrotoxicosis, there is an increase in *sex hormone-binding globulin* (SHBG) and a complex interaction with sex steroid hormone metabolism, resulting in changes in the levels of androgens and oestrogens. The net physiological result is an increase in *oestrogenic* activity, with *gynaecomastia* and a decrease in libido in ♂ presenting with thyrotoxicosis.

Non-thyroidal illness (sick euthyroid syndrome)

- Biochemistry:
  - Low T_4 and T_3.
  - Inappropriately normal/suppressed TSH.
- Tissue thyroid hormone concentrations are very low.
- Context—starvation.
  - Severe illness, e.g. ITU, severe infections, renal failure, cardiac failure, liver failure, end-stage malignancy.
- Thyroxine replacement is not indicated because there is no evidence that treatment provides benefit or is safe.

Atypical clinical situations

- *Thyrotoxicosis factitia* (usually unprescribed intake of exogenous thyroid hormone in non thyroid disease):
  - No thyroid enlargement.
  - Elevated free T_4 and suppressed TSH.
  - Depressed thyroid uptake on scintigraphy.
  - Low thyroglobulin differentiates from thyroiditis (which shows depressed uptake on scintigraphy but ↑ thyroglobulin) and all other causes of elevated thyroid hormones.
- *Struma ovarii* (ovarian teratoma containing hyperfunctioning thyroid tissue):
  - No thyroid enlargement.
  - Depressed thyroid uptake on scintigraphy.
  - Body scan after radioiodine confirms diagnosis.
- *Trophoblast tumours.* hCG has structural homology with TSH and leads to thyroid gland stimulation and usually mild thyrotoxicosis.
- *Hyperemesis gravidarum.* Thyroid function tests may be abnormal with a suppressed TSH (📖 see p. 44).
- *Choriocarcinoma of the testes* may be associated with gynaecomastia and thyrotoxicosis—measure hCG.

Thyrotoxicosis—aetiology

Epidemiology
- 10× more common in ♀ than in ♂ in the UK.
- Prevalence is approximately 2% of the ♀ population.
- Annual incidence is 3 cases per 1,000 ♀.

Definition of thyrotoxicosis and hyperthyroidism
- The term *thyrotoxicosis* denotes the clinical, physiological, and biochemical findings that result when the tissues are exposed to excess thyroid hormone. It can arise in a variety of ways (see Table 1.11). It is essential to establish a specific diagnosis, as this determines therapy choices and provides important information for the patient regarding prognosis.
- The term *hyperthyroidism* should be used to denote only those conditions in which hyperfunction of the thyroid leads to thyrotoxicosis.

Genetics of autoimmune thyroid disease (AITD)
- AITD consists of Graves's disease, Hashimoto's thyroiditis, atrophic autoimmune hypothyroidism, post-partum thyroiditis, and thyroid-associated ophthalmopathy, that appear to share a common genetic predisposition.
- There is a ♀ preponderance, and sex steroids appear to play an important role.
- Twin studies show ↑ concordance for Graves's disease and autoimmune hypothyroidism in monozygotic, compared to dizygotic, twins.
- It is estimated that genetic factors account for approximately 70% of the susceptibility for Graves's disease.
- Sib studies indicate that sisters and children of ♀ with Graves's disease have a 5–8% risk of developing Graves's disease or autoimmune hypothyroidism.
- On the background of a genetic predisposition, environmental factors are thought to contribute to the development of disease.
- A number of interacting susceptibility genes are thought to play a role in the development of disease—a complex genetic trait.
- CTLA-4 (cytotoxic T lymphocyte antigen-4) is associated with Graves's disease in Caucasian populations. In particular, the CT60 allele has a prevalence of 60% in the general population but is also the allele most highly associated with Graves's disease. These data emphasize the complex nature of genetic susceptibility and the likely interplay of environmental factors.
- Association of major histocompatibility complex (MHC) loci with Graves's disease has been demonstrated in some populations but not others. HLA-DR3 is associated with Graves's disease in whites. HLA-DQA1*0501 is associated in some populations, especially for men. However, the overall contribution of MHC genes to Graves's disease has been estimated to be only 10–20% of the inherited susceptibility.

Table 1.11 Classification of the aetiology of thyrotoxicosis

Associated with hyperthyroidism	
Excessive thyroid stimulation	Graves's disease, Hashitoxicosis
	Pituitary thyrotroph adenoma
	Pituitary thyroid hormone resistance syndrome (excess TSH) (🕮 see p. 50)
	Trophoblastic tumours producing hCG with thyrotrophic activity
Thyroid nodules with autonomous function	Toxic solitary nodule, toxic multinodular goitre
	Very rarely, thyroid cancer
Not associated with hyperthyroidism	
Thyroid inflammation	Silent and post-partum thyroiditis, subacute (de Quervain's) thyroiditis
	Drug-induced thyroiditis (amiodarone)
Exogenous thyroid hormones	Overtreatment with thyroid hormone
	Thyrotoxicosis factitia (thyroxine use in non-thyroidal disease)
Ectopic thyroid tissue	Metastatic thyroid carcinoma
	Struma ovarii (teratoma containing functional thyroid tissue)

Manifestations of hyperthyroidism

(See Box 1.2.)

> **Box 1.2 Manifestations of hyperthyroidism (all forms)**
> *Symptoms*
> - Hyperactivity, irritability, altered mood, insomnia.
> - Heat intolerance, ↑ sweating.
> - Palpitations.
> - Fatigue, weakness.
> - Dyspnoea.
> - Weight loss with ↑ appetite (weight gain in 10% of patients).
> - Pruritus.
> - ↑ stool frequency.
> - Thirst and polyuria.
> - Oligomenorrhoea or amenorrhoea, loss of libido, erectile dysfunction (50% of men may have sexual dysfunction).
>
> *Signs*
> - Sinus tachycardia, atrial fibrillation.
> - Fine tremor, hyperkinesia, hyperreflexia.
> - Warm, moist skin.
> - Palmar erythema, onycholysis.
> - Hair loss.
> - Muscle weakness and wasting.
> - Congestive (high output) heart failure, chorea, periodic paralysis (primarily in Asian ♂), psychosis (rare).

Investigation of thyrotoxicosis

(See Table 1.12.)
- Thyroid function tests—raised free T_4 and suppressed TSH (raised free T_3 in T_3 toxicosis).
- TSH receptor antibodies—see ▭ Table 1.6, p. 15. Also useful in the assessment of cessation of carbimazole and in pregnant women to assess the risk of fetal thyrotoxicosis.
- Radionucleotide thyroid scan if diagnosis uncertain (▭ see p. 17 but is seldom required.

Manifestations of Graves's disease

(in addition to those in Box 1.2)
- Diffuse goitre.
- Ophthalmopathy (▭ see Graves's ophthalmopathy, p. 54).
  - A feeling of grittiness and discomfort in the eye.
  - Retrobulbar pressure or pain, eyelid lag or retraction.
  - Periorbital oedema, chemosis,* scleral injection.*
  - Exophthalmos (proptosis).*
  - Extraocular muscle dysfunction.*
  - Exposure keratitis.*
  - Optic neuropathy.*

---

* Combination of these suggests congestive ophthalmopathy. Urgent action necessary if: corneal ulceration, congestive ophthalmopathy, or optic neuropathy (▭ see Graves's ophthalmopathy, p. 54).

Table 1.12 Tests which help to differentiate different causes of thyrotoxicosis

Cause	Thyroid iodine uptake	Thyroid parietal antibodies	Thyroid-stimulating immunoglobulin	Thyroglobulin
Graves's disease	↑	Usually positive	+	↑
Toxic nodular goitre	↑	–	–	↑
TSH-secreting pituitary adenoma	↑	–	–	↑
Hyperemesis gravidarum	↑	–	–	↑
Trophoblastic tumour	↑	–	–	↑
de Quervain's thyroiditis	↓	–	–	↑
Drugs, e.g. amiodarone	↓	Usually negative	–	↑
Struma ovarii	↓	–	–	↑
Thyrotoxicosis factitia	↓	–	–	↓

- Localized dermopathy (pretibial myxoedema, 🕮 see Graves's dermopathy, p. 62).
- Lymphoid hyperplasia.
- Thyroid acropachy (🕮 see Thyroid acropachy, p. 63).

Conditions associated with Graves's disease[1]

- Type 1 diabetes mellitus.
- Addison's disease.
- Vitiligo.
- Pernicious anaemia.
- Alopecia areata.
- Myasthenia gravis.
- Coeliac disease (4.5%).
- Other autoimmune disorders associated with the HLA-DR3 haplotype.

Reference

1. Boelaert K, Newby PR, Simmonds MJ, et al. (2010). Prevalence and relative risk of other autoimmune diseases in subjects with autoimmune thyroid disease. Am J Med **123**, 183.e1–9.

Medical treatment

In general, the standard policy in Europe is to offer a course of antithyroid drugs (ATD) first. In the USA, radioiodine is more likely to be offered as first-line treatment.

Aims and principles of medical treatment

- To induce remission in Graves's disease.
- Monitor for relapse off treatment, initially 6–8-weekly for 6 months, then 6-monthly for 2 years, and then annually thereafter or sooner if symptoms return.
- Use of a computerized thyroid follow-up register greatly facilitates monitoring and reduces the necessity for outpatient appointments.
- For relapse, consider definitive treatment, such as radioiodine or surgery. A second course of ATD almost never results in remission.

Choice of drugs—thionamides

- *Carbimazole*, which can be given as a once-daily dose, is usually the drug of first choice in the UK. Carbimazole is converted to methimazole by cleavage of a carboxyl side chain on first liver passage. It has a lower rate of side effects when compared with PTU (14 vs 52%).
- *Propylthiouracil* (PTU) should never be used as a first-line agent in either children or adults, with the possible exceptions of pregnant women and patients with life-threatening thyrotoxicosis. PTU use should be restricted to circumstances when neither surgery nor radioactive iodine is a treatment option in a patient who has developed a toxic reaction to carbimazole and antithyroid drug therapy is needed.
- During the first trimester of pregnancy, *propylthiouracil* is the preferred drug of choice because of the possible association of carbimazole with aplasia cutis.

Action of thionamides

- Thyroid hormone synthesis is inhibited by blockade of the action of thyroid peroxidase.
- Thionamides are especially actively accumulated in thyrotoxic tissue.
- Propylthiouracil also inhibits the deiodinase type 1 activity and thus may have advantages when given at high doses in severe thyrotoxicosis.

Dose and effectiveness

- 5mg of carbimazole is roughly equivalent to 50mg of propylthiouracil. Propylthiouracil has a theoretical advantage of inhibiting the conversion of T_4 to T_3, and T_3 levels decline more rapidly after starting the drug.
- 30–40% of patients treated with an ATD remain euthyroid 10 years after discontinuation of therapy. If hyperthyroidism recurs after treatment with an ATD, there is little chance that a second course of treatment will result in permanent remission. Young patients, smokers, those with large goitres, ophthalmopathy, or high serum

concentrations of thyrotropin receptor antibody at the time of diagnosis are unlikely to have a permanent remission.

- β-*adrenergic antagonists.* Propranolol 20–80mg 3× daily. Considerable relief from symptoms, such as anxiety, tremor, and palpitations, may be gained in the initial 4–8 weeks of treatment, before euthyroidism is achieved.

Atrial fibrillation

Should, if present, convert to sinus rhythm if no structural cardiac abnormality on echocardiography—otherwise, cardiovert after 4 months euthyroid. Consider use of aspirin or warfarin according to usual guidelines.

Side effects

- ATDs are generally well tolerated. Uncommonly, patients may complain of GI symptoms or an alteration in their sense of taste and smell.
- Agranulocytosis represents a potentially fatal, but rare, side effect of ATD, occurring in 0.1–0.5% of patients. It is less frequent with carbimazole than with propylthiouracil, and, because cross-reactivity of this reaction has been reported, one drug should never be substituted for the other after this reaction has been diagnosed. Agranulocytosis usually occurs within the first 3 months after initiation of therapy (97% within the first 6 months, especially on higher doses), but it is important to be aware of the documented cases, which have occurred (less frequently) a long time after starting treatment.
- As agranulocytosis occurs very suddenly and is potentially fatal, routine monitoring of FBC is thought to be of little use. Patients typically present with fever and evidence of infection, usually in the oropharynx, and *each patient should therefore receive written instructions to discontinue the medication and contact their doctor for a blood count should this situation arise.*
- Neutrophil dyscrasias occur more frequently in ♂ and are more often fatal in the elderly.
- Much more common are the allergic type reactions of rash, urticaria, and arthralgia, which occur in 1–5% of patients taking these drugs. These side effects are often mild and do not usually necessitate drug withdrawal, although one ATD may be substituted for another in the expectation that the second agent may be taken without side effects.
- Thionamides may cause cholestatic jaundice, and elevated serum aminotransferases have been reported as has fulminant hepatic failure.
- The frequency of PTU-related severe liver damage is approximately 0.1% in adults, of whom 10% will develop liver failure resulting in liver transplantation or death (1:10,000 incidence). Data for children suggest that the risk of drug-induced liver failure may be greater for children than for adults (1:1,000 incidence).
- All patients should be given written and verbal warnings about the potential side effects of thionamides.
- Rarely, anti-neutrophil cytoplasmic antibody (ANCA) –ve vasculitis develops with propylthiouracil therapy. It may cause arthralgia, skin lesions, glomerulonephritis, fever, and alveolar haemorrhage. Skin lesions include ulcers. Biopsy reveals vasculitis. Propylthiouracil should be stopped, and steroids may be needed.

Treatment regimen

Two alternative regimens are practised for Graves's disease: dose titration and block and replace.

Dose titration regime

- The $1°$ aim is to achieve a euthyroid state with relatively high drug doses and then to maintain euthyroidism with a low stable dose. The dose of carbimazole or propylthiouracil is titrated according to the thyroid function tests performed every 4–8 weeks, aiming for a serum free T_4 in the normal range and a detectable TSH. High serum TSH indicates the need for a dose reduction. TSH may remain suppressed for some weeks after normalization of thyroid hormone levels.
- The typical starting dose of carbimazole is 20–30mg/day. Higher doses (40–60mg) may be indicated in severe cases, with very high levels of FT_4.
- This regimen has a lower rate of side effects than the block and replace regimen.

The treatment is continued for 18 months, as this appears to represent the length of therapy which is generally optimal in producing the remission rate of up to 40% at 5 years after discontinuing therapy.

- Relapses are most likely to occur within the first year and may be more likely in the presence of a large goitre, ophthalmic Graves's disease, current smokers, and high T_4 level at the time of diagnosis, or the presence of TSH receptor antibodies at the end of treatment. Men have a higher recurrence rate than women.
- Patients with multinodular goitres and thyrotoxicosis always relapse on cessation of antithyroid medication, and definitive treatment with radioiodine or surgery is usually advised. Long-term thionamide therapy at low dose is also an option, particularly for the elderly.

Block and replace regimen

- After achieving a euthyroid state on carbimazole alone, carbimazole at a dose of 40mg daily, together with T_4 at a dose of 100 micrograms, can be prescribed. This is usually continued for 6 months.
- The main advantages are fewer hospital visits for checks of thyroid function and shorter duration of treatment.
- Most patients achieve a euthyroid state within 4–6 weeks of carbimazole therapy.
- During treatment, FT_4 values are measured 4 weeks after starting levothyroxine and the dose of levothyroxine altered, if necessary, in 25 micrograms increments to maintain FT_4 in the normal range. Most patients do not require any dose adjustment.
- The originally reported higher remission rate was not confirmed in a large prospective multicentre European trial when combination treatment was compared to carbimazole alone, but side effects were more common.[1]
- Relapses are most likely to occur within the first year.

Reference

1. Reinwein D, Benker G, Lazarus JH, *et al.* (1993). A prospective randomized trial of antithyroid drug dose in Graves's disease therapy. European Multicenter Study Group on Antithyroid Drug Treatment. *J Clin Endocrinol Metab* **76**, 1516–21.

Radioiodine treatment

(See Table 1.13.)

Indications

- Definitive treatment of multinodular goitre or adenoma.
- Relapsed Graves's disease.

Contraindications

- Young children because of the potential risk of thyroid carcinogenesis.
- Pregnant and lactating ♀.
- Situations where it is clear that the safety of other people cannot be guaranteed.
- *Graves's ophthalmopathy*. There is some evidence that Graves's ophthalmopathy may worsen after the administration of radioactive iodine, especially in smokers. In cases of moderate-to-severe ophthalmopathy, radioiodine may be avoided. Alternatively, steroid cover in a dose of 40mg prednisolone should be administered on the day of administering radioiodine, 30mg daily for the next 2 weeks, 20mg daily for the following 2 weeks, reducing to zero over subsequent 3 weeks. Lower steroid doses, e.g. starting with 20mg, may be effective. It is essential that euthyroidism is closely maintained following radioiodine to avoid worsening of ophthalmopathy.

Caveats

- The control of disease may not occur for a period of weeks or a few months.
- More than one treatment may be needed in some patients, depending on the dose given; 15% require a second dose, and a few patients require a third dose. The second dose should be considered only at least 6 months after the first dose.
- Compounds that contain iodine, such as amiodarone, block iodine uptake for a period of several months following cessation of therapy; iodine uptake measurements may be helpful in this instance in determining the activity required and the timing of radioiodine therapy.
- ♀ of childbearing age should avoid pregnancy for a minimum of 6 months following radioactive iodine ablation.
- Men should avoid fathering children for 4 months after radiation.
- The prevalence of hypothyroidism is about 50% at 10 years and continues to increase thereafter.

Side effects are rare

- Anterior neck pain caused by radiation-induced thyroiditis (1%).
- Transient rise (72h) in thyroid hormone levels which may exacerbate heart failure, if present. This aspect needs consideration in elderly patients.

Table 1.13 Recommended activity of radioiodine

Aetiology	Comments	Guide dose (MBq)
Graves's disease	First presentation; no significant eye disease Moderate goitre (40–50g)	400–600
Toxic multinodular goitre in older person	Mild heart failure; atrial fibrillation or other concomitant disease, e.g. cancer	500–800
Toxic adenoma	Usually mild hyperthyroidism	500
Severe Graves's disease with thyroid eye disease	Postpone radioiodine till eye disease stable Prednisolone 40mg to be administered at same time as radioiodine and for further 4–6 weeks (see 📖 Contraindications, p. 34)	500–800
Ablation therapy	Severe accompanying medical condition, such as heart failure; atrial fibrillation or other concurrent medical disorders (e.g. psychosis)	500–800

Data taken from The Use of Radioiodine in Benign Thyroid Disease. Royal College of Physicians, 2007.

Hypothyroidism after radioiodine

- After radioiodine administration, ATDs may be recommenced. The ATDs should be withdrawn gradually, guided by a 6–8-weekly thyroid function test. Early post-radioiodine hypothyroidism may be transient. TSH should be monitored initially, then annually after radioiodine to determine late hypothyroidism.
- In patients treated for autonomous toxic nodules, the incidence of hypothyroidism is lower since the toxic nodule takes up the radioactive iodine while the surrounding tissue will recover normal function once the hyperthyroidism is controlled.
- Mortality is not increased.

Cancer risk after radioiodine therapy

Radioiodine therapy for hyperthyroidism does not increase the overall risk of malignancy or thyroid cancer.

Clinical guidelines

The recommendation is to administer enough radioiodine to achieve euthyroidism, with the acceptance of a moderate rate of hypothyroidism, e.g. 15–20% at 2 years.

Instructions to patients before treatment

Discontinue ATDs 2–7 days before radioiodine administration since their effects last for 24h or more, although propylthiouracil has a prolonged radioprotective effect. ATDs may be recommenced 3–7 days after radioiodine administration without significantly affecting the delivered radiation dose.

Administration of radioiodine (see Table 1.13)

- Radioactive iodine-131 is administered orally as a capsule or a drink.
- There is no universal agreement regarding the optimal dose.
- A dose of 400–800MBq should be sufficient to cure hyperthyroidism in 90%.
- Most patients are treated with 400–600MBq as the first dose, and 600–800MBq if thyrotoxicosis persists 6–12 months after the first dose.

Outcomes of radioiodine treatment[1]

- In general, 50–70% of patients have restored normal thyroid function within 6–8 weeks of receiving radioiodine. Shrinkage of goitre occurs but is slower.

Instructions to patients after treatment

Precautions for patients following treatment with radioiodine are summarized in Table 1.14.

Table 1.14 Number of days to apply caution after radioiodine

Precaution	Administered activity of ^{131}I MBq			
	≤200	≤400	≤600	≤800
Avoid journeys on public transport >1h	0	0	0	6
Avoid places of entertainment or close contact with other people (duration 3h)	1	5	8	11
Stay off work when travel alone by private transport and work does not involve close contact with other people	0	0	0	0
Stay off work which involves prolonged contact with other people at a distance of 1m, e.g. bank cashier	8	13	16	18
Stay off work which involves close contact with other people, including pregnant ♀ or children, work of a radiosensitive nature, or commercial food production	11	17	20	22
Avoid non-essential close contact (<1m) with children, teenagers, pregnant women within the family	16*	22*	25*	27*
Avoid non-essential close contact and sleeping with another person	4	9	13	15

* These times need to be extended if the child concerned is young and needs a lot of close contact.

NB These apply only in the UK; they are less stringent in the USA.

Reference

1. Royal College of Physicians of London (2007). The use of radioiodine in benign thyroid disease. Royal College of Physicians, London.

Surgery

(Aspects of thyroid surgery are also covered see p. 606.)

Total thyroidectomy is now considered the operation of choice because of the risk of relapse with partial thyroidectomy. All such patients go home on T_4. See Box 1.3.

Indications

- Documented suspicious or malignant thyroid nodule by FNAC.
- Pregnant women who are not adequately controlled by ATDs or in whom serious allergic reactions develop while being treated medically. Thyroidectomy is usually performed in the second trimester.
- Patients:
  - Who reject or fear exposure to radiation.
  - With poor compliance to medical treatment.
  - In whom a rapid control of symptoms is desired.
  - With severe manifestations of Graves's ophthalmopathy, as total or near total thyroidectomy does not worsen eye manifestations (but carefully avoid post-operative hypothyroidism).
  - With relapsed Graves's disease.
  - With local compressive symptoms which may not improve rapidly with radioiodine whereas operation removes these symptoms in most patients.
  - With large thyroid glands and relatively low radioiodine uptake.

Preparation of patients for surgery

- ATDs should be used preoperatively to achieve euthyroidism.
- Propranolol may be added to achieve β-blockade, especially in those patients where surgery must be performed sooner than achieving euthyroid state.
- Potassium iodide, 60mg 3× daily, can be used during the preoperative period to prevent an unwanted liberation of thyroid hormones during surgery. Preoperatively, it should be given for 10 days. Operating later than this can be associated with exacerbation of thyrotoxicosis, as the thyroid escapes from the inhibitory effect of the iodide. In practice, it is rarely needed, as good control of thyrotoxicosis can be achieved with ATDs in the majority of patients.
- In the patient who appears to be non-compliant with ATDs and remains thyrotoxic prior to surgery, it may be necessary to admit them as an inpatient for supervised administration of high-dose ATDs, together with β-blockade, and measurement of FT_4 and FT_3 twice weekly. There is a risk of thyroid crisis or storm if a patient undergoes operation when thyrotoxic. Most patients can be rendered euthyroid within 2–4 weeks, and potassium iodide can be administered as above in this section to coincide with the timing of surgery.
- Additional measures are as for thyroid storm.

Box 1.3 Complications of thyroidectomy

Immediate
- Recurrent laryngeal nerve damage.
- Hypoparathyroidism.
- Thyroid crisis.
- Local haemorrhage, causing laryngeal oedema.
- Wound infection.

Late
- Hypothyroidism.
- Keloid formation.

Thyroid crisis (storm)

Thyroid crisis represents a rare, but life-threatening, exacerbation of the manifestations of thyrotoxicosis. It should be promptly recognized since the condition is associated with a significant mortality (30–50%, depending on series); see Box 1.4. Thyroid crisis develops in hyperthyroid patients who:

• Have an acute infection.
• Undergo thyroidal or non-thyroidal surgery or (rarely) radioiodine treatment.

Thyroid crisis should be considered in a very sick patient if there is:
• Recent history suggestive of thyrotoxicosis.
• Acute stressful precipitating factor, such as surgery.
• History of previous thyroid treatment.

Laboratory investigations

• Routine haematology may indicate a leukocytosis, which is well recognized in thyrotoxicosis, even in the absence of infection.
• The biochemical screen may reveal a raised alkaline phosphatase and mild hypercalcaemia.
• Thyroid function tests and thyroid antibodies should be requested, although treatment should not be delayed while awaiting the results.
• The levels of thyroid hormones will be raised, but may not be grossly elevated, and are usually within the range of uncomplicated thyrotoxicosis.

Treatment

General supportive therapy

• The patient is best managed in an intensive care unit where close attention can be paid to the cardiorespiratory status, fluid balance, and cooling.
• Standard anti-arrhythmic drugs can be used, including digoxin (usually in higher than normal dose) after correction for hypokalaemia.

If anticoagulation is indicated because of atrial fibrillation, then it must be remembered that thyrotoxic patients are very sensitive to warfarin.
• Chlorpromazine (50–100mg IM) can be used to treat agitation and, because of its effect in inhibiting central thermoregulation, it may be useful in treating the hyperpyrexia.
• Broad-spectrum antibiotics should be given if infection is suspected.

Box 1.4 Clinical signs suggestive of a thyroid storm

• Alteration in mental status.
• High fever.
• Tachycardia or tachyarrhythmias.
• Severe clinical hyperthyroid signs.
• Vomiting, jaundice, and diarrhoea.
• Multisystem decompensation: cardiac failure, respiratory distress, congestive hepatomegaly, dehydration, and prerenal failure.

Specific treatment
- Aim: to inhibit thyroid hormone synthesis completely.
  - Propylthiouracil 200–300mg 6-hourly via NG tube. Propylthiouracil is preferred because of its ability to block T_4 to T_3 conversion in peripheral tissues. There are no clinical data comparing propylthiouracil and carbimazole in this situation. ATDs should be commenced first.
- Potassium iodide, 60mg via NG tube 6-hourly, 6h *after* starting propylthiouracil, will inhibit thyroid hormone release.
- β-adrenergic blocking agents are essential in the management to control tachycardia, tremor, and other adrenergic manifestations:
  - Propranolol 160–480mg/day in divided doses or as an infusion at a rate of 2–5mg/h.
- Calcium channel blockers can be tried in patients with known bronchospastic disease where β-blockade is contraindicated.
- High doses of glucocorticoids are capable of blocking T_4 to T_3 conversion: prednisolone 60mg daily or hydrocortisone 400mg IM, 4× daily.
- Plasmapheresis and peritoneal dialysis may be effective in cases resistant to the usual pharmacological measures.
- Colestyramine (3g tds) reduces the enterohepatic circulation of thyroid hormones and may help improve thyrotoxicosis.

Subclinical hyperthyroidism

(See Box 1.5.)

- Values of thyroid hormones should be repeated to exclude non-thyroidal illness.
- Subclinical hyperthyroidism is defined as low serum thyrotropin (TSH) concentration in patients with normal levels of T_4 and T_3. Subtle symptoms and signs of thyrotoxicosis may be present.
- May be classified as endogenous in patients with thyroid hormone production associated with nodular thyroid disease or underlying Graves's disease; and as exogenous in those with low or undetectable serum thyrotropin concentrations as a result of treatment with levothyroxine.

There is epidemiological evidence that subclinical hyperthyroidism is a risk factor for the development of atrial fibrillation or osteoporosis.[1] Meta-analyses suggest a 41% increase in all-cause mortality.[2]

> **Box 1.5 Indications to treat subclinical hyperthyroidism**
> Consider treatment with:
> - TSH <0.1 (undetectable).
> - Atrial fibrillation.
> - Osteoporosis.

- The ↑ risk of fracture reported in older ♀ taking thyroid hormone disappears when those with a history of hyperthyroidism are excluded.
- In many patients with endogenous subclinical hyperthyroidism who do not have nodular thyroid disease or complications of excess thyroid hormone, treatment is unnecessary, but thyroid function tests should be performed every 6 months. In older patients with atrial fibrillation or osteoporosis that could have been caused or exacerbated by the mild excess of thyroid hormone, options include long-term, low-dose antithyroid drug therapy or ablative therapy with ^{131}I.
- In patients with exogenous subclinical hyperthyroidism, the dose of levothyroxine should be reduced, if possible, excluding those with prior thyroid cancer in whom thyrotropin suppression may be required. The dose of levothyroxine used for treating hypothyroidism may be reduced if the patient develops:
  - New atrial fibrillation, angina, or cardiac failure.
  - Accelerated bone loss.
  - Borderline high serum T_3 concentration.

Thyrotoxic hypokalaemic periodic paralysis

- More common in Asians (5–10% of all with thyrotoxicosis due to Graves's disease or multinodular goitre) (0.1–0.2% of non-Asian Europeans/North Americans).
- Thyrotoxic patients with periodic paralysis have been found to have higher sodium pump activity than those without paralytic episodes.
- Most common form of acquired periodic paralysis which is a muscle disease in the family of diseases called channelopathies.
- Usual age of onset 20–40 years, mostly ♂.
- Recurrent episodes of painless muscle weakness.
- Duration from minutes to days.
- Flaccid paralysis, usually spreading from legs proximally.
- Clinical manifestations of thyrotoxicosis may be few, and thus TSH should be checked in anyone presenting with periodic paralysis.
- Improves as thyrotoxicosis treated.
- Low serum potassium during attacks.
- CPK ↑ during recovery phase.
- Precipitated by carbohydrates, insulin, cold, vigorous exercise.
- Treatment with potassium replacement, usually by oral route, and treatment of thyrotoxicosis.
- Symptoms usually improve within 2–4h; full resolution in 24–48h.
- Non-selective β-blockers, such as propranolol (3mg/kg), help to prevent attacks until a euthyroid state is achieved.

References

1. Parle JV, Maisonneuve P, Sheppard MC, et al. (2001). Prediction of all-cause and cardiovascular mortality in elderly people from one low serum thyrotropin result: a 10-year cohort study. Lancet **358**, 861–5.
2. Vadiveloo T, et al. (2011). The Thyroid Epidemiology, Audit, and Research Study (TEARS): morbidity in patients with endogenous subclinical hyperthyroidism. J Clin Endocrinol Metab **96**, 1344.

Further reading

Rhee EP, et al. (2012). Case 4-2012—A 37-year-old man with muscle pain, weakness, and weight loss. New Engl J Med **366**, 553.

Thyrotoxicosis in pregnancy

(📖 also see p. 428 and Box 1.6.)

- Thyrotoxicosis occurs in about 0.2% of pregnancies.
- Graves's disease accounts for 90% of cases.
- Less common causes include toxic adenoma and multinodular goitre.
- Other causes are gestational hyperthyroidism (hyperemesis gravidarum) and trophoblastic neoplasia.
- Diagnosis of thyrotoxicosis during pregnancy may be difficult or delayed.
- Physiological changes of pregnancy are similar to those of hyperthyroidism.
- Total T_4 and T_3 are elevated in pregnancy because of an elevated level of TBG, but, with free hormone assays available, this is no longer a problem.
- Physiological features of normal pregnancy include an increase in basal metabolic rate, cardiac stroke volume, palpitations, and heat intolerance.
- Serum free T_3 concentrations remain within the normal range in most pregnant ♀; serum TSH concentration decreases during the first trimester.

Symptoms

- Hyperemesis gravidarum is the classic presentation (one-third is toxic). Tiredness, palpitations, insomnia, heat intolerance, proximal muscle weakness, shortness of breath, and irritability may be other presenting symptoms.
- Thyrotoxicosis may occasionally be diagnosed when the patient presents with pregnancy-induced hypertension or congestive heart failure.

Signs

- Failure to gain weight despite a good appetite.
- Persistent tachycardia with a pulse rate >90 beats/min at rest.
- Other signs of thyrotoxicosis as described previously.

Natural history of Graves's disease in pregnancy

There is aggravation of symptoms in the first half of the pregnancy; amelioration of symptoms in the second half of the pregnancy, and often recurrence of symptoms in the post-partum period.

Transient hyperthyroidism of gestational hyperthyroidism (hyperemesis gravidarum)

- The likely mechanism is a raised β-hCG level.
- β-hCG, LH, FSH, and TSH are glycoprotein hormones that contain a common α subunit and a hormone-specific β subunit. There is an inverse relationship between the serum levels of TSH and hCG, best seen in early pregnancy. There is also structural homology of the TSH and hCG receptors.

- Serum free T$_4$ concentration may be ↑ and the TSH levels suppressed in ♀ with hyperemesis gravidarum.
- Thyroid function tests recover after the resolution of hyperemesis.
- Pregnant ♀ with gestational hyperthyroidism (hyperemesis gravidarum) (which only accounts for two-thirds of hyperemesis) are not usually given ATD treatment but managed supportively with fluids, antiemetics, and nutritional support.
- There is no ↑ risk of thyrotoxicosis in subsequent pregnancies.
- Can be differentiated from Graves's disease by the absence of a goitre, antithyroid antibodies, or family history of Graves's disease, a history of other autoimmune phenomena, and a previous history of ophthalmic Graves's.

Management of Graves's disease in the mother

- Aim of treatment is alleviation of thyroid symptoms and normalization of tests in the shortest time. Patients should be seen every 4–8 weeks and TFTs performed. Serum free T$_4$ is the best test to follow the response to ATDs. Block and replace regimen should not be used, as this will result in fetal hypothyroidism.
- Both propylthiouracil (150mg bd) and carbimazole (10–20mg once daily) are effective in controlling the disease in pregnancy. Historically, propylthiouracil has been preferred in pregnancy because it is not associated with aplasia cutis and omphalocele, which may be the case for carbimazole. However, recent concern regarding hepatotoxicity of PTU, particularly in children, has led to recommendations that it should only be prescribed in the first trimester (check liver function monthly). A β-blocker (propranolol 20–40mg 6–8-hourly) is effective in controlling the hypermetabolic symptoms but should be used only for a few weeks until symptoms abate.
- The dosage of ATDs is frequently adjusted during the course of the pregnancy; therefore, thyroid tests should be done at 2–4 week intervals, with the goal of keeping free thyroid hormone levels in the upper third of the reference range.
- Thyroid tests may normalize spontaneously, with the progression of a normal pregnancy as a result of immunological changes.
- The use of iodides and radioiodine is contraindicated in pregnancy.
- Surgery is rarely performed in pregnancy. It is reserved for patients not responding to ATDs. If necessary, it is preferable to perform surgery in the second trimester.
- Breastfeeding mothers should be treated with the lowest possible dose of carbimazole rather than propylthiouracil in view of the concern regarding hepatotoxicity.

Pre-pregnancy counselling

- Hyperthyroid ♀ who want to conceive should attain euthyroidism before conception since uncontrolled hyperthyroidism is associated with an ↑ risk of congenital abnormalities (stillbirth and cranial synostosis are the most serious complications). See Box 1.6.
- There is no evidence that radioactive iodine treatment given to the mother (or father) 6 months or more before pregnancy has an adverse effect on the fetus or on an offspring in later life.

- Antithyroid medication requirements usually decrease during gestation; in about 50–60% of patients, the dose may be discontinued in the last few weeks of gestation.
- The risk of recurrent hyperthyroidism should be discussed with the patient.
- The rare occurrence of fetal and neonatal hyperthyroidism should be included during counselling sessions and the diagnosis of Graves's hyperthyroidism conveyed to the obstetrician and neonatologist.

Management of the fetus

- The hypothalamo–pituitary–thyroid axis is well developed at 12 weeks' gestation but remains inactive until 18–20 weeks. Circulating TSH receptor antibodies (TSH-RAB) in the mother can cross the placenta, and it is these, rather than the thyroid status of the mother, that cause neonatal thyrotoxicosis. The risk of hyperthyroidism to the neonate can be assessed by measuring TSH-RAB in the maternal circulation at the beginning of the third trimester. Antithyroglobulin antibody and thyroid peroxidase antibodies have no effect on the fetus.
- Long-term follow-up studies of children whose mothers received either carbimazole or propylthiouracil have not shown an ↑ incidence of any physical or psychological defects. The block and replace regimen using relatively high doses of carbimazole is contraindicated because the ATDs cross the placenta, but replacement T_4 does not, thus potentially rendering the fetus hypothyroid.
- Monitoring the fetal heart rate and growth rates are the standard means whereby fetal thyrotoxicosis may be detected. A rate >160 beats/min is suspicious of fetal thyrotoxicosis in the third trimester. Fetal thyrotoxicosis may complicate the latter part of the pregnancy of ♀ with Graves's disease, even if they have previously been treated with radioiodine or surgery, since TSH receptor antibodies may persist. If there is evidence of fetal thyrotoxicosis, the dose of the ATD should be ↑. If this causes maternal hypothyroidism, a small dose of T_4 can be added since, unlike carbimazole, T_4 crosses the placenta less. A paediatrician should be involved to monitor neonatal thyroid function and detect thyrotoxicosis.
- Hypothyroidism in the mother should be avoided because of the potential adverse effect on subsequent cognitive function of the neonate (see Box 1.6).
- If the mother has been treated with carbimazole, the post-delivery levels of T_4 may be low, and neonatal levels of T_4 may only rise to the thyrotoxic range after a few days. In addition, TSH is usually absent in neonates who subsequently develop thyrotoxicosis. Clinical indicators of neonatal thyrotoxicosis include low birthweight, poor weight gain, tachycardia, and irritability. Carbimazole can be given at a dose of 0.5mg/kg per day and withdrawn after a few weeks after the level of TSH-RAB declines.

Post-partum thyroiditis

- Defined as a syndrome of post-partum thyrotoxicosis or hypothyroidism in ♀ who were euthyroid during pregnancy.
- Post-partum thyroid dysfunction, which occurs in ♀ with autoimmune thyroid disease, is characterized in one-third by a thyrotoxic phase

Box 1.6 Potential maternal and fetal complications in uncontrolled hyperthyroidism in pregnancy

Maternal
- Pregnancy-induced hypertension
- Preterm delivery
- Congestive heart failure
- Thyroid storm
- Miscarriage
- Abruptio placentae
- Accidental haemorrhage

Fetal
- Hyperthyroidism
- Neonatal hyperthyroidism
- Intrauterine growth retardation
- Small-for-gestation age
- Prematurity
- Stillbirth
- Cranial synostosis

occurring in the first 3 months post-partum, followed by a hypothyroid phase that occurs 3–6 months after delivery, followed by spontaneous recovery. In the remaining two-thirds, a single-phase pattern or the reverse occurs.

- 5–7% of ♀ develop biochemical evidence of thyroid dysfunction after delivery. An ↑ incidence is seen in patients with type I diabetes mellitus (25%), other autoimmune diseases, in the presence of anti-TPO antibodies, and in the presence of a family history of thyroid disease.
- Hyperthyroidism due to Graves's disease accounts for 10–15% of all cases of post-partum thyrotoxicosis. In the majority of cases, hyperthyroidism occurs later in the post-partum period (>3–6 months) and persists.
- Providing the patient is not breastfeeding, a radioiodine uptake scan can differentiate the two principal causes of autoimmune thyrotoxicosis by demonstrating ↑ uptake in Graves's disease and low uptake in post-partum thyroiditis.
- Graves's hyperthyroidism should be treated with carbimazole. Thyrotoxic symptoms due to post-partum thyrotoxicosis are managed symptomatically using propranolol.
- One-third of affected ♀ with post-partum thyroiditis develop symptoms of hypothyroidism and may require T_4 for 6–12 months. There is a suggestion of an ↑ risk of post-partum depression in those with hypothyroidism.
- Histology of the thyroid in the case of post-partum thyroiditis shows lymphocytic infiltration with destructive thyroiditis and predominantly occurs at 16 weeks in ♀ with +ve antimicrosomal antibodies.
- There is an ↑ chance of subsequent permanent hypothyroidism in 25–30%. Patients with a history of post-partum thyroiditis should be followed up with annual TSH measurements.

Further reading

Lazarus JH (2012). Antithyroid drug treatment in pregnancy. *J Clin Endocrinol Metab* **97**, 2289–91.

Hyperthyroidism in children

Epidemiology
Thyrotoxicosis is rare before the age of 5 years. Although there is a progressive increase in incidence throughout childhood, it is still rare and accounts for <5% of all cases of Graves's disease.

Clinical features
- Behavioural abnormalities, hyperactivity, declining school performance may bring the child to medical attention. Features of hyperthyroidism are as described previously.
- Acceleration of linear growth is common in patients increasing in height percentiles on the growth charts. The disease may be part of McCune–Albright syndrome, and *café-au-lait* pigmentation, precocious puberty, and bony abnormalities should be considered during clinical examination.

Investigations
The cause of thyrotoxicosis in children is nearly always Graves's disease (with +ve TSH receptor antibodies), although thyroiditis and toxic nodules have been described, and a radioiodine scan may be useful if the diagnosis is not clear. Hereditary syndromes of thyroid hormone resistance, often misdiagnosed as Graves's disease, are now being increasingly recognized in children.

Treatment
ATDs represent the initial treatment of choice for thyrotoxic children. Therapy is generally started with carbimazole 250 micrograms/kg (initial dose 10mg/day). Since relapse after withdrawal of ATDs is common, definitive treatment with surgery or radioiodine should be offered. Hepatotoxicity with propylthiouracil can also occur in children.

Secondary hyperthyroidism

An elevated serum free T4 and non-suppressed serum TSH are characteristic of TSH-secreting adenomas or resistance to thyroid hormone. These conditions must be differentiated (see Table 1.15).

TSH-secreting pituitary tumours

- Estimated incidence 1 per million and <1% of all pituitary tumours.
- There are characteristically *elevated* serum free T_4 and T_3 concentrations and *non-suppressed* (inappropriately normal or frankly elevated) serum TSH levels.
- Approximately 25% of TSHomas co-secrete one or more other pituitary hormones; about 15% secrete growth hormone, 10% prolactin, and rarely gonadotrophins. Approximately 90% are macroadenomas (>1cm in diameter), and over two-thirds exhibit suprasellar extension, invasion, or both into adjacent tissues (📖 see p. 180).
- Patients with pure TSHomas present with typical symptoms and signs of thyrotoxicosis and the presence of a diffuse goitre. Patients may exhibit features of oversecretion of the other pituitary hormones, e.g. prolactin or growth hormone. Headaches, visual field defects, menstrual irregularities, amenorrhoea, delayed puberty, and hypogonadotrophic hypogonadism have also been reported. Careful establishment of the diagnosis is the key to treatment. Inappropriate treatment of such patients with subtotal thyroidectomy or radioiodine administration not only fails to cure the underlying disorder, but may be associated with subsequent pituitary tumour enlargement and an ↑ risk of invasiveness into adjacent tissues.
- Treatment options are:
  - Transphenoidal surgery.
  - Pituitary radiotherapy if surgical results are unsatisfactory or surgery is contraindicated or not desired.
  - Medical therapy with somatostatin analogues, such as octreotide or lanreotide, may be useful preoperatively and suppresses TSH secretion in 80% of the cases.

Resistance to thyroid hormones

- Patients with generalized resistance to thyroid hormone (GRTH) may present with mild hyperthyroidism, deaf mutism, delayed bone maturation, raised circulating thyroid hormone concentrations, non-suppressed TSH, and failure of TSH to decrease normally upon administration of supraphysiological doses of thyroid hormones. Most patients present with goitre or incidentally found abnormal TFTs. Treatment is determined by thyroid status.
- The estimated incidence is 1:50,000 live births.
- In selective pituitary resistance to thyroid hormones (PRTH), the thyroid hormone resistance is more pronounced in the pituitary; thus, the patient exhibits definite clinical manifestations of thyrotoxicosis.

- About 85% of thyroid hormone resistance syndromes result from mutations in the gene encoding TRβ, and their identification by gene sequencing can confirm the diagnosis. Mutant receptors have a reduced affinity for T_3 and are functionally deficient. It is usually inherited in an autosomal dominant pattern, with the affected individuals being heterozygous for the mutation.
- A subset of RTH receptors has been identified that are capable of inhibiting wild type receptor action. When co-expressed, the mutant proteins are able to inhibit the function of their wild type counterparts in a dominant –ve manner.
- Common features of patients with the thyroid hormone resistance syndromes include goitre (most commonly) and, less so, tachycardia, hyperkinetic behaviour, emotional disturbances, ear, nose, and throat infections, language disabilities, auditory disorders, low body weight, cardiac abnormalities, and subnormal intelligence quotients.

Treatment in RTH is not usually necessary. In PRTH, treatment may be needed, but this is uncommon. Chronic suppression of TSH secretion is with D T4, tri-iodothyroacetic acid, octreotide, or bromocriptine. If this is ineffective, thyroid ablation with radioiodine or surgery, with subsequent close monitoring of thyroid hormone status and pituitary gland size.

Table 1.15 Tests useful in the differential diagnosis of TSHomas, PRTH, and GRTH

Test	TSHomas	PRTH	GRTH
Clinical thyrotoxicosis	Present	Present	Absent
Family history	Absent	Present	Present
TSH response to TRH	No change	Increase	Increase
TSH response to T_3 (100 micrograms/day + β-blockers)	No change	Decrease	Decrease
SHBG	Elevated–92%[a]	Normal[b]	Normal
α subunit	Elevated–65%	2% elevated	
Pituitary MRI	Tumour–30% microadenoma[c]	Normal	Normal
Fall in TSH on octreotide LAR 20mg/month for 2 months	95%	No change	No change

[a] Not usually raised in mixed GH/TSH tumour.

[b] Peripheral markers of toxicosis sometimes affected (8% SHBG elevated).

[c] The best biochemical test is an elevated α subunit.

Further reading

Abalovich M, Amino N, Barbour LA, et al. (2007). Management of thyroid dysfunction during pregnancy and postpartum: an Endocrine Society Clinical Practice Guideline. *J Clin Endocrinol Metab* **92**(8 Suppl), S1–47.

Abraham P, Avenell A, McGeoch SC, et al. (2010). Antithyroid drug regimen for treating Graves's hyperthyroidism. *Cochrane Database Syst Rev* CD003420.

Bahn RS, Burch HB, Cooper DS, et al. (2011). Hyperthyroidism and other causes of thyrotoxicosis: management guidelines of the American Thyroid Association and American Association of Clinical Endocrinologists. *Thyroid* **21**, 593–646.

Bauer AJ (2011). Approach to the pediatric patient with Graves's disease: when is definitive therapy warranted? *J Clin Endocrinol Metab* **96**, 580–8.

Bonnema SJ, Hegedüs L (2012). Radioiodine therapy in benign thyroid diseases. *Endocr Rev* **33**, 920–80.

Brand OJ, Gough SC (2010). Genetics of thyroid autoimmunity and the role of the TSHR. *Mol Cell Endocrinol* **322**, 135–43.

Brent GP (2008). Graves's disease. *N Engl J Med* **358**, 2594–605.

Brent GA (2010). Environmental exposures and autoimmune thyroid disease. *Thyroid* **20**, 755–61.

Brix TH, Hegedüs L (2011). Twins as a tool for evaluating the influence of genetic susceptibility in thyroid autoimmunity. *Ann Endocrinol (Paris)* **72**, 103–7.

Cesur M, Bayram F, Temel MA, et al. (2008). Thyrotoxic hypokalaemic periodic paralysis in a Turkish population: three new case reports and analysis of the case series. *Clin Endocrinol (Oxf)* **68**, 143–152.

Clementi M, Di Gianantonio E, Cassina M, et al. (2010). Treatment of hyperthyroidism in pregnancy and birth defects. *J Clin Endocrinol Metab* **95**, E337–41.

Cooper DS, Rivkees SA (2009). Putting propylthiouracil in perspective. *J Clin Endocrinol Metab* **94**, 1881–2.

Franklyn JA (2009). Thyroid gland: Antithyroid therapy--best choice of drug and dose. *Nat Rev Endocrinol* **5**, 592–4.

Franklyn JA (2010). What is the role of radioiodine uptake measurement and thyroid scintigraphy in the diagnosis and management of hyperthyroidism? *Clin Endocrinol (Oxf)* **72**, 11–12

Metso S, Jaatinen P, Huhtala H, et al. (2007). Increased cardiovascular and cancer mortality after radioiodine treatment for hyperthyroidism. *J Clin Endocrinol Metab* **92**, 2190–6.

Pearce SH (2004). Spontaneous reporting of adverse reactions to carbimazole and propylthiouracil in the UK. *Clin Endocrinol* **61**, 589–94.

Ross DS (2011). Radioiodine therapy for hyperthyroidism. *N Engl J Med* **364**, 542–50.

Vanderpump MP (2011). Should we treat mild subclinical/mild hyperthyroidism? No. *Eur J Intern Med* **22**, 330–3.

Wiersinga WM (2011). Should we treat mild subclinical/mild hyperthyroidism? Yes. *Eur J Intern Med* **22**, 324–9.

Graves's ophthalmopathy

(See European Working Group on Graves's Ophthalmopathy, ⅏ http://www.EUGOGO.org.)

- An organ-specific autoimmune disorder characterized by swelling of the extraocular muscles, lymphocytic infiltration, late fibrosis, muscle tethering, and proliferation of orbital fat and connective tissue.
- The volume of both the extraocular muscles and retroorbital connective and adipose tissue is increased due to inflammation and the accumulation of hydrophilic glycosaminoglycans (GAG), principally hyaluronic acid, in these tissues. GAG secretion by fibroblasts is increased by activated T-cell cytokines, such as tumour necrosis factor (TNF) alpha and interferon gamma, implying that T-cell activation is an important part of this immunopathology. The accumulation of GAG causes a change in osmotic pressure, which, in turn, leads to a fluid accumulation and an increase in pressure within the orbit. These changes displace the eyeball forward and can also interfere with the function of the extraocular muscles and the venous drainage of the orbits.
- Clinically evident in ~20% of patients, but a further ~30% may have evidence on imaging. Most bilateral, but often asymmetrical, and 15% have unilateral disease.
- Most have mild self-limiting disease, but ~5% (more ♂ and the elderly) have severe disease that threatens sight. The natural history is variable, with spontaneous amelioration in 66%, no change in 20%, and worsening in 14%.
- Incidence higher in ♀ (except for severe disease where equal sex incidence). Prevalence decreasing (? associated with decreased smoking).
- Bimodal age distribution in ♀, with peak onsets between 40–44 years and 60–64 years. In ♂, a single peak incidence occurs at 65–69 years.
- There are two stages in the development of the disease, which can be recognized as an active inflammatory (dynamic) stage and a relatively quiescent static stage.
- The appearance of eye disease follows a different time course to thyroid dysfunction, and, in a minority, there is a lag period between the presentation of hyperthyroidism and the appearance of eye signs. 85% of patients develop Graves's disease within 18 months of Graves's ophthalmopathy developing (20% precede, 40% following).
- 5% of patients with Graves's ophthalmopathy have hypothyroidism, and 5% are euthyroid.
- High levels of TSH receptor antibodies identify high-risk patients.
- Current smokers (>20/day) are more likely to develop ophthalmopathy.
- Continuing smoking and uncontrolled hyperthyroidism or hypothyroidism moderately worsen Graves's ophthalmopathy.
- The role of an endocrinologist during a routine review of Graves's patients is to record accurately the clinical features of Graves's eye disease and to identify ocular emergencies, such as corneal ulceration, congestive ophthalmopathy, and optic neuropathy, which should be referred urgently to an ophthalmologist, preferably in a multidisciplinary clinic setting.

Clinical features

(See Box 1.7.)

- Retraction of eyelids is extremely common in thyroid eye disease. The margin of the upper eyelid normally rests about 2mm below the limbus, and retraction can be suspected if the lid margin is either level with or above the superior limbus, allowing the sclera to be visible. The lower lid normally rests at the inferior limbus, and retraction is suspected when the sclera shows above the lid.
- Proptosis or exophthalmos can result in failure of lid closure, increasing the likelihood of exposure keratitis and the common symptom of gritty eyes. This can be confirmed with fluorescein or Rose Bengal stain. As papilloedema can occur, fundoscopy should be performed. Proptosis may result in periorbital oedema and chemosis because the displaced orbit results in less efficient orbital drainage.
- Persistent visual blurring may indicate an optic neuropathy and requires urgent treatment.
- Severe conjunctival pain may indicate corneal ulceration, requiring urgent referral.

Investigation of proptosis

For details of the 'NOSPECS' classification, see ✆ http://www.EUGOGO. org and The European Group on Graves's Orbitopathy. However, NOSPECS is not always satisfactory for prospective objective assessment of orbital changes, and determining an overall activity score is sometimes more helpful. This is done by assigning one point for the presence of each of the following findings: spontaneous retrobulbar pain, pain on eye movement, eyelid erythema, conjunctival injection, chemosis, swelling of the carbuncle, and eyelid oedema.

Box 1.7 Assessment of severity of Graves's orbitopathy (GO)

Ocular involvement	Features
Mild GO	Minor lid retraction (<2mm)
	Mild soft tissue involvement
	Exophthalmos <3mm
	No or transient diplopia
	Mild corneal exposure
Moderate GO	Lid retraction (≥2mm)
	Moderate to severe soft tissue involvement
	Exophthalmos ≥3mm
	Diplopia
Sight-threatening GO	Optic neuropathy
	Corneal breakdown
	Congestive ophthalmopathy

- *Documentation using a Hertel exophthalmometer.* The feet of the apparatus are placed against the lateral orbital margin as defined by the zygomatic bones. The marker on the body of the exophthalmometer is then superimposed on the reflection of the contralateral one by adjusting the scale. The position of each cornea can be read off against the reflections on a millimetre scale as seen on the mirror of the apparatus. A normal result is generally taken as being <20mm (<18mm in Asians, <22mm in Afro-Caribbeans). A reading of 21mm or more is abnormal, and a difference of 2mm between the eyes is suspicious.
- *Soft tissue involvement.* Soft tissue signs and symptoms include conjunctival hyperaemia, chemosis, and foreign body sensation. The soft tissue changes can be 2° to exposure but are often seen in the absence of these aetiological factors.
- *CT or MRI scan of the orbit* demonstrates enlargement of the extraocular muscles, and this can be useful in cases of diagnostic difficulty. This is also more accurate for demonstration of proptosis.

Ophthalmoplegia

- Patients may complain of diplopia due to ocular muscle dysfunction caused by either oedema during the early active phase or fibrosis during the later phase. Assessment using a Hess chart may be helpful. Intraoptic pressure may increase on upgaze and result in compression of the globe by a fibrotic inferior rectus muscle. Ocular mobility may be restricted by oedema during the active inflammatory phase or by fibrosis during the fibrotic stage.
- The two most common findings are defective elevation caused by fibrotic contraction of the inferior rectus muscle and a convergence defect caused by fibrotic contraction of the medial rectus. Disorders of the medial rectus, superior rectus, and lateral rectus muscle produce typical signs of defective adduction, depression, and abduction, respectively.

Examining for possible optic neuropathy

- History of *poor vision*, a recent or *rapid change in vision*, or *poor colour vision* are reasons for prompt referral.
- A *visual acuity* of <6/18 warrants referral to an ophthalmologist. For *colour vision*, each eye should be evaluated by using a simple 15-plate Ishihara colour vision test. Colour vision is a subtle indicator of optic nerve function. Failure to identify >2 of the plates with either eye is an indication for referral. This is unhelpful in the 8% of ♂ who may be colour-blind.
- *Marcus Gunn pupil.* The 'swinging flashlight' test detects the presence of an *afferent pupillary defect* associated with optic nerve compression.

Medical treatment of Graves's ophthalmopathy

(See Box 1.8.)

Simple treatment for lid retraction

- Most patients do not require any treatment since clinical signs usually improve with treatment of hyperthyroidism or spontaneously with time (40%).
- Sunglasses help with photophobia and excess tears.
- In patients with significant lid retraction and exposure keratopathy, topical lubricants improve symptoms (surgery to reduce the vertical lid fissures can be considered when euthyroid).
- Botulinum toxin injection may reduce persistent upper lid retraction.
- Head elevation during sleep and diuretics may help congestion.

Acute treatment for active ophthalmopathy threatening sight

- Effectiveness is more likely in those with diplopia at neutral gaze and an inflammatory component to ophthalmoplegia.
- Glucocorticoids at high dose (60–80mg/day) improve ophthalmopathy in 60–75% of cases.
- Intravenous glucocorticoid pulse therapy has also been used and may have the advantage of fewer side effects than high oral doses of prednisolone (e.g. 0.5g methylprednisolone weekly for 6 weeks, followed by 0.25g weekly for 6 weeks, with monitoring of liver function tests ± PPIs and a bisphosphonate).
- The advantage of intravenous over oral glucocorticoid therapy was also demonstrated in a meta-analysis of four trials. Intravenous glucocorticoids were significantly better in reducing clinical activity scores; the advantage was mostly due to improvements in patients with severe ophthalmopathy. Adverse events were more common in patients receiving oral therapy, and high doses have been seen to induce liver failure.
- If high-dose oral prednisolone treatment—give for 2 weeks and then tapered gradually.
- Methylprednisolone intravenously is given at a maximum dose of 8g, as the risk of hepatic necrosis is seen at higher doses.
- Steroid-sparing agents used in long-term therapy include mycophenolate mofetil, azathioprine, and ciclosporin, but there are little data suggesting which is more effective.
- Urgent referral to an ophthalmologist is indicated for any suspicion of optic neuropathy or corneal ulceration. Multidisciplinary clinics are strongly advised.

Orbital radiotherapy

- Indications for lens-sparing orbital radiotherapy are similar to those for high-dose glucocorticoids.
- Radiotherapy works by killing retroorbital T cells.
- 20 Gray delivered over ten fractions is the standard regimen.
- Treatment with both radiotherapy and glucocorticoids is more effective than either alone.
- Effectiveness in 60% of cases <40 years.

Other medical therapies

- Selenium[1] may improve symptoms in patients with mild Graves's ophthalmopathy, as illustrated by the results of a randomized trial of selenium (100 micrograms bd), pentoxifylline (600mg bd), or placebo in 159 patients. After 6 months of treatment, eyelid aperture (37% vs 12%) and soft tissue signs (43% vs 32%) significantly improved in patients taking selenium vs placebo. Compared with placebo, selenium also significantly improved quality of life (both visual functioning and appearance scores), as assessed by the Graves's Ophthalmopathy Quality of Life Questionnaire (GO-QOL). Evaluation at 12 months confirmed the findings at 6 months.
- A number of reports have indicated that some patients with severe Graves's ophthalmopathy may respond to B cell depletion induced by rituximab, which is a monoclonal antibody directed against the B cell CD20 molecule. Rituximab induces a fall in TSH receptor antibody levels and depletion of B cells in the retroorbital tissues, not just the periphery. Although high doses of this antibody may be associated with severe side effects from profound immunosuppression, it is possible that much lower doses may be effective in Graves's ophthalmopathy to avoid such effects. This approach to the treatment of severe eye disease is currently undergoing larger trials; preliminary results from these trials suggest efficacy in some, but not all, patients.
- Other immunosuppressive regimens have no proven place in the general management of Graves's ophthalmopathy.
- Use of depot octreotide has been shown to be of no benefit in management.

Reference

1. Marcocci C, et al. (2011). Selenium and the course of mild Graves' orbitopathy. N Engl J Med **364**, 1920.

Surgical treatment of Graves's ophthalmopathy

(See Box 1.8.)

Surgery for decompression

- Orbital decompression may be indicated for urgent treatment of optic neuropathy.
- Posteromedial wall of orbit usually removed.
- Complications include dysmotility of the eye, blindness, orbital cellulitis, CSF leak, cerebral haematoma, obstruction to nasolacrimal flow, and anosmia.

Surgery for strabismus

- Should be performed after any necessary orbital decompression.
- Aims to allow correct binocular vision.
- Is performed when eyes are in a quiescent phase for at least 6 months after active disease.
- Involves alteration, loosening, or tightening of eye muscles, often over several operations, to improve binocular vision.

Eyelid surgery

Is the final stage of any surgical approach and aims to adjust upper and lower eyelid position to improve comfort and appearance.

Box 1.8 Treatment of Graves's ophthalmopathy

General measures

- Stop smoking.
- Dark glasses, with eye protection.
- Control thyroid function to maintain strict euthyroidism.
- Prisms for diplopia.
- Consider selenium supplements.

Specific measures

Problem	Treatment
Grittiness	Artificial tears and simple eye ointment
Eyelid retraction	Tape eyelids at night to avoid corneal damage Surgery if risk of exposure keratopathy
Proptosis	Head elevation during sleep
	Diuretics
	Systemic steroids
	Radiotherapy
	Orbital decompression
Ophthalmoplegia	Prisms in the acute phase
	Orbital decompression
	Orbital muscle surgery
Optic neuropathy	Systemic steroids
	Radiotherapy
	Orbital decompression

Graves's dermopathy

- This is a rare complication of Graves's thyrotoxicosis (0.5%). It is usually pretibial in location (99%) and hence called *pretibial myxoedema*.
- Associated with ophthalmopathy (97%) and acropachy (18%).
- It typically appears as raised, discoloured, and indurated lesions on the front or back of the legs or on the dorsum of the feet and has occasionally been described in other areas, including the hands and the face.
- The lesions are due to localized accumulation of *glycosaminoglycans*. It is now recognized that there is a lymphocytic infiltrate. Lesions are characteristically asymptomatic, but they can also be pruritic and tender. They can be very disfiguring.
- *Treatment*. Usually not treated. Potent topical fluorinated steroids, such as fluocinolone acetonide, may be effective (4–8 weeks), not only in the treatment of localized pain and tenderness, but also in some resolution of the visible skin signs. Surgery may worsen the condition.
- 25% remit completely; 50% are chronic on no therapy. A beneficial effect of topical steroids on remission rates is unproven.

Thyroid acropachy

- This is the rarest manifestation of Graves's disease.
- It presents as clubbing of the digits and subperiosteal new bone formation. The soft tissue swelling is similar to that seen in localized myxoedema and consists of glycosaminoglycan accumulation.
- Patients almost inevitably have Graves's ophthalmopathy or pretibial myxoedema. If not, an alternative cause of clubbing should be looked for.
- It is typically painless, and there is no effective treatment.

Further reading

Bahn RS (2010). Graves's ophthalmopathy. *N Engl J Med.* **362**, 726–38.

Banga JP, Nielsen CH, Gilbert JA, et al. (2008). Application of new therapies in Graves's disease and thyroid-associated ophthalmopathy: animal models and translation to human clinical trials. *Thyroid* **18**, 973–81.

Bartalena L (2010). What to do for moderate-to-severe and active Graves's orbitopathy if glucocorticoids fail? *Clin Endocrinol (Oxf).* **73**, 149–52.

European Group on Graves's orbitopathy (EUGOGO) (2008). Consensus statement of the European Group on Graves's orbitopathy (EUGOGO) on management of GO. *Eur J Endocrinol.* **158**, 273–85.

Hegedüs L, Smith TJ, Douglas RS, et al. (2011). Targeted biological therapies for Graves's disease and thyroid-associated ophthalmopathy. Focus on B-cell depletion with Rituximab. *Clin Endocrinol (Oxf).* **74**, 1–8.

Marcocci C, Kahaly GJ, Krassas GE, et al. (2011). Selenium and the course of mild Graves's orbitopathy. *N Engl J Med.* **364**, 1920–31.

Schwartz KM, Fatourechi V, Ahmed DD, et al. (1992). Dermopathy of Graves's disease (pretibial myxedema): long-term outcome. *J Clin Endocrinol Metab* **87**, 438–46.

Stiebel-Kalish H, Robenshtok E, Hasanreisoglu M, et al. (2009). Treatment modalities for Graves's ophthalmopathy: systematic review and metaanalysis. *J Clin Endocrinol Metab.* **94**, 2708–16.

Träisk F, Tallstedt L, Abraham-Nordling M, et al. (2009). Thyroid-associated ophthalmopathy after treatment for Graves's hyperthyroidism with antithyroid drugs or iodine-131. *J Clin Endocrinol Metab.* **94**, 3700–7.

The European Group on Graves's Orbitopathy (2006). Clinical assessment of patients with Graves's orbitopathy: recommendations to generalists, specialists and clinical researchers. *Eur J Endocrinol* **155**, 387–9.

Zang S, Ponto KA, Kahaly GJ (2011). Clinical review: Intravenous glucocorticoids for Graves's orbitopathy: efficacy and morbidity. *J Clin Endocrinol Metab.* **96**, 320–32.

Multinodular goitre and solitary adenomas

Background

Nodular thyroid disease denotes the presence of single or multiple palpable or non-palpable nodules within the thyroid gland.

- Prevalence rates range from 5–50%, depending on the population studied and sensitivity of detection methods. Prevalence increases linearly with age, exposure to ionizing radiation, and iodine deficiency.
- Clinically apparent thyroid nodules are evident in ~5% of the UK population.
- Incidence of thyroid nodules is about 4× more in ♀.
- Thyroid nodules always raise the concern of cancer, but <5% are cancerous.

Clinical evaluation

- An asymptomatic thyroid mass may be discovered either by a clinician on routine neck palpation or by the patient during self-examination.
- History should concentrate on:
  - An enlarging thyroid mass.
  - A previous history of radiation, especially childhood head and neck irradiation.
  - A family history of thyroid cancer.
  - The development of hoarseness or dysphagia.
- Nodules are more likely to be malignant in patients <20 or >60 years.
- Thyroid nodules are more common in ♀ but more likely to be malignant in ♂.
- The risk of malignancy is similar in a patient with a single or multiple nodules. Thus, a dominant nodule in a multinodular goitre should be evaluated as if it were a single nodule.
- Physical findings suggestive of malignancy include a firm or hard, non-tender nodule, a recent history of enlargement, fixation to adjacent tissue, and the presence of regional lymphadenopathy.
- *Pemberton's sign* is facial erythema and jugular venous distension on raising the arms. It is a sign of superior vena caval obstruction caused by a substernal mass.
- A hot nodule on a radioisotope scan makes malignancy less likely.
- See Box 1.9 for aetiology of thyroid nodules and Box 1.10 for aetiology of goitre.

Box 1.9 Aetiology of thyroid nodules

Common causes
- Colloid nodule.
- Cyst.
- Lymphocytic thyroiditis.
- Benign neoplasms:
  - Hürthle cell.
  - Follicular.
- Malignancy:
  - Papillary.
  - Follicular.

Uncommon causes
- Granulomatous thyroiditis.
- Infections.
- Malignancy:
  - Medullary.
  - Anaplastic.
  - Metastatic.
  - Lymphoma.

Clinical features raising the suspicion of thyroid malignancy
- Age (childhood or elderly).
- Short history of enlarging nodule.
- Local symptoms, including dysphagia, stridor, or hoarseness.
- Previous exposure to radiation.
- +ve family history of thyroid cancer or MEN syndrome.
- Gardner's syndrome (familial large intestinal polyposis).
- Familial polyposis coli.
- Cowden syndrome (autosomal, dominantly inherited multiple hamartomas and breast, thyroid, and other tumours) 📖 p. 584.
- Lymphadenopathy.
- History of Hashimoto's disease (↑ incidence of lymphoma).
- High serum TSH.

Investigations
- FNAC (📖 see p. 20).
- Serum TSH concentration.
- Respiratory flow loop, especially for a large goitre possibly causing tracheal obstruction.
- CT scan or MRI if there are concerns about retrosternal goitre or tracheal compression.

Treatment

Toxic multinodular goitre or nodule

Anti thyroid drugs (ATDs)
ATDs are effective in controlling the hyperthyroidism but are not curative. As the hot nodules are autonomous, the condition will recur after stopping the drugs. Carbimazole is useful treatment to gain control of the disease in preparation for surgery or as long-term treatment in those patients unwilling to accept radioiodine or surgery.

Radioiodine
- This form of treatment is often considered as first choice for definitive treatment. ^{131}I is preferentially accumulated in hot nodules but not in normal thyroid tissue which, because of the thyrotoxic state, is non-functioning.
- Radioiodine treatment commonly induces a euthyroid state, as the hot nodules are destroyed and the previously non-functioning follicles gradually resume normal function. A dose of 500–800MBq for small-to-medium and 600 or 800MBq for medium-to-large goitres is recommended.

Surgery
- The aim of surgery is to remove as much of the nodular tissue as possible and, if the goitre is large, to relieve local symptoms. Post-operative follow-up should involve checks of thyroid function.
- Goitre recurrence, although rare, does occasionally occur.

Non-toxic multinodular goitre
Surgery
- Is the preferred treatment for patients with:
  - Local compression symptoms.
  - Cosmetic disfigurement.
- Solitary nodule with FNAC suspicious of malignancy.

Radioiodine
- Radioiodine may be particularly indicated in elderly patients in whom surgery is not appropriate. It may require admission. Up to 50% shrinkage of goitre mass has been reported in recent studies.
- Hypothyroidism following radioiodine is relatively infrequent but is still recognized.

Medical treatment
Use of T_4 to suppress TSH is associated with risk of cardiac arrhythmias and bone loss. T_4 is useful only if TSH is detectable but is not generally indicated.

Box 1.10 Aetiology of goitre
- Autoimmune thyroid disease.
- Sporadic.
- Endemic (iodine deficiency, dietary origins).
- Pregnancy.
- Drug-induced (ATDs, lithium, amiodarone).
- Thyroiditis syndromes.

Pathology

- Thyroid nodules may be described as *adenomas* if the follicular cell differentiation is enclosed within a capsule; *adenomatous* when the lesions are circumscribed but not encapsulated.
- The most common benign thyroid tumours are the nodules of multinodular goitres (colloid nodules) and follicular adenomas. The oncogene changes accounting for these benign thyroid nodules are not well delineated. Multinodular goitres are occasionally familial, which means that the patient has at least one germline mutation. One familial form of non-toxic multinodular goitre has been linked to DNA markers on chromosome 14q, but the aetiologic gene is not known. Follicular adenomas are clonal, and approximately 25% of sporadic follicular adenomas have a hemizygous deletion of a chromosome region containing PTEN (MMAC1), the tumour suppressor gene in which germline defects cause Cowden syndrome (see 📖 p. 584).
- Autonomously functioning thyroid adenomas (or nodules) are benign tumours that produce thyroid hormone. Clinically, they present as a single nodule that is hyperfunctioning ('hot') on thyroid radionuclide scan, sometimes causing hyperthyroidism. Many of these tumours are caused by somatic mutations in genes that code for the TSH receptor and α subunit of the guanyl nucleotide stimulatory protein (Gs).
- Activating mutations of the TSH receptor produce constitutive activation of adenylyl cyclase in the absence of TSH. The thyroid follicular cell with this TSH receptor mutation divides and produces thyroid hormone without TSH stimulation, eventually becoming clinically recognized as a hot nodule. Among patients with an autonomously functioning thyroid adenoma, the frequency of TSH receptor mutations in the adenoma varies from ~5% to 80%. Since the mutations are scattered throughout the receptor, studies of the entire receptor are most likely to identify a mutation. In rare families, germline mutations in the TSH receptor cause hereditary hyperthyroidism, initially with a diffuse goitre but ultimately with a nodular goitre with multiple hot nodules.

Thyroid nodules in pregnant women

- Increase in size during gestation.
- Increase in number.
- Need FNA as higher risk of malignancy.
- Can be operated upon in second trimester or post-partum.

Further reading

Bahn RS, Castro MR (2011). Approach to the patient with nontoxic multinodular goiter. *J Clin Endocrinol Metab* **96**, 1202–12.

Boelaert K (2009). The association between serum TSH concentration and thyroid cancer. *Endocr Relat Cancer* **16**, 1065–72.

Eszlinger M, Jaeschke H, Paschke R (2007). Insights from molecular pathways: potential pharmacologic targets of benign thyroid nodules. *Curr Opin Endocrinol Diabetes Obes* **14**, 393–7.

Fast S, Bonnema SJ, Hegedüs L (2011). Radioiodine therapy of benign non-toxic goitre. Potential role of recombinant human TSH. *Ann Endocrinol (Paris)* **72**, 129–35.

Lueblinghoff J, Eszlinger M, Jaeschke H, et al. (2011). Shared sporadic and somatic thyrotropin receptor mutations display more active in vitro activities than familial thyrotropin receptor mutations. *Thyroid* **21**, 221–9.

Thyroiditis

Background

Inflammation of the thyroid gland often leads to a transient thyrotoxicosis followed by hypothyroidism. Overt hypothyroidism caused by autoimmunity has two main forms: *Hashimoto's (goitrous) thyroiditis* and *atrophic thyroiditis*. See Tables 1.16 and 1.17.

Table 1.16 Causes and characteristics of thyroiditis

Cause	Characteristic features
Autoimmune thyroiditis (Hashimoto's)	Grossly lymphocytic and fibrotic hypothyroidism or thyrotoxicosis
Post-partum thyroiditis	Lymphocytic thyroiditis, transient thyrotoxicosis or hypothyroidism
Drug-induced	Amiodarone and interferon alfa
Subacute (de Quervain's)	Thought to be viral in origin, multinuclear giant cells
Riedel's thyroiditis	Extensive fibrosis of the thyroid
Radiation thyroiditis	Radiation injury, transient thyrotoxicosis
Pyogenic (rare)	*Staphylococcus aureus*, streptococci, *Escherichia coli*, tuberculosis, fungal

Table 1.17 Clinical presentation of thyroiditis

Form of thyroiditis	Clinical presentation	Thyroid function
Suppurative (acute)	Painful, tender thyroid, fever	Usually normal
Subacute (de Quervain's)	Painful anterior neck, arthralgia, antecedent upper respiratory tract infection, generalized malaise	Early thyrotoxicosis, occasionally late hypothyroidism
Autoimmune	Hashimoto: goitre Atrophic: no goitre	Usually hypothyroid Sometimes euthyroid Rarely early thyrotoxicosis
Riedel's	Hard, woody consistency of thyroid	Usually normal

Chronic autoimmune (atrophic or Hashimoto's) thyroiditis

(See Tables 1.16 and 1.17.)

- *Hashimoto's thyroiditis.* Characterized by a painless, variably-sized goitre with rubbery consistency and an irregular surface. The normal follicular structure of the gland is extensively replaced by lymphocytic and plasma cell infiltrates, with the formation of lymphoid germinal centres. The patient may have normal thyroid function or subclinical or overt hypothyroidism. Occasionally, patients present with thyrotoxicosis in association with a thyroid gland that is unusually firm and with high titres of circulating antithyroid antibodies.
- *Atrophic thyroiditis.* Probably indicates end-stage thyroid disease. These patients do not have goitre and are antibody +ve. Biochemically, the picture is that of frank hypothyroidism.

Investigations

Investigations which are useful in establishing a diagnosis of Hashimoto's thyroiditis include:

- Testing of thyroid function.
- Thyroid antibodies (antithyroglobulin antibodies +ve in 20–25% and antithyroperoxidase antibodies in >90%).
- Occasionally, a thyroid biopsy to exclude malignancy in patients who present with a goitre and dominant nodule.

Prognosis

The long-term prognosis of patients with chronic thyroiditis is good because hypothyroidism can easily be corrected with T_4 and the goitre is not usually of sufficient size to cause local symptoms. In the atypical situation where Hashimoto's thyroiditis presents with rapidly enlarging goitre and pain, a short course of prednisolone at a dose of 40mg daily may prove helpful.

Any unusual increase in size of the thyroid in patients known to suffer from Hashimoto's thyroiditis should be investigated with an FNA and, possibly later, a biopsy since there is an association between this condition and thyroid lymphoma (rare, but risk ↑ by a factor of 70).

Other types of thyroiditis

Silent thyroiditis

Associated with transient thyrotoxicosis or hypothyroidism. A significant percentage of patients have a personal or family history of autoimmune thyroid disease. It may progress to permanent hypothyroidism. There is a depressed radionuclide uptake.

Post-partum thyroiditis

 also see pp. 46, 432. Thyroid dysfunction occurring within the first 6 months post-partum. Prevalence ranges from 5% to 7%. Post-partum thyroiditis develops in 30–52% of ♀ who have +ve thyroid peroxidase (TPO) antibodies. Most patients have a complete remission, but some may progress to permanent hypothyroidism. It is thrice as common in patients with type 1 diabetes mellitus.

Chronic fibrosing (Riedel's) thyroiditis

A rare disorder characterized by intense fibrosis of the thyroid gland and surrounding structures, leading to induration of the tissues of the neck. May be associated with mediastinal and retroperitoneal fibrosis, salivary gland fibrosis, sclerosing cholangitis, lacrimal gland fibrosis, and parathyroid gland fibrosis leading to hypoparathyroidism. Patients are usually euthyroid. Main differential diagnosis is thyroid neoplasia.

Management

Corticosteroids are usually ineffective. Surgery may be required to relieve obstruction and to exclude malignancy. Tamoxifen may be of benefit.

Pyogenic thyroiditis

- Rare. Usually anteceded by a pyogenic infection elsewhere. Characterized by tenderness and swelling of the thyroid gland, redness and warmth of the overlying skin, and constitutional signs of infection.
- Piriform sinus infection should be excluded. Excision of tract is preferable to incision and drainage.
- Treatment consists of antibiotic therapy and incision and drainage if a fluctuant area within the thyroid should occur.

Subacute thyroiditis (granulomatous, giant cell, or de Quervain's thyroiditis)

- Viral in origin. Symptoms include pronounced asthenia, malaise, pain over the thyroid, or pain referred to lower jaw, ear, or occiput. Less commonly, the onset is acute, with fever, pain over the thyroid, and symptoms of thyrotoxicosis. Characteristically, signs include exquisite tenderness and nodularity of the thyroid gland. There is characteristically an elevated ESR/CRP and a depressed radionuclide (^{99m}Tc can be used) uptake. Biochemically, the patient may be initially thyrotoxic, though later the patient may become hypothyroid (15%).

- In mild cases, non-steroidal anti-inflammatory agents and paracetamol offer symptom relief. In severe cases, glucocorticoids (prednisolone 20–40mg/day) are effective. Propranolol can be used to control associated thyrotoxicosis. Treatment can be withdrawn when T_4 returns to normal. T_4 replacement is required if the patient becomes hypothyroid. Treatment with carbimazole or propylthiouracil is not indicated.

Drug-induced thyroiditis

Causes include:

- Amiodarone.
- Lithium.
- Interferon alfa (15% develop thyroid peroxidase antibodies and/or thyroid dysfunction).
- Interleukin 2.

Further reading

Costelloe SJ, Wassef N, Schulz J, et al. (2010). Thyroid dysfunction in a UK hepatitis C population treated with interferon-alpha and ribavirin combination therapy. *Clin Endocrinol (Oxf)* **73**, 249–56.

Fatourechi MM, Hay ID, McIver B, et al. (2011). Invasive fibrous thyroiditis (Riedel thyroiditis): the Mayo Clinic experience, 1976-2008. *Thyroid* **21**, 765–72.

Lazarus JH, Hall R, Othman S, et al. (1996). The clinical spectrum of postpartum thyroid disease. *QJM* **89**, 429–35.

Paes JE, Burman KD, Cohen J, et al. (2010). Acute bacterial suppurative thyroiditis: a clinical review and expert opinion. *Thyroid* **20**, 247–55.

Pearce EN, Farwell AP, Braverman LE (2003). Thyroiditis. *New Engl J Med* **348**, 2646–55.

Premawardhana LD, Parkes AB, Ammari F, et al. (2000). Postpartum thyroiditis and long-term thyroid status: prognostic influence of thyroid peroxidase antibodies and ultrasound echogenicity. *J Clin Endocrinol Metab* **85**, 71–5.

Weetman AP (2004). Autoimmune thyroid disease. *Autoimmunity* **37**, 337–40.

Weetman AP (2011). Diseases associated with thyroid autoimmunity: explanations for the expanding spectrum. *Clin Endocrinol (Oxf)* **74**, 411–18.

Hypothyroidism

Background

Hypothyroidism results from a variety of abnormalities that cause insufficient secretion of thyroid hormones (see Table 1.18). The commonest cause is autoimmune thyroid disease. *Myxoedema* is severe hypothyroidism in which there is accumulation of hydrophilic mucopolysaccharides in the ground substance of the dermis and other tissues, leading to thickening of the facial features and a doughy induration of the skin. See Box 1.11 for pitfalls with the thyroid function tests in non-thyroidal illness.

Epidemiology

- High TSH (>5.0) in 7.5% of ♀ and 2.5% of ♂ >65 years, 1.7% overt hypothyroidism, 13.7% subclinical hypothyroidism (Whickham Survey, UK).
- Incidence higher in whites than Hispanics or African-American populations.
- Incidence higher in areas of high iodine intake.
- An elevated TSH is associated with higher serum lipid concentrations, which may be an additional reason to initiate therapy.

Clinical picture

Adult

- Insidious, non-specific onset.
- Fatigue, lethargy, constipation, cold intolerance, muscle stiffness, cramps, carpal tunnel syndrome, menorrhagia, later oligo- or amenorrhoea.
- Slowing of intellectual and motor activities.
- ↓ appetite and weight gain.
- Dry skin; hair loss.
- Deep hoarse voice, ↓ visual acuity.
- Obstructive sleep apnoea.

Myxoedema

- Dull expressionless face, sparse hair, periorbital puffiness, macroglossia.
- Pale, cool skin that feels rough and doughy.
- Enlarged heart (dilation and pericardial effusion).
- Megacolon/intestinal obstruction.
- Cerebellar ataxia.
- Prolonged relaxation phase of deep tendon reflexes.
- Peripheral neuropathy.
- Encephalopathy.
- Hyperlipidaemia.
- Hypercarotenaemia (also caused by hyperlipidaemia, diabetes mellitus, anorexia, and porphyria).
- Psychiatric symptoms, e.g. depression, psychosis.
- Marked respiratory depression with ↑ arterial PCO_2.
- Hyponatraemia from impaired water excretion and disordered regulation of vasopressin secretion.

Myxoedema coma

- Predisposed to by cold exposure, trauma, infection, administration of central nervous system depressants.

Table 1.18 Classification of the causes of hypothyroidism

	TSH	Free T$_4$
Non-goitrous	↑	↓
Post-ablative (radioiodine, surgery)		
Congenital development defect		
Atrophic thyroiditis		
Post-radiation (e.g. for lymphoma)		
Goitrous	↑	↓
Chronic thyroiditis (Hashimoto's thyroiditis)		
Transient, 2–8 weeks (de Quervain's thyroiditis)		
Iodine deficiency		
Drug-elicited (amiodarone, aminosalicylic acid, iodides, phenylbutazone, lithium, aminoglutethimide, interferon alfa, thalidomide, sunitinib, rifampicin, stavudine)		
Haemochromatosis		
Heritable biosynthetic defects		
Maternally transmitted (antithyroid agents, iodides)		
Pituitary	↓	↓
Panhypopituitarism		
Isolated TSH deficiency Drugs (bexarotene)		
Hypothalamic	↓	↓
Neoplasm		
Infiltrative (sarcoidosis)		
Congenital defects		
Infection (encephalitis)		
Self-limiting	↑	↓
Following withdrawal of suppressive thyroid therapy		
Subacute thyroiditis and chronic thyroiditis with transient hypothyroidism		
Post-partum thyroiditis		

Box 1.11 Pitfalls with the thyroid function tests in non-thyroidal illness

- TSH suppressed in hospitalized patients with acute illness.
- Dopamine and steroids may suppress TSH, e.g. in critically ill patients.
- TSH increase during recovery from acute illness.
- TSH may fall during first trimester of pregnancy (hCG).
- TSH inhibited by subcutaneous octreotide.
- Anorexia nervosa is associated with low TSH and FT_4.
- Heterophilic antibodies, including rheumatoid factor, may falsely elevate TSH.
- Adrenal insufficiency may be associated with a raised TSH which reverses on treatment with glucocorticoids.

Subclinical hypothyroidism

- This term is used to denote raised TSH levels in the presence of normal concentrations of free thyroid hormones.
- Treatment is indicated if the biochemistry is sustained in patients with a past history of radioiodine treatment for thyrotoxicosis or +ve thyroid antibodies as, in these situations, progression to overt hypothyroidism is almost inevitable (at least 5% per year of those with +ve antithyroid peroxidase antibodies).
- Two samples should be taken 2–3 months apart to distinguish from non-thyroidal illness.
- The reference range for serum TSH rises with age.
- There is controversy over the advantages of T_4 treatment in patients with −ve thyroid antibodies and no previous radioiodine treatment.
- If treatment is not given, follow-up with annual thyroid function tests is important.
- There is no generally accepted consensus of when patients should receive treatment. Some authorities suggest treatment when serum TSH is >10mU/L because of ↑ rate of progression to overt hypothyroidism. Below that, if the TSH is raised, treatment is geared to the individual patient.
- Increased incidence of cardiovascular risk, probably greater if <65 years old.
- There is some evidence that women with autoimmune thyroiditis are more likely to have an increased risk of recurrent miscarriage, although it is not known whether the risk is related to thyroid autoimmunity or to subtle thyroid failure. In this situation, there may be an advantage to giving thyroxine if TSH is between 2.5 and 5mU/L.
- Acceleration of thyroid hormone metabolism during pregnancy can lead to hypothyroidism in women with a limited thyroid hormone reserve. If untreated, mild hypothyroidism can lead to subtle impairment of subsequent childhood neuropsychological development. Early correction of maternal hypothyroxinaemia is recommended, aiming to maintain serum TSH in the lower half of the reference range prior to conception, if possible.

Management

- If serum TSH is >10mU/L, then levothyroxine is indicated.
- If serum TSH is mildly increased between 4–10mU/L and the patient is TPO antibody +ve, an annual check of serum TSH is recommended, with commencement of levothyroxine once serum TSH >10mU/L.
- If the patient is thyroid antibody −ve, then ensuring a check of serum TSH every 3–5 years is all that is required.
- If the patient with a serum TSH 4–10mU/L has symptoms consistent with hypothyroidism and the TSH elevation persists, then a 3–6 months' therapeutic trial of levothyroxine appears justified. If the patient feels improved by therapy, it is reasonable to continue treatment.

- If the patient with serum TSH 4–10U/L does not have symptoms and the serum TSH level appears stable with +ve TPO antibodies, the annual risk of progression to overt hypothyroidism is 4% per year, and so an annual serum TSH surveillance strategy is warranted. If the TPO antibodies are −ve, then 3-yearly serum TSH surveillance is recommended, with a risk of progression to overt hypothyroidism of 3% per year.
- The exception to the above is in *neonates and children*, pregnancy, or in someone trying to conceive when a mildly increased serum TSH should always be treated, as it is associated with adverse outcomes for both mother and fetus.
- Recent data suggest that levothyroxine treatment for those with *serum TSH 5–10U/L* may also now be justified in subjects <65 years and in those older subjects with documented evidence of heart failure on echocardiography.

Treatment of hypothyroidism

Note that patients in the UK with hypothyroidism are entitled to a medical exemption certificate for prescription charges.

- Thyroid hormone replacement with synthetic levothyroxine remains the treatment of choice in primary hypothyroidism. See Table 1.19 for excipient content in case of intolerance.
- Levothyroxine with a long half-life enables the patient to take two doses at once if a dose is omitted.
- Normal metabolic state should be restored gradually, as a rapid increase in metabolic rate may precipitate cardiac arrhythmias.
- The average replacement dose is 1.6–1.8 micrograms/kg/day.
- To avoid iatrogenic subclinical disease, fasting ingestion of levothyroxine is best either in the morning or the evening.
- In the younger patients, start levothyroxine at 50–100 micrograms. In the elderly with a history of ischaemic heart disease, an initial dose of levothyroxine 25–50 micrograms can be ↑ by 25 micrograms increments at 4-week intervals until normal metabolic state and TSH is attained.
- Optimum dose is determined by clinical criteria, the objective of treatment being to restore serum TSH to the normal range.
- TSH should be checked only 6 weeks after any dose change. Once stabilized, TSH should be checked on an annual basis. Patients should stay on the same brand of levothyroxine as far as is possible—otherwise, TSH should be checked at 2 months.
- Muscle problems may take up to 6 months to fully recover.
- It is estimated that 5% of hypothyroid patients remain symptomatic in spite of levothyroxine replacement and normal serum TSH concentrations. Possible causes include awareness of a chronic disease, presence of associated autoimmune diseases, and thyroid autoimmunity *per se* (independent of thyroid function).
- In those patients who remain symptomatic and in whom serum TSH remains towards the upper end of the reference range, it is usual practice for the dose of levothyroxine to be increased slightly to target a serum TSH at the lower end of the reference range (≤2.5mU/L). Whether or not such small changes in serum TSH within the reference range are associated with symptoms is uncertain.
- Patients with iatrogenic hyperthyroidism (serum TSH <0.03U/L) have a significantly increased risk of arrhythmia and fractures.
- In most trials, combination levothyroxine-T_3 therapy does not appear to be superior to levothyroxine monotherapy for the management of hypothyroid symptoms. In three trials, patients preferred combined therapy to levothyroxine monotherapy; however, in one of those studies, patients were given doses of thyroid hormone which resulted in mild hyperthyroidism. In general, clinical trials of combination levothyroxine-T_3 therapy have not successfully replicated physiological T_4-T_3 production. Forty micrograms of T_3 is approximately equivalent to 0.125mg of T_4.
- One study has suggested that a small group of patients with a polymorphism in D2 may benefit from levothyroxine-T_3 therapy.

Table 1.19 Excipient content of generic levothyroxine tablets

Excipient	Goldshield	Norton/IVAX (manufactured by Goldshield)	Cox/Alpharma (50 + 100 micrograms only)*	APS/Berk (50 + 100 micrograms only)*	CP Pharmaceuticals (only make 25 micrograms)	Hillcross 25 micrograms	Hillcross 50/100 micrograms
Thyroxine	✓	✓	✓	✓	✓	✓	✓
Lactose	✓	✓	✓	✓	✓	✓	✓
Sucrose			✓		✓	✓	
Dextrin				✓			
Maize starch	✓	✓	✓	✓	✓	✓	✓
Magnesium stearate	✓	✓	✓	✓	✓	✓	
Pre-gelatinized maize starch			✓				✓
Stearic acid	✓		✓				✓
Water	✓ (50 + 100 micrograms)	✓	✓				✓
Sodium citrate	✓						
Powdered acacia	✓						

* 25 microgram tablets made by Goldshield.

Hillcross: 25 micrograms are manufactured by CP Pharmaceuticals; 50 and 100 micrograms are manufactured by Alpharma.

Norton/IVAX: 25, 50, and 100 micrograms are manufactured by Goldshield.

Data from Drug Information department of each manufacturer, August 2004.

- Dessicated animal thyroid extracts (e.g. thyroid Armour) contain an excessive amount of T_3 and are not consistent with normal physiology.
- In patients with 2° hypothyroidism, free T_4 is the most useful parameter to follow.
- Dose requirements can increase by 25–50% in pregnancy due to the increase in thyroid-binding globulin (TBG). Recent data have shown that mild maternal hypothyroidism in the first trimester is associated with slightly impaired cognitive function in offspring. Thus, it is now recommended to routinely ↑ levothyroxine dose by 25 micrograms in any ♀ on replacement therapy when she learns she is pregnant.

Management of myxoedema coma

- Identify and treat concurrent precipitating illness.
- Antibiotic therapy after blood cultures.
- Management of hypothermia by passive external rewarming.
- Manage in intensive treatment unit if comatose.
- Give warm humidified oxygen by face mask. Mechanical ventilation needed if hypoventilating.
- Aim for slow rise in core temperature (0.5°C/h).
- Cardiac monitor for supraventricular arrhythmias.
- Correct hyponatraemia (mild fluid restriction), hypotension (cautious volume expansion with crystalloid or whole blood), and hypoglycaemia (glucose administration).
- Monitor rectal temperature, oxygen saturation, BP, CVP, and urine output hourly.
- Take blood samples for thyroid hormones, TSH, and cortisol before starting treatment. If hypocortisolaemic, administer glucocorticoids.
- Thyroid hormone replacement: no consensus has been reached. The following is an accepted regimen:
  - T_4 300–500 micrograms IV or by NG tube as a starting dose, followed by 50–100 micrograms daily until oral medication can be taken.
  - If no improvement within 24–48h, T_3 10 micrograms IV 8-hourly or 25 micrograms IV 8-hourly can be given in addition to above.
- Give hydrocortisone 50–100mg 6–8-hourly in case of cortisol deficiency.

Management of persistently elevated TSH despite thyroxine replacement

(See Fig. 1.2).
- As levothyroxine has a narrow therapeutic index, the margin between over- and underdosing can be small.
- Elevated TSH despite thyroxine replacement is common, most usually due to lack of compliance.
- If TSH still elevated when levothyroxine dose at 1.6 micrograms/kg/day or higher, careful questioning of compliance is needed.
- Consider malabsorption.
- Consider other drugs that may interfere with levothyroxine absorption (see Box 1.12).

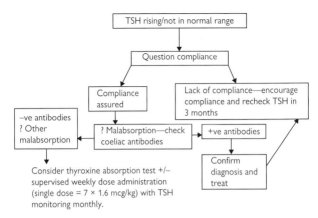

Fig. 1.2 Suggestions for investigations of elevated TSH despite levothyroxine replacement therapy to >1.6 micrograms/kg/day.

Box 1.12 Interference with absorption of thyroxine

- Coeliac disease.
- Drugs: ↑ clearance of thyroxine—rifampicin, phenytoin, phenobarbital, carbamazepine, imatinib; ↓ absorption of thyroxine—calcium salts, ferrous sulfate, aluminium hydroxide, colestyramine, omeprazole, sucralfate.
- Atrophic gastritis in *Helicobacter pylori* infection (↓ T_4 by 30%).

Congenital hypothyroidism

Incidence—about 1 in 3,500–4,000 neonates. All neonates should be screened. There is an inverse relationship between age at diagnosis and intelligence quotient (IQ) in later life. In iodine-replete areas, 85% of the cases are due to sporadic developmental defects of the thyroid gland (thyroid dysgenesis), such as the arrested migration of the embryonic thyroid (ectopic thyroid) or a complete absence of thyroid tissue (athyreosis). The remaining 15% have thyroid dyshormonogenesis defects transmitted by an autosomal recessive mode of inheritance. See Box 1.13 for clinical features.

Thyroid hormone dysgenesis

- Caused by inborn errors of thyroid metabolism. The disorders may be autosomal recessive, indicating single protein defects.
- Can be caused by inactivation of the TSH receptor, abnormalities of the thyroid transcription factors TTF1, TTF2, and PAX8, or due to defects in iodide transport, organification (peroxidase), coupling, deiodinase, or thyroglobulin synthesis.
- In a large proportion of patients with congenital hypothyroidism, the molecular background is unknown.

Pendred's syndrome

Characterized by overt or subclinical hypothyroidism, goitre, and moderate-to-severe sensorineural hearing impairment. The prevalence varies between 1 in 15,000 and 1 in 100,000. There is a partial iodide organification defect detected by ↑ perchlorate discharge. Thyroid hormone synthesis is only mildly impaired and so may not be detected by neonatal thyroid screening.

Box 1.13 Clinical features and congenital hypothyroidism

The following features are late sequelae of congenital hypothyroidism and, with routine screening now available, should never be seen nowadays.

- Physiological jaundice.
- Goitre.
- Hoarse cry, feeding problems, constipation, somnolence.
- Delay in reaching normal milestones of development, short stature.
- Coarse features with protruding tongue, broad flat nose, widely set eyes.
- Sparse hair and dry skin, protuberant abdomen with umbilical hernia.
- Impaired mental development, retarded bone age.
- Epiphyseal dysgenesis, delayed dentition.

Laboratory tests

- Neonatal screening by measurement of serum TSH.
- Imaging procedure: ultrasonography or ^{123}I scintigraphy.
- Measurement of serum thyroglobulin and low molecular weight iodopeptides in urine to discriminate between the various types of defects.
- Measurement of neonatal and maternal autoantibodies as an indication of possible transient hypothyroidism.

Treatment

Irrespective of the cause of congenital hypothyroidism, early treatment is essential to prevent cerebral damage. Sufficient T_4 should be given to maintain the TSH in the normal range.

Further reading

Biondi B, Cooper DC (2008). The clinical significance of subclinical thyroid dysfunction. *Endocr Rev* **29**, 76–131.

Escobar-Morales HF, Botella-Carretero JI, Escobar del Rey F, et al. (2005). Treatment of hypothyroidism with combinations of levothyroxine plus liothyronine. *J Clin Endocrinol Metab* **90**, 4949–54.

Flynn RW, Bonellie SR, Jung RT, et al. (2010). Serum thyroid-stimulating hormone concentration and morbidity from cardiovascular disease and fractures in patients on long-term thyroxine therapy. *J Clin Endocrinol Metab* **95**, 186–93.

Garber JR, Cobin RH, Gharib H, et al. (2012). Clinical practice guidelines for hypothyroidism in adults. *Thyroid* **22**, 1–32.

Grozinsky-Glasberg S, Fraser A, Nahshoni E, et al. (2006). L. Thyroxine-triiodothyronine combination therapy versus thyroxine monotherapy for clinical hypothyroidism: meta-analysis of randomized controlled trials. *J Clin Endocrinol Metab* **91**, 2592–9.

Grüters A, Krude H (2007). Update on the management of congenital hypothyroidism. *Horm Res* **68**(Suppl 5), 107–111.

Hennemann G, Docter R, Visser TJ, et al. (2004). Thyroxine plus low-dose, slow-release triiodothyronine replacement in hypothyroidism: proof of principle. *Thyroid* **14**, 271–5.

Nygaard B, Jensen EW, Kvetny J, et al. (2009). Effect of combination therapy with thyroxine (T4) and 3,5,3'-triiodothyronine versus T4 monotherapy in patients with hypothyroidism, a double-blind, randomised cross-over study. *Eur J Endocrinol* **161**, 895–902.

Okosieme OE, Belludi G, Spittle K, et al. (2011). Adequacy of thyroid hormone replacement in a general population. *QJM* **104**, 395–401.

Roberts CG, Ladenson PW (2004). Hypothyroidism. *Lancet* **363**, 793–803.

Rodondi N, den Elzen WP, Bauer DC, et al. (2010). Subclinical hypothyroidism and the risk of coronary heart disease and mortality. *JAMA* **304**, 1365–74.

Royal College of Physicians (2011). The diagnosis and management of primary hypothyroidism. Royal College of Physicians, London.

Taylor PN, Panicker V, Sayers A, et al. (2011). A meta-analysis of the associations between common variation in the PDE8B gene and thyroid hormone parameters, including assessment of longitudinal stability of associations over time and effect of thyroid hormone replacement. *Eur J Endocrinol* **164**, 773–80.

Vaidya B, Pearce SH (2008). Management of hypothyroidism. *BMJ* **337**, a801.

Vanderpump MP (2010). How should we manage patients with mildly increased serum thyrotrophin concentrations? *Clin Endocrinol (Oxf)* **72**, 436–40.

Amiodarone and thyroid function

Background

- Amiodarone has a high concentration of iodine (39% by weight). It is a benzofuranic derivative, and its structural formula closely resembles that of thyroxine. On a dose of amiodarone between 200 and 600mg daily, 7–21mg iodine is made available each day. The optimal daily iodine intake is 150–200 micrograms. Amiodarone is distributed in several tissues from where it is slowly released. In one study, terminal elimination half-life of amiodarone averaged 52.6 days, with a standard deviation of 23.7 days.
- Abnormalities of thyroid function occur in up to 50% of patients (see Table 1.20).
- In the UK and USA, 2% of patients on amiodarone develop thyrotoxicosis and about 13% develop hypothyroidism.
- Patients residing in areas with high iodine intake develop amiodarone-induced hypothyroidism (AIH) more often than amiodarone-induced thyrotoxicosis (AIT), but AIT occurs more frequently in regions with low iodine intake.
- AIT can present several months after discontinuing the drug because of its long half-life.
- Hypothyroidism is commoner in ♀ and in patients with thyroid autoantibodies.
- Thyroid function tests should be monitored initially prior and then every 6 months in patients taking amiodarone.
- Other side effects and complications occur (see Table 1.22).
- Dronedarone is a non-iodinated benzofuran derivative with multichannel blocking effects and anti-adrenergic properties. Although it is an antagonist of $TR\alpha_1$ and $TR\beta_1$ isoforms, it has little impact on thyroid hormones.

Pathogenesis

- The high iodine content of amiodarone may inhibit thyroglobulin iodination and thyroid hormone synthesis and release, causing AIH (Wolff–Chaikoff effect), or lead to iodine-induced hyperthyroidism in susceptible individuals (Jod-Basedow phenomenon).
- Amiodarone also inhibits monodeiodination of T_4, thus decreasing T_3 production, and blocks T_3 binding to nuclear receptors.
- Thyrotoxicosis resulting from iodine excess, and therefore ↑ hormone synthesis, is referred to as *AIT type I*. Thyrotoxicosis due to a direct toxic effect of amiodarone (thyroiditis) is referred to as *AIT type II* (see Table 1.21).
- Drug-induced destructive thyroiditis results in leakage of thyroid hormones from damaged follicles into the circulation and, like subacute thyroiditis, can be followed by a transient hypothyroid state before euthyroidism is restored.

Table 1.20 Thyroid function tests in clinically euthyroid patients after administration of amiodarone

Tests	1–3 months	>3 months
Free T_3	Decreased	Remains slightly decreased but within normal range
TSH	Transient increase	Normal
Free T_4	Modest increase	Slightly increased compared to pretreatment values, may be in normal range or slightly increased
Reverse T_3	Increased	Increased

Table 1.21 Characteristics of AIT (some patients have a mixed form, and classification is not always possible)

	AIT type I (10%)	AIT type II (90%)
Aetiology	Iodine toxicity	Thyroiditis
Signs of clinical thyroid disease	Yes	No
Goitre	Frequent	Infrequent
Thyroid antibodies	Positive	Negative
Radioiodine uptake	Normal	Decreased
Thyroglobulin	Normal or slightly elevated	Very elevated
Late hypothyroidism	No	Possible
Vascularity (Doppler)	Increased/normal	Reduced

Diagnosis and treatment

(See Table 1.22.)

- After chronic administration of amiodarone, a steady state is achieved, typically reflected in mild elevation of free T_4 and reduction in free T_3. Thus, in clinically euthyroid patients on amiodarone, a slightly elevated T_4 is neither indicative of hyperthyroidism nor is a low T_3 indicative of hypothyroidism.
- Hyperthyroidism is indicated by significantly ↑ free T_4, together with elevated free T_3 and suppressed serum TSH.
- Hypothyroidism is indicated by elevation of TSH, with low serum free T_4. Levothyroxine replacement is almost always considered for those with serum TSH >20U/L. If serum TSH is between 5 and 20U/L, the value of levothyroxine replacement can be judged on clinical grounds, such as abnormality of diastolic function, which can be reversible.
  If serum free T_4 is below the reference range, then levothyroxine replacement is usually indicated.

- Discontinuation of amiodarone does not always control the thyrotoxic state because of its long half-life (particularly in the obese) due to its very high volume of distribution and fat solubility.
- Numerous complex published algorithms exist for management, but, since classification into type I and type II is often difficult (see Table 1.22), in practice, most patients are treated with ATDs ± glucocorticoids (see Table 1.23).
- There is often reluctance amongst endocrinologists to use relatively high-dose glucocorticoid therapy, particularly in an elderly patient group with significant comorbidities who may often present asymptomatically with a mild, and often self-limiting, disease, but evidence exists that early use of glucocorticoid therapy is safe and effective in patients with AIT type II.
- If there is doubt as to whether a patient has AIT type I or type II, a regimen of 40mg of carbimazole and 40mg of prednisolone daily for 2 weeks, followed by measurement of serum T_3 does seem a reasonable initial strategy. If there is a reduction in serum T_3 by >50%, compared to pretreatment levels, then carbimazole is stopped, as the diagnosis of AIT type II is suggested. Prednisolone can then be continued in a tapering dose, reducing course over 2–3 months, according to the clinical and biochemical response. If there is no change in serum T_3 levels following initial treatment, prednisolone can be stopped and carbimazole is continued, as the assumption is that the predominant diagnosis is AIT type I.
- Radioiodine is not usually effective because of reduced uptake by the thyroid gland, reflecting the iodine load associated with the drug.
- Surgery remains a very successful form of treatment, with euthyroidism being restored within a matter of days. Achieving preoperative euthyroidism may be difficult, however.
- Cardiac function may be compromised by propranolol used in combination with amiodarone since this may produce bradycardia and sinus arrest.
- Potassium perchlorate inhibits iodide uptake by the thyroid gland, reduces intrathyroidal iodine, and renders thionamides more effective. It can be given as a 1g daily dose, together with carbimazole, a regimen shown to restore euthyroidism in a large percentage of patients with both type I and type II AIT. In small case studies, a combination of potassium perchlorate and carbimazole has been effective while treatment with amiodarone was continued.
- See Box 1.14 for treatment of amiodarone-induced hypothyroidism.

Box 1.14 Treatment of amiodarone-induced hypothyroidism

Underlying thyroid abnormality (usually Hashimoto's thyroiditis)
- Amiodarone therapy can be continued.
- Add thyroxine replacement therapy.

Apparently normal thyroid
- Discontinue amiodarone, if possible, and follow up for restoration of euthyrodism.
  - If amiodarone cannot be withdrawn, start thyroxine replacement therapy.

Table 1.22 Side effects and complications of amiodarone therapy

Side effect	Incidence (%)
Corneal microdeposits	100
Anorexia and nausea	80
Photosensitivity, blue/grey skin discoloration	55–75
Ataxia, tremors, peripheral neuropathy	48
Deranged liver function tests	25
Abnormal thyroid function tests	14–18
Interstitial pneumonitis	10–13
Cardiac arrhythmias	2–3

Table 1.23 Treatment of amiodarone-induced thyrotoxicosis

	Type I AIT	Type II AIT
Step 1: Aim to restore euthyroidism	Carbimazole up to 40mg/day or propylthiouracil 400mg/day, in combination, if necessary, with potassium perchlorate 1g/day for 16–40 days If possible, discontinue amiodarone*	Discontinue amiodarone, if possible* Prednisolone 40mg/day In mixed forms, add carbimazole or propylthiouracil as in type I AIT
Step 2: Definitive treatment	Radioiodine treatment or thyroidectomy	Follow-up for possible spontaneous progression to hypothyroidism

* If amiodarone cannot be withdrawn and medical therapy is unsuccessful, consider total thyroidectomy.

Further reading

Bogazzi F, Bartalena L, Dell'Unto E, *et al.* (2007). Proportion of type 1 and type 2 amiodarone-induced thyrotoxicosis has changed over a 27-year period in Italy. *Clin Endocrinol (Oxf)* **67**, 533–7.

Bogazzi F, Bartalena L, Martino E (2010). Approach to the patient with amiodarone-induced thyrotoxicosis. *J Clin Endocrinol Metab* **95**, 2529–35.

Bogazzi F, Tomisti L, Rossi G, *et al.* (2009). Glucocorticoids are preferable to thionamides as first-line treatment for amiodarone-induced thyrotoxicosis due to destructive thyroiditis: A matched retrospective cohort study. *J Clin Endocrinol Metab* **94**, 3757–62.

Franklyn JA, Gammage MD (2007). Treatment of amiodarone-associated thyrotoxicosis. *Nat Clin Pract Endocrinol Metab* **3**, 662–6.

Han T, Williams GR, Vanderpump MP (2009). Benzofuran derivatives and the thyroid. *Clin Endocrinol (Oxf)* **70**, 2–13.

Loy M, Perra E, Mellis A, *et al.* (2007). Color-flow doppler sonography in the differential diagnosis and management of amiodarone-induced thyrotoxicosis. *Acta Radiol* **48**, 628–34.

Tanda ML, Piantanida E, Lai A, *et al.* (2008). Diagnosis and management of amiodarone-induced thyrotoxicosis: similarities and differences between North American and European thyroidologists. *Clin Endocrinol (Oxf)* **69**, 812–18.

Epidemiology of thyroid cancer

- Clinical presentation of thyroid cancer is usually as a solitary thyroid nodule or increasing goitre size (see Tables 1.24 and 1.25).
- Although thyroid nodules are common, clinically detectable thyroid cancer is rare. It accounts for <1% of all cancer and <0.5% of cancer deaths.
- The incidence of thyroid cancer is increasing, with the majority of the increase attributable to an increase in incidence of papillary thyroid cancer measuring ≤2cm.
- Papillary thyroid microcarcinomas (diameter <1cm) are found in up to one-third of adults at post-mortem in population-based studies.
- Thyroid cancers are commonest in adults aged 40–50 and rare in children and adolescents.
- ♀ are affected more frequently than ♂.

Table 1.24 Classification of thyroid cancer

Cell of origin	Tumour type	Frequency (%)
Differentiated:		
Papillary		>80
Follicular		10
Undifferentiated (anaplastic)		1–5
C cells	Medullary	5–10
Lymphocytes	Lymphoma	1–5

Table 1.25 Comparison of papillary, follicular and anaplastic carcinomas (Ca) of the thyroid

Characteristic	Papillary Ca	Follicular Ca	Anaplastic Ca
Age at presentation (years)	30–50 (mean 44)	40–50	60–80
Spread	Lymphatic	Haematogenous	Haematogenous
Prognosis	Good	Good	Poor
Treatment	Initially: near total thyroidectomy Post-operative TSH suppression High-risk patient: ^{131}I remnant ablation Post-operative total body radioiodine scan + thyroglobulin measurement	Initially: near total thyroidectomy Post-operative TSH suppression ^{131}I remnant ablation Post-operative total body radioiodine scan + thyroglobulin measurement	Total thyroidectomy with lymph node clearance Chemotherapy with doxorubicin and cisplatin External beam irradiation

Aetiology of thyroid cancer

(See Tables 1.26 and 1.27.)

Irradiation

- There does not appear to be a threshold dose of external irradiation for thyroid carcinogenesis; doses of 200–500cGy seem to produce thyroid cancer at a rate of about 0.5%/year.
- There is no evidence that therapeutic or diagnostic ^{131}I administration can induce thyroid cancer, although there is a small increase in death rates from thyroid cancer after ^{131}I. At present, it is unclear whether this is due to an effect of ^{131}I or part of the natural history of the underlying thyroid disease.
- External irradiation at an age <20 years is associated with an ↑ risk of thyroid nodule development and thyroid cancer (most commonly papillary). The radioactive fallout from the Chernobyl nuclear explosion in 1986 resulted in a 4.7-fold increase in thyroid cancer in the regions of Belarus from 1985 to 1993, including a 34-fold increase in children. Children aged <10 years were the most sensitive to radiation-induced carcinogenesis, and the minimal latent period for thyroid cancer development after exposure is as short as 4 years. The vast majority of these cancers were papillary carcinomas, many of which have characteristic solid or solid follicular microscopic appearance.
- The risk is greater for ♀ and when irradiation occurs at a younger age.
- There is a latency of at least 5 years, with maximum risk at 20 years following exposure, though this was not seen following the Chernobyl disaster.

Other environmental factors

Most investigators agree that iodine supplementation has resulted in a decrease in the incidence of follicular carcinoma.

Genetic syndromes and oncogenes

- Non-overlapping genetic alterations, including *BRAF* and *RAS* point mutations and *RET/PTC* and *PAX8/PPAR*γ rearrangements, are found in >70% of papillary and follicular thyroid carcinomas.
- *RET/PTC1* proto-oncogene abnormalities in the long arm of chromosome 10 are associated with some papillary tumours (5–30%), especially after irradiation (60–80%). It is similar to the abnormality associated with medullary thyroid carcinoma in MEN2A.
- Post-Chernobyl tumours are characterized by frequent occurrence of chromosomal rearrangements, such as *RET/PTC*, whereas point mutations of *BRAF* and other genes are much less common in this population.
- *BRAF* mutations may be more aggressive, with higher rates of extrathyroidal extension, lymph node metastases, and clinically apparent recurrence.
- The tumour suppressor gene *p53* has been found to be mutated in some dedifferentiated cancers.

Table 1.26 TNM staging system for papillary and follicular thyroid carcinoma

Stage	Age <45 years	Age >45 years
I	Any T, any N, M0	T1, N0, M0
II	Any T, any N, M1	T2, N0, M0
III		T3, N0, M0 or any T1–3, N1a, M0
IVA		T1–3, N1b, M0 or T4a, any N, M0 N, M0
IVB		T4b, any N, M0
IVC		Any T, any N, M1

Primary tumour (T): T1, tumour ≤ 2cm limited to the thyroid; T2, tumour > 2 to ≤ 4cm limited to the thyroid; T3, tumour > 4cm limited to the thyroid or any tumour with minimal extrathyroidal extension (e.g. extension to sternothyroid muscle or perithyroidal soft tissues); T4a, tumour of any size with extension beyond the thyroid capsule and invading any of the following: subcutaneous soft tissues, larynx, trachea, oesophagus, recurrent laryngeal nerve; T4b, tumour invading prevertebral fascia, mediastinal vessels, or encases carotid artery.

Lymph nodes (N): To classify as N0 or N1, at least six lymph nodes should be examined at histology. Otherwise, the tumour is classified as Nx. N0, no regional lymph node metastasis; N1a, metastases in pretracheal and paratracheal, including prelaryngeal and Delphian lymph nodes; N1b, metastases in other unilateral, bilateral, or contralateral cervical or upper mediastinal lymph nodes.

Distant metastases (M): M0, no distant metastasis; M1, distant metastasis.

Reproduced from Wass, J, Oxford Textbook of Endocrinology and Diabetes, 2011, with permission from OUP.

Table 1.27 Risk categorization for thyroid cancer follow-up

Very low risk	Tumour 1cm	N0, M0
Low risk	Tumour 2–4cm	N0, M0
High risk	T3, T4	N0, M0

- Overexpression of the *RAS* and *PTTG* oncogenes is also found in papillary thyroid cancers and have been found to be markers for adverse prognosis.
- c-*myc* mRNA expression has been correlated with histological markers of papillary cancer aggression.
- The use of these and other emerging molecular markers will likely improve the diagnosis of malignancy in thyroid nodules as well as facilitate more individualized operative and post-operative management.

Papillary microcarcinoma of the thyroid (PMC)

- PMC is defined by WHO as a tumour focus of 1.0cm or less in diameter. It is detected coincidentally on histopathological examination of the thyroid following resection of multinodular goitre or any thyroid resected.

- Autopsy studies show:
  - Prevalence ranges from 1% to 35.6%.
  - No significant difference in the prevalence rates of PMC has been demonstrated between the sexes.
  - PMC rarely progresses to clinically apparent thyroid cancer with advancing age.
  - PMC can be multifocal.
  - Cervical lymph node metastasis from PMC ranges from 4.3% to 18.2%.
  - Lymph node metastasis was most often associated with multifocal tumours.
- Although exposure to irradiation increases the likelihood of developing papillary thyroid cancer, the tumours will usually be >1.0cm in diameter and thus not PMC.
- Follow-up studies suggest that PMC is a slow-growing lesion which rarely spreads to distant sites and which carries a good prognosis.
- The recommendations for treatment of PMC vary widely:
  - The low morbidity and long survival mean that collection of randomized prospective data has never been performed, and comparisons of therapies are based on retrospective studies.
  - The treatment of PMC should not cause more morbidity than the disease process itself.
  - Surgical treatment recommendations range from simple excision to ipsilateral lobectomy.
  - With adjuvant therapy, the consensus is routine use of T_4, but not the use of radioiodine, as there is no difference in the recurrence rate. There is some evidence to keep TSH below the reference range, but robust data are not available.

Papillary thyroid carcinoma

- Constitutes almost >80% of all thyroid cancers.
- Commoner in ♀ (3:1).
- Rare in childhood; peaks occur in second and third decades and again in later life (bimodal frequency).
- Incidence: 3–5 per 100,000 population.

Pathology

- Slow-growing, usually non-encapsulated, may spread through the thyroid capsule to structures in the surrounding neck, especially regional lymph nodes. Multifocal in 30% of cases.
- Recognized variants are follicular, papillary, dorsal, columnar cell, tall cell, and diffuse sclerosing.
- *Histology.* The tumour contains complex branching papillae that have a fibrovascular core covered by a single layer of tumour cells.
- Nuclear features include:
  - Large size with pale-staining, 'ground glass' appearance (*orphan Annie-eye nucleus*).
  - Deep nuclear grooves.
- The characteristic and pathognomonic cytoplasmic feature is the 'psammoma body' which is a calcified, laminated, basophilic, stromal structure.
- It is confined to the neck in over 95% of cases, although 15–20% have local extrathyroidal invasion. Metastases (1–2% of patients) occur via lymphatics to local lymph nodes and, more distantly, to lungs.
- Several prognostic scoring systems are in use, none of which permits definitive decisions to be made for individual patients.
- Low risk—TNM stage I (under 45, no metastases, tumour size <2cm, who may not need RAI ablation) (See Tables 1.26 and 1.27).

Management

Primary treatment—surgery

- Should be performed by an experienced thyroid surgeon at a centre with adequate case load to maintain surgical skills.
- In general, as near total thyroidectomy as possible should be performed.
- Clinically evident cervical lymph node metastasis is best treated with radical modified neck dissection, with preservation of sternocleidomastoid muscle, spinal accessory nerve, and internal jugular vein.

Adjuvant therapy—radioiodine therapy

- Post-operative radioiodine therapy is advised in the high-risk patient with differentiated thyroid cancer. After surgery in a low-risk group, some thyroidologists argue that ^{131}I is not required. A dose of 3.1GBq is used for thyroid ablation. A whole body scan done 4–6 months after administration of 150MBq ^{131}I helps to determine the presence of any residual disease. In the presence of metastasis, a dose of approximately 5.5–7.4GBq radioiodine is used. Liothyronine should be administered for 4–6 weeks in place of levothyroxine. It is then omitted for 10 days prior to the scan, allowing TSH to rise. A low-iodine diet for 2 weeks increases the effective specific activity of the administered iodine. Exogenous TSH is an alternative to T_3 cessation.

- The patient should be isolated until residual dose meter readings indicate <30MBq.
- Chronic suppression of serum TSH levels to <0.10mU/L is standard practice in patients with differentiated thyroid carcinoma. Inhibition of TSH secretion reduces recurrence rate, as TSH stimulates growth of the majority of thyroid cancer cells.

Patients are followed up with thyroglobulin levels. After effective treatment, thyroglobulin levels are undetectable. A trend of ↑ thyroglobulin values should be investigated with a radioiodine uptake scan. Liothyronine (T_3) is substituted for T_4 4–6 weeks before the scan and omitted for 10 days immediately beforehand. As above exogenous TSH can also be used.

Thyroglobulin

- A very sensitive marker of recurrence of thyroid cancer.
- Secreted by the thyroid tissue.
- After total thyroidectomy and radioactive iodine ablation, the levels of thyroglobulin should be <0.27 micrograms/L.
- Measurement of thyroglobulin levels could be made difficult in the presence of antithyroglobulin antibodies, which should be checked.
- Coming off thyroid hormones or giving recombinant TSH increases the sensitivity of thyroglobulin to detect recurrence, but this may not affect survival rates.

Recurrent disease/distant metastases

- In the case of recurrence, treatment employs all methods used in 1° and adjuvant therapy.
- Surgery for local metastases.
- Radioactive iodine for those tumours with uptake.
- External radiotherapy is indicated in non-resectable tumours that do not take up [131]I.
- Bony and pulmonary metastases (usually osteolytic) may be treated with [131]I.
- Unfortunately, only 50% of metastases concentrate [131]I.
- External beam radiation is given to patients who have gross residual disease after attempted surgery and radioiodine. Radiation therapy may be of value in controlling local disease. If thyroidectomy is not possible, it is given alone for palliation.
- Due to the low efficacy of traditional cytotoxic chemotherapies, consensus guidelines now recommend consideration of clinical trials of novel agents when patients require therapy for progressive, locally advanced, or metastatic differentiated thyroid cancer.
- Tyrosine kinase inhibitors (TKIs) (e.g. sorafenib, sunitinib, pazopanib, gefitinib) have been of interest for the treatment of advanced differentiated thyroid cancer, given the oncogenic roles of mutations in the serine kinase *BRAF* and tyrosine kinases *RET* (in the mutated fusion protein *RET/PTC*) and *RAS* and the contributory roles of tyrosine

kinases in growth factor receptors, such as the vascular endothelial growth factor receptor (VEGFR).
- Partial responses are reported in approximately 15–30% of patients. Complete responses are absent, and no study has evaluated survival.
- Side effects that are common to all of the VEGF-targeted TKIs include hypertension, renal toxicity, bleeding, myelosuppression, arterial thromboembolism, cardiotoxicity, thyroid dysfunction (typically hypothyroidism), cutaneous toxicity, including hand-foot skin reaction, delayed wound healing, hepatotoxicity, and muscle wasting.
- Selumetinib, a selective mitogen-activated protein kinase (MAPK) pathway antagonist, increases iodine uptake in a subgroup of patients refractory to radioiodine.

Recombinant TSH
- Avoids morbidity of hypothyroidism during T_3/T_4 withdrawal.
- Necessary for patients with TSH deficiency (hypopituitarism) and thyroid carcinoma.
- Comparable thyroglobulin rise but slightly reduced ^{131}I scan sensitivity compared to thyroid hormone withdrawal.
- Give 0.9mg of recombinant TSH on day 1 and 2, and measure thyroglobulin on day 5.
- For serum thyroglobulin testing, serum thyroglobulin should be obtained 72h after final injection of recombinant TSH.

Follicular thyroid carcinoma (FTC)

- Constitutes 10% of all thyroid cancers.
- Mean patient age in most studies is 50 years.
- Commoner in ♀ (2:1).
- Relatively more common in endemic goitre areas.

Pathology

- Follicular carcinoma is a neoplasm of the thyroid epithelium that exhibits follicular differentiation and shows capsular or vascular invasion.
- Differentiation of benign follicular adenoma from encapsulated low-grade or minimally invasive tumours can be impossible to diagnose, particularly for the cytopathologist, and surgery is usually necessary for a follicular adenoma.
- FTC may be minimally invasive or widely invasive.
- Metastases (15–20% cases) are more likely to be spread by haematogenesis to the lung and bones and less likely to local lymph nodes.
- Hürthle cell carcinoma is an aggressive type of follicular tumour with a poor prognosis because it fails to concentrate ^{131}I.

Treatment

As for papillary thyroid carcinoma, 📖 see p. 96.

Follow-up of papillary and FTC

- This should be lifelong—recurrences occur, at least, to 25 years (see Fig. 1.3).
- Follow-up usually involves an annual clinical review, with clinical examination for the presence of suspicious lymph nodes and measurements of serum TSH (to ensure adequate TSH suppression to <0.1mU/L) and thyroglobulin.
- Serum thyroglobulin should be undetectable in patients with total thyroid ablation. However, detectable levels may be seen for up to 6 months after thyroid ablation. A trend of ↑ thyroglobulin level requires investigations with ^{131}I uptake scan (off thyroid hormones or with TSH stimulation) and other imaging modalities, such as US of the neck, CT scan of the lungs, or bone scans. Thyroglobulin antibodies must be checked, as there may be interactions with thyroglobulin assays.
- TSH-stimulated thyroglobulin levels can be avoided in patients with thyroglobulin levels <0.27 micrograms/L.
- Isolated lymph node metastases can occasionally be associated with normal thyroglobulin. Stopping thyroid hormone replacement, or using recombinant TSH, before the measurement of thyroglobulin can increase sensitivity of detecting persistent recurrent disease.
- Detectable thyroglobulin and absent uptake on radioiodine uptake scan may be due to dedifferentiation of the tumour and failure to take up iodine. In patients with serum thyroglobulin >10ng/mL and a negative radioiodine scan, (18F)-2-fluoro-2-deoxy-D-glucose PET may be useful. Metastatic lesions with high avidity for glucose in PET imaging, measured by elevated standard uptake values, are associated with resistance to radioiodine therapy and worse prognosis.

For patients with differentiated thyroid cancer (DTC) who undergo subtotal thyroidectomy or total thyroidectomy without RAI:
- Follow periodic thyroglobulin (Tg) and perform US.
- Rising Tg over time is suspicious.

For DTC patients after undergoing total thyroidectomy and remnant ablation, the following schedule is recommended:

6–12 months

- Clinical examination, serum TSH, free thyroxine, neck US, Tg, and thyroglobulin antibodies while on T_4.
- If the neck US is suspicious for lymph nodes or nodules >5–8mm, send for biopsy for cytology and Tg wash.
  - If biopsy +ve, send for compartment dissection.
  - If biopsy −ve, monitor size of lymph nodes or nodules.
- If the US is −ve and TgAb are −ve, send for rhTSH or thyroxine withdrawal (THW) Tg stimulation and diagnostic RAI WBS.
- If −ve WBS but stimulated Tg >5–10, send for neck/check CT or PET/CT.
- If imaging −ve, consider repeat ^{131}I therapy.

- If imaging +ve, consider surgery, ^{131}I therapy, EBRT, clinical trial, or tyrosine kinase inhibitor therapy.
- If −ve WBS and stimulated Tg <5–10, monitor Tg and neck US. If Tg rising, consider repeat ^{131}I therapy.
- If +ve WBS, consider repeat ^{131}I therapy.
- If the US is −ve but TgAb is +ve, follow TgAb and neck US.

Years 2–10
- Clinical examination, measurements of serum free thyroxine, TSH, and thyroglobulin annually.
- Neck ultrasonography every 1–2 years or less frequently in low-risk patients with no evidence of disease.
- Thyrogen-stimulated Tg and WBS if serum Tg increases or there is other evidence of recurrence.

Years 11–20
- Clinical examination and measurements of serum free thyroxine, TSH, and thyroglobulin annually.
- Neck ultrasonography every 1–3 years or less frequently in low-risk patients with no evidence of disease.
- Thyrogen-stimulated Tg and WBS if serum Tg increases or there is other evidence of recurrence.

Years 21+
- Clinical examination and measurements of serum free thyroxine, TSH, and thyroglobulin annually.
- Neck ultrasonography every 3–5 years or less frequently in low-risk patients with no evidence of disease.
- Thyrogen-stimulated Tg and radioiodine imaging if serum Tg increases or there is other evidence of recurrence.

See Box 1.15 for thyroid cancer in children.

Thyroid cancer and pregnancy
- The natural course of thyroid cancer developing during pregnancy may be different from that in non-pregnant ♀.
- Any ♀ presenting with a thyroid nodule in pregnancy appears to have an ↑ risk for thyroid cancer.
- Evaluation should be undertaken with FNAC. Radioiodine scan is contraindicated.
- Lesions <2cm diameter or any lesion appearing after 24 weeks' gestation should be treated with TSH suppression and further evaluations carried out post-partum.
- If FNAC is suspicious or diagnostic, operation should be performed at the earliest safe opportunity—generally, the second trimester or immediately post-partum.
- ^{131}I ablation should be scheduled for the post-partum period and the mother advised to stop breastfeeding.
- Avoid pregnancy for 6 months after any ^{131}I ablation.

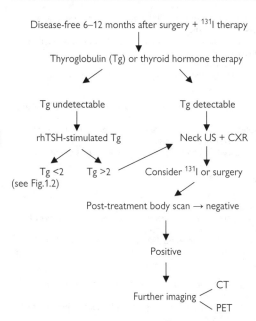

Disease-free 6–12 months after surgery + ^{131}I therapy

Thyroglobulin (Tg) or thyroid hormone therapy

Tg undetectable

rhTSH-stimulated Tg

Tg <2   Tg >2
(see Fig.1.2)

Tg detectable

Neck US + CXR

Consider ^{131}I or surgery

Post-treatment body scan → negative

Positive

Further imaging   CT
                     PET

Fig. 1.3 Algorithm for follow-up of low-risk cases of papillary thyroid cancer.

Box 1.15 Thyroid cancer in children
- Uncommon, with an incidence of 0.2–5 per million per year.
- >85% are papillary but with more aggressive behaviour than in adults (local invasion and distant metastases are commoner).
- Recently, an ↑ incidence in children in Belarus and Ukraine has been reported following the Chernobyl nuclear accident in 1986. *RET* oncogene rearrangements are common in these tumours.
- Management is similar to that in adults.
- Various studies report an overall recurrence rate of 0–39%; disease-free survival of 80–93% and disease-specific mortality of 0–10%.
- Evidence is currently lacking on the independent risks or benefits of radioactive iodine or extensive surgery.
- Many investigators recommend lifelong follow-up with a combination of thyroglobulin and radionuclide scanning.

Medullary thyroid carcinoma (MTC)

also see MEN type 2, 📖 p. 592.
- Accounts for 5–10% of all thyroid cancers.
- Should be managed by a dedicated regional service.

Presentation
- Lump in neck.
- Systemic effects of calcitonin—flushing/diarrhoea.

Diagnosis
- FNAC.
- Comprehensive family history and screening in search for features of MEN-2 is needed.
- Pathology specimens show immunostaining for calcitonin and staining for amyloid.

Management
- Baseline plasma calcitonin.
- Baseline biochemical investigations for phaeochromocytoma and hyperparathyroidism.
- Genetic screening.
- Staging with thoracoabdominal CT/MRI.
- MIBG and pentavalent ^{99m}Tc DMSA scintigraphy may also be used.

Treatment
- Total thyroidectomy and central node dissection is the 1° treatment modality.
- Germline *RET* mutation carriers should ideally undergo thyroidectomy before 5 years of age.

Adjuvant therapy
- Radioiodine and TSH suppression do not play a role.
- External radiotherapy has been shown to be of little benefit.
- For patients with metastatic tumours at least 2cm in diameter, growing by at least 20% per year, or for patients with symptoms related to multiple metastatic foci that cannot be alleviated with surgery or external beam radiotherapy, systemic chemotherapy with a TKI (vandetanib), as part of a clinical trial, should be considered.
- Therapeutic MIBG may help in some cases.

Follow-up
All patients should have lifelong follow-up at the dedicated regional service.

Anaplastic (undifferentiated) thyroid cancer

- Rare.
- Peak incidence: seventh decade; ♀:♂ = 1:1.5.
- Characterized by rapid growth of a firm/hard, fixed tumour.
- Often infiltrates local tissue, such as larynx and great vessels, and so does not move on swallowing. Stridor and obstructive respiratory symptoms are common.
- Aggressive, with poor long-term prognosis—7% 5-year survival rate and a mean survival of 6 months from diagnosis.
- Optimal results occur, following total thyroidectomy. This is usually not possible and external irradiation is used, sometimes in association with chemotherapy.

Lymphoma

- Uncommon.
- Almost always associated with autoimmune thyroid disease (Hashimoto's thyroiditis). Occurs more commonly in ♀ and in patients aged >40 years.
- Characterized by rapid enlargement of the thyroid gland.
- May be limited to thyroid gland or part of a more extensive systemic lymphoma (usually non-Hodgkin's lymphoma).
- Treatment with radiotherapy alone or chemotherapy, if more extensive, often produces good results.

Further reading

American Thyroid Association Guidelines Task Force (2009). Medullary thyroid cancer: management guidelines of the American Thyroid Association. *Thyroid* **19**, 565–612.

American Thyroid Association (ATA) Guidelines Taskforce on Thyroid Nodules and Differentiated Thyroid Cancer (2009). Revised American Thyroid Association management guidelines for patients with thyroid nodules and differentiated thyroid cancer. *Thyroid* **19**, 1167–214.

Aschebrook-Kilfoy B, Ward MH, Sabra MM, *et al.* (2011). Thyroid cancer incidence patterns in the United States by histologic type, 1992-2006. *Thyroid* **21**, 125–34.

Bogsrud TV, Hay ID, Karantanis D, *et al.* (2011). Prognostic value of 18F-fluorodeoxyglucose-positron emission tomography in patients with differentiated thyroid carcinoma and circulating antithyroglobulin autoantibodies. *Nucl Med Commun* **32**, 245–51.

British Thyroid Association and Royal College of Physicians (2007). Guidelines for the management of thyroid cancer (Perros P, ed). Report of the Thyroid Cancer Guidelines Update Group. Royal College of Physicians, London. Available at: ◌ http://www.british-thyroid-association.org/news/Docs/Thyroid_cancer_guidelines_2007.pdf.

Hay ID (2007). Management of patients with low-risk papillary thyroid carcinoma. *Endocr Pract* **13**, 521–33.

Hay I, Wass JAH (2008). *Clinical Endocrine Oncology*, 2nd edn, pp.109–71. Blackwell-Wiley, Massachussetts.

Kloos RT, Eng C, Evans D, *et al.* (2009). Medullary thyroid cancer: management guidelines of the American Thyroid Association. *Thyroid* **19**, 565–612.

Nikiforov YE (2006). Radiation-induced thyroid cancer: what we have learned from Chernobyl. *Endocr Pathol* **17**, 307–17.

Nikiforov YE, Nikiforova MN (2011). Molecular genetics and diagnosis of thyroid cancer. *Nat Rev Endocrinol* **7**, 569–80.

Paschke R, Hegedüs L, Alexander E, *et al.* (2011). Thyroid nodule guidelines: agreement, disagreement and need for future research. *Nat Rev Endocrinol* **7**, 354–61.

Sherman SI (2011). Targeted therapies for thyroid tumors. *Mod Pathol* **24**(Suppl 2), S44–52.

Smallridge RC (2012). Approach to the patient with anaplastic thyroid carcinoma. *J Clin Endocrinol Metab* **97**, 2566–72.

Pituitary

Anatomy and physiology of anterior pituitary gland

Anatomy

The pituitary gland is centrally located at the base of the brain in the sella turcica within the sphenoid bone. It is attached to the hypothalamus by the pituitary stalk and a fine vascular network. The cavernous sinuses are on either side of the sella, lateral and superior to the sphenoid sinuses, and comprise important neurovascular structures, including the cavernous segments of the internal carotid arteries and the cranial nerves III, IV, V, and VI. The optic chiasm is located superiorly, separated from the pituitary by the suprasellar cistern and the diaphragma sellae (see Fig. 2.1). The pituitary measures around 13mm transversely, 9mm anteroposteriorly, and 6mm vertically and weighs approximately 100mg. It increases during pregnancy to almost twice its normal size, and it decreases in the elderly.

The anterior pituitary gland receives most of its blood supply from the hypothalamo-hypophyseal portal system (primary plexus, long portal venous system, and secondary plexus), which originates from the capillary plexus of the median eminence and superior stalk derived from the terminal ramifications of the superior and inferior hypophyseal arteries. This system carries blood and hypophysiotropic hormones down to the stalk. The remainder of the blood supply is through the pituitary capsular vessels originating from the superior hypophyseal arteries. The venous drainage from the anterior pituitary is through the cavernous sinuses into the petrosal sinuses and the internal jugular veins.

Physiology

(See Table 2.1.)

Prolactin (PRL) secretion[*]

Single chain polypeptide. Pulsatile secretion in a circadian rhythm with around 14 pulses/24h, and a superimposed bimodal 24h pattern of secretion with a nocturnal peak during sleep and a lesser peak in the evening.

Growth hormone (GH) secretion[*]

Single chain polypeptide. Pulsatile secretion—usually undetectable in the serum, apart from 5 to 6 90min pulses/24h that occur more commonly at night. The secretion is modified by age and sex.

LH/FSH secretion

Glycoprotein hormones, with α chain common to LH and FSH (also TSH and hCG), but β chain specific for each hormone. Pulsatile secretion determined by the frequency and amplitude of GnRH secretion.

Thyroid-stimulating hormone (TSH) secretion

Glycoprotein with α chain common to LH and FSH (also TSH and hCG), but β chain specific for each hormone. Pulsatile secretion with 9 ± 3 pulses/24h and ↑ amplitude of pulses at night.

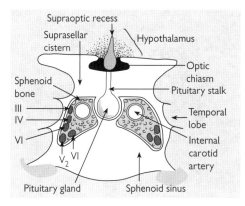

Fig. 2.1 The pituitary gland. Reproduced with permission from Weatherall DJ, Ledingham JGG, and Warrell DA (eds) (1996). Oxford Textbook of Medicine, 3rd edn. Oxford University Press: Oxford.

Adrenocorticotrophic hormone (ACTH)[*]
Single chain polypeptide cleaved from pro-opiomelanocortin (POMC). Circadian rhythm of secretion, beginning to rise from 3 a.m. to a peak before waking in the morning and gradually falling thereafter.

Posterior pituitary
📖 see p. 208.

[*] Concentrations ↑ with stress: NB venepuncture.

Table 2.1 Anterior pituitary gland physiology

Cell type (hormone)	% pituitary	+ve regulation	−ve regulation	Targets	Effects
Somatotropes (growth hormone, GH)	45–50	Growth hormone-releasing hormone (GHRH)	Insulin-like growth factor (IGF-1) and somatostatin	Liver, cartilage, muscle, fat, skin	Linear and somatic growth Metabolism (lipids, proteins, carbohydrates)
Lactotropes (prolactin, PRL)	15–25 (↑ in pregnancy)	Thyrotropin-releasing hormone (TRH) and oestrogen	Dopamine	Breast	Lactation
Gonadotropes (luteinizing hormone and follicle-stimulating hormone, LH/FSH)	10–15	Gonadotrophin-releasing hormone (GnRH), oestrogen—late follicular phase of menstrual cycle	Oestrogen Progesterone Testosterone Inhibin (FSH only)	Gonads	Sex steroid production Folliculogenesis and ovulation (♀) Spermatogenesis (♂)
Thyrotropes (thyroid-stimulating hormone, TSH)	5–10	TRH	T_4, T_3 somatostatin	Thyroid	Thyroid hormone production
Corticotropes (adrenocorticotrophin, ACTH)	15–20	Corticotrophin-releasing hormone (CRH)	Cortisol	Adrenal gland	Glucocorticoid and DHEA production

Reproduced from Draznin and Epstein, Oxford American Handbook of Endocrinology and Diabetes (2011), with permission of OUP.

Imaging

Background

- Magnetic resonance imaging (MRI) currently provides the optimal imaging of the pituitary gland.
- Computed tomography (CT) scans may still be useful in demonstrating calcification in tumours (e.g. craniopharyngiomas) and hyperostosis in association with meningiomas or evidence of bone destruction.
- Plain skull radiography may show evidence of pituitary fossa enlargement but has been superseded by MRI.

MRI appearances

(See Fig. 2.2.)

- T_1-weighted images demonstrate cerebrospinal fluid (CSF) as dark grey and brain as much whiter. This imaging is useful for demonstrating anatomy clearly. The normal posterior pituitary gland appears bright white (due to neurosecretory granules and phospholipids) on T_1-weighted images, in contrast to the anterior gland which is of the same signal as white matter. The bony landmarks have low signal intensity on MRI, and air in the sphenoid sinus below the fossa shows no signal. Fat in the dorsum sellae may shine white. T_2-weighted images may sometimes be used to characterize haemosiderin and fluid contents of a cyst.
- IV gadolinium compounds are used for contrast enhancement. Because the pituitary and pituitary stalk have no blood–brain barrier, in contrast to the rest of the brain, the normal pituitary gland enhances brightly following gadolinium injection. Contrast enhancement is particularly useful for the demonstration of cavernous sinus involvement and of microadenomas.
- The normal pituitary gland has a flat or slightly concave upper surface. In adolescence or pregnancy, the surface may become slightly convex.

Pituitary adenomas

On T_1-weighted images, pituitary adenomas are of lower signal intensity than the remainder of the normal gland. The size and extent of the pituitary adenomas are noted in addition to the involvement of other structures, such as invasion of the cavernous sinus, erosion of the fossa, and relations to the optic chiasm. Larger tumours may show low-intensity areas compatible with necrosis or cystic change or higher intensity signal due to haemorrhage. The presence of microadenomas may be difficult to demonstrate. Contrast enhancement, asymmetry of the gland, or stalk position can be helpful in such cases.

Neuroradiological classification

📖 see p. 184.

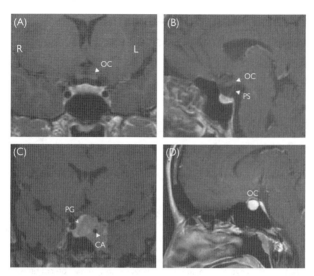

Fig. 2.2 Normal and abnormal pituitary MRI images. (A) Normal coronal, post-contrast T1 image showing optic chiasm (OC). (B) Normal sagittal image showing pituitary stalk (PS) and OC. (C) Pituitary macroadenoma with evidence of pituitary gland (PG) compression, left cavernous sinus invasion, and encroachment of carotid artery (CA). (D) Rathke's cleft cyst—bright T1 image, consistent with mucinous, proteinaceous, or blood products. Reproduced from Draznin and Epstein, Oxford American Handbook of Endocrinology and Diabetes (2011), with permission of OUP.

Craniopharyngiomas

These appear as intra- and/or suprasellar masses with cystic and/or solid components. A solid lesion appears as iso- or hypointense relative to the brain on pre-contrast T_1-weighted images, shows enhancement following gadolinium administration, and is usually of mixed hypo- or hyperintensity on T_2-weighted sequences. A cystic element is usually hypointense on T_1- and hyperintense on T_2-weighted sequences. Protein, cholesterol, and methaemoglobin may cause high signal on T_1-weighted images. Calcification is present in 45–57%, better visualized by CT or plain skull X-ray.

Further reading

Naidich MJ, Russell EJ (1999). Current approaches to imaging of the sellar region and pituitary. *Endocrinol Metab Clin N Am* **28**, 45.

Pituitary function—dynamic tests: insulin tolerance test (ITT)

Indications
- Assessment of ACTH reserve.
- Assessment of GH reserve.

Physiology
IV insulin is used to induce hypoglycaemia (glucose <2.2mmol/L with signs of glycopenia), which produces a standard stress causing ACTH and GH secretion.

Contraindications
- 9 a.m. serum cortisol <100nmol/L.
- Untreated hypothyroidism.
- Abnormal ECG.
- Ischaemic heart disease.
- Seizures.
- Glycogen storage disease.

Note that patients should discontinue oral oestrogen replacement for 6 weeks before the test, as ↑ CBG will make the cortisol results difficult to interpret. Progesterone and transdermal oestrogen may be continued.
  See Box 2.1 for procedure.

Response
- In the presence of inadequate hypoglycaemia (glucose >2.2mmol/L), the test cannot be interpreted.
- A normal cortisol response (peak cortisol >450nmol/L) demonstrates the ability to withstand stress (including major surgery) without requiring glucocorticoid cover. Subnormal cortisol response requires glucocorticoid replacement treatment (📖 see Glucocorticoids, p. 128).
- Severe GH deficiency in adults is diagnosed if peak GH <3 micrograms/L, and, in the appropriate clinical situation (📖 see p. 130), GH replacement therapy may be recommended. In children, the secretory capacity of GH is higher, and a cut-off of 10 micrograms/L is used.

Box 2.1 Procedure

- Continued medical surveillance is essential throughout.
- Patient is fasted overnight. Weight is checked.
- Insert cannula. Check basal (time 0) glucose, cortisol, and GH.
- Administer IV soluble insulin 0.15U/kg (occasionally, 0.2–0.3U/kg needed in untreated Cushing's syndrome and acromegaly because of ↑ insulin resistance).
- Measure glucose, GH, and cortisol at 30, 45, 60, 90, and 120min. Repeat insulin dose if a bedside stick test for glucose does not show hypoglycaemia at 45min.
- During the procedure, pulse rate, blood pressure, and manifestations of hypoglycaemia should be recorded.
- Test is terminated if prolonged hypoglycaemia—may need to administer 25mL of 25% glucose and IV 100mg hydrocortisone after sampling for cortisol and GH.
- Ensure patient eats lunch and has normal glucose before discharge.

Glucagon test

Indications
- Assessment of ACTH reserve.
- Assessment of GH reserve.

Physiology
Glucagon leads to release of insulin, which then leads to GH and ACTH release. The response may be 2° to the drop in glucose seen after the initial rise following glucagon injection or may relate to the nausea induced by glucagon.

Contraindications
- Phaeochromocytoma or insulinoma, glycogen storage disease, and severe hypocortisolaemia.
- Often unreliable in patients with diabetes mellitus.
- Note that patients should discontinue oral oestrogen replacement for 6 weeks before the test, as ↑ CBG will make the cortisol results difficult to interpret.

Response
- The normal response is a rise in glucose to a maximum at 90min. The cut-offs for cortisol and GH are those of the ITT.
- This is a less reliable test than the ITT, as 20% of normal individuals may fail to respond.

See Box 2.2 for procedure.

> **Box 2.2 Procedure**
> The test is performed at 9 a.m. following an overnight fast. Basal GH and cortisol are measured, then 1mg (1.5mg if the patient weighs >90kg) glucagon is administered SC. The injection may cause nausea, abdominal pain, and vomiting. Samples for GH, cortisol, and glucose are checked from 90min, every 30min, until 240min.

ACTH stimulation test

Short Synacthen® test (tetracosactide test).

Indication
• Assessment of adrenal cortical function.
• Assessment of ACTH reserve.

Physiology
The rationale of its use is that chronic underexposure of the adrenal glands to ACTH (following prolonged corticosteroid therapy or due to hypothalamic–pituitary disease) will result in a blunted cortisol response to exogenously administered ACTH. Furthermore, a lack of cortisol rise following administration of ACTH demonstrates adrenal cortical disease. Prolonged ACTH administration will lead to cortisol secretion in ACTH deficiency but not in 1° adrenal disease.

See Box 2.3 for procedure.

Response
The post-stimulation cortisol should rise to >450nmol/L at 30min. This is an unreliable test of ACTH reserve within 6 weeks of an insult, e.g. surgery to the pituitary.

Box 2.3 Procedure

• The test can be done at any time of the day; the response is not time-dependent.
• Synacthen® is administered 250 micrograms IM, and cortisol is measured at 0, 30, and 60min. When this test is used to measure ACTH reserve, only the 0 and 30min values are required. The dose may also be given IV with identical results.
• Note that patients should discontinue oestrogen replacement for 6 weeks before the test, as ↑ CBG will make the cortisol results difficult to interpret.

Arginine test[1]

Indication

Second-line test for assessment of GH reserve.

Physiology

Arginine leads to GH release.

Contraindications

None.

See Box 2.4 for procedure.

Response

A normal response is a rise in GH to >15–20mU/L.

Box 2.4 Procedure

- Fast from midnight, and administer 0.5g/kg (max 30g) arginine IV in 100mL normal saline over 30min from time 0 (9 a.m.).
- Sample glucose and GH at 0, 30, 60, 90, and 120min.

Reference

1. Corneli G, Di Somma C, Baldelli R, et al. (2005). The cut-off limits of the GH response to GH-releasing hormone–arginine test related to body mass index. *European Journal of Endocrinology*, **153**, 257–64.

Clomifene test

Indications
Assessment of gonadotrophin deficiency (e.g. Kallmann's syndrome).

Physiology
Clomiphene has mixed oestrogen and antioestrogenic effects. The basis of
the test is competitive inhibition of oestrogen binding at the hypothalamus
and pituitary gland, leading to ↑ LH and FSH after 3 days.

Contraindications
• Avoid in those with liver disease.
• May transiently worsen depression.

See Box 2.5 for procedure.

Response
• The normal response is a doubling of gonadotrophins by day 10,
  usually rising beyond the normal range.
• In hypothalamic or pituitary disease, no gonadotrophin rise is seen.
  Prepubertal patients may show a fall in gonadotrophins.
• Ovulation is presumed if day 21 progesterone is >30nmol/L.

hCG test

Indications

To examine Leydig cell function, 📖 see Clinical assessment, p. 402.

> **Box 2.5 Procedure**
> - Advise patient of possible side-effects—visual disturbance (peripheral flickering of vision)—and also of possible ovulation in ♀ (contraceptive advice).
> - Measure LH and FSH on days 0, 4, 7, and 10. In ♀, measure day 21 progesterone to detect whether ovulation has occurred.
> - Administer clomifene 3mg/kg (max 200mg/day) in divided doses for 7 days.

TRH test

Indications
- Differentiation of pituitary TSH and hypothalamic TRH deficiency.
- Differentiation of TSH-secreting tumour from thyroid hormone resistance (☐ see Table 1.15, p. 51).

See Box 2.6 for procedure.

Response
- Normal response is a rise in TSH by >2mU/L to >3.4mU/L, with a maximum at 20min and lower values at 60min.
- A delayed peak (60min rather than 20min) is typically found in hypothalamic disease.

Box 2.6 Procedure
- Administer TRH 200 micrograms IV to supine patient.
- Measure T_4 and TSH at time 0, and TSH at 20 and 60min.
- Note occasional reports of pituitary tumour haemorrhage. TRH induces a rise in blood pressure.

Hypopituitarism

Definition

Hypopituitarism refers to either partial or complete deficiency of anterior and/or posterior pituitary hormones and may be due to 1° pituitary disease or to hypothalamic pathology which interferes with the hypothalamic control of the pituitary.

Causes

- Pituitary tumours.
- Parapituitary tumours—craniopharyngiomas, meningiomas, secondary deposits (e.g. breast, lung), chordomas, gliomas.
- Radiotherapy—pituitary, cranial, nasopharyngeal.
- Pituitary infarction (apoplexy), Sheehan's syndrome.
- Infiltration of the pituitary gland—sarcoidosis, lymphocytic hypophysitis, haemochromatosis, Langerhans cell histiocytosis, Erdheim–Chester disease, Wegener's (ANCA-positive, 1% pituitary involvement, diabetes insipidus commonest).
- Empty sella.
- Infection—tuberculosis, pituitary abscess.
- Trauma (including traumatic brain injury).
- Subarachnoid haemorrhage.
- Isolated hypothalamic-releasing hormone deficiency, e.g. Kallmann's syndrome due to GnRH deficiency.
- Genetic causes.
- Mutations of genes encoding transcription factors, including HESX1 (homeobox gene expressed in embryonic stem cells 1), LHX3 (Lim-domain homeobox gene 3), LHX4 (Lim-domain homeobox gene 4), PROP-1 (Prophet of Pit1), POU1F1 (Pou domain, class 1, transcription factor 1).
- Russell viper envenomation.

Features

(See Table 2.2.)

- The clinical features depend on the type and degree of the hormonal deficits, and the rate of its development, in addition to whether there is intercurrent illness. In the majority of cases, the development of hypopituitarism follows a characteristic order, with secretion of GH, then gonadotrophins being affected first, followed by TSH and ACTH secretion at a later stage. PRL deficiency is rare, except in Sheehan's syndrome associated with failure of lactation. ADH deficiency is virtually unheard of with pituitary adenomas but may be seen rarely with infiltrative disorders and trauma.
- The majority of the clinical features are similar to those occurring when there is target gland insufficiency. There are important differences, e.g. lack of pigmentation and normokalaemia in ACTH deficiency in contrast to ↑ pigmentation and hyperkalaemia (due to aldosterone deficiency) in Addison's disease.
- NB *Houssay phenomenon*. Amelioration of diabetes mellitus in patients with hypopituitarism due to reduction in counter-regulatory hormones.

Apoplexy

Apoplexy refers to infarction of the pituitary gland due to either haemorrhage or ischaemia. It occurs most commonly in patients with pituitary adenomas, usually macroadenomas, but other predisposing conditions include post-partum (Sheehan's syndrome), radiation therapy, diabetes mellitus, anticoagulant treatment, disseminated intravascular coagulopathy, and reduction in intracranial pressure. It is a medical emergency, and rapid hydrocortisone replacement can be lifesaving.

It may present with a syndrome which is difficult to differentiate from any other intracranial haemorrhage, with sudden onset headache, vomiting, meningism, visual disturbance, and cranial nerve palsy. The diagnosis is based on the clinical features and pituitary imaging which shows high signal on T_1- and T_2-weighted images (📖 see p. 112). It should be managed by a pituitary multidisciplinary team. It has been suggested that early surgery (within 8 days) provides the optimal chance for neurological recovery. However, some patients may be managed conservatively if the patient has no significant visual or other neurological manifestations.

After apoplexy, pituitary tumour regrowth may occur (11% at 7 years), so follow-up surveillance is necessary.

Empty sella syndrome

An enlarged pituitary fossa, which may be 1° (due to arachnoid herniation through a congenital diaphragmatic defect) or 2° to surgery, radiotherapy, or pituitary infarction. The majority of patients have normal pituitary function. Hypopituitarism (and/or hyperprolactinaemia) is found in <10%.

Traumatic brain injury (TBI)

- Associated with subarachnoid haemorrhage and skull base fractures.
- May be seen with moderate-to-severe head trauma.
- Most common deficiencies—GH and gonadotrophins (10–15%).
- Best assessed 6–12 months after trauma.

Table 2.2 Main manifestations of hypopituitarism

Hormone deficiency	Clinical features
GH	Adult GHD (📖 see p. 130)
	Reduced exercise capacity, reduced lean body mass, impaired psychological well-being, ↑ cardiovascular risk
LH/FSH	Anovulatory cycles, oligo/amenorrhoea, dyspareunia in ♀
	Erectile dysfunction and testicular atrophy, loss of 2° sexual hair (often after many years) in ♂
	Reduced libido, infertility, osteoporosis in both sexes
ACTH	As in Addison's disease, except lack of hyperpigmentation, absence of hyperkalaemia (📖 see p. 128)
TSH	As in 1° hypothyroidism (📖 see p. 74)
PRL	Failure of lactation
ADH	Polyuria and polydipsia

Sheehan's syndrome

Haemorrhagic infarction of the enlarged post-partum pituitary gland causing hypopituitarism, following severe hypotension usually due to blood loss, e.g. post-partum haemorrhage. It can be fatal, and survivors require life replacement therapy. Improvement in obstetric care has made this a rare occurrence in the developed world.

Investigations of hypopituitarism

The aims of investigation of hypopituitarism are to biochemically assess the extent of pituitary hormone deficiency and also to elucidate the cause.

Basal hormone levels

Basal concentrations of the anterior pituitary hormone, as well as the target organ hormone, should be measured, as the pituitary hormones may remain within the normal range despite low levels of target hormone. Measurement of the pituitary hormone alone does not demonstrate that the level is inappropriately low, and the diagnosis may be missed.

- LH and FSH, and testosterone (9 a.m.) or oestradiol.
- TSH and thyroxine.
- 9 a.m. cortisol.
- PRL.
- IGF-1 (NB May be normal in up to half of GHD, depending on age).

See Box 2.7 for dynamic tests.

Posterior pituitary function

- It is important to assess and replace corticotroph function before assessing posterior pituitary hormone production because ACTH deficiency leads to reduced GFR and the inability to excrete a water load, which may, therefore, mask diabetes insipidus (DI).
- Plasma and urine osmolality are often adequate as baseline measures. However, in patients suspected to have DI, a formal fluid deprivation test should usually be performed (🕮 see Box 2.31, p. 213).

Investigation of the cause

- Pituitary imaging—MRI ± contrast.
- Investigation of hormonal hypersecretion if a pituitary tumour is demonstrated.
- Investigation of infiltrative disorders, (🕮 see Parasellar inflammatory conditions, pp. 192–3), e.g. serum and CSF ACE, ferritin, hCG, aFP.
- Occasionally, biopsy of a lesion found on imaging is required.

Box 2.7 Dynamic tests

- Dynamic tests, such as the ITT (🕮 see Insulin tolerance test, p. 114) or glucagon test (🕮 see Glucagon test, p. 116) if the ITT is contraindicated, are used to assess cortisol and GH reserve.
- Some centres use the short Synacthen® test to assess ACTH reserve, using the 0 and 30min values of cortisol (🕮 see ACTH stimulation test, p. 117). There are few false –ves using this investigation, and it is simpler to perform than the former tests but gives no measure of GH reserve. It is important to note that falsely normal results occur when hypopituitarism is of recent onset because the test relies on the fact that ACTH deficiency causes atrophy of the adrenal cortex and, therefore, a delayed response to Synacthen®. Less than 6 weeks of ACTH deficiency may allow a 'normal' adrenal response.

Treatment of hypopituitarism

Treatment involves adequate and appropriate hormone replacement (📖 see p. 127, p. 128, and p. 130) and management of the underlying cause.

Isolated defects of pituitary hormone secretion

Rarely, patients have isolated insufficiency of only one anterior pituitary hormone. The aetiology of these disorders is largely unknown, although loss of hypothalamic control may play a role; an autoimmune pathology has been suggested in some and genetic mutations in others. Examples include:

- GnRH deficiency (Kallman's syndrome—congenital GnRH deficiency ± anosmia).
- Isolated ACTH deficiency.
- *Pit1* gene mutation (leads to isolated GH, PRL, and TSH deficiency).
- *Prop1* gene mutation (leads to isolated GH, PRL, TSH, and gonadotrophin deficiency).

Further reading

De Marinis L, *et al.* (2005). Primary empty sella. *J Clin Endocrinol Metab* **90**, 5471–7.

Glynn N, Agha A (2013). Which patient requires neuroendocrine assessment following traumatic brain injury, when and how. *Clin Endocrinol* **78**, 17–20.

Pal A, *et al.* (2011). Pituitary apoplexy in non-functioning pituitary adenomas: long term follow up is important because of significant numbers of tumour recurrences. *Clin Endocrinol* **75**, 501.

Rajasekaran S (2011). UK guidelines for the management of pituitary apoplexy.*Clini Endocrinol* **74**, 9.

Toogood AA, Stewart PM (2008). Hypopituitarism: clinical features, diagnosis, and management. *Endocrinol Metab Clin North Am* **37**, 235–61.

Anterior pituitary hormone replacement

Background

Anterior pituitary hormone replacement therapy is usually performed by replacing the target hormone rather than the pituitary or hypothalamic hormone that is actually deficient. The exceptions to this are GH replacement (📖 see Growth hormone replacement therapy in adults, p. 130) and when fertility is desired (📖 see Management, p. 396).

See Table 2.3 for usual doses.

Thyroid hormone replacement

This is discussed in the section on 1° hypothyroidism (📖 see p. 80).

Monitoring of therapy

- In contrast to replacement in 1° hypothyroidism, the measurement of TSH cannot be used to assess adequacy of replacement in TSH deficiency due to hypothalamo–pituitary disease. Therefore, monitoring of treatment in order to avoid under- and over-replacement should be via both clinical assessment and by measuring free thyroid hormone concentrations, which should be in the middle/upper part of the normal range.
- FT_4 should be monitored before ingestion of daily thyroxine tablets.
- T_4 requirements should be reassessed when additional replacement with other pituitary hormones becomes necessary. Thus, GH therapy, when added, can cause a reduction of FT_4 or unmask previously undiagnosed hyperthyroidism.

Sex hormone replacement

📖 see Hormone replacement therapy, p. 346; Androgen replacement therapy, p. 378.

Oestrogen/testosterone administration is the usual method of replacement, but gonadotrophin therapy is required if fertility is desired (📖 see p. 410).

Table 2.3 Usual doses of hormone replacement therapy

Hydrocortisone	10mg on waking, 5mg at lunchtime, and 5mg early evening or twice daily regimens with a usual total dose of 15–20mg/day
or	
Prednisolone	3mg on waking and 2mg early evening (usual total dose 5–7.5mg/day)
Levothyroxine	100–150 micrograms/day
GH	0.2–0.6mg/day for adults (0.4–1.0IU)
Oestrogens/testosterone	Depends on formulation

Glucocorticoids

Replacement therapy

Patients with ACTH deficiency usually need glucocorticoid replacement only and do not require mineralocorticoids, in contrast to patients with Addison's disease.

The normal production rate of cortisol is 9.9 ± 2.7mg/day. The glucocorticoid most commonly used for replacement therapy is *hydrocortisone*. It is rapidly absorbed, with a short half-life (90–120min). *Prednisolone* and *dexamethasone* can occasionally be used for glucocorticoid replacement. The longer half-lives of these two drugs make them useful where sustained ACTH suppression is required in, for example, congenital adrenal hyperplasia (CAH). Dexamethasone is useful when monitoring endogenous production, as it is not detected in most cortisol assays. Cortisol acetate was previously used for glucocorticoid replacement therapy but requires hepatic conversion to active cortisol.

Monitoring of replacement

This is important to avoid over-replacement which is associated with ↑ BP, elevated glucose and insulin, and reduced bone mineral density (BMD). Under-replacement leads to the non-specific symptoms, as seen in Addison's disease (🕮 see p. 266). A clinical assessment is important, but biochemical monitoring, using plasma and urine cortisol (UFC) measurements, is used by many endocrinologists. The aim is to keep the UFC within the reference range. Many centres use plasma cortisol measurements on a hydrocortisone day curve (see Box 2.8). The aim is to keep the plasma cortisol between 150 and 300nmol/L, avoiding nadirs of <50nmol/L predose. Conventional replacement (20mg hydrocortisone/24h) may overtreat patients with partial ACTH deficiency.

Safety

Patients should be encouraged to wear a MedicAlert, indicating that they are cortisol-deficient, to carry a steroid card, and to keep a vial of parenteral hydrocortisone at home to be administered in emergency situations.

Equivalent oral glucocorticoid doses

1mg hydrocortisone is equivalent to:
- 1.5mg cortisol acetate.
- 0.2mg prednisolone.
- 0.0375mg dexamethasone.
- 4mg prednisolone ≡ 20mg hydrocortisone ≡ 0.75 mg dexamethasone.

Box 2.8 Hydrocortisone day curve

There are various protocols for this test, ranging from a 3-point curve to detect under-replacement (used with 24h UFC to detect over-replacement)—serum cortisol checked at 9 a.m., 12.30 p.m. (before the lunchtime dose), and 5 p.m. (pre-evening dose)—to more frequent sampling to detect over- and under-replacement. This involves serum cortisol at time 0, then administration of the morning dose of hydrocortisone. Plasma cortisol is then checked at 30min, 1, 2, 3, and 5h (pre-lunchtime dose specimen), and 7 and 9h (pre-evening dose), followed by samples at 10 and 11h.

- Oral oestrogen therapy should be stopped 6 weeks before the test, as ↑ CBG, leading to higher cortisol values, will make the test uninterpretable.
- This test is only valid for hydrocortisone replacement. Prednisolone or dexamethasone replacement can only be monitored clinically.

Acute/severe intercurrent illness

- *Mild disease without fever.* No change in glucocorticoid replacement.
- *Pyrexial illness.* Double replacement dose for duration of fever.
- *Vomiting or diarrhoea.* Parenteral therapy 100mg IM (from GP/trained relative; useful for patient to have vial of hydrocortisone at home with instruction sheet for emergency administration by suitable, trained personnel).
- *Severe illness/operation.* Parenteral therapy with IM hydrocortisone 50–100mg 6-hourly (e.g. 72h for major surgery, 24h for minor surgery). An alternative is a continual IV infusion of 1–3mg/h hydrocortisone.

Further reading

Persani L (2012). Central hypothyroidism: pathogenic, diagnostic and therapeutic challenges. *J Clin Endocrinol Metab* **97**, 3068–78.

Growth hormone (GH) replacement therapy in adults

Background

There is now a considerable amount of evidence that there are significant and specific consequences of GH deficiency (GHD) in adults and that many of these features improve with GH replacement therapy. GH replacement for adults has now been approved in many countries.

Definition

It is important to differentiate between adult and childhood onset GHD.

- Although *childhood onset* GHD occurs 2° to structural lesions, such as craniopharyngiomas and germinomas, and following treatment, such as cranial irradiation, the commonest cause in childhood is an isolated variable deficiency of GH-releasing hormone (GHRH) which may resolve in adult life because of maturation of the hypothalamo–somatotroph axis. It is, therefore, important to retest patients with childhood onset GHD when linear growth is completed (50% recovery of this group).
- *Adult onset.* GHD usually occurs 2° to a structural pituitary or parapituitary condition or due to the effects of surgical treatment or radiotherapy.

Prevalence

- Adult onset GHD 1/10,000.
- Adult GHD due to adult and childhood onset GHD 3/10,000.

Benefits of GH replacement

- Improved QoL and psychological well-being.
- Improved exercise capacity.
- ↑ lean body mass and reduced fat mass.
- Prolonged GH replacement therapy (>12–24 months) has been shown to increase BMD, which would be expected to reduce fracture rate.
- There are, as yet, no outcome studies in terms of cardiovascular mortality. However, GH replacement does lead to a reduction (~15%) in cholesterol. GH replacement also leads to improved ventricular function and ↑ left ventricular mass.

NICE guidelines for GH replacement

Adult criteria

- Severe GHD—GH <9mU/L.
- Impaired QoL (AGHDA QoL score >/= 11).
- Treatment for other pituitary hormone deficiencies.

Reassessment of treatment after 9 months' treatment (3-month dose titration, followed by 6-month therapeutic trial)—GH discontinued if improvement in AGHDA <7.

Young adults (up to 25 years)
- GH discontinued for 3 months at completion of linear growth (<2cm/year) and GH status reassessed.
- If severe GH deficiency confirmed, GH continued at adult dose until age 25 years (peak bone mass).
- Age 25 and above—adult criteria apply.

Diagnosis

The diagnosis of GHD depends on appropriate biochemical testing in the presence of an appropriate clinical context. The latter is important because distinguishing 'partial GHD' from physiological causes of reduced GH secretion, such as obesity or ageing and pathological causes, e.g. hypercortisolaemia in Cushing's syndrome, can be problematic. In these situations, GHD can be diagnosed when there is supportive evidence, such as pituitary disease and other anterior pituitary hormone deficiencies.

Who should be tested?

As the features of GHD may be non-specific and biochemical tests can be misleading in certain clinical situations, such as obesity, investigation of GHD should only be performed in the following groups of patients:
- Patients with hypothalamo–pituitary disease (GHD occurs early in hypopituitarism and is almost invariable in patients with other anterior pituitary hormone deficiencies).
- Patients who had childhood onset GHD.
- Patients who have received cranial irradiation.

Investigation of GH deficiency

Dynamic tests of GH secretion
- ITT is most widely used test. Peak GH <10mU/L (3 micrograms/L) is diagnostic of severe GHD (see 📖 p. 114).
- Alternative tests, if the ITT is contraindicated, include a combination of GHRH (1 microgram/kg) and arginine (0.5g/kg) IV over 30min (see 📖 p. 118).
- A second confirmatory dynamic biochemical test is recommended, particularly in patients who have suspected isolated GH deficiency.

A single GH dynamic test is sufficient to diagnose GHD in patients with two or three pituitary hormonal defects.

IGF-1
IGF-1 concentrations may remain within the age-matched reference range despite severe GHD in up to 50% of patients and, therefore, do not exclude the diagnosis, and reduced IGF-1 is seen in a number of conditions.
   For causes of lowered IGF-1 levels, see Box 2.9.

Abnormalities in adult GH deficiency
- Stimulated GH <10mU/L (3 micrograms/L).
- Low or low-normal IGF-1 (IGF-1 may be normal in up to 50%, depending on age).
- ↓ BMD.
- ↑ insulin resistance.
- Dyslipidaemia (↑ LDL).
- Impaired cardiac function.

Clinical features of GH deficiency
- Impaired well-being.
- Reduced energy and vitality (depressed mood, ↑ social isolation, ↑ anxiety).
- Reduced muscle mass and impaired exercise capacity.
- ↑ central adiposity (↑ waist/hip ratio) and ↑ total body fat.
- ↓ sweating and impaired thermogenesis.
- ↑ cardiovascular risk.
- ↑ fracture risk (osteoporosis).

> **Box 2.9 Causes of lowered IGF-1 levels**
> - GHD.
> - Malnutrition.
> - Poorly controlled diabetes mellitus.
> - Hepatic disease.
> - Renal disease.
> - Severe intercurrent illness.

Treatment of GH deficiency

All patients with GHD should be considered for GH replacement therapy. In particular, patients with impaired QoL, reduced mineral density, an adverse cardiovascular risk profile, and reduced exercise capacity should be considered for treatment.

Dose

See Box 2.10.

- Unlike paediatric practice, where GH doses are determined by body weight and surface area, most adult endocrinologists use dose titration, using serial IGF-1 measurements, to increase the dose of GH until the IGF-1 level approaches the middle to upper end of the age-matched IGF-1 reference range. This reduces the likelihood of side effects, mainly related to fluid retention, which were frequently observed in the early studies of GH replacement in adults when doses equivalent to those used in paediatric practice were used.
- The normal production of GH is 200–500 micrograms/day in an adult. Current recommendations are a starting dose of 150–300 micrograms/day. The maintenance dose is usually 200–600 micrograms/day. The dose in ♀ is often higher than for age-matched ♂ (particularly if the female is on oral oestrogens).

Monitoring of treatment

- A clinical examination, looking for reduction in overall body weight (a good response is loss of 3–5kg in 12 months) and reduced waist/hip ratio. BP may fall in hypertensive patients because of reduction in peripheral systemic vascular resistance.
- IGF-1 is monitored to avoid over-replacement, aiming to keep values within the age-matched reference range. During dose titration, IGF-1 should be measured every 1–2 months. Once a stable dose is reached, IGF-1 should be checked at least once a year.
- The adverse effects experienced with GH replacement usually resolve with dose reduction and tend to be less frequent with the lower starting doses used in current practice.
- GH treatment may be associated with impairment of insulin sensitivity, and therefore markers of glycaemia should be monitored.
- Lipids should be monitored annually. BMD should be monitored every 2 years, particularly in those with ↓ BMD.
- It may be helpful to monitor QoL using a questionnaire, such as the AGHDA (adult GHD assessment) questionnaire.

Box 2.10 GH starting doses, according to age	
Age (years)	Dose (micrograms/day)
<30	400–500
30–60	300
>60	100–200

- As the long-term safety and efficacy of GH replacement in adults is, as yet, unknown, it is recommended that patients receiving GH therapy should remain under the care of an endocrinologist. There are large databases of patients receiving GH in order to monitor and determine these questions regarding long-term benefits and safety, particularly with regard to cardiovascular risk.

GH therapy in special situations

- *Pregnancy.* There are currently no data on GH replacement in pregnancy.
- *Critical illness.* There is no good evidence for a beneficial effect of GH replacement during critical illness. Patients should continue GH replacement during non-severe illness, but many endocrinologists would suggest that GH should be discontinued in patients who are severely ill, e.g. those receiving major surgery or on ITU.
- *Cardiac failure.* GH treatment has recently been suggested as a potential therapy in dilated cardiomyopathy. Longer term data are required in this group of patients.

Adverse effects of GH replacement

See Box 2.11 for contraindications
- Sodium and water retention.
  - Weight gain.
  - Carpal tunnel syndrome.
- Hyperinsulinaemia.
- Arthralgia (possibly due to intra-articular cartilage swelling).
- Myalgia.
- Benign intracranial hypertension (resolves on stopping treatment).
- No data suggest that GH therapy affects tumour development (no evidence from long-term studies in children of ↑ risk of recurrence with GH treatment; insufficient long-term data in adults). No evidence of ↑ risk of tumour recurrence in adolescents and adults following childhood malignancy.

Box 2.11 Contraindications to GH replacement

- Active malignancy.
- Benign intracranial hypertension.
- Pre-proliferative/proliferative retinopathy in diabetes mellitus.

Further reading

Carroll PV, Christ ER, Bengtsson BA, *et al.* (1998). GH deficiency in adulthood and the effects of GH replacement: a review. *J Clin Endocrinol Metab* **83**, 382–95.

Molitch ME, Clemmons DR, Malozowski S, Merriam GR, Vance ML (2011). Endocrine Society. Evaluation and treatment of adult growth hormone deficiency: an Endocrine Society clinical practice guideline. *J Clin Endocrinol Metab* **96**, 1587–609.

Pituitary tumours

Epidemiology
- Pituitary adenomas are the most common pituitary disease in adults and constitute 10–15% of primary brain tumours.
- Approximately 10% of individuals harbour incidental tumours, most commonly microadenomas.
- The incidence of clinically apparent pituitary disease is 1 in 10,000.
- Pituitary carcinoma is very rare (<0.1% of all tumours) and is most commonly ACTH- or prolactin-secreting.

See Table 2.4.

Classification
Size
- Microadenoma <1cm.
- Macroadenoma >1cm.

Functional status (clinical or biochemical)
- Prolactinoma 35–40%.
- Non-functioning 30–35%.
- Growth hormone (acromegaly) 10–15%.
- ACTH adenoma (Cushing's disease) 5–10%.
- TSH adenoma <5%.

Pathogenesis
The mechanism of pituitary tumourigenesis remains largely unclear. Pituitary adenomas are monoclonal, supporting the theory that there are intrinsic molecular events leading to pituitary tumourigenesis. However, the mutations (e.g. p53) found in other tumour types are only rarely found. A role for hormonal factors and, in particular, the hypothalamic hormones in tumour progression is also a suggested hypothesis.

Table 2.4 Approximate relative frequencies of pituitary tumours

Tumour type	Mean prevalence[1] (per 100,000)	Annual incidence
Clinically overt pituitary adenomas	72	1–2/100,000
Acromegaly 12%	9	4 cases/million
Cushing's syndrome 7%	1	2 cases/million
Non-functioning adenoma 25%	22	6 cases/million
Prolactinomas 49%	44	10 cases/million (if hyper-prolactinaemia is considered, then higher incidence)

TSHomas <1%.

Mortality

Pituitary disease is associated with an increased mortality, predominantly due to vascular disease. This may be due to oversecretion of GH or ACTH, hormone deficiencies or excessive replacement (e.g. of hydrocortisone). Radiotherapy of the pituitary is also associated with an increased mortality (especially cerebrovascular). Craniopharyngioma patients have a particularly increased mortality.

Reference

1. Fernandez, *et al.* (2010). Prevalence of pituitary adenomas: a community-based, cross-sectional study in Banbury (Oxfordshire, UK). *Clin Endocrinol (Oxf)* **72**, 377.

Molecular mechanisms of pituitary tumour pathogenesis

Activation of oncogenes

- *Gsα mutation* found in up to 40% GH-secreting tumours (less in non-Caucasians) and also described in a minority of NFAs and ACTH-secreting tumours.
- *Ras mutation* found in aggressive tumours and mainly pituitary carcinomas. ? role in malignant transformation.
- *Pituitary tumour transforming gene (PTTG)* has recently been described and found to be overexpressed in pituitary tumours. Its role in tumour pathogenesis is, as yet, uncertain.

Inactivation of tumour suppressor genes (TSG)

- *MEN-1 gene* loss of heterozygosity (LOH) at 11q13 had been previously demonstrated in up to 20% sporadic pituitary tumours; however, the expression of the *MEN-1* gene product menin is not downregulated in the majority of sporadic pituitary tumours.
- *Retinoblastoma gene.* Mutations in mice lead to intermediate lobe corticotroph adenomas; however, no mutations have been demonstrated in human pituitary adenomas.

Cyclins and modulators of cyclin activity

- Mutations of the cyclin-dependent kinases p27 and p18 are rare in human pituitary tumours (unlike tumours in mice). p27 may be translationally downregulated, and p16 may be transcriptionally silenced by methylation of its gene. Cyclin D1 overexpression may be an early step in pituitary tumourigenesis, as it is commonly found in different tumour types.
- Mutations are rare in pituitary tumours.

Alterations in receptor and growth factor expression (e.g. TGF, activin, bFGF)

No consistent patterns have emerged.

Further reading

Asa SL, Ezzat S (1998). The cytogenesis and pathogenesis of pituitary adenomas. *Endocr Rev* **19**, 798–827.

Sherlock M, *et al.* (2010). Mortality in patients with pituitary disease. *Endocr Rev* **31**, 301–42.

Prolactinomas

Epidemiology

- Prolactinomas are the commonest functioning pituitary tumour.
- Post-mortem studies show microadenomas in 10% of the population.
- During life, microprolactinomas are commoner than macroprolactinomas, and there is a ♀ preponderance of microprolactinomas.

Pathogenesis

Unknown. Occur in 20% of patients with MEN-1 (prolactinomas are the commonest pituitary tumour in MEN-1 and may be more aggressive than sporadic prolactinomas). Malignant prolactinomas are very rare and may harbour *RAS* mutations.

Clinical features

Hyperprolactinaemia (microadenomas and macroadenomas)

- Galactorrhoea (up to 90% ♀, <10% ♂).
- Disturbed gonadal function in ♀ presents with menstrual disturbance (up to 95%)—amenorrhoea, oligomenorrhoea, or with infertility and reduced libido.
- Disturbed gonadal function in ♂ presents with loss of libido and/ or erectile dysfunction. Presentation with reduced fertility and oligospermia or gynaecomastia is unusual.
- Hyperprolactinaemia is associated with a long-term risk of ↓ BMD.
- Hyperprolactinaemia inhibits GnRH release, leading to ↓ LH secretion. There may be a direct action of PRL on the ovary to interfere with LH and FSH signalling which inhibits oestradiol and progesterone secretion and also follicle maturation.

Mass effects (macroadenomas only)

- Headaches and visual field defects (uni- or bitemporal field defects).
- Hypopituitarism.
- Invasion of the cavernous sinus may lead to cranial nerve palsies.
- Occasionally, very invasive tumours may erode bone and present with a CSF leak or 2° meningitis.

For causes of hyperprolactinaemia, see Box 2.12.

Box 2.12 Causes of hyperprolactinaemia

- Physiological:
  - Pregnancy.
  - Sexual intercourse.
  - Nipple stimulation/suckling.
  - Neonatal.
  - Stress.
- Pituitary tumour:
  - Prolactinomas.
  - Mixed GH/PRL-secreting tumour.
  - Macroadenoma compressing stalk.
  - Empty sella.
- Hypothalamic disease—mass compressing stalk (craniopharyngioma, meningioma, neurofibromatosis).
- Infiltration—sarcoidosis, Langerhans cell histiocytosis.
- Stalk section—head injury, surgery.
- Cranial irradiation.
- Drug treatment:
  - Dopamine receptor antagonists (metoclopramide, domperidone).
  - Neuroleptics* (perphenazine, flupentixol, fluphenazine, haloperidol, thioridazine, chlorpromazine, trifluoperazine, risperidone, sulpiride).
  - Antidepressants (tricyclics, selective serotonin reuptake inhibitors, monoamine oxidase inhibitors, sulpiride, amisulpride, imipramine, clomipramine, amitriptyline, pargyline, clorgiline).
  - Cardiovascular drugs—verapamil, methyldopa, reserpine.
  - Opiates.
  - Cocaine.
  - Protease inhibitors—e.g. ritonavir, indinavir, zidovudine.
  - Oestrogens.
  - Others—bezafibrate, omeprazole, H_2 antagonists.
- Metabolic:
  - Hypothyroidism—TRH increases PRL.
  - Chronic renal failure—reduced PRL clearance.
  - Severe liver disease—disordered hypothalamic regulation.
- Other:
  - PCOS—can make differential diagnosis of menstrual problems difficult.
  - Chest wall lesions—zoster, burns, trauma (stimulation of suckling reflex).
- No cause found:
  - 'Idiopathic' hyperprolactinaemia.

* Quetiapine, clozapine, aripiprazole, and olanzapine are antipsychotics, with little or no effect on prolactin (lower binding affinity to D2 receptors).

Investigations of prolactinomas

Serum PRL

- The differential diagnosis of elevated PRL is shown in Box 2.12. Note that the stress of venepuncture may cause mild hyperprolactinaemia, so 2–3 levels should be checked, preferably through an indwelling cannula after 30min.
- Serum PRL <2,000mU/L is suggestive of a tumour—either a microprolactinoma or a non-functioning macroadenoma compressing the pituitary stalk, with loss of dopamine inhibitory tone to the lactotroph and subsequent hyperprolactinaemia.
- Serum PRL >4,000mU/L is diagnostic of a macroprolactinoma.
- *Hook effect.* This occurs where the assay utilizes antibodies recognizing two ends of the molecule. One is used to capture the molecule and one to label it. If PRL levels are very high, it may be bound by one antibody but not by the other. Thus, above a certain concentration, the signal will reduce, rather than increase, and very high PRL levels will be spuriously reported as normal or only slightly raised.

Thyroid function and renal function

Hypothyroidism and chronic renal failure are causes of hyperprolactinaemia.

Imaging

- *MRI.* Microadenomas usually appear as hypointense lesions within the pituitary on T_1-weighted images. Negative imaging is an indication for contrast enhancement with gadolinium. Stalk deviation or gland asymmetry may also suggest microadenoma.
- Macroadenomas are space-occupying tumours, often associated with bony erosion and/or cavernous sinus invasion.

Macroprolactin ('big' PRL)

Occasionally, aggregate forms (150–170kDa) of PRL are detected in the circulation. Although these are measurable in the prolactin assay, they do not interfere with reproductive function but may be found in 10% of patients referred. Typically, there is hyperprolactinaemia with regular ovulatory menstrual cycles. Assays for macroprolactin are available, using PEG (polyethylene glycol) precipitation, where low recovery of PRL demonstrates the presence of macroprolactin, or gel filtration chromatography (gold standard).

Hyperprolactinaemia and drugs

(📖 see p. 141, Box 2.12)

Antipsychotic agents are the most likely psychotropic agents to cause hyperprolactinaemia. If dose reduction is not possible or not effective, then an MRI to exclude a prolactinoma and treatment of hypogonadism may be indicated. Where dopamine antagonism is the mechanism of action of the drug, then dopamine agonists may reduce efficacy. Drug-induced increases in PRL are usually <3,000mU/L.

'Idiopathic' hyperprolactinaemia

When no cause is found following evaluation, as described on 📖 p. 141, the hyperprolactinaemia is designated idiopathic but, in many cases, is likely to be due to a tiny microprolactinoma which is not demonstrable on current imaging techniques. In other cases, it may be due to alterations in hypothalamic regulation. Follow-up of these patients shows that, in one-third, PRL levels return to normal; in 10–15%, there is a further increase in PRL, and, in the remainder, PRL levels remain stable.

Treatment of prolactinomas

Aims of therapy

- *Microprolactinomas.* Restoration of gonadal function.
- *Macroprolactinomas.*
  - Reduction in tumour size and prevention of tumour expansion.
  - Restoration of gonadal function.
- Although microprolactinomas may expand in size without treatment, the vast majority do not. Therefore, although restoration of gonadal function is usually achieved by lowering PRL levels, ensuring adequate sex hormone replacement is an alternative if the tumour is monitored in size.
- Macroprolactinomas, however, will continue to expand and lead to pressure effects. Definitive treatment of the tumour is, therefore, necessary.

Drug therapy—dopamine agonists

- Dopamine agonist treatment (📖 see Dopamine agonists, p. 204) leads to suppression of PRL in most patients, with 2° effects of normalization of gonadal function and termination of galactorrhoea. Tumour shrinkage occurs at a variable rate (from 24h to 6–12 months) and extent and must be carefully monitored. Continued shrinkage may occur for years. Slow chiasmal decompression will correct visual field defect in the majority of patients, and immediate surgical decompression is not necessary. Lack of improvement of visual fields, despite tumour shrinkage, makes improvement with surgery unlikely. Restoration of other hormonal axes may occur with tumour shrinkage.
- *Cabergoline* is more effective in normalization of PRL in microprolactinoma (83% compared with 59% on bromocriptine), with fewer side effects than *bromocriptine*.
- Although cabergoline in higher doses used for Parkinson's disease can cause right-sided cardiac fibrosis, there is no evidence for this using the lower doses necessary for the control of PRL levels (see Box 2.13).
- Dopamine agonist resistance (see Box 2.14) may occur when there are reduced numbers of D2 receptors.
- Tumour enlargement following initial shrinkage on treatment is usually due to non-compliance. A rare possibility, however, is carcinoma.

Drug therapy—oestrogens

Oestrogen replacement, rather than dopamine agonist therapy, may be appropriate in ♀ with idiopathic hyperprolactinaemia or microprolactinomas where fertility and galactorrhoea are not issues. Small short-term series suggest no evidence of tumour enlargement. However, individual cases where tumour enlargement has occurred make monitoring of PRL important.

Surgery

📖 see Transsphenoidal surgery, p. 196.

- Since the introduction of dopamine agonist treatment, transsphenoidal surgery is indicated only for patients who are resistant to, or intolerant of, dopamine agonist treatment. The cure rate for macroprolactinomas treated with surgery is poor (30%), and, therefore, drug treatment is first-line in tumours of all size. Occasionally, surgery may be required for patients with CSF leak 2° to an invasive macroprolactinoma. Cure rates for microprolactinomas treated with surgery are >80%, but the risk of hypopituitarism (GH-deficient in 25%) and recurrence (4% at 5 years) makes this a second-line option.

- Bromocriptine given for more than a month may make the tumour fibrous.
- The surgical management of a CSF leak can be very difficult in patients with very invasive tumours. Tumour shrinkage with dopamine agonists will either precipitate or worsen the leak, with the subsequent risk of meningitis. There is no evidence for the long-term use of prophylactic antibiotics in this group, but patients at risk should be informed of the warning symptoms and advised to seek expert medical attention urgently.

Radiotherapy
📖 see Technique, p. 200.
- Standard pituitary irradiation leads to slow reduction (over years) of PRL in the majority of patients. While waiting for radiotherapy to be effective, dopamine agonist therapy is continued but should be withdrawn on a biannual basis at least to assess if it is still required.

Box 2.13 Cabergoline and cardiac valvulopathy
- Cabergoline, but not bromocriptine, is a 5-hydroxytryptamine 2B (5-HT2B) receptor agonist.
- High doses of cabergoline (e.g. 3mg/day for ≥6 months in Parkinson's patients) have been associated with valvular heart disease (aortic, mitral, and tricuspid regurgitations) via a 5-HT2B target effect.
- The risk of cardiac valvulopathy appears to be low in prolactinoma patients on standard doses of cabergoline (<2mg/week).
- For patients requiring higher cabergoline doses, annual clinical cardiac exams are warranted, and consideration should be given to periodic echocardiograms.

Reproduced from Draznin and Epstein, Oxford American Handbook of Endocrinology and Diabetes (2011), with permission of OUP.

Box 2.14 Dopamine agonist resistance
- *Definition.* Failure to normalize prolactin. Failure to decrease tumour size to <50%.
- Occurs with 24% treated with bromocriptine, 13% with pergolide, and 11% with cabergoline.
- D2 receptors are reduced in number but not efficacy.
- Treatment options include switching dopamine agonist, increasing dose of dopamine agonist, surgery, fertility treatment, or oestrogen replacement (± DXR (pituitary radiotherapy) for macroprolactinomas).

- Radiotherapy is not indicated in the management of patients with microprolactinomas. It is useful in the treatment of macroprolactinomas once the tumour has been shrunken away from the chiasm, only if the tumour is resistant.

Prognosis

(See Box 2.15.)
- The natural history of microprolactinomas is difficult to assess. However, they are a common post-mortem incidental finding, and <7% show any increase in tumour size. It has been demonstrated that hyperprolactinaemia in approximately one-third of ♀ will resolve, particularly after the menopause or pregnancy. This shows that patients receiving dopamine agonist treatment for microprolactinoma should have treatment withdrawn intermittently to assess the continued requirement for it, and certainly the dose may be titrated downwards over time.
- There are few data on dopamine agonist withdrawal in macroprolactinomas in the absence of definitive treatment (radiotherapy or surgery). There are data suggesting that cautious attempts at dose reduction could be considered after 5 years if the PRL is normal and the MRI shows no tumour, but it seems that the majority have a recurrence of hyperprolactinaemia (60–80%) but to levels lower than pretreatment values.
- It seems, at present, that there is no increase in the risk of breast cancer.

Management of prolactinomas in pregnancy

📖 see Prolactinoma in pregnancy, p. 437.

Box 2.15 Dopamine resistance of prolactinoma
- Definition:
  - Failure to normalize prolactin on dopamine agonist therapy.
  - Failure to decrease tumour size by 50% or more.
- Frequency:
  - Bromocriptine 24%.
  - Pergolide 13%.
  - Cabergoline 11%.
- Cause:
  - D2 receptors on tumour decreased in number: normal affinity.
- Treatment:
  - Switch dopamine agonist.
  - Increase dose of dopamine agonist.
  - Transsphenoidal surgery.
  - Clomifene gonadotrophins for fertility.
  - Oestrogen replacement therapy ± DXR for macroadenoma.

Further reading

Barber T, et al. (2011). Recurrence of hyperprolactinaemia following discontinuation of dopamine agonist therapy in patients with prolactinoma occurs commonly especially in macroprolactoinoma. Clin Endocrinol **75**, 819–24.

Bevan JS, Webster J, Burke CW, et al. (1992). Dopamine agonists and pituitary tumour shrinkage. Endocrinol Rev **13**, 220–40.

Casaneuva FF, Molitch ME, Schlechte JA, et al. (2006). Guidelines of the Pituitary Society for the diagnosis and management of prolactinomas. Clin Endocrinol **65**, 265–73.

Dekkers OM, Lagro J, Burman P, Jørgensen JO, Romijn JA, Pereira AM (2011). Recurrence of hyperprolactinaemia after withdrawal of dopamine agonists: systematic review and meta-analysis. J Clin Endocrinol Metab **95**, 43–51.

Karavitaki N, Thanabalasingham G, Shore HC (2006). Do the limits of serum prolactin in disconnection hyperprolactinaemia need re-definition? A study of 226 patients with histologically verified non-functioning pituitary macroadenoma. Clin Endocrinol **65**, 524–9.

Melmed S, et al. (2011). Diagnosis and treatment of hyperprolactinaemia: an Endocrine Society Clinical practice guideline. J Clin Endocrinol Metab **96**, 273–88.

Molitch ME (1985). Pregnancy and the hyperprolactinaemic woman. New Engl J Med **312**, 1364–70.

Molitch ME (1992). Pathologic hyperprolactinaemia. Endocrinol Metabo Clin N Am **21**, 877–910.

Molitch ME (2002). Medical management of prolactinomas. Pituitary **5**, 55–65.

Molitch ME (2003). Dopamine resistance of prolactinomas. Pituitary **6**, 19–27.

Molitch ME (2008). Drugs and prolactin. Pituitary **11**, 209–18.

Suliman SG, Gurlek A, Byrne JV (2007). Non-surgical cerebrospinal fluid rhinorrhoea in invasive macroprolactinoma: incidence, radiological and clinicopathological features. J Clin Endocrinol Metab **92**, 3829–35.

Definition of acromegaly

Acromegaly is the clinical condition resulting from prolonged excessive GH and hence IGF-1 secretion in adults. GH secretion is characterized by blunting of pulsatile secretion and failure of GH to become undetectable during the 24h day, unlike normal controls.

Epidemiology of acromegaly

- Rare. Equal sex distribution.
- Prevalence 40–86 cases/million population. Annual incidence of new cases in the UK is 4/million population.
- Onset is insidious, and there is, therefore, often a considerable delay between onset of clinical features and diagnosis. Most cases are diagnosed at 40–60 years. Typically, acromegaly occurring in an older patient is a milder disease, with lower GH levels and a smaller tumour.

Pituitary gigantism

The clinical syndrome resulting from excess GH secretion in children prior to fusion of the epiphyses.
- Rare.
- ↑ growth velocity without premature pubertal manifestations should arouse suspicion of pituitary gigantism.
- *Differential diagnosis.* Marfan's syndrome, neurofibromatosis, precocious pubertal disorders, cerebral gigantism (large at birth with accelerated linear growth and disproportionately large extremities—associated normal IGF-1 and GH).
- Arm span > standing height is compatible with eunuchoid features and suggests onset of disease before epiphyseal fusion (pituitary gigantism).

Causes of acromegaly

- *Pituitary adenoma* (>99% of cases). Macroadenomas 60–80%, microadenomas 20–40%. Local invasion is common, but frank carcinomas are very rare.
- *GHRH secretion:*
  - Hypothalamic secretion.
  - Ectopic GHRH, e.g. carcinoid tumour (pancreas, lung) or other neuroendocrine tumours.
  - Pituitary shows global enlargement. Somatroph hyperplasia seen on histology.
- *Ectopic GH secretion.* Very rare (e.g. pancreatic islet cell tumour, lymphoreticulosis).
- There has been some progress on the molecular pathogenesis of the GH-secreting pituitary adenomas—as mutations of the Gsα are found in up to 40% of tumours. This leads to an abnormality of the G protein that usually inhibits GTPase activity in the somatotroph.
- Gene mutations have been shown in some young patients with acromegaly who also have large tumours (familial isolated pituitary adenoma) in whom a family history should be sought.

Associations of acromegaly

- *MEN-1*. Less common than prolactinomas (📖 see MEN type 1, p. 586).
- *Carney complex*. AD, spotty cutaneous pigmentation, cardiac and other myxomas, and endocrine overactivity, particularly Cushing's syndrome due to nodular adrenal cortical hyperplasia and GH-secreting pituitary tumours in <10% of cases. Mainly due to activating mutations of protein kinase A (📖 see p. 583).
- *McCune–Albright syndrome* (📖 see p. 576). Caused by somatic mosaicism for the gsp mutation.
- *Familial isolated pituitary adenomas:*
  - Existence of two or more cases of acromegaly or gigantism in a family that does not exhibit MEN-1 or Carney complex.
  - Autosomal dominant.
  - Most have acromegaly, but acromegaly and prolactinoma families exist as rarely as do NFA families.
  - 30–50% cases have a mutation in the *AIP* gene (tumour suppressor gene).
  - Early-onset disease (<30 years).
  - Poor response to somatostatin analogues.
  - Take a careful family history, especially in acromegalic patients with a large pituitary tumour presenting below the age of 30 years, and consider screening for *AIP*.
- See Box 2.25 for causes of macroglossia.

Box 2.25 Macroglossia—causes

- Acromegaly.
- Hypothyroidism.
- Beckwith–Wiedemann syndrome (macrosomia, visceromegaly)— associated with hypoglycaemia and malignancies.
- Simpson–Golabi–Behmel syndrome (macrosomia and renal skeletal abnormalities).
- Tongue amyloidoses (primary or secondary to myeloma).
- Mucopolysaccharidoses/lysosomal storage disease.
- Focal tongue lesions, e.g. haemorrhage.
- Down's syndrome.
- Hyperinsulinaemia.

Clinical features of acromegaly

The clinical features arise from the effects of excess GH/IGF-1, excess PRL in some (as there is co-secretion of PRL in a minority (30%) of tumours or, rarely, stalk compression), and the tumour mass.

Symptoms
- ↑ sweating—>80% of patients.
- Headaches—independent of tumour effect.
- Tiredness and lethargy.
- Joint pains.
- Change in ring or shoe size.

Signs
- *Facial appearance.* Coarse features, oily skin, frontal bossing, enlarged nose, deep nasolabial furrows, prognathism, and ↑ interdental separation.
- *Deep voice*—laryngeal thickening.
- *Tongue enlargement*—macroglossia (see 📖 p. 209).
- *Musculoskeletal changes.* Enlargement of hands and feet, degenerative changes in joints lead to osteoarthritis. Generalized myopathy.
- *Soft tissue swelling.* May lead to entrapment neuropathies, such as carpal tunnel syndrome (40% of patients).
- *Goitre and other organomegaly*—liver, heart, kidney.

NB Fabry's disease causes thickening of the lips.

Complications
- Hypertension (40%).
- Insulin resistance and impaired glucose tolerance (40%)/diabetes mellitus (20%).
- Obstructive sleep apnoea—due to soft tissue swelling in nasopharyngeal region.
- ↑ risk of colonic polyps and colonic carcinoma—extent currently considered controversial.
- Ischaemic heart disease and cerebrovascular disease.
- Congestive cardiac failure and possible ↑ prevalence of regurgitant valvular heart disease.

Effects of tumour
- Visual field defects.
- Hypopituitarism.

Investigations of acromegaly

Oral glucose tolerance test (OGTT)

- In acromegaly, there is failure to suppress GH to <0.33 micrograms/L in response to a 75g oral glucose load. In contrast, the normal response is GH suppression to undetectable levels.
- *False +ves.* Chronic renal and liver failure, malnutrition, diabetes mellitus, heroin addiction, adolescence (due to high pubertal GH surges).

Random GH

Not useful in the diagnosis of acromegaly as, although normal healthy subjects have undetectable GH levels throughout the day, there are pulses of GH which are impossible to differentiate from the levels seen in acromegaly. However, in untreated patients, a random GH <0.33 micrograms/L practically excludes the diagnosis.

IGF-1

Useful in addition to the OGTT in differentiating patients with acromegaly from normals, as it is almost invariably elevated in acromegaly, except in severe intercurrent illness. It has a long half-life, as it is bound to binding proteins, and reflects the effect of GH on tissues. However, abnormalities of GH secretion may remain while IGF-1 is normal.

MRI

MRI usually demonstrates the tumour (98%) and whether there is extrasellar extension, either suprasellar or into the cavernous sinus.

Pituitary function testing

(also see Insulin tolerance test (ITT), p. 114.) Serum PRL should be measured, as some tumours co-secrete both GH and PRL.

Serum calcium

Some patients are hypercalciuric due to ↑ 1,25-DHCC, as GH stimulates renal 1α-hydroxylase. There may be an ↑ likelihood of renal stones due to hypercalcaemia as well as hypercalciuria (which occurs in 80%). Rarely, hypercalcaemia may be due to associated MEN-1 and hyperparathyroidism.

GHRH

Occasionally, it is not possible to demonstrate a pituitary tumour, or the pituitary gland MRI reveals global enlargement and histology reveals hyperplasia. A serum GHRH, in addition to radiology of the chest and abdomen, may then be indicated to identify the cause, usually a GHRH-secreting carcinoid of lung or pancreas.

GH day curve (GHDC)

- GH taken at 4–5 time points during the day.
- This is used to assess response to treatment following surgery or radiotherapy and also to assess GH suppression on somatostatin analogues in order to determine whether an increase in dose is required.
- It does not have a role in the diagnosis of acromegaly, but, in acromegaly, GH is detectable in all samples in contrast to normal. The degree of elevation of GH is relevant to the response to all forms of treatment; the higher the GH, the less frequent treatment is effective by surgery, drugs, or radiotherapy. See Box 2.26 for differential diagnosis.

Note on GH and IGF-I assays

- To improve standardization, it is recommended that the GH reference preparation should be a recombinant 22kDa hGH; presently, 88/624.
- There is currently no acceptable IGF-1 reference preparation.

Box 2.26 Differential diagnosis of elevated GH

- Pain.
- Pregnancy.
- Puberty.
- Adolescence if tall.
- Stress.
- Chronic renal failure.
- Chronic liver failure.
- Heart failure.
- Diabetes mellitus.
- Malnutrition.
- Prolonged fast.
- Severe illness.
- Heroin addiction.

Management of acromegaly

The management strategy depends on the individual patient and also on the tumour size. Lowering of GH is essential in all situations (see Fig. 2.7).

Transsphenoidal surgery

(🕮 also see Transsphenoidal surgery, p. 196.)
- This is usually the first line for treatment in most centres.
- Reported cure rates vary: 40–91% for microadenomas and 10–48% for macroadenomas, depending on surgical expertise.
- A GHDC should be performed following surgery to assess whether 'safe' levels of GH and IGF-1 have been attained. If the mean GH is <2.5 micrograms/L, then the patient can be followed up with annual IGF-1 and/or GH assessment. If safe levels of GH have not been achieved, then medical treatment and/or radiotherapy is indicated.
- Surgical debulking of a large macroadenoma should be undertaken, even if cure is not expected, because this lowers GH levels and improves the cure rate with subsequent somatostatin analogues.

Tumour recurrence following surgery

This is defined as tumour regrowth and increase in GH levels, leading to active acromegaly following post-operative normalization of GH levels. Using the definition of post-operative cure as mean GH <2.5 micrograms/L, the reported recurrence rate is low (6% at 5 years).

Radiotherapy

(🕮 also see Technique, p. 200.)
- This is usually reserved for patients following unsuccessful transsphenoidal surgery, only occasionally is it used as 1° therapy. The largest fall in GH occurs during the first 2 years, but GH continues to fall after this. However, normalization of mean GH may take several years and, during this time, adjunctive medical treatment (usually with somatostatin analogues) is required. With a starting mean GH >25 micrograms/L, it takes, on average, 6 years to achieve mean GH <2.5 micrograms/L, compared with 4 years with a starting mean GH <25 micrograms/L.
- After radiotherapy, somatostatin analogues should be withdrawn on an annual basis to perform a GHDC to assess progress and identify when mean GH <2.5 micrograms/L and, therefore, radiotherapy has been effective and somatostatin analogue treatment is no longer required.
- Radiotherapy can induce GH deficiency which may need GH therapy.

Definition of cure

- Controlled disease is, most recently, defined as a random GH <1 micrograms/L or nadir GH <0.4 micrograms/L on GTT + normal age-related IGF-1.

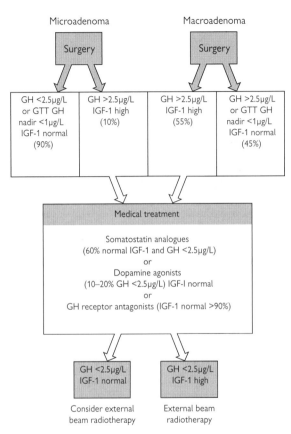

Fig. 2.7 Treatment paradigms in acromegaly. Reproduced with permission from Wass J (2001). *Handbook of Acromegaly*, p.81. BioScientifica Ltd.

- In treated patients, there is an approximately 25% discordance of GH and IGF-1. The management of this situation is unclear, but if there are symptoms, it should probably be treated.

Colonic polyps and acromegaly

- ↑ incidence of *colonic polyps and colonic carcinoma* has been reported by many groups. Both retrospective and prospective studies have demonstrated that 9–39% of acromegalic patients studied have colonic polyps and 0–5% have been shown to have colonic carcinoma.

- *Mechanism.* IGF-1 and/or GH are implicated, as both may stimulate colonic mucosal turnover. However, some studies have failed to demonstrate a direct relationship between serum levels and polyps/carcinoma.
- *Importance.* Patients with acromegaly are probably at slightly ↑ risk and, therefore, need screening for polyps. All patients aged >40 years should have routine colonoscopy, and those with polyps or persistently active acromegaly should receive 5-yearly repeat colonoscopy. Agreement has not been reached though on the frequency of follow-up colonoscopy.

Drug treatment

Somatostatin analogues
(📖 also see Somatostatin analogues, p. 204.)
- Somatostatin analogues lead to suppression of GH secretion in 20–60% of patients with acromegaly. At least 40% of patients are complete responders, and somatostatin analogues will lead to normalization of GH (<2.5 micrograms/L) and IGF-1. However, some patients are partial responders, and although somatostatin analogues will lead to lowering of mean GH, they do not suppress to normal despite dose escalation.
- Acute response to these drugs is assessed by measuring GH at hourly intervals for 6h, following the injection of 50–100 micrograms octreotide SC. This predicts long-term response.
- Depot preparations lanreotide Autogel® and octreotide LAR® are available. Octreotide LAR® 20mg IM is administered every 4 weeks, with dose alterations either down or up to 10–30mg every 3 months. Lanreotide Autogel® 90mg (deep SC) is administered every 28 days, with dose alteration either down to 60mg or up to 120mg every 3 months. Patients can be taught to self-administer lanreotide.
- These drugs may be used as 1° therapy where the tumour does not cause mass effects or in patients who have received surgery and/or radiotherapy who have elevated mean GH.
- Pasireotide stimulates somatostatin receptors 2 and 5, and treatment may increase the response rate in patients with acromegaly, but glucose tolerance declines and patients may develop diabetes mellitus.

Dopamine agonists
(📖 also see Dopamine agonists, p. 204.)

These drugs do lead to lowering of GH levels but, very rarely, lead to normalization of GH or IGF-1 (<30%). They may be helpful, particularly if there is coexistent secretion of PRL, and, in these cases, there may be significant tumour shrinkage. Cabergoline has recently been shown to be more effective than bromocriptine and may lead to IGF-1 normalization in up to 30%. A lower pretreatment IGF-1 favours a good response.

GH receptor antagonists (pegvisomant) 📖 p. 206
Indicated for somatostatin non-responders. Liver function tests should be monitored 6-weekly for 6 months. MRI of the pituitary is indicated 6-monthly in case of pituitary enlargement (5%). Therapy may be continued with octreotide or lanreotide to decrease the frequency of pegvisomant injections (e.g. pegvisomant 10mg daily and lanreotide). Normalization of

IGF-1 in >90% of patients is reported. More data on the effect on tumour size are required, as GH rises during treatment. GH levels cannot, therefore, be used to guide treatment, and IGF-1 is used to monitor therapy. Monitoring of liver biochemistry is necessary for safety.

Mortality data of acromegaly

- Mortality in untreated patients is double that of the normal population.
- Major causes include cardiovascular, cerebrovascular, and respiratory disease. More effective treatment has now ↑ life expectancy.

Further reading

Alexopoulou O, *et al.* (2008). Divergence between growth hormone and insulin-like growth factor-I concentrations in the follow-up of acromegaly. *J Clin Endocrinol Metab* **93**, 1324–30.

Bates AS, Van't Hoff W, Jones JM, *et al.* (1993). An audit of outcome of treatment in acromegaly. *QJM* **86**, 293–9.

Bevan JS, Atkin SL, Atkinson AB, *et al.* (2002). Primary medical therapy for acromegaly: an open, prospective, multicenter study of the effects of subcutaneous and intramuscular slow-release ocreotide on growth hormone, insulin-like growth factor-I, and tumor size. *J Clin Endocrinol Metab* **87**, 4554–63.

Chahal, AS, *et al.* (2011). AIP mutation in pituitary adenomas in the 18th century and today. *N Engl J Med* **364**, 43–50.

Daly AF, *et al.* (2007). Aryl hydrocarbon receptor-interacting protein gene mutations in familial isolated pituitary adenomas: analysis in 73 families. *J Clin Endocrinol Metab* **92**, 1891–6.

Dekkers OM, *et al.* (2008). Mortality in acromegaly: a metaanalysis. *J Clin Endocrinol Metab* **93**, 61–7.

Giustina A, *et al.* (2010). A consensus on criteria for cure of acromegaly. *J Clin Endocrinol Metab* **95**, 3141–8.

Jenkins PJ, Bates P, Carson MN, *et al.* (2006). Conventional pituitary irradiation is effective in lowering serum growth hormone and insulin-like growth factor-I in patients with acromegaly. *J Clin Endocrinol Metab* **91**, 1239–45.

Karavitaki N, *et al.* (2008). Surgical debulking of pituitary macroadenomas causing acromegaly improves control by lanreotide. *Clin Endocrinol (Oxf)* **68**, 970–5.

Melmed S (2006). Medical progress: acromegaly. *N Engl J Med* **55**, 2558–73.

Melmed S, Casanueva FF, Cavagnini F, *et al.* (2002). Guidelines for acromegaly management. *J Clin Endocrinol Metab* **87**, 4054–8.

Orme SM, McNally RJQ, Cartwright RA, *et al.* (1998). Mortality and cancer incidence in acromegaly: a retrospective cohort study. *JCEM* **83**, 2730–4.

Sandret L, *et al.* (2011). Place of cabergoline in acromegaly: a meta-analysis. *J Clin Endocrinol Metab* **96**, 1322–5.

Trainer PJ, Drake WM, Katznelso L, *et al.* (2000). Treatment of acromegaly with the growth hormone-receptor antagonist pegvisomant. *N Engl J Med* **342**, 1171–7.

Wass JAH (ed.) (2009). *Acromegaly*. BioScientifica: Bristol.

Definition of Cushing's disease

Cushing's syndrome is an illness resulting from excess cortisol secretion, which has a high mortality if left untreated. There are several causes of hypercortisolaemia which must be differentiated, and the commonest cause is iatrogenic (oral, inhaled, or topical steroids). It is important to decide whether the patient has true Cushing's syndrome rather than pseudo-Cushing's associated with depression or alcoholism. Secondly, ACTH-dependent Cushing's must be differentiated from ACTH-independent disease (usually due to an adrenal adenoma or, rarely, carcinoma—📖 see p. 250). Once a diagnosis of ACTH-dependent disease has been established, it is important to differentiate between pituitary-dependent (Cushing's disease) and ectopic secretion.

Epidemiology of Cushing's disease

- Rare; annual incidence approximately 2/million.
- Commoner in ♀ (♀:♂, 3–15:1).
- Age—most commonly, 20–40 years.

Pathophysiology of Cushing's disease

- The vast majority of Cushing's syndrome is due to a pituitary ACTH-secreting corticotroph microadenoma. The underlying aetiology is ill understood.
- Occasionally, corticotroph adenomas reach larger sizes (macroadenomas) and rarely become invasive or malignant. The tumours typically maintain some responsiveness to the usual feedback control factors that influence the normal corticotroph (e.g. high doses of glucocorticoids and CRH). However, this may be lost, and the tumours become fully autonomous, particularly in Nelson's syndrome.
- NB Crooke's hyaline change is a fibrillary appearance seen in the non-tumourous corticotroph associated with elevated cortisol levels from any cause.

For causes of Cushing's syndrome, see Box 2.27.

> **Box 2.27 Causes of Cushing's syndrome**
> - Pseudo-Cushing's syndrome:
>   - Alcoholism <1%.
>   - Severe depression 1%.
> - ACTH-dependent:
>   - Pituitary adenoma 68% (Cushing's disease).
>   - Ectopic ACTH syndrome 12%.
>   - Ectopic CRH secretion <1%.
> - ACTH-independent:
>   - Adrenal adenoma 10%.
>   - Adrenal carcinoma 8%.
>   - Nodular (macro- or micro-) hyperplasia 1%.
>   - Carney complex (📖 see p. 583).
> - Exogenous steroids, including skin creams, e.g. clobetasol.

Clinical features of Cushing's disease

The features of Cushing's syndrome are progressive and may be present for several years prior to diagnosis. A particular difficulty may occur in a patient with cyclical Cushing's where the features and biochemical manifestations appear and disappear with a variable periodicity. Features may not always be florid, and clinical suspicion should be high.

- *Facial appearance*—round plethoric complexion, acne and hirsutism, thinning of scalp hair.
- *Weight gain*—truncal obesity, buffalo hump, supraclavicular fat pads.
- *Skin*—thin and fragile due to loss of SC tissue, purple striae on abdomen, breasts, thighs, axillae (in contrast to silver, healed post-partum striae), easy bruising, tinea versicolor, occasionally pigmentation due to ACTH.
- Proximal *muscle weakness*.
- *Mood disturbance*—labile, depression, insomnia, psychosis.
- *Menstrual disturbance*.
- *Low libido and impotence*.
- There is a high incidence of venous thromboembolism (careful during surgery).
- Overall mortality greater than of general population (by a factor of 6).
- *Growth arrest* in children.

Associated features

- Hypertension (>50%) due to mineralocorticoid effects of cortisol (cortisol overwhelms the renal 11β-hydroxysteroid dehydrogenase enzyme protecting the mineralocorticoid receptor from cortisol). Cortisol may also increase angiotensinogen levels.
- Impaired glucose tolerance/diabetes mellitus (30%).
- Osteopenia and osteoporosis (leading to fractures of spine and ribs).
- Vascular disease due to metabolic syndrome.
- Susceptibility to infections.

Investigations of Cushing's disease

Does the patient have Cushing's syndrome?

Outpatient tests

- *2–3× 24h urinary free cortisol.* This test can be useful for outpatient screening—however, the false −ve rate of 5–10% means that it should not be used alone. (Fenofibrate, carbamazepine, and digoxin may lead to false +ves, depending on assay, and reduced GFR <30mL/min may lead to false −ves.) In children: correct for body surface area. Mild elevation occurs in pseudo-Cushing's and normal pregnancy.
- *Overnight dexamethasone suppression test.* Administration of 1mg dexamethasone at midnight is followed by a serum cortisol measurement at 9 a.m. Cortisol <50nmol/L makes Cushing's unlikely. (NB False +ves with poor dexamethasone absorption or hepatic enzyme induction). The false −ve value is 2% of normal individuals but rises to <20% in obese or hospitalized patients.
- If both the above tests are normal, Cushing's syndrome is unlikely.

Inpatient tests

- *Midnight cortisol.* Loss of circadian rhythm of cortisol secretion is seen in Cushing's syndrome, and this is demonstrated by measuring a serum cortisol at midnight (patient must be asleep for this test to be valid and ideally after 48h as an inpatient). In normal subjects, the cortisol at this time is at a nadir (<50nmol/L), but in patients with Cushing's syndrome, it is elevated. Late-night salivary cortisol may be promising, particularly in those with possible cyclical Cushing's (see Box 2.28).
- *Low-dose dexamethasone suppression test.* Administration of 0.5mg dexamethasone 6-hourly (30 micrograms/kg/day) for 48h at 9 a.m., 3 p.m., 9 p.m., and 3 a.m. should lead to complete suppression of cortisol to <50nmol/L in normal subjects (30 micrograms/kg/day). Serum cortisol is measured at time 0 and 48h (day 2).
- Interfering conditions should be considered with all dexamethasone testing: ↓ dexamethasone absorption, hepatic enzyme inducers (e.g. phenytoin, carbamazepine, and rifampicin), and ↑ CBG.

Pseudo-Cushing's

- Patients with pseudo-Cushing's syndrome will also show loss of diurnal rhythm and lack of low-dose suppressibility. However, alcoholics return to normal cortisol secretory dynamics after a few days' abstinence in hospital. Severe depression can be more difficult to differentiate, particularly since this may be a feature of Cushing's syndrome itself.
- Typically, patients with pseudo-Cushing's show a normal cortisol rise with hypoglycaemia (tested using ITT) whereas patients with true Cushing's syndrome show a blunted rise. However, this is not 100% reliable, as up to 20% of patients with Cushing's syndrome (especially those with cyclical disease) show a normal cortisol rise with hypoglycaemia.

Box 2.28 Cyclical Cushing's

A small group of patients with Cushing's syndrome have alternating normal and abnormal cortisol levels on an irregular basis. All causes of Cushing's syndrome may be associated with cyclical secretion of cortisol. Clearly, the results of dynamic testing can only be interpreted when the disease is shown to be active (elevated urinary cortisol secretion and loss of normal circadian rhythm and suppressibility on dexamethasone).

* The combined dexamethasone suppression test–CRH test (0.5mg dexamethasone 6-hourly for 48h, starting at 12 p.m., followed by ovine CRH 1 microgram/kg IV at 8 a.m.) (2h after last dose of dexamethasone) may be helpful, as patients with pseudo-Cushing's are thought to be under chronic CRH stimulation, thus showing a blunted response to CRH after dexamethasone suppression (cortisol 15min after CRH >38nmol/L in Cushing's and <38nmol/L in pseudo-Cushing's).
* IV desmopressin 10 micrograms increases ACTH in 80–90% with Cushing's but rarely in patients with pseudo-Cushing's.
* No screening tests are fully capable of distinguishing all cases of Cushing's syndrome from normal individuals/pseudo-Cushing's (see Table 2.8).

What is the underlying cause?

ACTH

(See Table 2.9.)

* Once the presence of Cushing's syndrome has been confirmed, a serum basal ACTH should be measured to differentiate between ACTH-dependent and ACTH-independent aetiologies (see Fig. 2.8). ACTH may not be fully suppressed in some adrenal causes of Cushing's; however, ACTH >4pmol/L is suggestive of an ACTH-dependent aetiology.
* The basal ACTH is, however, of very little value in differentiating between pituitary-dependent Cushing's syndrome and ectopic Cushing's syndrome, as there is considerable overlap between the two groups, although patients with ectopic disease tend to have higher ACTH levels (see Fig. 2.8).

Serum potassium

A rapidly spun potassium is a useful discriminatory test, as hypokalaemia <3.2mmol/L is found in almost 100% of patients with ectopic secretion of ACTH but in <10% of patients with pituitary-dependent disease.

High-dose dexamethasone suppression test

The high-dose dexamethasone suppression test is performed in an identical way to the low-dose test but with 2mg doses of dexamethasone (120 micrograms/kg/day). In Cushing's disease, the cortisol falls by >50% of the basal value. In ectopic disease, there is no suppression. However, approximately 10% of cases of ectopic disease, particularly those due to carcinoid tumours, show >50% suppression, and 10% of patients with Cushing's disease do not suppress.

Table 2.8 Screening tests for Cushing's syndrome

Test	False +ves	False –ves	Sensitivity
24h urinary free cortisol	1%	5–10%	95%
Overnight 1mg dexamethasone suppression test	2% normal 13% obese 23% hospital inpatients	2%	
Midnight cortisol	?	0	100%
Low-dose dexamethasone suppression test	<2%	2%	98%

Table 2.9 Investigation of ACTH-dependent Cushing's syndrome

Test	Pituitary-dependent disease (% with this finding)	Ectopic disease (% with this finding)
Serum potassium <3.2mmol/L	10	100
Suppression of basal cortisol to >50% on high-dose dexamethasone suppression test	90	10
Exaggerated rise in cortisol on CRH test	95	<1

Reproduced from Besser M and Thorner GM (1994). *Clinical Endocrinology 2nd edn.* Mosby. Copyright Elsevier, with permission.

Corticotrophin-releasing hormone test (see Fig. 2.9)
The administration of 100 micrograms of CRH IV (side effects: transient flushing; very rarely, apoplexy reported) leads to an exaggerated rise in cortisol (14–20%) and ACTH (35–50%) in 95% of patients with pituitary-dependent Cushing's syndrome. There are occasional reports of patients with ectopic disease who show a similar response.

Inferior petrosal sinus sampling (see Fig. 2.10)
- Bilateral simultaneous inferior petrosal sinus sampling with measurement of ACTH centrally and in the periphery in the basal state and following stimulation with IV CRH (100 micrograms) allows differentiation between pituitary-dependent and ectopic disease. A central to peripheral ratio of >2 prior to CRH is very suggestive of pituitary-dependent disease, and >3 following CRH gives a diagnostic accuracy approaching 90–95% for pituitary-dependent disease. The test should be performed when cortisol levels are elevated.
- The accurate lateralization of a tumour using the results from inferior petrosal sinus sampling (IPSS) is difficult, as differences in blood flow and catheter placement, etc. will affect the results.
- Brainstem vascular events and deep vein thrombosis are rare complications. *apoplexy, groin haematoma*

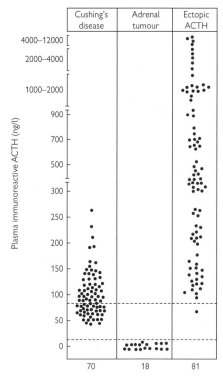

Fig. 2.8 Plasma ACTH levels (9 a.m.) in patients with pituitary-dependent Cushing's disease, adrenal tumours, and ectopic ACTH secretion. From Besser M and Thorner GM (1994). *Clinical Endocrinology 2nd edn.* Mosby.

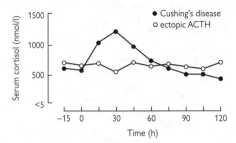

Fig. 2.9 CRH test in pituitary-dependent and ectopic disease. In the patient with pituitary-dependent disease, the characteristic marked plasma cortisol rise after an IV bolus of 100 micrograms of CRH is seen. Serum cortisol levels are unaltered in the patient with ectopic ACTH secretion. Reproduced from Besser M and Thorner GM (1994). *Clinical Endocrinology, 2nd edn.* Mosby. Copyright Elsevier, with permission.

Pituitary imaging
MRI, following gadolinium enhancement which significantly increases the pickup rate, localizes corticotroph adenomas in up to 80% of cases. However, it should be remembered that at least 10% of the normal population harbour microadenomas and, therefore, the biochemical investigation of these patients is essential, as a patient with an ectopic source to Cushing's syndrome may have a pituitary 'incidentaloma'.

Other pituitary function
Hypercortisolism suppresses the thyroidal, gonadal, and GH axes, leading to lowered levels of TSH and thyroid hormones as well as reduced gonadotrophins, gonadal steroids, and GH.

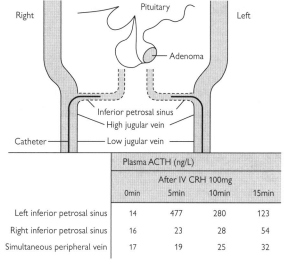

	Plasma ACTH (ng/L)			
	After IV CRH 100mg			
	0min	5min	10min	15min
Left inferior petrosal sinus	14	477	280	123
Right inferior petrosal sinus	16	23	28	54
Simultaneous peripheral vein	17	19	25	32

Fig. 2.10 Simultaneous bilateral inferior petrosal sinus and peripheral vein sampling for ACTH. The ratio of >3 between the left central and peripheral vein confirm a diagnosis of Cushing's disease. Reproduced from Besser M and Thorner GM (1994). *Clinical Endocrinology, 2nd edn.* Mosby. Copyright Elsevier, with permission.

Treatment of Cushing's disease

Transsphenoidal surgery

(📖 also see Transsphenoidal surgery, p. 196.)
- This is the first-line option in most cases. Selective adenomectomy gives the greatest chance of cure, with a reported remission rate of up to 90%. However, strict criteria of a post-operative cortisol of <50nmol/L lead to lower cure rates but much lower recurrence rates (<10% compared with up to 50% in those with detectable post-operative cortisol). This should be the current definition of successful surgery, as the long-term outcome is significantly better in this group of patients.
- Delayed normalization (1–2 months) of cortisol after surgery can occur.
- Complications of surgery may be higher in these patients, as their preoperative general status and the condition of the tissues are poorer than other patients who are referred for surgery.
- Cushing's is associated with a hypercoagulable state, with increased cardiovascular thrombotic risks.
- Risk of relapse lasts for at least 10 years and is higher in Cushing's disease than for other secreting adenomas (13% at 5 years).

Pituitary radiotherapy

(📖 also see p. 200.) This is usually administered as second-line treatment, following unsuccessful transsphenoidal surgery. As control of cortisol levels may take months to years, medical treatment to control cortisol levels, while waiting for cortisol levels to fall, is essential. A more rapid response to radiotherapy is seen in childhood.

Adrenalectomy

- This used to be the favoured form of treatment. It successfully controls cortisol hypersecretion in the majority of patients. Occasionally, a remnant is left and leads to recurrent hypercortisolaemia.
- Nelson's syndrome may occur in up to 30% of patients (see Box 2.29). The administration of prophylactic radiotherapy ↓ the likelihood of this complication. Careful follow-up of these patients is, therefore, essential to allow prompt treatment of the tumour. These tumours are associated with marked increase in ACTH, and associated pigmentation is common. Loss of normal responsiveness to glucocorticoids is characteristic and, therefore, biochemical monitoring should be performed at least 6 months first and then annually by measuring a basal ACTH and rechecking it 1 and 2h after the morning dose of glucocorticoid (ACTH curve).
- Bilateral adrenalectomy may still be indicated when pituitary surgery, radiotherapy, and medical treatment have failed to control the disease. It is also helpful in Cushing's syndrome due to ectopic disease when the ectopic source remains elusive or inoperable. Laparoscopic surgery minimizes morbidity and complications.

Box 2.29 Nelson's syndrome
- Occurs in patients with Cushing's disease, following adrenalectomy.
- Hyperpigmentation and an enlarging (often invasive) pituitary tumour, associated with markedly elevated ACTH levels.
- Usually within 2 years of adrenalectomy.
- Overall incidence is 50% at 10 years. However, if pituitary adenoma visible at time of adrenalectomy, incidence is 80% at 3 years. MRI and ACTH monitoring are important for at least 6 years post-adrenalectomy and should be initiated 6 months after adrenalectomy.

Peri- and post-operative management following transsphenoidal surgery for Cushing's disease
- Perioperative hydrocortisone replacement is given in the standard way, as it is assumed that the patient will become cortisol-deficient after successful removal of the tumour.
- After 3–4 days, the evening steroid replacement is omitted and 9 a.m. cortisol and ACTH checked the following day and 24h later after withholding steroids. Undetectable cortisol (<50nmol/L) is suggestive of cure, and glucocorticoid replacement is commenced. Cortisol 50–300nmol/L is compatible with resolution of symptoms, and a day curve should be performed. Patients with levels >300nmol/L should be considered for re-exploration and/or radiotherapy.
- Antithrombotic prophylaxis should be considered, as Cushing's is associated with a hypercoagulable state.

Medical treatment

(See Table 2.10.)

- This is indicated during the preoperative preparation of patients or while awaiting radiotherapy to be effective or if surgery or radiotherapy are contraindicated.
- Inhibitors of steroidogenesis: *metyrapone* is usually used first-line, but *ketoconazole* should be used as first-line in children, as it is unassociated with ↑ adrenal metabolites. There is also a suggestion that ketoconazole may have a direct action on the corticotroph as well as lowering cortisol secretion.
- Disadvantage of these agents inhibiting steroidogenesis is the need to increase the dose to maintain control, as ACTH secretion will increase as cortisol concentrations decrease.
- Steroidogenesis inhibitors may be used with glucocorticoid replacement regimen to completely inhibit cortisol or with an aim for *partial* inhibition of cortisol production.
- The dose of these drugs needs to be titrated against the cortisol results from a day curve (cortisol taken at 9 a.m., 12 noon, 3 p.m., 6 p.m.), aiming for a mean cortisol of 150–300nmol/L, as this approximates the normal production rate.
- Response rates for drugs that reduce ACTH/CRH synthesis/release, e.g. somatostatin agonists (pasireotide affecting SSTR5 and 2), bromocriptine, valproate, and cyproheptadine, are variable. Pasireotide improves urinary cortisol to normal in about 30%, but carbohydrate tolerance may worsen.
- Successful treatment (surgery or radiotherapy) of Cushing's disease leads to cortisol deficiency and, therefore, glucocorticoid replacement therapy is essential. In addition, patients who have undergone bilateral adrenalectomy require fludrocortisone. These patients should all receive instructions for intercurrent illness and carry a MedicAlert bracelet and steroid card.

Table 2.10 Drug treatment of Cushing's syndrome

Drug	Dose	Action	Side effects
Metyrapone	1–6g/day (usually given in four divided doses)	11β-hydroxylase inhibitor	Nausea ↑ androgenic and mineralocorticoid precursors lead to hirsutism and hypertension
Ketoconazole	400–1,600mg/day given 6–8h. First-line in children NB Avoid if taking H$_2$ antagonists, as acid required to metabolize active compound	Direct inhibitor of P450 enzymes at several different sites Needs gastric acid for absorption	Abnormalities of liver function (usually reversible 1 in 15,000) Gynaecomastia Testosterone ↓. Irregular menses Not effective with proton pump inhibitors
Mitotane (o-p-DDD)	4–12g/day (begin at 0.5–1g/day and gradually increase dose)	Inhibits steroidogenesis at the side chain cleavage, 11- and 18-hydroxylase, and 3β-hydroxysteroid dehydrogenase Adrenolytic Half-life 18–159 days	Nausea and vomiting Cerebellar disturbance Somnolence Hypercholesterolaemia NB May increase clearance of steroids—replacement dosage may need to be ↑ ↑ liver enzymes ↑ lipids NB May be teratogenic. Avoid if fertility desired Avoid concurrent spironolactone—interferes with action
Aminoglutethimide	0.5–2.0g/day	Inhibits steroidogenesis at 🔲 p. 450 side chain cleavage enzyme.	Rash 10% ↓ T$_4$ ↑ hepatic enzymes
Mifepristone	400–1,000mg	Glucocorticoid antagonist	Amenorrhoea Hypokalaemia (progesterone and androgen receptor antagonist)
Etomidate	0.3mg/kg/h. Useful when parenteral treatment is required	Inhibits side chain cleavage and 11β-hydroxylase	Need steroid replacement with this dose
Pasireotide	900mg daily 25% get a normal 24h urine cortisol	Binds SSTR5 and 2	Nearly 50% need glucose-lowering medications because of insulin suppression

Follow-up of Cushing's disease

Successful treatment for Cushing's disease leads to a cortisol that is undetectable (<50nmol/L) following surgery. (This is due to the total suppression of cortisol production from the normal corticotrophs in Cushing's disease.) An undetectable post-operative cortisol leads to a significantly higher chance of long-term cure compared to the patients who have post-operative cortisol between 50–300nmol/L.

- The aim of follow-up is:
  - To detect recurrent Cushing's.
- After successful surgery, the adrenals are suppressed.
- Therefore, patients need to have regular assessment of cortisol production off glucocorticoid replacement. When cortisol is detectable following surgery, recurrent disease must be excluded (low-dose dexamethasone suppression). If recurrence is excluded, it is then important to document the adequacy of the stress response once weaned off glucocorticoid replacement (ITT).

Prognosis of Cushing's disease

- Untreated disease leads to an approximately 30–50% mortality at 5 years, owing to vascular disease and ↑ susceptibility to infections.
- Treated Cushing's syndrome has a good prognosis. Patients who have an undetectable post-operative cortisol are very unlikely to recur (0–20%) whereas 50–75% recur if the post-operative cortisol is detectable.
- Although the physical features and severe psychological disorders associated with Cushing's improve or resolve within weeks or months of successful treatment, more subtle mood disturbance may persist for longer. Adults may also have impaired cognitive function. In addition, it is likely that there is an ↑ cardiovascular risk.
- Osteoporosis will usually resolve in children but may not improve significantly in older patients. Bone mineral density, therefore, requires monitoring and may need specific treatment. *Alendronic acid* has been shown to be effective therapy, leading to improved bone mineral density in patients with Cushing's syndrome and osteoporosis.
- Hypertension has been shown to resolve in 80% and diabetes mellitus in up to 70%.
- Recent data suggests that mortality even with successful treatment of Cushing's is increased significantly.

Cushing's syndrome in children

In a series of 59 patients aged 4–20 years, the following factors were found:

Causes
- Pituitary-dependent disease 85%.
- Adrenal disease 10%.
- Ectopic ACTH secretion 5%.

Initial presentation
- Excessive weight gain 90%.
- Growth retardation 83%.

Below the age of 5 years, adrenal causes are common. In neonates and young children, McCune–Albright syndrome should be considered whereas, in late childhood and early adolescence, ACTH independence may suggest Carney complex (📖 also see Carney complex, p. 583).

Treatment
- Transsphenoidal surgery is used as first-line therapy in pituitary-dependent Cushing's in children as in adults and is usually successful.
- Radiotherapy cures up to 85% children, and this may be considered first-line in some patients. Ketoconazole is the preferred medical therapy in this age group, as it is not associated with ↑ adrenal androgens.
- The long-term management of children with Cushing's syndrome requires careful attention to growth, as growth failure is a very common presentation of this condition. Post-operatively or after radiotherapy, GH therapy may restore growth and final height to normal.

Further reading
Assié G, Bahurel H, Coste J, et al. (2007). Corticotroph tumor progression after adrenalectomy in Cushing's disease: a reappraisal of Nelson's syndrome. J Clin Endocrinol Metab **92**, 172–9.

Colao A, et al. (2012). A 12-month phase 3 study of pasireotide in Cushing's disease. N Engl J Med **366**, 914–24.

Florez JC, Shepard J-AO, Kradin RL (2013). Ectopic ACTH syndrome. New England J Med **368**, 2116–36.

Isidori AM, Kaltsas GA, Pozza C, et al. (2006). The ectopic adrenocorticotropin syndrome: clinical features, diagnosis, management, and long-term follow-up. J Clin Endocrinol Metab **91**, 371–7.

Magiakou MA, Mastorakos G, Oldfield EH, et al. (1994). Cushing's syndrome in children and adolescents. N Engl J Med **331**, 629–36.

Newell-Price J, Morris DG, Drake WM, et al. (2002). Optimal response criteria for the human CRH test in the differential diagnosis of ACTH-dependent Cushing's Syndrome. J Clin Endocrinol Metab **87**, 1640–5.

Newell-Price J, Trainer P, Besser M, et al. (1998). The diagnosis and differential diagnosis of Cushing's syndrome and pseudo-Cushing's states. Endocrinol Rev **19**, 647–72.

Nieman LK (2002). Medical management of Cushing's disease. Pituitary **5**, 77–82.

Nieman LK, Biller BM, Findling JW, et al. (2008). The diagnosis of Cushing's syndrome. An Endocrine Society clinical practice guideline. JCEM **93**, 1526–40.

Ntali G, Asimakopoulou A, Siamatras T, et al. (2013). Mortality in Cushing's syndrome: Systematic Analysis of a Large Series with Prolonged Follow-up. Eur J Endocrinol **169**, 715–23.

van der Pas R, Leebeek FW, Hofland LJ, et al. (2013). Hypercoagulability in Cushing's syndrome: prevalence, pathogenesis and treatment. Clin Endocrinol **78**(4), 481–8.

Preda VA, et al. (2012). Etomidate in the management of hypercortisolaemia in Cushing's syndrome: a review. Eur J Endocrinol **167**, 137–43.

Tritos NA, et al. (2011). Care 40-2011: A 52-year-old man with weakness, infections, and enlarged adrenal glands. N Engl J Med **365**, 2520–30.

Non-functioning pituitary tumours

Background
These pituitary tumours are unassociated with clinical syndromes of anterior pituitary hormone excess.

Epidemiology
- Non-functioning pituitary tumours (NFA) are the commonest pituitary macroadenoma. They represent around 28% of all pituitary tumours.
- There is an equal sex distribution, and the majority of cases present in patients aged >50 years.
- 50% enlarge, if left untreated, at 5 years.

Pathology
- Despite the fact that NFAs are unassociated with hormone production, they may immunostain for:
  - Glycoprotein hormones (most commonly gonadotrophins)—LH, FSH, the α or β subunits of TSH.
  - ACTH (silent corticotroph adenomas), or
  - Be −ve on immunostaining—either null cell tumours or oncocytomas (characteristically contain multiple mitochondria on electron microscopy).
- Tumour behaviour is variable, with some tumours behaving in a very indolent, slow-growing manner and others invading the sphenoid and cavernous sinus.
- K1 67 >3% is a potential marker for aggression.

Clinical features
Mass effects
- Visual field defects (uni- or bitemporal quadrantanopia or hemianopia).
- Headache.
- Ophthalmoplegia (III, IV, and VI cranial nerves—rarely).
- Optic atrophy (rarely, following long-term optic nerve compression).
- Apoplexy (rarely).

Hypopituitarism
📖 also see Hypopituitarism, p. 122.
At diagnosis, approximately 50% of patients are gonadotrophin-deficient.

Incidental finding
An NFA may be detected on the basis of imaging performed for other reasons.

Investigations
- *Pituitary imaging.* MRI/CT demonstrates the tumour and/or invasion into the cavernous sinus or supraoptic recess.
- *Visual fields assessment.* Abnormal in up to two-thirds of cases.
- *PRL.* Essential to exclude a PRL-secreting macroadenoma (📖 see p. 142).
  - Mild elevation (<3,000mU/L usually 2,000mU/L) may occur secondary to stalk compression
- *Pituitary function.* Assessment for hypopituitarism (📖 see Pituitary function—dynamic tests, pp. 114–20).

Management

Surgery

(Aspects of pituitary surgery are also covered on 📖 p. 196.)
- The initial definitive management in virtually every case is surgical. This removes mass effects and may lead to some recovery of pituitary function in around 10%. The majority of patients can be operated on successfully via the transsphenoidal route.
- Close follow-up is necessary after surgery, as tumour regrowth can only be detected using pituitary imaging and visual field assessment.

Radiotherapy

- The use of post-operative radiotherapy remains controversial. Some centres advocate its use for every patient following surgery; others reserve its use for those patients who have had particularly invasive or aggressive tumours removed or those with a significant amount of residual tumour remaining (e.g. in the cavernous sinus).
- The regrowth rate at 10 years without radiotherapy approaches 45%, and there are no good predictive factors for determining which tumours will regrow. However, administration of post-operative radiotherapy reduces this regrowth rate to <10%. As discussed in 📖 Complications, p. 76, however, there are sequelae to radiotherapy—with a significant long-term risk of hypopituitarism and a possible ↑ risk of visual deterioration and malignancy in the field of radiation.

Medical treatment

- Unlike the case for GH- and PRL-secreting tumours, medical therapy for NFAs is usually unhelpful, although there have been reports of the somatostatin agonist octreotide leading to tumour shrinkage and/or visual field improvement in some cases.
- Hormone replacement therapy is required to treat any hypopituitarism (📖 see p. 127).
- Visual field defects at diagnosis may improve following surgery in the majority, and improvement may continue for a year following tumour debulking.

Prediction of regrowth of NFAs?

No markers that provide certainty. However, the following have been suggested as useful markers to raise suspicion of aggressive behaviour:
- Younger age.
- Preoperative cavernous sinus invasion and post-operative suprasellar extension.
- Atypical features on histology (elevated mitotic index, MIB-1 labelling index >3%, and macronucleoli).

Biochemical markers for NFAs?

- The majority of patients lack a hormone marker—despite approximately half immunostaining positively for gonadotrophins and containing secretory granules at the EM level.
- A minority of patients have elevated circulating FSH/LH levels (📖 see Gonadotrophinomas, p. 178).

Follow-up

(See Fig. 2.3.)

- Patients who have not received post-operative irradiation require careful, long-term follow-up with serial pituitary imaging and visual field assessment. The optimal protocol is still not known, but an accepted practice is to image in the first 3 months following surgery, and then reimage annually for 5 years, and biannually thereafter. Tumour recurrence has been reported at up to 15 years following surgery, and, therefore, follow-up needs to be long-term. The amount of post-operative tumour remnant predicates recurrence risk. Thus, with an empty sella post-operatively, the 10-year recurrence is around 6%. With an intrasellar remnant, it is 50% and with an extrasellar remnant 90%.
- Patients who have received post-operative radiotherapy, require follow-up with annual visual field assessment and imaging only if a deterioration is noted.
- Dopamine agonists may decrease recurrences, but this needs a proper prospective study.

Prognosis

Patients with NFAs have a good prognosis once the diagnosis and appropriate treatment, including replacement of hormone deficiency, is performed. The main concern is the risk of tumour regrowth, with subsequent visual failure. As mentioned earlier, the administration of radiotherapy, although not without potential complications itself, significantly reduces this risk. Non-irradiated patients require very close follow-up in order to detect regrowth and perform repeat surgery or administer radiotherapy.

Post-Operative Assessment of NFA	
Immediately	Cortisol – replace if <500nmol/L
6 weeks	Pituitary function
	Thyroxine/TSH
	prolactin
	GH/IGF-I
	cortisol – synacthen + ITT if necessary
	LH/FSH, T/E2
	osmolalities
Replace	Hydrocortisone, thyroxine, gonadal steroids, GH, DHEA
3 months	MRI pituitary
	Consider radiotherapy
Yearly	MRI if no radiotherapy at least to 5 years

Fig. 2.3 Follow-up of non-functioning pituitary adenomas.

Further reading

Dekkers OM, Pereira AM, Romijn JA (2008). Treatment and follow-up of nonfunctioning pituitary macroadenomas. *J Clin Endocrinol Metab* **93**, 3717–26.

Karavitaki N, et al. (2007). What is the natural history of nonoperated nonfunctioning pituitary adenomas? *Clin Endocrinol (Oxf)* **67**, 938–43.

Karavitaki N, Thanabalasingham G, Shore HC, et al. (2006). Do the limits of serum prolactin in disconnection hyperprolactinaemia need re-definition? A study of 226 patients with histologically verified non-functioning pituitary macroadenoma *Clin Endocrinol (Oxf)* **65**, 524–9.

Reddy R, et al. (2011). Can we ever stop imaging in surgically treated and radiotherapy-naive patients with non-functioning pituitary adenoma? *Eur J Endocrinol* **165**, 739–74.

Gonadotrophinomas

Background

These are tumours that arise from the gonadotroph cells of the pituitary gland and produce FSH, LH, or the α subunit. They are often indistinguishable from other non-functioning pituitary adenomas, as they are usually silent and unassociated with excess detectable secretion of LH and FSH, although studies demonstrate gonadotrophin/α subunit secretion *in vitro*. Occasionally, however, these tumours do produce detectable excess hormone *in vivo*.

Clinical features

- Gonadotrophinomas present in the same manner as other non-functioning pituitary tumours, with mass effects and hypopituitarism (📖 see p. 122).
- The rare FSH-secreting gonadotrophinomas may lead to macroorchidism in ♂.
- May cause ovarian hyperstimulation in premenopausal females.

Investigations

The secretion of FSH and LH from these tumours is usually undetectable in the plasma. Occasionally, elevated FSH and, more rarely, LH are measured. This finding is often ignored, particularly in post-menopausal ♀.

Management

These tumours are managed as non-functioning tumours. The potential advantage of FSH/LH secretion from a functioning gonadotrophinoma is that it provides a biochemical marker of presence of tumour for follow-up.

Thyrotrophinomas

Epidemiology

These are rare tumours, comprising approximately 1% of all pituitary tumours. The diagnosis may be delayed because the significance of an unsuppressed TSH in the presence of elevated free thyroid hormone concentrations may be missed. Approximately one-third of cases in the literature have received treatment directed at the thyroid in the form of radioiodine treatment or surgery before diagnosis. Unlike 1° hyperthyroidism, thyrotrophinomas are equally common in ♂ and ♀; 5% are associated with MEN-1.

Tumour biology and behaviour

- The majority are macroadenomas (90%) and secrete only TSH, often with α subunit in addition, but some co-secrete GH (55%) and/or PRL (15%).
- The pathogenesis of thyrotoxicosis in the presence of normal TSH levels is poorly understood, but there are reports of secretion of TSH with ↑ bioactivity, possibly due to changes in post-translational hormone glycosylation.
- The observation that prior thyroid ablation is associated with deleterious effects on the size of the tumour suggests some feedback control and is similar to the aggressive tumours seen in Nelson's syndrome after bilateral adrenalectomy has been performed for Cushing's disease. Thyrotropin-secreting pituitary carcinoma has been very rarely reported.
- 5% are associated with MEN-1.

Clinical features

(🕮 see p. 28.)
- Clinical features of *hyperthyroidism* are usually present but often milder than expected, given the level of thyroid hormones. In mixed tumours, hyperthyroidism may be overshadowed by features of *acromegaly*.
- *Mass effects.* Visual field defects and hypopituitarism.

Investigations

(🕮 see also pp. 11, 125.)
- *TSH is inappropriately normal or elevated.* The range of TSH that has been described is <1–568mU/L, and one-third of untreated patients had TSH in the normal range. There is no correlation between TSH and T_4.
- *Free thyroid hormones.* Elevated in 65% of patients.
- *α subunit (raised in 65%).* Typically, patients have an ↑α subunit:TSH molar ratio (>1) (81%).
- *Other anterior pituitary hormone levels.* PRL and/or GH may be elevated in mixed tumours (an OGTT may be indicated to exclude acromegaly).
- *SHBG.* Elevated into the hyperthyroid range.
- *TRH test.* Absent TSH response to stimulation with TRH (useful to differentiate TSH-secreting tumours from thyroid hormone resistance where the TSH response is normal or exaggerated).

- *T$_3$ suppression test* (lack of suppression of TSH following 100 micrograms/day for 10 days).
- *Thyroid antibodies.* In contrast to Graves's disease, the incidence of thyroid antibodies is similar to that in the general population.
- *Pituitary imaging.* MRI scan will demonstrate a pituitary tumour (macroadenoma) in the majority of cases (90%).

Causes of an elevated FT$_4$ in the presence of an inappropriately unsuppressed TSH

(📖 see p. 11.)

- TSH-secreting tumour.
- Thyroid hormone resistance.
- Amiodarone therapy.
- Inherited abnormalities of thyroid-binding proteins.

Management

Medical treatment

Somatostatin analogues

- Medical treatment with the somatostatin agonists octreotide and lanreotide is successful in the majority of patients in suppressing TSH secretion and leading to tumour shrinkage. In one study, octreotide reduced TSH secretion in almost all patients treated and normalized thyroid hormone levels in 73% of patients. There was partial tumour shrinkage in 40%.
- Drug therapy is useful in the preoperative preparation of these patients to ensure that they are fit for general anaesthetic and also while waiting for radiotherapy to be effective.

Surgery

- Surgery leads to cure in approximately one-third of patients, as judged by apparent complete removal of tumour mass and normalization of thyroid hormone levels, with another third improved with normal thyroid hormone levels but incomplete removal of the adenoma.
- Microadenomas are cured in higher proportions.

Radiotherapy

Radiotherapy is useful, following unsuccessful surgery, and leads to a gradual (over years) reduction in TSH.

Antithyroid medication

Treatment with antithyroid drugs has been associated with ↑ TSH in approximately 60% of patients reported. It should be avoided, if possible, and the more appropriate somatostatin agonist therapy utilized.

Further reading

Beck-Peccoz P, Brucker-Davis F, Persani L, *et al.* (1996). Thyrotropin-secreting pituitary tumours. *Endocr Rev* **17**, 610–38.

Chanson P, Weintraub BD, Harris AG (1993). Octreotide therapy for thyroid stimulating hormone-secreting pituitary adenomas. *Ann Intern Med* **119**, 236–40.

Pituitary incidentalomas

Definition

The term incidentaloma refers to an incidentally detected lesion that is unassociated with hormonal hyper- or hyposecretion and has a benign natural history.

The increasingly frequent detection of these lesions with technological improvements and more widespread use of sophisticated imaging has led to a management challenge—which, if any, lesions need investigation and/or treatment, and what is the optimal follow-up strategy (if required at all)?

Epidemiology

- Autopsy studies have shown that 10–20% of pituitary glands unsuspected of having pituitary disease harbour pituitary adenomas. Approximately half the tumours stain for PRL, and the remainder is –ve on immunostaining.
- Imaging studies using MRI demonstrate pituitary microadenomas in approximately 10% of normal volunteers.
- Incidentally detected macroadenomas have been reported when imaging has been performed for other reasons. However, these are not true incidentalomas, as they are often associated with visual field defects and/or hypopituitarism.
- Clinical significant pituitary tumours are present in about 1 in 1,000 patients.

Natural history

Incidentally detected microadenomas are very unlikely (<10%) to increase in size whereas larger incidentally detected meso- and macroadenomas are more likely (40–50%) to enlarge. Thus, conservative management in selected patients may be appropriate for microadenomas which are incidentally detected as long as careful follow-up imaging is in place and patients are truly asymptomatic. Macroadenomas should be treated, if possible.

Clinical features

By definition, a patient with an incidentaloma should be asymptomatic. Any patient who has an incidentally detected tumour should have visual field assessment and a clinical review to ensure that this is not the initial presentation of Cushing's syndrome, acromegaly, or a prolactinoma.

Investigations

- Aims:
  - Exclude any hormone hypersecretion from the tumour.
  - Detect hypopituitarism.
- Investigation of hypersecretion of hormones should include measurement of PRL, IGF-1 and an OGTT if acromegaly is suspected, 24h urinary free cortisol and overnight dexamethasone suppression test, and thyroid function tests (unsuppressed TSH in the presence of elevated T_4).
- Others suggest that this approach is unnecessary, but, with limited data, most endocrinologists would perform investigations as above.

Management

- All extrasellar macroadenomas (incidentally detected but, by definition, not true incidentalomas) require definitive treatment.
- Tumours with excess hormone secretion require definitive treatment.
- Mass <1cm diameter—repeat MRI at 1, 2, and 5 years.
- Mass >1cm diameter—repeat MRI at 6 months, 1, 2, and 5 years.

Further reading

Fernando A, Karavitaki N, Wass JA (2010) Prevalence of pituitary adenomas: a community-based cross-sectional study in Banbury, Oxfordshire (UK) *Clin Endocrinol* **72**, 377–82.

Frida PU, *et al.* (2011). Pituitary incidentaloma: an Endocrine Society clinical practice guideline. *Clin Endocrinol Metab.* **96**, 894–904.

Karavitaki N, Collison K, Halliday J, *et al.* (2007). What is the natural history of nonoperated non-functioning pituitary adenomas? *Clin Endocrinol (Oxf)* **67**, 938–43.

Molitch ME (1997). Pituitary incidentalomas. *End Met Clin North America* **26**, 725–40.

Pituitary carcinoma

Definition
Pituitary carcinoma is defined as a 1° adenohypophyseal neoplasm with craniospinal and/or distant systemic metastases (see Table 2.5 for types).

Epidemiology
These are extremely rare tumours, and only approximately 60 cases have been reported in the world literature.

Pathology and pathogenesis
- The initial tumours and subsequent carcinomas show higher proliferation indices than the majority of pituitary adenomas. They are also likely to demonstrate p53 positivity and have an ↑ mitotic index. However, histology is unable to reliably distinguish between benign invasive pituitary adenomas and carcinomas.
- The aetiology of these tumours is unknown, but the adenoma–carcinoma sequence is followed in ACTH-secreting tumours: pituitary adenoma causing Cushing's disease, followed by locally invasive adenoma (Nelson's syndrome), leading to pituitary carcinoma.
- Metastatic spread outside the CNS is via lymphatic and vascular routes while intra-CNS spread is via local invasion and tumour seeding.

Features
Virtually all pituitary carcinomas initially present as invasive pituitary macroadenomas. After a variable interval of time (mean 6.5 years), the majority presents with local recurrence. There is a tendency to systemic (liver, lymph nodes, lungs, and bones), rather than craniospinal, metastases, but metastases do not usually predominate in the clinical picture.

Neuroradiological classification of pituitary adenomas (modified Hardy criteria)
- Grade 1—microadenoma.
- Grade 2—macroadenoma with or without suprasellar extension.
- Grade 3—locally invasive tumour with bony destruction and tumour in the cavernous or sphenoid sinus.
- Grade 4—spread within the CNS or extracranial dissemination.

Grades 3 and 4 are termed 'invasive'.

Treatment
Treatment involves surgery, radiotherapy, and medical treatment. As mass effects often predominate, initial debulking surgery may provide relief. It may need to be repeated to maintain local control. Some advocate a transsphenoidal route as less likely to disseminate tumour.

Radiotherapy or medical treatment provides palliation only. Radiotherapy has been reported to be successful, in some cases, in controlling growth and occasionally leading to regression. Stereotactic radiosurgery may play a role. Medical treatment with dopamine agonists for malignant prolactinomas and acromegaly has been reported, with varying results. Many pituitary carcinomas are dedifferentiated and, therefore,

Table 2.5 Types of pituitary carcinoma

Type	Proportion of reported cases (%)
PRL	30
ACTH	28
GH	2
Non-functioning	30

NB Many 'non-functioning' carcinomas were reported prior to routine measurement of PRL or routine immunostaining, and, therefore, the true incidence of PRL-producing carcinomas may be higher.

escape from control. Various chemotherapy regimes have been reported, with occasional success (e.g. CCNU, 5FU and folinic acid or cisplatin, procarbazine, lomustine, and vincristine). Temozolomide has also recently been used (📖 see p. 206) and may be effective but further controlled trials are needed.

Prognosis

Most patients die within a year of diagnosis.

Further reading

Kaltsas GA, Grossman AB (1998). Malignant pituitary tumours. *Pituitary* **1**, 69–81.
McCormack AI, Wass JA, Grossman AB (2011). Aggressive pituitary tumours: the role of temozolomide and the assessment of MGMT status. *Eur J Clin Invest* **41**(10):1133–48.
Pernicone PJ, Scheithauer BW, Sebo TJ, *et al.* (1997). Pituitary carcinoma. *Cancer* **79**, 804–12.

Pituitary metastases

Incidence
0.1–28% autopsy series; <1% found at transsphenoidal surgery.

Epidemiology
Equal sex distribution. Age >60 (occasionally younger).

Features
Diabetes insipidus in almost 100%. Symptomatic pituitary failure and cranial nerve defects less common. Often difficult to differentiate neuroradiologically from other pituitary mass lesions (adenoma, cyst, or inflammatory pituitary mass). Many do not have symptoms, as features of end-stage malignancy predominate. Disconnection hyperprolactinaemia may be a feature, and very rare cases of endocrine hyperfunction related to metastasis within a primary adenoma have been reported (see Box 2.16).

Diagnosis
Histology is required to confirm.

Treatment
- Of 1° tumour where possible.
- Management of endocrine symptoms.
- Decompression may be indicated for visual field defects.

Prognosis
Mean survival 6–7 months.

Box 2.16 Primary tumours associated with pituitary metastases

- Breast.
- Lung.
- GI.
- Prostate.
- Kidney.

Breast and lung primary tumours account for two-thirds of pituitary metastases.

Craniopharyngiomas and perisellar cysts

(See Box 2.17 for Rathke's cleft cysts.)

Prevalence and epidemiology
- 0.065/1,000.
- Any age; only 50% present in childhood (<16 years).

Pathology
- Tumour arising from squamous epithelial remnants of craniopharyngeal duct.
- Histology may be either adamantinomatous or squamous papillary.
- Cyst formation and calcification are common.
- Benign tumour, although infiltrates surrounding structures.

Features
- Raised intracranial pressure.
- Visual disturbance.
- Hypothalamo–pituitary disturbance.
- Growth failure in children.
- Precocious puberty and tall stature are less common.
- Anterior and posterior pituitary failure, including DI.
- Weight gain.

Other perisellar cysts
- Arachnoid.
- Epidermoid.
- Dermoid.

Investigations
- MRI/CT (CT may be helpful to evaluate bony erosion).
- Visual field assessment.
- Anterior and posterior pituitary assessment (see p. 114 and p. 212).

Management
(See Fig. 2.4.)
- Gross total removal is the aim of treatment, as this is associated with a significantly lower recurrence rate. This may be via a transfrontal or transsphenoidal route. If total removal cannot be safely achieved, adjuvant radiotherapy is beneficial in reducing recurrence.
- Restoration of pituitary hormone deficiencies is extremely unlikely following surgery.
- Cystic lesions may be treated with aspiration alone, although radiotherapy reduces the likelihood of reaccumulation.

Prognosis
- Craniopharyngiomas are associated with ↓ survival (up to 5× the mortality of the general population).
- Recurrence following initial treatment may present early or several decades following initial treatment. Childhood and adult onset lesions behave similarly.

Box 2.17 Rathke's cleft cysts

Pathology

Derived from the remnants of Rathke's pouch, lined by epithelial cells (ciliated cuboidal/columnar epithelium, compared with squamous for craniopharyngiomas) and filled with fluid.

Features

Usually asymptomatic although may present with headache and amenorrhoea and, rarely, hypopituitarism and hydrocephalus.

Investigation

CT/MRI—variable enhancement.

Management

- Decompression if symptomatic.
- Recurrence is not as rare as originally thought.

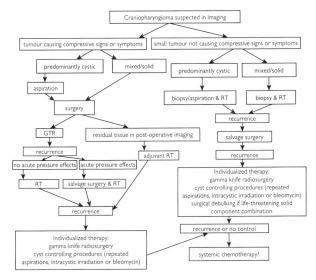

Fig. 2.4 Treatment algorithm for craniopharyngiomas. Reproduced with permission from Karavitaki N, Cudlip S, Adams CB, Wass JA (2006). Craniopharyngiomas. Endocr Rev 27 (4), pp.371–97. Epub 2006 Mar 16, copyright 2006, The Endocrine Society.

Further reading

Karivitaki N, Cudlip S, Adams CB, et al. (2006). Craniopharyngiomas. *Endocr Rev* **27**, 371–93.

Trifanescu R, et al. (2011). Outcome in surgically treated Rathke's cleft cysts: long-term monitoring needed. *Eur J Endocrinol* **165**, 33–7.

Trifanescu R, et al. (2012). Rathke's cleft cysts. *Clin Endocrinol (Oxf)* **76**, 51–60.

Parasellar tumours

Meningiomas

- Suprasellar meningiomas arise from the tuberculum sellae or the chiasmal sulcus.
- Usually present with a chiasmal syndrome where loss of visual acuity occurs in one eye, followed by reduced acuity in the other eye.
- Differentiation from a 1° pituitary tumour can be difficult where there is downward extension into the sella.
- MRI is the imaging of choice. T_1-weighted images demonstrate meningiomas as isodense with grey matter and hypointense with respect to pituitary tissue, with marked enhancement after gadolinium.
- Cerebral angiography also demonstrates a tumour blush.
- Management is surgical and may also be complicated by haemorrhage, as these are often very vascular tumours. They are relatively radioresistant, but inoperable or partially removed tumours may respond. As they are slow-growing, a conservative approach with regular imaging may be appropriate.
- Associations include type 2 neurofibromatosis (📖 p. 578).

Clivus chordomas

- Rare. Arise from embryonic crest cells of the notochord.
- May present with cranial nerve palsies (III, VI, IX, X) or pyramidal tract dysfunction.
- Anterior and posterior pituitary hypofunction is reported.
- Often invasive and relentlessly progressive.
- Treatment is surgical, followed by radiotherapy in some cases, although they are relatively radioresistant. Data on radiosurgery are not yet available, but this may be considered.

Hamartomas

- Non-neoplastic overgrowth of neurones and glial cells.
- Rare. May present with seizures—typically gelastic (laughing).
- May release GnRH leading to precocious puberty or, very rarely, GHRH leading to disorders of growth or acromegaly.
- Appear as homogeneous, isointense with grey matter, pedunculated or sessile non-enhancing tumours on T_1-weighted MRI scans.

Management

Tumours do not enlarge, and, therefore, treatment is of endocrine consequences—most commonly, precocious puberty.

Ependymomas

- Intracranial ependymomas typically affect children and adolescents.
- Pituitary insufficiency may follow craniospinal irradiation.
- Occasionally, third ventricle tumours may interfere with hypothalamic function.

Further reading

Whittle IR, Smith C, Navoo P, *et al.* (2004). Meningiomas. *Lancet* **363**, 1535–43.

Parasellar inflammatory conditions

Neurosarcoidosis

Pituitary and hypothalamus may be affected by meningeal disease. Most patients with hypothalamic sarcoidosis also have involvement outside the CNS.

Features

Hypopituitarism and DI, in addition to hypothalamic syndrome of absent thirst, somnolescence, and hyperphagia.

Investigations

- Serum and CSF ACE may be raised.
- CSF examination may reveal a pleocytosis, oligoclonal bands, and low glucose.
- MRI may demonstrate additional enhancement, e.g. meningeal.
- Gallium scan may reveal ↑ uptake in lacrimal and salivary glands.

Management

- High doses of glucocorticoids (60–80mg prednisolone) for initial treatment. Subsequent treatment with 40mg/day is often required for several months. Pulsed methylprednisolone may also be useful. Steroid-sparing agents, such as azathioprine, may be helpful.
- Management of hormonal deficiency can be very difficult, particularly in the context of absent thirst and poor memory.

Langerhans cell histiocytosis

- >50% of cases occur in children.
- Most frequent endocrine abnormalities are DI and growth retardation due to hypothalamic infiltration by Langerhans cells or involvement of the meninges adjacent to the pituitary. Rarely, hyperprolactinaemia and panhypopituitarism develop. In adults, DI may precede the bone and soft tissue abnormalities, making diagnosis difficult.

Management

The role of radiotherapy is controversial, with some workers reporting improvement and others questioning the efficacy. If radiotherapy is used, rapid institution of treatment appears to be important (within 10 days of diagnosis). High-dose glucocorticoids can lead to transient improvement, but chemotherapy does not alter the course of DI, although it may lead to temporary regression of lesions.

Wegener's granulomatosis

- Systemic vasculitis, affecting mainly 30–50 year olds.
- Necrotizing vasculitis, affecting lungs and kidneys in 85% (cavitating nodules infiltrates).
- Pituitary involvement 1%.
- Present with diabetes insipidus and hyperprolactinaemia.
- High titres of anti-neutrophil cytoplasmic antibody (ANCA).
- Treated with glucocorticoids and/or cyclophosphamide.

Tuberculosis

TB may present as a tuberculoma which may compromise hypothalamic or pituitary function. DI is common. Most patients have signs of TB elsewhere but not invariably so. Transsphenoidal biopsy is, therefore, sometimes required. An alternative strategy is antituberculous treatment with empirical glucocorticoid treatment.

Further reading

Freda PU, Post KD (1999). Differential diagnosis of sellar masses. *Endocrinol Metabol Clin N Am* **28**, 81.

Lymphocytic hypophysitis

Background
This is a rare inflammatory condition of the pituitary.

Epidemiology
Lymphocytic hypophysitis occurs more commonly in ♀ and usually presents during late pregnancy or the first year thereafter.

Pathogenesis
Ill understood—probably autoimmune. Approximately 25% of cases of lymphocytic hypophysitis have been associated with other autoimmune conditions—Hashimoto's thyroiditis in the majority but also pernicious anaemia.

There is a recent association with ipilimumab, immunostimulating agent a monoclonal antibody against cytotoxic T lymphocyte antigen 4 (CTLA4).

Pathology
* Somatotroph and gonadotroph function are more likely to be preserved than corticotroph or thyrotroph function, unlike the findings in hypopituitarism due to a pituitary tumour. The posterior pituitary is characteristically spared so that DI is not part of the picture, but there are occasional reports of coexistent or isolated DI, presumably because of different antigens.
* Lymphocytic hypophysitis has occasionally involved the cavernous sinus and extraocular muscles.
* Light microscopy typically reveals a lymphoplasmacytic infiltrate, occasionally forming lymphoid follicles, with variable destruction of parenchyma and fibrosis.

Clinical features
* Mass effects, leading to headache and visual field defects.
* Often a temporal association with pregnancy.
* Hypopituitarism (ACTH and TSH deficiency, less commonly gonadotrophin and GH deficiency).
* Posterior pituitary involvement and cavernous sinus involvement occur less commonly.
* See Box 2.18 for classification.

Investigations
* Investigation of hypopituitarism is essential and may not be thought of because gonadotrophin secretion often remains intact, leaving the potentially life-threatening ACTH deficiency unsuspected.
* MRI shows an enhancing mass, with variably loss of hyperintense bright spot of neurohypophysis, thickening of pituitary stalk, and enlargement of the neurohypophysis. Suprasellar extension often appears tongue-like along the pituitary stalk. There may be central necrosis but no calcification.
* Biopsy of the lesion is often required but may be avoided in the presence of typical features.

Box 2.18 Classification of hypophysitis
- Acute:
  - Bacterial infections.
- Chronic:
  - Lymphocytic hypophysitis.
  - Xanthomatous—characterized by lipid-laden macrophages.
- Granulomatous:
  - Tuberculosis.
  - Sarcoidosis.
  - Syphilis.
  - Giant cell—? variant of lymphocytic hypophysitis.

- The presence of antipituitary antibodies has been investigated by some groups and shown to be variably present. This is, however, a research tool and an unreliable marker.

Treatment
- Most often, no specific treatment is necessary. There is anecdotal evidence only of the effectiveness of immunosuppressive doses of glucocorticoids—e.g. prednisolone 60mg/day for 3 months and progressive reduction for 6 months. This has been reported to be associated with reduction in the mass and gradual recovery of pituitary function. However, relapse after discontinuing therapy is also reported.
- Spontaneous recovery may also occur.
- Surgery has also been used to improve visual field abnormalities.

Natural history
Variable—some progress rapidly to life-threatening hypopituitarism while others spontaneously regress.

Relationship to other conditions
Lymphocytic hypophysitis remains an ill-understood condition but has been suggested to be the underlying cause of other conditions, such as isolated ACTH deficiency and the empty sella syndrome.

Further reading
Caturegli P, Newschaffer C, Olivi A, et al (2005). Autoimmune hypophysitis. *Endocr Rev* **26**, 599–614.

Thodou E, Asa SL, Kontogeorgos G, et al. (1995). Clinical case seminar: lymphocytic hypophysitis: clinicopathological findings. *J Clin Endocrinol Metab* **80**, 2302–11.

Surgical treatment of pituitary tumours

Transsphenoidal surgery

This is currently the favoured technique for pituitary surgery and is first-line for virtually every case. It is preferred to the previously used technique of craniotomy because there is minimal associated morbidity as a result of the fact that the cranial fossa is not opened and there are, therefore, no immediate sequelae due to direct cerebral damage (particularly frontal lobe) and no long-term risk of epilepsy. There is reduced duration of hospital stay and improved cure rates, as there is better visualization of small tumours. Unfortunately, the technique may be inadequate to deal with very large tumours with extensive suprasellar extension. In these situations, craniotomy is required if adequate debulking is not possible following the transsphenoidal approach. See Box 2.19 for indications for surgery. See Table 2.6 for complications.

Preparation for transsphenoidal surgery

Pretreatment before surgery

- Pretreatment with *metyrapone* or *ketoconazole* to improve the condition of patients with Cushing's syndrome is often given for at least 6 weeks. This allows some improvement in healing and also improves the general state of the patient.
- Patients with macroprolactinomas will, in the majority of cases, have received treatment with dopamine agonists in any case, and surgery is usually indicated for resistance or intolerance. There is a risk of tumour fibrosis, with long-term (>6 months) dopamine agonist therapy with bromocriptine.

Immediately preoperative

- Immediate preoperative treatment requires appropriate anterior pituitary hormone replacement. In particular, a decision as to whether perioperative glucocorticoid treatment is required. The majority of microadenomas will not require perioperative hydrocortisone, but patients with Cushing's syndrome will require peri- and post-operative glucocorticoid treatment. Patients with macroadenomas and an intact preoperative pituitary–adrenal axis do not usually require perioperative steroids, but those who are deficient or whose reserve has not been tested need to be given perioperative glucocorticoids. TSH deficiency should be corrected with levothyroxine. Ensure the patient is not taking aspirin.
- Prophylactic antibiotics are started in some centres the night before surgery to reduce the chances of meningitis.

Complications

(See also Box 2.20 and Table 2.6.)

- Patients should be informed about the possible complications of transsphenoidal surgery prior to consent. The commonest complications are DI, which may be transient or permanent (5% and 0.1%, respectively; often higher in Cushing's disease and prolactinoma), and the development of new anterior pituitary hormonal deficiencies (uncommon with microadenomas; approximately 10% of TSA for macroadenomas).
- Other complications include meningitis, CSF leak, visual deterioration, haemorrhage (rare), and transient hyponatraemia, usually 7 days post-operatively.

Box 2.19 Indications for pituitary surgery

- Non-functioning pituitary adenoma.
- GH-secreting adenoma.
- ACTH-secreting tumour.
- Nelson's syndrome. (see Box 2.29, p. 169)
- Prolactinoma—if patient dopamine agonist-resistant or -intolerant.
- Recurrent pituitary tumour.
- Gonadotrophin-secreting tumour.
- TSH-secreting adenoma.
- Craniopharyngioma.
- Pituitary biopsy to define diagnosis, e.g. hypophysitis, pituitary metastases.
- Chordoma.
- Rathke's cleft cyst.
- Arachnoid cyst.

Box 2.20 Post-operative disorders of fluid balance

- Acute post-operative transient DI.
- SIADH.
- Triphasic response: initial DI due to axon shock (hours to days), followed by antidiuretic phase due to uncontrolled release of ADH from damaged posterior pituitary (2–14 days), followed by DI due to depletion of ADH.
- Transient hyponatraemia (isolated second phase) at 5–10 days post-operatively, usually mild and self-limiting.

Table 2.6 Complications of transsphenoidal surgery

Complications of any surgical procedure	Anaesthetic-related
	Venous thrombosis and pulmonary embolism
Immediate	Haemorrhage
	Hypothalamic damage
	Meningitis
Permanent	Visual deterioration or loss
	Cranial nerve damage (e.g. oculomotor nerve palsies)
	Hypopituitarism
	DI
	SIADH
Transient	DI
	CSF rhinorrhoea
	Meningitis
	Visual deterioration
	Cerebral salt wasting

Cerebral salt wasting

A rare, but important, complication of transsphenoidal surgery, more commonly seen after subarachnoid haemorrhage, is cerebral salt wasting syndrome (CSW). This typically occurs at day 5–10 post-operatively and is associated with, often massive, urinary salt loss and hypovolaemia. It needs to be differentiated from SIADH which may also occur at this stage (often using central venous pressure measurement to demonstrate hypovolaemia in CSW compared with euvolaemia in SIADH). The management of CSW involves the administration of saline whereas fluid restriction is indicated for SIADH.

Transfrontal craniotomy

Indications
- Pituitary tumours with major suprasellar and lateral invasion where transsphenoidal surgery is unlikely to remove a significant proportion of the tumour.
- Parasellar tumours, e.g. meningioma.

Complications
- In addition to the complications of transsphenoidal surgery, brain retraction can lead to cerebral oedema or haemorrhage.
- Manipulation of the optic chiasm may lead to visual deterioration.
- Vascular damage.
- Damage to the olfactory nerve.

Perioperative management
Similar to that for patients undergoing transsphenoidal surgery (☐ see Transsphenoidal surgery, p. 196).

Post-operative management
- Recovery is typically slower than after transsphenoidal surgery.
- Prophylactic anticonvulsants are administered for up to 1 year.
- The DVLA must be advised of surgery and relevant regulations to be followed.

Further reading
Laws ER, Thapar K (1999). Pituitary surgery. *Endocrinol Metab Clin N Am* **28**, 119.

Pituitary radiotherapy

Indications
(□ see Box 2.21.)
- Pituitary radiotherapy is an effective treatment used to reduce the likelihood of tumour regrowth following surgery, to further shrink a tumour, and to treat persistent hormone hypersecretion (usually after surgical resection or non-successful medical treatment).
- Pituitary radiotherapy is usually only administrable once in a lifetime.

Technique
(See Box 2.22 for focal forms of radiotherapy.)
- Conventional external beam 3-field radiotherapy is able to deliver a beam of ionizing irradiation accurately to the pituitary fossa.
- Accurate targeting requires head fixation in a moulded plastic shell to keep the head immobilized. The fields of irradiation are based on simulation using MRI or CT scanning, and the volume is usually the tumour margins plus 0.5cm in all planes. The preoperative tumour volume is used for planning whereas the post-drug (dopamine agonist) shrinkage films are used for prolactinomas. There are three portals— two temporal and one anterior.
- The standard dose is 4500cGy in 25 fractions over 35 days, but 5,000 cGy may be used for relatively 'radioresistant' tumours, such as craniopharyngiomas.

Efficacy
Radiotherapy is effective in reducing the chance of pituitary tumour regrowth. Comparison of non-functioning tumour recurrence following surgery and radiotherapy compared with surgery alone shows that radiotherapy is effective in reducing the likelihood of regrowth (see Fig. 2.5).

Box 2.21 Indications for pituitary radiotherapy

Tumour	Aim of treatment
Non-functioning pituitary adenoma	To shrink residual mass or reduce likelihood of regrowth
GH/PRL/ACTH-secreting tumour	To reduce persistent hormonal hypersecretion and shrink residual mass
Craniopharyngioma	To reduce likelihood of regrowth
Recurrent tumour	To shrink mass and reduce likelihood of regrowth.

Box 2.22 Focal forms of radiotherapy

Stereotactic radiosurgery uses focused radiation to deliver a precise dose of radiation:

- Gamma knife 'radiosurgery'—ionizing radiation from a cobalt 60 source delivered by convergent collimated beams.
- Linear accelerator focal radiotherapy—photons focused on a stationary point from a moving gantry.
- Potential advantages are that a single high dose of irradiation is given which can be sharply focused on the tumour, with minimal surrounding tissue damage.
- Long-term data are required to demonstrate endocrine efficacy, but it may have a particular role in recurrent or persistent tumours which are well demarcated and surgically inaccessible, e.g. in the cavernous sinus.
- Potential limitations include proximity to the optic chiasm.

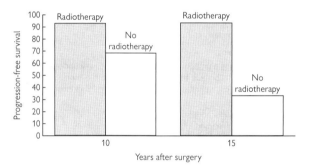

Fig. 2.5 Recurrence rates following radiotherapy. Modified from Gittoes NJL, Bates AS, Tse W, et al. (1998). Radiotherapy for non-functioning pituitary tumours. Clin Endocrinol 48, 331–7. With permission from Wiley Blackwell.

Complications of pituitary radiotherapy

Short term
- Nausea.
- Headache.
- Temporary hair loss at radiotherapy portals of entry.

Hypopituitarism (see Fig. 2.6)
- Anterior pituitary hormone deficiency occurs due to the effect of irradiation on the normal pituitary or the hypothalamus, leading to reduced hypothalamic-releasing hormone secretion. The total dose of irradiation is one of the main determinants of the speed, incidence, and extent of hypopituitarism (see Table 2.7).
- The onset of hypopituitarism is gradual, and the order of development of deficiency is as for any other cause of developing hypopituitarism—namely, GH first, followed by gonadotrophin and ACTH, followed finally by TSH. Posterior pituitary deficiencies are very rare, but 2° temporary mild hyperprolactinaemia may be seen after about 2 years which gradually returns to normal.

Visual impairment
- The optic chiasm is particularly radioresistant but may undergo damage thought to be due to vascular damage to the blood supply. Visual deterioration typically occurs within 3 years of irradiation and is progressive.
- The literature suggests that the risk is greatest with high total and daily doses. A standard total dose of 4,500cGy and daily dose of 180cGy appear to pose very little, if any, risk to the chiasm.
- Our practice is to avoid administration of radiotherapy, where possible, when the chiasm is under pressure from residual tumour.

Radiation oncogenesis
- There is controversy as to whether pituitary irradiation leads to the development of second tumours. There have been reports of sarcomas, gliomas, and meningiomas developing in the field of irradiation after 10–20 years. However, there are also reports of gliomas and meningiomas occurring in non-irradiated patients with pituitary adenomas. A retrospective review of a large series of patients given pituitary irradiation suggested a risk of second tumour of 1.9% by 20 years after irradiation when compared to the normal population (but not patients with pituitary tumours).
- Subtle changes in neurocognition have also been suggested.

Table 2.7 Development of new hypopituitarism at 10 years following pituitary radiotherapy

	No previous surgery	Previous surgery
Gonadotrophin deficiency	47%	70%
ACTH deficiency	30%	54%
Thyrotrophin deficiency	16%	38%

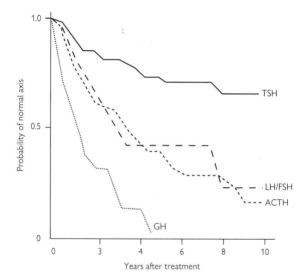

Fig. 2.6 Life-table analysis, indicating the probability of developing pituitary hormone deficiencies after conventional radiation therapy. Reproduced with permission from Littley MD, Shalet SM, Beardwell CG, Ahmed, SR, et al. (1989). Q J Med 70:145–160.

Further reading

Brada M, Ford D, Ashley S, et al. (1992). Risk of second brain tumour after conservative surgery and radiotherapy for pituitary adenoma. *BMJ* **304**, 1343–6.

Jackson IMD, Noren G (1999). Role of gamma knife therapy in the management of pituitary tumours. *Endocrinol Metab Clin N Am* **28**, 133.

Jones A (1991). Radiation oncogenesis in relation to treatment of pituitary tumours. *Clin Endocrinol* **35**, 379.

Loeffler JS, Shih HA (2011). Radiation therapy in the management of pituitary adenomas. *J Clin Endocrinol Metab* **96**, 1992–2003.

Minniti G, et al. (2005). Risk of second brain tumor after conservative surgery and radiotherapy for pituitary adenoma: update after an additional 10 years. *J Clin Endocrinol Metab* **90**, 800–4.

Plowman PN (1999). Pituitary adenoma radiotherapy. *Clin Endocrinol* **51**, 265–71.

Drug treatment of pituitary tumours

Dopamine agonists
(See Box 2.23 for uses.)

Types
- *Bromocriptine*—the first ergot alkaloid to be used, short-acting, taken daily. Usually administered orally, although vaginal and IM formulations can be used and may reduce GI intolerance.
- *Quinagolide*—non-ergot, longer-acting, taken daily.
- *Cabergoline*—ergot derivative, long-acting, taken once or twice a week.
- *Less commonly used*—pergolide and lisuride.

Mechanism of action
Activation of D2 receptors.

Side effects
Commonly at initiation of treatment
- Nausea.
- Postural hypotension.

Less common
- Headache, fatigue, nasal stuffiness, constipation, abdominal cramps, and a Raynaud-like phenomenon in hands.
- Very rarely, patients have developed hallucinations and psychosis (usually at higher doses).
- Side effects may be minimized by slow initiation of therapy (e.g. 1.25mg bromocriptine or 250 micrograms cabergoline), taking medication before going to bed and taking the tablets with food.

Somatostatin analogues
(See Box 2.24 for uses.)

Mechanism of action
- Since the half-life of somatostatin is very short, longer-acting analogues were synthesized—octreotide and lanreotide. These have a half-life of 110min in the circulation, and inhibit GH secretion 45× more actively than native somatostatin, with none of the rebound hypersecretion that occurs with somatostatin.
- The somatostatin analogues act predominantly on somatostatin receptors 2 and 5. Unlike dopamine agonists, somatostatin analogues do not lead to dramatic tumour shrinkage, but some shrinkage is still seen in the majority of tumours.

Types
- Octreotide LAR® (10–30mg IM) administered every 4–6 weeks.
- Lanreotide Autogel® (60–120mg IM) administered every 28 days.
- SC octreotide (50–200 micrograms) administered usually 3× daily.
- Paireotide is a new somatostatin analogue which has increased affinity for somatostatin receptor 5. It is licensed for use in Cushing's disease.

Box 2.23 Uses of dopamine agonists

Hyperprolactinaemia (📖 see p. 144)

- D2 receptor stimulation leads to inhibition of PRL secretion and reduction in cell size, leading to tumour shrinkage. The PRL often falls before significant tumour shrinkage is seen.
- Problems may arise when patients are either intolerant of the medication or resistant. Cabergoline appears to be better tolerated than bromocriptine, and it is often worth trying an alternative in the case of intolerance, although true intolerance is probably a class effect. Dopamine agonist resistance macro- > microadenomas (10–25% patients) may be due to differences in receptor subtype (e.g. loss of D2 receptors) or possibly altered intracellular signalling.

GH-secreting tumours

- Although administration of L-dopa to normal individuals leads to acute increase in GH due to hypothalamic dopamine and noradrenaline synthesis and inhibition of somatostatin secretion, >50% of patients with GH-secreting tumours given dopamine agonists have a fall in GH. Dopamine acts directly on somatotroph tumours to inhibit GH release.
- Patients with acromegaly often need larger doses of dopamine agonist than patients with prolactinomas e.g. cabergoline 3mg/week. Tumour shrinkage is most likely if there is concomitant secretion of PRL from the tumour. Dopamine agonists are currently usually reserved for second-line drug therapy in patients who are somatostatin analogue-resistant or as a co-prescription with somatostatin analogues in patients with mixed GH- and PRL-secreting tumours.

Pregnancy

Bromocriptine is licensed for use in pregnancy, but cabergoline is not licensed in the UK, although it has not thus far been associated with any ↑ teratogenicity.

Box 2.24 Uses of somatostatin analogues

- Acromegaly.
- Carcinoid tumours.
- Pancreatic neuroendocrine tumours.
- TSH-secreting pituitary tumours.

Side effects
- *Gallstones.* At least 20–30% of patients develop gallstones or sludge on octreotide (thought, by most, to antedate stone formation), but only 1%/year develop symptoms. The incidence is unknown on octreotide LAR® or lanreotide. Symptoms may particularly occur if somatostatin analogue therapy is withdrawn.
- GI due to inhibition of motor activity and secretion, leading to nausea, abdominal cramps, and mild steatorrhoea. These usually settle with time.
- Injection site pain obviated by allowing vial to warm to room temperature before injecting.
- Hair loss (<10%).

Growth hormone receptor antagonist

Pegvisomant—newly developed treatment for acromegaly.

Mechanism of action
- Binds to GH receptor and induces internalization but blocks receptor signalling, leading to reduction in IGF-1 (but not GH) production.
- Studies suggest that it is the most potent available medical therapy. Normalization of IGF-1 in >90% treated patients.

Usage
- May be used with somatostatin analogues to decrease frequency of injections.

Problems
- High cost.
- Further data required on the effects on pituitary tumour growth.
- Occasional deterioration in liver biochemistry.
- IGF-1 used to monitor effectiveness of treatment.

Temozolomide
- Is an alkylating chemotherapeutic agent effective in glioblastoma and neuroendocrine tumours.
- It has been successfully used to treat pituitary carcinoma and invasive and aggressive pituitary adenomas.
- Response may be predicated by O-6-methylguanine DNA methyltransferase (MGMT) staining, which is lower in responders.

Further reading

McCormack AI, *et al.* (2011). Aggressive pituitary tumours: the role of temozolomide and the assessment of MGMT status. *Eur J Clin Invest* **41**, 1133–48.

Sandret L, Maison P, Chanson P (2011). Place of cabergoline in acromegaly: a meta-analysis. *J Clin Endocrinol Metab* **96**, 1327–35.

Sherlock M, Woods C, Sheppard MC (2011). Medical therapy in acromegaly. *Nat Rev Endocrinol* **7**, 291–300.

Trainer PJ, *et al.* (2000). Treatment of acromegaly with the growth hormone–receptor antagonist pegvisomant. *N Engl J Med* **342**, 1171–7.

Posterior pituitary

Physiology and pathology

The posterior lobe of the pituitary gland arises from the forebrain and comprises up to 25% of the normal adult pituitary gland. It produces arginine vasopressin and oxytocin. Both hormones are synthesized in the hypothalamic neurons of the supraoptic and paraventricular nuclei and migrate as neurosecretory granules to the posterior pituitary before release into the circulation. The hormones are unbound in the circulation, and their half-life is short.

Oxytocin

- Oxytocin has no known role in ♂. It may aid contraction of the seminal vesicles.
- In ♀, oxytocin contracts the pregnant uterus and also causes breast duct smooth muscle contraction, leading to breast milk ejection during breastfeeding. Oxytocin is released in response to suckling and also to cervical dilatation during parturition. However, oxytocin deficiency has no known adverse effect on parturition or breastfeeding.
- There are several, as yet, ill-understood features of oxytocin physiology. For example, osmotic stimulation may also lead to oxytocin secretion. Oxytocin may play a role in the ovary and testis, as ovarian luteal cells and testicular cells have both been shown to synthesize it, although its subsequent role is not known.

Vasopressin and neurophysin

- Arginine vasopressin is the major determinant of renal water excretion and, therefore, fluid balance. Its main action is to reduce free water clearance.
- Vasopressin is a nonapeptide and derives from a large precursor with a signal peptide and a neurophysin. The vasopressin gene is located on chromosome 20 and is closely linked to the oxytocin gene. Vasopressin travels to the posterior pituitary and undergoes cleavage as it travels. Neurophysin is released with vasopressin but has no further role after acting as a carrier protein in the neurons.
- Release of vasopressin occurs in response to changes in osmolality detected by osmoreceptors in the hypothalamus. Large changes in blood volume (5–10%) also influence vasopressin secretion. Many substances modulate vasopressin secretion, including the catecholamines and opioids.
- The main site of action of vasopressin is in the collecting duct and the thick ascending loop of Henle where it increases water permeability so that solute-free water may pass along an osmotic gradient to the interstitial medulla. Vasopressin in higher concentrations has a pressor effect. It also acts as an ACTH secretagogue synergistically with CRH.

Diabetes insipidus (DI)

Definition

DI is defined as the passage of large volumes (>3L/24h) of dilute urine (osmolality <300mOsm/kg).

Classification

Cranial

Due to deficiency of circulating arginine vasopressin (antidiuretic hormone).

Nephrogenic

Due to renal resistance to vasopressin.

Primary polydipsia

- Polyuria due to excessive drinking.
- In addition to suppressed levels of vasopressin due to low plasma osmolality, there may be impaired renal effectiveness because of washout of solute and, therefore, reduced urine-concentrating ability.

Features

- *Adults*—polyuria, nocturia, and thirst.
- *Children*—polyuria, enuresis, and failure to thrive.
- NB Clinical syndrome of cranial DI may be masked by cortisol deficiency as a result of failure to excrete a water load.
- Syndrome may worsen in pregnancy due to placental breakdown (vasopressinase) of circulating vasopressin.

See Box 2.30 for causes of DI.

Box 2.30 Causes of DI

Cranial

10% vasopressin cells should be sufficient to keep the urine volume <4L/day.

Familial

- Autosomal dominant (vasopressin gene).
- DIDMOAD syndrome (DI, diabetes mellitus, optic atrophy, deafness).

Acquired

- Trauma—head injury, neurosurgery.
- Tumours—craniopharyngiomas, pituitary infiltration by metastases.
- Inflammatory conditions—sarcoidosis, tuberculosis, Langerhans cell histiocytosis, lymphocytic hypophysitis, Wegener's granulomatosis.
- Infections—meningitis, encephalitis.
- Vascular—Sheehan's syndrome, sickle cell disease.
- Idiopathic.

Nephrogenic

Familial

- X-linked recessive—vasopressin receptor gene.
- Autosomal recessive—aquaporin-2 gene.

Acquired

- Drugs—lithium, demeclocycline.
- Metabolic—hypercalcaemia, hypokalaemia, hyperglycaemia.
- Chronic renal disease.
- Post-obstructive uropathy.

Primary polydipsia

- Psychological.

Investigations of DI

Diagnosis of type of DI
- Confirm large urine output (>3L/day).
- Exclude diabetes mellitus and renal failure (osmotic diuresis).
- Check electrolytes. Hypokalaemia and hypercalcaemia (nephrogenic DI).
- Fluid deprivation test (see Box 2.31) and assessment of response to vasopressin.
- Occasionally, further investigations are required, particularly when only partial forms of the condition are present.
- Measurement of plasma vasopressin, osmolality, and thirst threshold:
  - In response to infusion of 0.05mL/kg/min 5% hypertonic saline for 2h for cranial DI (no ↑ vasopressin).
  - In response to fluid deprivation for nephrogenic DI (vasopressin levels rise, with no ↑ urine osmolality).
- An alternative is a therapeutic trial of desmopressin, with monitoring of sodium and osmolality.

Investigation of the cause
- MRI head:
  - Looking for tumours (e.g. hypothalamic, pineal, or infiltration).
  - May demonstrate loss of bright spot of posterior pituitary gland.
- Serum ACE (sarcoidosis) and tumour markers, e.g. βhCG (pineal germinoma).
- Differential diagnosis of pituitary stalk lesions. Includes congenital, inflammatory (sarcoid, langerhans, lymphocytic hypophysitis, Wegener's) and neoplastic (craniopharyngioma, metastases, germinoma).

Box 2.31 Fluid deprivation test

1. Patient is allowed fluids overnight. If psychogenic polydipsia suspected, consider overnight fluid deprivation to avoid morning overhydration.
2. Patient is then deprived of fluids for 8h or until 5% loss of body weight if earlier. Weigh patient hourly.
3. Plasma osmolality is measured 4-hourly and urine volume and osmolality every 2h.
4. The patient is then given 2 micrograms IM desmopressin with urine volume and urine and serum osmolality measured over the next 4h.
5. In partial diabetes insipidus and possible psychogenic polydipsia, the fluid deprivation can be continued, measuring plasma and urine osmolalities until there is 30mOsm/kg increase in urine osmolality between three consecutive samples, noting precautions above (Miller & Moses modified test).

Results

If serum osmolality >305mOsm/kg, the patient has DI and the test is stopped (see Table 2.11).

Table 2.11 Urine osmolality (mOsm/kg)

Diagnosis	After fluid deprivation	After desmopressin
Cranial DI	<300	>800
Nephrogenic DI	<300	<300
1° polydipsia	>800	>800
Partial DI or polydipsia	300–800	<800

Treatment of DI

Maintenance of adequate fluid input

In patients with partial DI and an intact thirst mechanism, drug therapy may not be necessary if the polyuria is mild (<4L/24h).

Drug therapy

Desmopressin

- Vasopressin analogue, acting predominantly on the V2 receptors in the kidney, with little action on the V1 receptors of blood vessels. It thus has reduced pressor activity and ↑ antidiuretic efficacy, in addition to a longer half-life than the native hormone.
- Drug may be administered in divided doses, orally (100–1,000 micrograms/day), intranasally (10–40 micrograms/day), parenterally (SC, IV, IM) (0.1–2 micrograms/day) or buccally. There is wide variation in the dose required by an individual patient.
- Monitoring of serum sodium and osmolality is essential, as hyponatraemia or hypo-osmolality may develop.

Lysine vasopressin

- The antidiuretic hormone of the pig family.
- Not used very often, as its effects are short-lived (1–3h) and it may retain pressor activity. Intranasal administration. Dose 5–20U/day.

Chlorpropamide (100–500mg/day) and carbamazepine enhance the action of vasopressin on the collecting duct.

Nephrogenic DI

- Correction of underlying cause (metabolic or drugs).
- High doses of desmopressin (e.g. up to 5 micrograms IM) can be effective.
- Maintenance of adequate fluid input.
- Thiazide diuretics and prostaglandin synthase inhibitors (decrease the action of prostaglandins which locally inhibit the action of vasopressin in the kidney), e.g. indometacin, can be helpful.

Polydipsic polyuria

Management is difficult. Treatment of any underlying psychiatric disorder is important.

Further reading

Fenske W, Allolio B (2012). Clinical review: Current state and future perspectives in the diagnosis of diabetes insipidus: a clinical review. *J Clin Endocrinol Metab* **97**, 3426–37.

Loh JA, Verbalis JG. (2008). Disorders of water and salt metabolism associated with pituitary disease. *Endocrinol Metab Clin North Am* **37**, 213–34.

Turcu AF, Erickson BJ, Lin E et al. (2013). Pituitary stalk lesions: The Mayo Clinic Experience. *J Clin Endocrinol Metab* **98**(5):1812–18.

Hyponatraemia

(See Table 2.12; for causes, see Box 2.32.)

Incidence
- 1–6% hospital admissions Na <130mmol/L.
- 15–22% hospital admissions Na <135mmol/L.

Box 2.32 Causes of hyponatraemia
Excess water (dilutional)
- Excess water intake.
- ↑ water reabsorption (cirrhosis, congestive cardiac failure, nephrotic syndrome).
- Reduced renal excretion of a water load (SIADH, glucocorticoid deficiency).

Salt deficiency
- Renal loss (salt-wasting nephropathy—tubulointerstitial nephritis, polycystic kidney disease, analgesic nephropathy, recovery phase of acute tubular necrosis, relief of bilateral ureteric obstruction).
- Non-renal loss (skin, GI tract [bowel sequestration, high fistulae]).
- Renal sodium conservation of sodium is efficient and, therefore, low salt intake alone never causes sodium deficiency.

Pseudohyponatraemia
- Lipids, proteins (e.g. paraproteinaemia).
- Sodium only in aqueous phase of plasma; therefore, depending on assay, total sodium concentration may be spuriously low if concentrations of lipid or protein are high.

Solute
- Glucose, mannitol, ethanol.
- Addition of solute confined to the ECF causes water to shift from the ICF, lowering ECF sodium concentration.

Sick cell syndrome
- Symptomless hyponatraemia at 120–130mmol/L.
- True clinically apparent hyponatraemia is associated with either excess water or salt deficiency. The other causes can usually be easily excluded.

Table 2.12 Hyponatraemia investigations

Hypovolaemic		Euvolaemic		Hypervolaemic	
NaU <20mmol/L	NaU >20mmol/L	NaU <20mmol/L	NaU >20mmol/L Serum osmolality <270mOsm/kg	NaU <20mmol/L	NaU >20mmol/L Serum osmolality <270mOsm/kg
			Urine osmolality >100mOsm/kg		Urine osmolality >100mOsm/kg
Non-renal sodium loss	Renal sodium loss	Depletional ECF loss with inappropriate fluid replacement	Distal dilution	Excess water	
? GIT loss	? Salt-losing nephropathy		SIADH	Cirrhosis	SIADH
? Skin loss	? Mineralocorticoid deficiency		GC deficiency	Nephrotic syndrome CCF	

GC = glucocorticoid

Features

- Depend on the underlying cause and also on the rate of development of hyponatraemia. May develop once sodium reaches 115mmol/L or earlier if the fall is rapid. Level at 100mmol/L or less is life-threatening.
- Features of excess water are mainly neurological because of brain injury and depend on the age of the patient and rate of development. They include confusion and headache, progressing to seizures and coma. In hypervolaemic forms of excess water (where the fluid is confined to the ECF, e.g. cardiac failure, nephrotic syndrome, and cirrhosis), oedema and fluid overload are apparent. In contrast, in the syndromes of excess water associated with SIADH, the fluid is distributed throughout the ECF and ICF and there is no apparent fluid overload. Salt deficiency presents with features of hypovolaemia, with tachycardia and postural hypotension.

Investigations

(See Table 2.12.)
- Urinary sodium is very helpful in differentiating the underlying cause.
- Assess volume status.
- Other investigations as indicated, e.g. serum and urine osmolality, cortisol, thyroid function, liver biochemistry, serum electrophoresis.

Treatment

Salt deficiency (renal or non-renal)
- Increase dietary salt.
- May need IV normal saline if dehydrated.

Excess water (cirrhosis, nephrotic syndrome, CCF)
- Fluid restriction to 500–750mL/24h.
- Occasionally, hypertonic (3%) saline (513mmol/L) may be required in patients with acute symptomatic hyponatraemia. The appropriate infusion rate can be calculated from the formula:

Rate of sodium replacement (mmol/h) = total body water (60% of body weight) × desired correction rate (0.5–1mmol/h).

For example, for a 70kg ♂:

$$Na^+ = 60\% \times 70kg \times 1mmol/h = 42mmol/h$$

$$= 42 \times \frac{1000}{513} = 82mL/h \text{ of } 3\% \text{ saline}$$

- Rapid normalization (faster than 0.5mmol/h) of sodium may be associated with central pontine myelinolysis.

SIADH
📖 see Syndrome of inappropriate ADH (SIADH), p. 220.

Neurosurgical hyponatraemia
- Injudicious fluids.
- Diuretics.
- Drugs, e.g. carbamazepine, opiates.
- SIADH.
- Glucocorticoid deficiency.
- Cerebral salt wasting.

Unexplained hyponatraemia
- Common in elderly (↑ ADH release in response to ↑ osmolality and less effective suppression of ADH).
- ↑ risk of hyponatraemia with SSRIs.

Syndrome of inappropriate ADH (SIADH)

Definition
SIADH is a common cause of hyponatraemia. It is clinically normovolaemic hyponatraemia since the ↑ water is distributed through all compartments. (NB The elderly are more prone to SIADH, as they are unable to suppress ADH as efficiently and, therefore, investigation is probably only necessary if Na <130mmol/L in this group.) See Box 2.33 for causes.

Criteria for diagnosis
- Hyponatraemia and hypotonic plasma (osmolality <270mOsm/kg).
- Hyperproteinaemia and hyperlipidaemia may cause hyponatraemia but not hypotonic plasma.
- Inappropriate urine osmolality >100mOsm/kg.
- Excessive renal sodium loss (>30mmol/L, often >50mmol/L).
- Absence of clinical evidence of hypovolaemia or of volume overload.
- Normal renal, adrenal, and thyroid function (all must be excluded).
- NB Fluid restriction may reduce sodium loss.
- Differentiate from cerebral salt-wasting (🕮 see Transsphenoidal surgery, p. 198).

See Box 2.33 for causes of SIADH.

Types of SIADH
- Type 1—erratic excess ADH secretion, unrelated to plasma osmolality commonest (40%), associated (not exclusively) with tumours.
- Type 2—'reset osmostat': patients autoregulate around a lower serum osmolality.
- Chest and CNS disease.
- Type 3—'leaky osmostat', normal osmoregulation until plasma hypotonicity develops when vasopressin secretion continues.
- Type 4—normal osmoregulated vasopressin secretion, possible receptor defect, or alternative antidiuretic hormone.

Investigation of aetiology of SIADH
- Plasma and serum osmolalities and biochemistry.
- Thyroid function tests.
- Synacthen® test.
- Chest X-ray.
- Optional or if not explained—MRI head, imaging of chest/abdomen, HIV serology, bronchoscopy, lumbar puncture.

Treatment
- Treatment of the underlying cause.
- Fluid restriction to 500–750mL/24h.
- If the problem is not temporary and fluid restriction long-term can be difficult for the patient, drug treatment may be tried. *Demeclocycline* may be effective by inducing partial nephrogenic DI. New specific vasopressin antagonists are under trial (e.g. tolvaptan) (see Box 2.34).

Box 2.33 Causes of SIADH

- Tumours.
  - Small cell lung carcinoma, thymoma, lymphoma, leukaemia, sarcoma, mesothelioma.
- Chest disease.
  - Infections (pneumonia, tuberculosis, empyema).
  - Pneumothorax.
  - Asthma.
  - Cystic fibrosis.
  - Positive pressure ventilation.
- CNS disorders.
  - Pituitary, macroadenoma.
  - Infections (meningitis, encephalitis, abscess).
  - Head injury.
  - Guillain–Barré.
  - Vascular disorders (subarachnoid haemorrhage, cerebral thrombosis).
  - Psychosis.
  - Brain tumour.
- Drugs.
  - Chemotherapy (vincristine, vinblastine, cyclophosphamide).
  - Psychiatric drugs (phenothiazines, MAOI).
  - Carbamazepine.
  - Clofibrate.
  - Chlorpropamide.
- Metabolic.
  - Hypothyroidism.
  - Glucocorticoid deficiency.
  - Acute intermittent porphyria.
- Idiopathic.

NB The elderly are more prone to SIADH, as they are less able to suppress AVP.

Box 2.34 Tolvaptan

- Competitive vasopressin receptor 2 antagonist.
- Used for resistant hyponatraemia.
- Great care should be taken to avoid overrapid correction of sodium levels.
- Side effects include thirst, dry mouth, and urination.
- Only rarely indicated.

- In an emergency, saline infusion may be required, e.g. 100mL 3% over 15/30min IV twice daily—great care is required, as rapid overcorrection of hyponatraemia may cause central pontine myelinolysis (demyelination). This can be avoided if the rate of sodium correction does not exceed 0.5mmol/L per hour.

Further reading

Ellison DH, Berl T (2007). Clinical practice. The syndrome of inappropriate antidiuresis. *N Engl J Med* **356**, 2064–71.

Eating disorders

Anorexia nervosa

Features

- Typical presentation is a ♀ aged <25 with weight loss, amenorrhoea, and behavioural changes.
- There is a long-term risk of severe osteoporosis associated with >6 months of amenorrhoea. There is loss of bone mineral content and bone density, with little or no recovery after resolution of the amenorrhoea. Bone loss occurs at 2.5% per annum.

Endocrine abnormalities

- Deficiency of GnRH, low LH and FSH, normal PRL, and low oestrogen in ♀ or testosterone in ♂.
- Elevated circulating cortisol (usually non-suppressible with dexamethasone).
- Low normal thyroxine, reduced T_3, and normal TSH.
- Elevated resting GH levels.
- In addition, it is common to find various metabolic abnormalities, such as reduced magnesium, zinc, phosphorus, and calcium levels, in addition to hyponatraemia, hypoglycaemia, and hypokalaemia.
- Weight gain leads to a reversion of the prepubertal LH secretory pattern to the adult-like secretion. Administration of GnRH in a pulsatile pattern leads to normalization of the pituitary–gonadal axis, demonstrating that the 1° abnormality is hypothalamic.

Management

- The long-term treatment of these patients involves treatment of the underlying condition and then management of osteoporosis, although many patients will refuse oestrogen replacement.
- Resumption of menstrual function is important for recovery of spine bone mineral density (BMD). Weight gain is important for hip BMD recovery. Oral contraceptives do not help BMD recovery.

Bulimia

Features

- Typically occurs in ♀ who are slightly older than the group with anorexia nervosa. Weight may be normal, and patients often deny the abnormal eating behaviour. Patients gorge themselves, using artificial means of avoiding excessive weight gain (laxatives, diuretic abuse, vomiting). This may be a cause of 'occult' hypokalaemia.
- These patients may, or may not, have menstrual irregularity. If menstrual irregularity is present, this is often associated with inadequate oestrogen secretion and anovulation.

Further reading

Miller KK, Lee EE, Lawson EA, et al. (2006). Determinants of skeletal loss and recovery in anorexia nervosa. J Clin Endocrinol Metab **91**, 2931–7.

Hypothalamus

Pathophysiology

- The hypothalamus releases hormones that act as releasing hormones at the anterior pituitary gland. It produces dopamine that inhibits PRL release from the anterior pituitary gland. It also synthesizes arginine vasopressin and oxytocin (🕮 see p. 208).
- The commonest syndrome to be associated with the hypothalamus is abnormal GnRH secretion, leading to reduced gonadotrophin secretion and hypogonadism. Common causes are stress, weight loss, and excessive exercise. Management involves treatment of the cause, if possible. Administration of pulsatile GnRH is usually effective at reversing the abnormality but rarely undertaken.

Hypothalamic syndrome

Uncommon but may occur due to a large tumour, following surgery for a craniopharyngioma, or due to infiltration from, for example, Langerhans cell histiocytosis. The typical features are hyperphagia and weight gain, loss of thirst sensation, DI, somnolence, problems with temperature control, and behaviour change. Management can be challenging, e.g. DI with the loss of thirst sensation may require the prescription of regular fluid, in addition to desmopressin, and monitoring with daily weights and fluid balance as a routine. See Box 2.35 for metabolic effects.

Box 2.35 Metabolic effects of hypothalamic mass lesions

- Appetite:
  - Hyperphagia and obesity.
  - Anorexia.
- Thirst:
  - Adipsia.
  - Compulsive drinking.
- Temperature:
  - Hyperthermia.
  - Hypothermia.
- Somnolence and coma.

Pineal gland

Physiology

- The pineal gland lies behind the third ventricle, is highly vascular, and produces melatonin and other peptides.
- During daylight, light-induced hyperpolarization of the retinal photoreceptors inhibits signalling and the pineal gland is quiescent.
- Darkness stimulates the gland, and there is synthesis and release of melatonin.
- Melatonin levels are usually low during the day, rise during the evening, peak at midnight, and then decline independent of sleep.
- Exposure to darkness during the day does not increase melatonin secretion.

Jet lag

- It is claimed that pharmacological doses of melatonin can reset the body clock.
- Studies have suggested that melatonin may reduce the severity or duration of jet lag. There are few safety data, and currently melatonin does not have a product licence in the UK.

Pineal and intracranial germ cell tumours

- *Incidence.* 0.5–3% intracranial neoplasms.
- *Epidemiology.* ♂ > ♀. All ages. Two-thirds present between age 10 and 21 years.
- Germ cell tumours are now classified as germinomas or non-germinomatous germ cell tumours (choriocarcinoma, teratoma). The latter term includes the tumours previously called 'true' pinealomas.

Features

- Raised intracranial pressure (compression of cerebral aqueduct), headache, and lethargy.
- Visual disturbance (pressure on quadrigeminal plate).
- Parinaud's syndrome (paralysis of upward gaze, convergent nystagmus, Argyll–Robertson pupils).
- Ataxia.
- Pyramidal signs.
- Hypopituitarism.
- DI.
- Sexual precocity in boys (excess hCG secretion mimics LH, leading to Leydig cell testosterone secretion or related to space-occupying mass).

Investigations

- Imaging of craniospinal axis MRI/CT (may detect second tumour/ metastases).
- CSF examination.
- Tumour markers (hCG, alpha fetoprotein).
- Cytology.
- Biopsy if tumour markers unhelpful.
- Pituitary function assessment.

Management
- External beam radiotherapy—standard therapy is to irradiate the whole craniospinal axis.
- Germinomas are exquisitely radiosensitive.
- Chemotherapy may be indicated, e.g. vincristine, etoposide, carboplatin.
- Craniospinal irradiation cures the majority of patients (90%).

Prognosis

Excellent for germinomas (70–85% 5-year survival), but non-germinomatous germ cell tumours have a worse prognosis (15–40% 5-year survival).

Further reading

Hussaini M, *et al.* (2009). Pineal gland tumors: experience from the SEER database. *J Neuro Oncol* **94**, 351–8.

Adrenal

Anatomy

The normal adrenal glands weigh 4–5g. The cortex represents 90% of the normal gland and surrounds the medulla. The arterial blood supply arises from the renal arteries, aorta, and inferior phrenic artery. Venous drainage occurs via the central vein into the inferior vena cava on the right and into the left renal vein on the left. See Figs. 3.1 and 3.2.

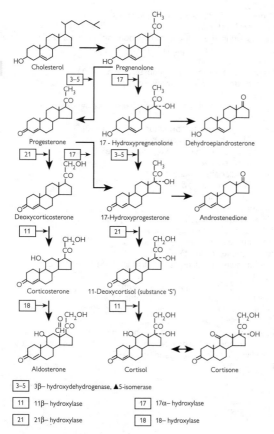

3–5	3β– hydroxydehydrogenase, ▲5-isomerase

11	11β– hydroxylase	17	17α– hydroxylase
21	21β– hydroxylase	18	18– hydroxylase

Fig. 3.1 Pathways and enzymes involved in synthesis of glucocorticoids, mineralocorticoids, and adrenal androgens from a cholesterol precursor. Reproduced from Besser M and Thorner GM (1994). *Clinical Endocrinology 2nd edn.* Mosby. With permission from Elsevier.

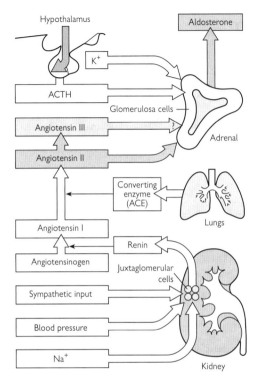

Fig. 3.2 Physiological mechanisms governing the production and secretion of aldosterone. Reproduced from Besser GM and Thorner M (1994). *Clinical Endocrinology 2nd edn.* Mosby. With permission from Elsevier.

Physiology

Glucocorticoids

Glucocorticoid (cortisol 10–20mg/day) (see Table 3.1) production occurs from the zona fasciculata, and adrenal androgens arise from the zona reticularis. Both of these are under the control of ACTH, which regulates both steroid synthesis and also adrenocortical growth.

Mineralocorticoids

Mineralocorticoid (aldosterone 100–150 micrograms/day) (see Table 3.1) synthesis occurs in zona glomerulosa, predominantly under the control of the renin–angiotensin system (see Fig. 3.2), although ACTH also contributes to its regulation.

Androgens

The adrenal gland (zona reticularis and zona fasciculata) also produces sex steroids in the form of dehydroepiandrosterone (DHEA) and androstenedione. The synthetic pathway is under the control of ACTH.

Urinary steroid profiling provides quantitative information on the biosynthetic and catabolic pathways. Profiling can be useful in:
• Mineralocorticoid hypertension.
• Polycystic ovary syndrome.
• Congenital adrenal hyperplasia.
• Steroid-producing tumours.
• Precocious puberty/virilization.
• Hirsutism.

Pathophysiology

Urine steroid profile useful in:
• Mineralocortoid hypertension (↓K).
• Polycystic ovary syndrome.
• Congenital adrenal hyperplasia.
• Cushing's Syndrome.
• Androgen resistance.

Table 3.1 Adrenal cortex steroid production

Adrenal cortex	Cortisol	Aldosterone	DHEA	DHEAS
Production rate/24h	10	100 micrograms	10mg	25mg
Half-life	80min	20min	20min	9h
Control	ACTH	Renin	ACTH	ACTH

Further reading

Taylor NF (2006). Urinary steroid profiling. *Method Mol Biol* **324**, 159–75.

Imaging

Computed tomography (CT) scanning

CT is the most widely used modality for imaging the adrenal glands. It is able to detect masses >5mm in diameter. It can be useful in differentiating between different adrenal pathologies, in particular by identifying benign adrenal tumours with high fat content (adrenocortical adenoma, adreno-myelolipoma), as indicated by pre-contrast tumour density of less than 10HU (Hounsfield units) (see Fig. 3.3).

Magnetic resonance imaging (MRI)

MRI can also reliably detect adrenal masses >5–10mm in diameter and, in some circumstances, provides additional information to CT, in particular by determining signal loss in opposed phase, T_2-weighted sequences. Rapid signal loss is indicative of a benign tumour whereas malignant tumours, and also phaeochromocytomas, show a delay or lack in signal loss.

Ultrasound (US) imaging

US detects masses >20mm in diameter, but normal adrenal glands are not usually visible, except in children. Body morphology and bowel gas can provide technical difficulties.

Normal adrenal

Normal adrenal cortex is assessed by measuring limb thickness and is considered enlarged at >5mm approximately the thickness of the diaphragmatic crus nearby.

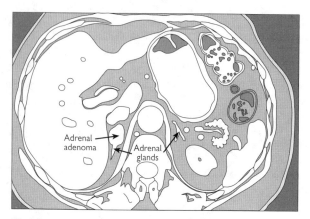

Fig. 3.3 Typical appearance of adrenal adenoma on CT scan.

Radionucleotide imaging

- *[123]Iodine-metaiodobenzylguanidine* (MIBG) is a guanethidine analogue, concentrated in some phaeochromocytomas, paragangliomas, carcinoid tumours, and neuroblastomas, and is useful diagnostically. A different isotope ^{131}I-MIBG may be used therapeutically, e.g. in malignant phaeochromocytomas, when the diagnostic imaging shows uptake.
- *[75]Se 6β-selenomethyl-19-norcholesterol*. This isotope is concentrated in functioning steroid synthesizing tissue and has, in the past, been used to image the adrenal cortex. However, high resolution CT and MRI have largely replaced it in localizing functional adrenal adenomas.
- *[123]Iodo-metomidate* is an isotope that is derived from etomidate, which is a known 11β-hydroxylase (CYP11B1) inhibitor. Metomidate binds CYP11B1, which is specifically expressed in the adrenal gland, and thus iodo-metomidate SPECT can identify adrenocortical tissue.

Positron emission tomography (PET)

PET can be useful in locating tumours and metastases. Radiopharmaceuticals for specific endocrine tumours are being developed, e.g. ^{11}C-metahydroxyephedrine for phaeochromocytoma—combined with CT (PET-CT), it may offer particular value in localizing occult neuroendocrine tumours. ^{11}C-metomidate PET-CT has recently been shown to be of value for the lateralization of aldosterone-producing adrenal masses.

Venous sampling

Adrenal vein sampling (AVS) (📖 p. 244) can be useful to lateralize an adenoma or to differentiate an adenoma from bilateral hyperplasia. It is technically difficult—particularly, catheterizing the right adrenal vein because of its drainage into the IVC. There is no widespread agreement on the exact protocol, e.g. consecutive or concurrent adrenal vein catherization, with and without concurrent or preceding ACTH stimulation. Usually, samples are drawn from the vena cava, superior and inferior to the renal veins, and separately from both adrenal veins, with subsequent determination of plasma aldosterone and serum cortisol levels (correct localization of the catheter in the adrenal vein is only confirmed when cortisol >3-fold of vena cava cortisol). AVS is of particular value in lateralizing small aldosterone-producing adenomas that cannot easily be visualized on CT or MRI.

Further reading

Boland GW (2011). Adrenal imaging: from Addison to algorithms. *Radiol Clin North Am* **49**, 511–28.
Guest P (2011). Imaging of the adrenal gland. In: Wass JAH, Stewart PM (eds.) *Oxford textbook of endocrinology*, pp. 763–73. Oxford University Press, Oxford.
Hahner S, Sundin A (2011). Metomidate-based imaging of adrenal masses. *Horm Cancer* **2**, 348–53.
Pacak K, Eisenhofer G, Goldstein DS (2004). Functional imaging of endocrine tumors: role of positron emission tomography. *Endocr Rev* **25**, 568–80.

Mineralocorticoid excess: definitions

The majority of cases of mineralocorticoid excess are due to excess aldosterone production, which may be 1° or 2°, and are typically associated with hypertension and hypokalaemia.

- *Primary hyperaldosteronism* is a disorder of autonomous aldosterone hypersecretion with suppressed renin levels.
- *Secondary hyperaldosteronism* occurs when aldosterone hypersecretion occurs 2° to elevated circulating renin levels. This is typical of heart failure, cirrhosis, or nephrotic syndrome but can also be due to renal artery stenosis and, occasionally, a very rare renin-producing tumour (reninoma).
- Other mineralocorticoids may occasionally be the cause of this syndrome (see Box 3.1).

Box 3.1 Causes of mineralocorticoid excess

Primary hyperaldosteronism
- Conn's syndrome (aldosterone-producing adrenal adenoma) 35%.
- Bilateral adrenal hyperplasia 60%.
- Glucocorticoid-remediable aldosteronism (GRA) <1%.
- Aldosterone-producing adrenal carcinoma <1%.

Secondary hyperaldosteronism
- Renal artery stenosis.
- Renal hypoperfusion.
- Cirrhosis.
- Congestive cardiac failure.
- Nephrotic syndrome.
- Renin-secreting tumour.

Other mineralocorticoid excess syndromes
- Apparent mineralocorticoid excess (📖 see p. 248).
- Liquorice ingestion (📖 see p. 249) (inhibits II β HSD2) ↓ aldosterone, ↓ renin, ↓ K⁻ found in sweets, chewing tobacco, cough mixtures, herbal medicines.
- Deoxycorticosterone and corticosterone (📖 see p. 249).
- Ectopic ACTH secretion (📖 see p. 164).
- Congenital adrenal hyperplasia (📖 see p. 320).
- Exogenous mineralocorticoids.

'Pseudoaldosteronism' due to abnormal renal tubular transport
- Bartter's syndrome (📖 see p. 259).
- Gitelman's syndrome (📖 see p. 260).
- Liddle's syndrome (📖 see p. 258).

Primary aldosteronism

Epidemiology

Primary hyperaldosteronism is present in around 10% of hypertensive patients. It is the most prevalent form of secondary hypertension. The most common cause is bilateral adrenal hyperplasia (see Table 3.2).

Pathophysiology

Aldosterone causes renal sodium retention and potassium loss. This results in expansion of body sodium content, leading to suppression of renal renin synthesis. The direct action of aldosterone on the distal nephron causes sodium retention and loss of hydrogen and potassium ions, resulting in a hypokalaemic alkalosis, although serum potassium may not be significantly reduced and may be normal in up to 50% of cases.

Aldosterone has pathophysiological effects on a range of other tissues, causing cardiac fibrosis, vascular endothelial dysfunction, and nephrosclerosis.

Clinical features

- Moderately severe hypertension, which is often resistant to conventional therapy. There may be disproportionate left ventricular hypertrophy.
- Hypokalaemia is usually asymptomatic. Occasionally, patients may present with tetany, myopathy, polyuria, and nocturia (hypokalaemic nephrogenic diabetes insipidus) due to severe hypokalaemia.
- There may be an association with osteoporosis.

Table 3.2 Causes of primary hyperaldosteronism

Condition	Relative frequency	Age	Pathology
Aldosteronoma (Conn's adenoma)	35%	3rd–6th decade	Benign, adenoma, <2.5cm diameter, yellow because of high cholesterol content
Idiopathic hyperaldosteronism (bilateral adrenal hyperplasia)	60%	Older than Conn's, ♂ > ♀	Macronodular or micronodular hyperplasia
Adrenal carcinoma	Rare	5th–7th decade (occasionally young)	Tumour >4cm in diameter—often larger, may be evidence of local invasion
Glucocorticoid-suppressible hyperaldosteronism	Rare	Childhood	Chimeric crossover between CYP11B1 and CYP11B2 genes results in an ACTH-responsive aldosterone synthase

Conn's syndrome—aldosterone-producing adenoma

Very high levels of the enzyme aldosterone synthase are expressed in tumour tissue. Recently, inactivating mutations in the potassium channel KCJN5 have been identified as the cause of disease in approximately 40% of aldosterone-producing adrenal adenomas. Very rarely, Conn's adenomas may be part of the MEN-1 syndrome.

Bilateral adrenal hyperplasia (bilateral idiopathic hyperaldosteronism)

This is the most common form of 1° hyperaldosteronism in adults. Hyperplasia is more commonly bilateral than unilateral and may be associated with micronodular or macronodular hyperplasia. Note, however, that CT-demonstrable nodules have a prevalence of 2% in the general population, including hypertensive patients without excess aldosterone production. The pathophysiology is not known, although aldosterone secretion is very sensitive to circulating angiotensin II. The pathophysiology of bilateral adrenal hyperplasia is not understood, and it is possible that it represents an extreme end of the spectrum of low renin essential hypertension.

Glucocorticoid-remediable aldosteronism (GRA)

This is a rare autosomal dominantly inherited condition due to the presence of a chimeric gene (8q22) containing the 5′ sequence, which determines regulation of the 11β-hydroxylase gene (*CYP11B1*) coding for the enzyme catalysing the last step in cortisol synthesis, and the 3′ sequence from the aldosterone synthase gene (*CYP11B2*) coding for the enzyme catalysing the last step in aldosterone synthesis. This results in the expression of aldosterone synthase in the zona fasciculata as well as the zona glomerulosa, and aldosterone secretion comes under ACTH control. Glucocorticoids are the treatment of choice and lead to suppression of ACTH and suppression of aldosterone production.

• Early hypertension and family history.
• Hybrid steroids (18OHcortisol and 18oxocortisol) elevated.

Aldosterone-producing carcinoma

Rare and usually associated with excessive secretion of other corticosteroids (cortisol, androgen, oestrogen). Hypokalaemia may be profound and aldosterone levels very high. A tumour larger than 2.5cm associated with aldosterone excess has to be treated as suspicious.

Screening

Indications

- Patients resistant to conventional antihypertensive medication (i.e. not controlled on three agents).
- Hypertension associated with hypokalaemia (potassium <3.7mmol/L, irrespective of thiazide use). NB: ↓ K only present in 40%.
- Hypertension developing before age of 40 years.
- Adrenal incidentaloma.

Method

- Give oral supplements of potassium to control hypokalaemia; screening and confirmation should be carried out in the normokalaemic situation.
- There is no need to stop all concomitant antihypertensive medication for the first screening by paired plasma aldosterone and plasma renin measurements; the only medication that must be stopped are mineralocorticoid receptor antagonists (spironolactone, eplerenone) that must be stopped 4 weeks prior to diagnostic tests.
- *Measure aldosterone:renin ratio.*
  - A high ratio is suggestive of 1° hyperaldosteronism (aldosterone (pmol/L)/plasma renin activity (ng/mL/h) >750 or aldosterone (ng/dL)/plasma renin activity (ng/mL/h) >30–50). Note that newer assays that measure renin mass (rather than activity) will require the development of different cut-offs.
- Test results should be interpreted, having the effects of antihypertensive drugs in mind (see Table 3.3); β-blockers can cause false +ves while ACE/AT1R blockers can cause false –ves in borderline cases. In doubt, the test can be repeated off these drugs; BP can be controlled using doxazosin or calcium antagonists. False –ve results can also occur in patients with chronic renal failure due to upregulated plasma renin.

Confirmation of diagnosis

Confirmation of autonomous aldosterone production is made by demonstrating failure to suppress aldosterone in face of sodium/volume loading. This can be achieved by a number of mechanisms after optimizing test conditions as described.

- Test of choice—*saline infusion test*:
  - Administer 2L normal saline over 4h.
  - Measure plasma aldosterone at 0, 2, 3, and 4h.
  - Aldosterone fails to suppress to <140pmol/L (140–280 equivocal) in 80–90% of 1° aldosteronism.
  - Most used test; caution in patients with fluid overload and/or evidence of heart failure.
- *Fludrocortisone suppression test:*
  - Give fludrocortisone 100 micrograms 6-hourly for 4 days.
  - Measure plasma aldosterone basally and on last day.
  - Aldosterone fails to suppress in 1° aldosteronism.
  - Caveat: difficult to execute in hypokalaemic, hypertensive patients.

Table 3.3 Interpreting test results of aldosterone/renin ratios

Antihypertensive	Effect on renin	Effect on aldosterone	Net effect on ARR
β-blockers	↓	↑	↑
α1-blockers	→	→	→
α2-sympathomimetics	→	→	→
ACE inhibitors	↑	↓	↓
AT1R blockers	↑	↓	↓
Calcium antagonists	→	→	→
Diuretics	(↑)	(↑)	→/(↓)

- *Dietary sodium loading test:*
  - Patients are given instructions antagonists to take a diet with a high sodium content (sufficient to raise the sodium intake to 200mmol per day for 3 days. If necessary, this can be achieved by adding supplemental sodium chloride tablets).
  - It is important to ensure that potassium is maintained as normal during this period, and potassium supplementation may also be required.
  - Failure to suppress aldosterone in 1° aldosteronism.
  - Caveat: cumbersome to execute, limited diagnostic value in populations with a high background sodium intake.
- Other tests, such as the captopril suppression test, are described but are of lesser value in this circumstance, lacking appropriate sensitivity or specificity in the diagnosis of 1° aldosteronism.
- A number of tests have been described that are said to differentiate between the various subtypes of 1° aldosteronism (solitary Conn's adenoma; bilateral adrenal hyperplasia; GRA). However, none of these are sufficiently specific to influence management decisions, and more specific investigations (imaging and adrenal vein sampling) are necessary if there is doubt. Additional tests, such as postural response of aldosterone and the measurement of urinary 18-hydroxycortisol, have been largely superseded because of this. Diagnosis of GRA is best made using a specific genetic test, rather than on the ability of dexamethasone (0.5mg 6-hourly for 3 days) to suppress aldosterone; the diagnosis is confirmed by genetic analysis (chimeric crossover between *CYP11B1* (11β-hydroxylase) and *CYP11B2* (aldosterone synthase) promoter regions that brings CYP11B2 under the regulatory control of ACTH).

Localization and confirmation of differential diagnosis

CT/MRI scan

CT and MRI scanning are of value in identifying adrenal nodules >5mm diameter. It should be noted, however, that the frequency of adrenal incidentalomas rises with age and, for this reason, it is prudent to consider adrenal vein sampling if in doubt.

- In bilateral adrenal hyperplasia, both glands can appear enlarged or normal in size.
- Macronodular hyperplasia may result in identifiable nodules on imaging.
- A mass >4cm in size is suspicious of carcinoma but is unusual in Conn's syndrome.
- NB In essential hypertension, nodules are described.

Adrenal vein sampling

Is indicated in patients with bilateral adrenal changes and in older patients (age >50) with 1° aldosteronism who have an apparent solitary adenoma on scanning, as the incidence of adrenal nodules rises with age (3–4% at 40 years, 70–80% at 70 years). The procedure should only be undertaken in patients in whom surgery is feasible and desired.

Catheterization of the adrenal veins may not be necessary if there is a unilateral adrenal mass (>10mm) plus a potassium 3.5 on presentation, as this predicts an adenoma.

Aldosterone measurements from both adrenal veins allow a gradient between the two sides to be identified in the case of unilateral disease. It is the gold standard for differentiation between uni- and bilateral aldosterone production, but cannulating the right adrenal vein is technically difficult as it drains directly into the inferior vena cava. Cortisol measurements must also be taken concomitantly with aldosterone to confirm successful positioning within the adrenal veins and should be more than thrice a peripheral sample (central/peripheral ratio >3).

Adrenal vein sampling should be carried out in specialist centres only; centres with <20 procedures per year have been shown to have poor success rates for bilateral catheterization of the adrenal vein (8–10%), thus producing mostly non-informative results, whereas experienced centres achieve around 70%.

Radiolabelled scanning

The iodocholesterol test has low sensitivity/specificity and offers no advantage over a high resolution CT or MRI with, where necessary, adrenal vein sampling. Recent data with ^{11}C-metomidate scanning are promising but warrant further confirmation prior to widespread use.

Treatment

Surgery

- Laparascopic adrenalectomy is the treatment of choice for aldosterone-secreting adenomas and is associated with lower morbidity than open adrenalectomy.
- Surgery is not indicated in patients with idiopathic hyperaldosteronism, as even bilateral adrenalectomy may not cure the hypertension.
- Presurgical spironolactone treatment may be used to correct potassium stores before surgery.
- The BP response to treatment with spironolactone (50–400mg/day) before surgery can be used to predict the response to surgery of patients with adenomas.
- Hypertension is cured in about 70%.
- If it persists (more likely in those with long-standing hypertension and increased age), it is more amenable to medical treatment.
- Overall, 50% become normotensive in 1 month and 70% within 1 year.
- Adrenal carcinoma. Open surgery and post-operative adrenolytic therapy with *mitotane* is usually required, but the prognosis is usually poor (📖 see Treatment, p. 252).

Medical treatment

Medical therapy remains an option for patients with bilateral disease and those with a solitary adrenal adenoma who are unlikely to be cured by surgery, who are unfit for operation, or who express a preference for medical management.

- The mineralocorticoid receptor antagonist *spironolactone* (50–400mg/day; once daily administration) has been used successfully for many years to treat the hypertension and hypokalaemia associated with bilateral adrenal hyperplasia and idiopathic hyperaldosteronism profile.
- There may be a delay in response of hypertension of 4–8 weeks. However, combination with other antihypertensive agents (ACEI and calcium channel blockers) is usually required.
- Spironolactone also interacts with the androgen and the progesterone receptor, which contributes to its side effect. Side effects are common—particularly, gynaecomastia and impotence in ♂, menstrual irregularities in ♀, and GI effects.
- *Eplerenone* (50–200mg/day; twice daily administration) is a mineralocorticoid receptor antagonist without antiandrogen effects and hence greater selectivity and less side effects than spironolactone.
- Alternative drugs include the potassium-sparing diuretics *amiloride* and *triamterene*. Amiloride may need to be given in high dose (up to 40mg/day) in 1° aldosteronism, and monitoring of serum potassium is essential. Calcium channel antagonists may also be helpful.
- Glucocorticoid-remediable aldosteronism can be treated with low-dose *dexamethasone* (0.25–0.5mg on going to bed). If needed, spironolactone and/or amiloride can be added.

Further reading

Allolio B, Hahner S, Weismann D, *et al.* (2004). Management of adrenocortical carcinoma. *Clin Endocrinol* **60**, 273–8.

Espiner EA, Ross DG, Yandle TG, *et al.* (2003). Predicting surgically remedial primary aldosteronism: role of adrenal scanning, posture testing, and adrenal vein sampling *J Clin Endocrinol Metab* **88**, 3637–44.

Funder JW, *et al.* (2008). Case detection, diagnosis, and treatment of patients with primary aldosteronism: an Endocrine Society clinical practice guideline. *J Clin Endocrinol Metab* **93**, 3266–81.

Ganguly A (1998). Primary aldosteronism. *N Engl J Med* **339**, 1828–33.

Mulatero P (2002). Drug effects on aldosterone/plasma renin activity ratio in primary aldosteronism. *Hypertension* **40**, 897–902.

Young WF (2007). Primary aldosteronism—renaissance of a syndrome. *Clin Endocrinol* **66**, 607–18.

Excess other mineralocorticoids

Epidemiology

Occasionally, the clinical syndrome of hyperaldosteronism is not associated with excess aldosterone. This can be due either to an increase in an alternative mineralocorticoid or due to ↑ mineralocorticoid effect of cortisol.

These conditions are rare.

Apparent mineralocorticoid excess (AME)

- The mineralocorticoid receptor has an equal affinity for cortisol and aldosterone, but there is a 100-fold excess of circulating cortisol over aldosterone.
- The mineralocorticoid receptor is usually protected from the effects of stimulation by cortisol by the 11β-hydroxysteroid type 2 dehydrogenase enzyme, which converts cortisol to cortisone.
- In AME, there is a deficiency of the 11β-hydroxysteroid dehydrogenase (HSD) enzyme type 2. This can be caused either by inactivating mutations in the corresponding gene encoded on chromosome 16q22 or due to exogenous intake of substances that inhibit 11β-HSD2, such as liquorice.
- Congenital absence (autosomal recessive) of the enzyme or inhibition of its activity allows cortisol to stimulate the receptor and leads to severe hypertension.

Type 1 is seen predominantly in children, presenting with failure to thrive, thirst, polyuria, and severe hypertension, which can lead to brain haemorrhage in childhood or adolescence. The urinary cortisol over cortisone metabolites ratio (tetrahydrocortisol + allo-tetrahydrocortisol/tetrahydrocortisone) is raised to 10× normal.

Type 2 is a milder form that may be a cause of hypertension in adolescence/early adulthood.

However, multiple mutations have been found in the 11β-HSD2 gene for both types, and some authors believe there is a spectrum of disease: mild forms may present with salt-sensitive hypertension.

Biochemistry

- Suppression of renin and aldosterone.
- Hypokalaemic alkalosis.
- Urinary free cortisol/cortisone ratio ↑.
- Ratio of urinary tetrahydrocortisol and allo-tetrahydrocortisol to tetrahydrocortisone is raised (>10×) in type 1 but is normal in type 2.
- Confirm with genetic testing (HSD11B2 gene).

Treatment

- Dexamethasone leads to suppression of ACTH secretion, reduced cortisol concentrations, and lowered BP in 60%. It has a much lower affinity for the mineralocorticoid receptor.
- Other antihypertensive agents are often required.
- One patient with hypertensive renal failure was cured with a renal transplant.

Liquorice ingestion

- Liquorice contains glycyrrhetinic acid which is used as a sweetener.
- It inhibits the action of 11β-HSD2, which allows circulating cortisol to get increased access to the mineralocorticoid receptor causing hypertension.
- Liquorice can be found in sweets, chewing tobacco, cough mixtures, and some herbal medicines.

Ectopic ACTH syndrome

(□ see p. 164.)

In the syndrome of ectopic ACTH and generally in very severe Cushing's cases, the 11β-HSD2 protection is overcome because of high cortisol secretion rates, which saturate the enzyme, leading to impaired conversion of cortisol to cortisone. Therefore, cortisol has greater access to the mineralocorticoid receptor in the kidney, which results in hypokalaemia and hypertension.

Deoxycorticosterone (DOC) excess

Two forms of congenital adrenal hyperplasia (□ see p. 320) are associated with excess production of deoxycorticosterone (DOC), as they result in inhibition of enzymes downstream of DOC and thus lead to its accumulation. DOC acts as an agonist at the mineralocorticoid receptor, resulting in hypertension with suppression of renin.

- 17α-hydroxylase (CYP17A1) deficiency.
- 11β-hydroxylase (CYP11B1) deficiency.

Glucocorticoid replacement to inhibit ACTH is effective treatment for these conditions.

Adrenal tumours, in particular adrenocortical carcinomas, rarely secrete excessive amounts of deoxycorticosterone. This may be concomitant with excessive aldosterone production, but occasionally it may occur in an isolated fashion.

Adrenal Cushing's syndrome

Definition and epidemiology

- Cushing's syndrome results from chronic excess cortisol and is described in Chapter 2 (🕮 see Cushing's disease, p. 158).
- The causes may be classified as ACTH-dependent and ACTH-independent. This section describes ACTH-independent Cushing's syndrome, which is due to adrenal tumours (benign and malignant), and is responsible for 10–15% cases of Cushing's syndrome.
- Adrenal tumours causing Cushing's syndrome are commoner in ♀. The peak incidence is in the fourth and fifth decade.
- Causes and relative frequencies of adrenal Cushing's syndrome in adults:
  - Adrenal adenoma 10%.
  - Adrenal carcinoma 2%.
  - Bilateral micronodular adrenal hyperplasia <1%.
  - Bilateral macronodular hyperplasia <1%.

Pathophysiology

- Benign adrenocortical adenomas (ACA) are usually encapsulated and <4cm in diameter. They are usually associated with pure glucocorticoid excess.
- Adrenocortical carcinomas (ACC) are usually >6cm in diameter, although they may be smaller, and are not infrequently associated with local invasion and metastases at the time of diagnosis. Adrenal carcinomas are characteristically associated with the excess secretion of several hormones; most frequently found is the combination of cortisol and androgen (precursors); occasionally, they may be associated with mineralocorticoid or oestrogen secretion.
- Bilateral adrenal hyperplasia may be micronodular (<1cm diameter) or macronodular (>1cm), but increasingly mixed cases of combined micro- and macronodular hyperplasia are observed.
- ACTH-dependent Cushing's results in bilateral adrenal hyperplasia, thus one has to firmly differentiate between ACTH-dependent and independent causes of Cushing's before assuming bilateral adrenal hyperplasia as the primary cause of disease.
- The majority of cases of ACTH-independent bilateral macronodular adrenal hyperplasia (AIMAH) do not have an identifiable cause.
- Abnormal expression of receptors that would not normally be expressed in the adrenal has been described as the cause of disease, including gastric inhibitory peptide (GIP), vasopressin, β-adrenoceptor, human chorionic gonadotrophin (hCG)/luteinizing hormone (LH), and serotonin receptors.
- Several 'food-dependent' Cushing's syndrome cases have been described due to ectopic GIP receptor expression.
- Carney complex (🕮 see Carney complex, p. 583) is an autosomal dominant condition characterized by a variable penetrance of atrial myxomas, spotty skin pigmentation (hyperlentiginosis), peripheral nerve tumours, and endocrine disorders, including Sertoli cell

tumours and Cushing's syndrome due to primary pigmented nodular adrenal disease (PPNAD), which can be micro- or macronodular in appearance. PPNAD, in the context of Carney complex, has been shown to be caused by mutations in the *PRKAR1A* gene that encodes a regulatory subunit of protein kinase A (PKA), which is a key regulator of the adrenal ACTH response.

- McCune–Albright syndrome 🕮 p. 576 can be associated with polyostotic fibrous dysplasia, unilateral *café-au-lait* spots, precocious puberty, and ACTH-independent Cushing's with bilateral macronodular adrenal hyperplasia, caused by activating mutations in the *GNAS-1* gene that encodes the GSalpha protein, which is a key component of the transmembrane signal transduction cascade of the ACTH receptor. *GNAS-1* mutations have also been found in bilateral macronodular adrenal hyperplasia without other features of McCune–Albright's.
- Recent work has described phosphodiesterase (PDE) 11A and 8B mutations in patients with bilateral micronodular adrenal hyperplasia and ACTH-independent Cushing's.

Clinical features

- The clinical features of ACTH-independent Cushing's syndrome are as described in 🕮 Clinical features, p. 160 in Chapter 2, Cushing's disease.
- It is important to note that, in patients with adrenal carcinoma, there may also be features related to excessive androgen production in ♀ and also a relatively more rapid time course of development of the syndrome.

Investigations

- Once the presence of Cushing's syndrome is confirmed (🕮 see Clinical features, p. 160), subsequent investigation of the cause depends on whether ACTH is suppressed (ACTH-independent) or measurable/elevated (ACTH-dependent).
- Patients with ACTH-independent Cushing's syndrome do not suppress cortisol to <50% basal on high-dose dexamethasone testing and fail to show a rise in cortisol and ACTH following administration of CRH. (The latter test is often important when patients have borderline/low ACTH to differentiate pituitary-dependent disease from adrenal.)
- ACTH-independent causes are adrenal in origin, and the mainstay of further investigation is adrenal imaging by CT, which allows excellent visualization of the adrenal glands and their anatomy.

Treatment of adrenal Cushing's syndrome

(📖 see Treatment, p. 168.)

Adrenal adenoma

- Unilateral adrenalectomy (normally laparoscopic) is curative.
- Post-operative temporary adrenal insufficiency ensues because of long-term suppression of ACTH and the contralateral adrenal gland requiring glucocorticoid replacement for up to 2 years.
- Steroid cover is, therefore, required.

Adrenal carcinoma

(See Table 3.4 for staging classification.)

- Treatment of adrenocortical carcinoma (ACC) should be carried out in a specialist centre, with expert surgeons, oncologists, and endocrinologists with extensive expertise in treating ACC. This improves survival.
- The primary approach is surgical, aiming at complete removal of the primary tumour without capsule violation; in case of stage III disease with invasion of adjacent organs or venous thrombosis, a radical surgical approach with *en bloc* resection and removal of tumour thrombus, if necessary, in collaboration with vascular and cardio-thoracic surgeons is beneficial. Single metastases can also be approached surgically (lung, liver) or by radiofrequency ablation (liver). Surgical debulking can be helpful, even in metastatic disease, in case of florid and difficult-to-control Cushing's, but needs to be carefully weighed against the resulting delay in initiating chemotherapy.
- Disease-free and total survival is defined by tumour stage and the presence or absence of capsule violation or invasion. Histopathology is notoriously difficult, as it insufficiently differentiates between benign and malignant tumours. The most predictive marker for recurrence of disease after successful and apparently complete removal of the primary tumour is the proliferation index marker Ki67 (high risk of recurrence in patients with Ki67 >10%), but one regularly observes patients with Ki67 of 1%, indicative of benign disease, who later present with recurrence/metastasis. The majority of recurrences occur within 2–3 years of the removal of the primary tumour.
- Post-operative adjuvant treatment with the adrenolytic agent *mitotane* (*ortho-para* DDD) has been shown to prolong survival in high-risk patients. It should be given for 2 years. Mitotane treatment should be monitored by experienced physicians; it is invariably associated with the development of glucocorticoid deficiency, requiring permanent glucocorticoid replacement. Due to the induction of the major drug-metabolizing enzyme CYP3A4 by mitotane, a significant amount of hydrocortisone is immediately inactivated. Thus, patients

Table 3.4 European Network for the Study of Adrenal Tumours (ENSAT) staging classification for adrenocortical carcinoma

ENSAT stage	TNM stage	TNM definitions
I	T1, N0, M0	T1, tumour ≤5cm
		N0, no positive lymph node
		M0, no distant metastases
II	T2, N0, M0	T2, tumour >5cm
		N0, no positive lymph node
		M0, no distant metastases
III	T1–T2, N1, M0	N1, positive lymph node(s)
	T3–T4, N0–N1, M0	M0, no distant metastases
		T3, tumour infiltration into surrounding tissue
		T4, tumour invasion into adjacent organs *or* venous tumour thrombus in vena cava or renal vein
IV	T1–T4, N0–N1, M1	M1, presence of distant metastases

on mitotane treatment require glucocorticoid replacement with an increased dose, e.g. hydrocortisone 20–20–10mg. There are other important drug interactions with mitotane caused by induction of CYP3A4 (e.g. statins, benzodiazepines, opioid analgesias, oestrogen, and macrolide antibiotics). Monitoring of drug levels is mandatory to ensure that concentrations within the therapeutic range (14–20 micrograms/mL) are achieved in a timely fashion. Plasma mitotane level monitoring also limits unwanted side effects, including neurotoxic effects ('trouble talking, trouble walking') that usually occur when plasma levels increase above 20–25 micrograms/mL but resolve within days to weeks after transiently stopping mitotane treatment. Other possible side effects include diarrhoea, fatigue, allergic skin rashes, and moderate elevation of liver transaminases.
- Other drugs may be required to control cortisol hypersecretion (e.g. *metyrapone, ketoconazole, in extreme cases non-anaesthetic doses of etomidate*).
- Mitotane also represents the first-line treatment in metastatic adrenal cancer. In patients with metastatic disease occurring on mitotane treatment or in patients with rapidly progressive disease, cytotoxic chemotherapy should be initiated. First choice is the so-called Berruti regimen (cisplatin, etoposide, doxorubicin, and continued mitotane treatment). Newer treatments options, such as PI3 kinase inhibitors and IGF receptor antagonists, are currently under investigation.

Bilateral adrenal hyperplasia

- Bilateral adrenalectomy is curative. Lifelong glucocorticoid and mineralocorticoid treatment is required. In some cases of bilateral macronodular adrenal hyperplasia, there is a dominant, larger adrenal nodule on one side, and it has been described that unilateral adrenalectomy can lead to resolution of Cushing's for a number of years, but ultimately removal of the remaining adrenal may be necessary if Cushing's reoccurs due to further nodules developing.
- Medical treatment may be possible for some of the rare cases with aberrant receptors, e.g. octreotide for GIP-dependent disease.

Prognosis

- Adrenal adenomas, which are successfully treated with surgery, have a good prognosis, and recurrence is unlikely. The prognosis depends on the long-term effects of excess cortisol before treatment—in particular, atherosclerosis and osteoporosis.
- The prognosis for adrenal carcinoma is very poor despite surgery. Reports suggest a 5-year survival of 22% and median survival time of 14 months, but recent data have shown that survival significantly improves when patients are managed in a specialist centre and receive mitotane treatment.

Subclinical Cushing's syndrome

- Describes a subset of 5–10% of patients with an adrenal incidentaloma with signs of autonomous glucocorticoid production, which, however, is insufficient to produce clinically overt Cushing's syndrome.
- Urinary free cortisol measurement may be within the normal range, but there is a failure to sufficiently suppress with low-dose dexamethasone, and ACTH may be low or suppressed.
- An associated ↑ risk of diabetes mellitus, osteoporosis, and hypertension has been reported.
- Current data are insufficient to indicate the superiority of a surgical or non-surgical approach to management.
- Hypoadrenalism post-adrenalectomy has been reported due to suppression of the contralateral adrenal gland. Perioperative steroid cover is, therefore, required with re-evaluation post-operatively.

Further reading

Allolio B, Fassnacht M (2006). Clinical review: Adrenocortical carcinoma: clinical update. *J Clin Endocrinol Metab* **91**, 2027–37.

Fassnacht M, et al. (2012). Combination chemotherapy in advanced adrenocortical carcinoma. *N Engl J Med* **366**, 2189–97.

Kroiss M (2011). Drug interactions with mitotane by induction of CYP3A4 metabolism in the clinical management of adrenocortical carcinoma. *Clin Endocrinol (Oxf)* **75**, 585–91.

Lacroix A, N'Diaye N, Tremblay J, et al. (2001). Ectopic and abnormal hormone receptors in adrenal Cushing's syndrome. *Endocr Rev* **22**, 75–110.

Terzolo M, Angeli A, Fassnacht M, et al. (2007). Adjuvant mitotane treatment for adrenocortical carcinoma. *N Engl J Med* **356**, 2372–80.

Adrenal surgery

Adrenalectomy

Open adrenalectomy may still be necessary for large and complex pathology. However, laparoscopic adrenalectomy (first performed in 1992) has become the procedure of choice for removal of most adrenal tumours. Retrospective comparisons with open approaches suggest reduced hospital stay and analgesic requirements and lower post-operative morbidity. This may be improved even further by the recently introduced retroperitoneoscopic approach. However, there are few long-term outcome data on this technique. It is most useful in the management of small (<6cm) benign adenomas. Laparoscopic bilateral adrenalectomy, although technically demanding, offers a useful approach to patients with macronodular hyperplasia and in selected patients with ACTH-dependent Cushing's syndrome where alternative therapeutic options are not appropriate.

Preoperative preparation of patients
- Cushing's—metyrapone or ketoconazole (🕮 see p. 170).
- Phaeochromocytoma—α- and β-blockade (🕮 see p. 294).

Perioperative management
See Box 3.2.

Box 3.2 Perioperative management of patients undergoing adrenalectomy

Adrenal cortical tumours (benign and malignant)/bilateral adrenalectomy for Cushing's syndrome.

• Perioperative glucocorticoid cover is required in all patients who fail to adequately suppress serum cortisol in the 1mg overnight dexamethasone suppression test. If in doubt, replace, as even 'silent' adenomas may be associated with subclinical excess cortisol and hence suppression of the contralateral adrenal gland.

• Hydrocortisone is given as for pituitary surgery—100mg IM with the premedication and then continued every 6h for 24–48h, until the patient can take oral medication and is eating and drinking.

• This is changed to oral hydrocortisone at double replacement dose—20mg on waking, 10mg at lunchtime, and 10mg at 5 p.m., and mineralocorticoid replacement commenced if bilateral adrenalectomy has been performed (100 micrograms fludrocortisone daily). Electrolytes and BP guide adequacy of treatment. Normal replacement hydrocortisone (e.g. 10, 5, 5mg) can be commenced when the patient is recovered and may be omitted altogether if the patient did not have preoperative evidence of Cushing's syndrome/suppression of the contralateral gland/bilateral adrenalectomy. Mineralocorticoid replacement is only required in patients who have had bilateral adrenalectomy.

• A short Synacthen® test (off hydrocortisone for at least 24h) is performed after at least 2 weeks to demonstrate adequate function of the contralateral adrenal. However, in patients with ACTH-independent Cushing's syndrome, it may take up to 2 years for full recovery of the contralateral adrenal gland and thus the first assessment by SST should be done only after 4–6 months.

• The exception is patients undergoing adrenalectomy for mineralocorticoid-secreting tumours. These patients do not usually require perioperative glucocorticoid replacement, but preoperative amiloride or spironolactone allows recovery of potassium stores and control of hypertension prior to surgery.

Further reading

Dudley NE, Harrison BJ (1999). Comparison of open posterior versus transperitoneal laparoscopic adrenalectomy. *Br J Surg* **86**, 656–60.

McCallum R, Connell JMC (2001). Laparoscopic adrenalectomy. *Clin Endocrinol* **55**, 435–6.

Wells SA, Merke DP, Cutler GB, *et al.* (1998). The role of laparoscopic surgery in adrenal disease. *J Clin Endocrinol Metab* **83**, 3041–9.

Renal tubular abnormalities

Background

Bartter's syndrome and Gitelman's syndrome are both associated with hypokalaemic alkalosis and the activation of the renin–angiotensin system but without hypertension—in contrast, BP tends to be low in these conditions. Liddle's syndrome is associated with hypokalaemic alkalosis and hypertension but low renin and aldosterone levels.

Liddle's syndrome

A rare autosomal dominant (AD) condition with variable penetrance that is caused by mutations in the gene encoding for the epithelial sodium channel (ENaC), usually by mutations in the gene encoding the β or γ subunit of ENaC, which is highly selective and located in the distal nephron. This leads to constitutive activation of sodium transport, independent of circulating mineralocorticoids; consequently, 2° activation of the sodium/potassium exchange occurs.

Features

Hypokalaemia and hypertension.

Investigation

• Hypokalaemic alkalosis.
• Suppressed renin and aldosterone levels.
• See Table 3.5.

Treatment

Hypertension responds to amiloride (doses up to 40mg/day) but not spironolactone because amiloride acts on the sodium channel directly whereas spironolactone acts on the mineralocorticoid receptor.

Bartter's syndrome

Cause

Loss of function of the bumetanide-sensitive Na–K–2Cl co-transporter in the thick ascending limb of the loop of Henle. Mutations in three genes have been reported to account for the phenotype—these encode regulatory ion channels (*NKCC2*; *ROMK*; *CLCNKB*). Inactivation of the co-transporter leads to salt wasting, activation of the renin–angiotensin system, and ↑ aldosterone which leads to ↑ sodium reabsorption at the distal nephron and causes hypokalaemic alkalosis. Reabsorption of calcium also occurs in the thick ascending loop, and thus inactivation leads to hypercalciuria. The lack of associated hypertension is thought to be due to ↑ prostaglandin production from the renal medullary interstitial tissue in response to hypokalaemia.

- Rare (~1/million) autosomal recessive hypokalaemic metabolic alkalosis associated with salt wasting and normal or reduced BP.
- Usually present at an early age (<5 years).

Features

- Intravascular volume depletion.
- Seizures.
- Tetany.
- Muscle weakness.

There is also an antenatal variant which is a life-threatening disorder of renal tubular hypokalaemic alkalosis and hypercalciuria.

Investigations

- Hypokalaemic alkalosis.
- ↑ PRA and aldosterone.
- Hypercalciuria.

Treatment

Potassium replacement. Potassium-sparing diuretics may be helpful. However, they are usually inadequate in correcting hypokalaemia. Prostaglandin synthase inhibitors (NSAIDs), e.g. indometacin 2–5mg/kg per day or ibuprofen, may be required.

Gitelman's syndrome

Cause
- Loss of function in the thiazide-sensitive Na–Cl transporter of the distal convoluted tubule (DCT) due to mutations in the *SCL12A3* gene that encodes it (located on chromosome 16q13). This leads to salt wasting, hypovolaemia, and metabolic alkalosis.
- Hypovolaemia leads to activation of the renin–angiotensin system and ↑ aldosterone levels.
- Hypokalaemic alkalosis, in conjunction with hypocalciuria and hypomagnesaemia.
- Present at older ages without overt hypovolaemia (essentially, a less severe phenotype of Bartter's syndrome).

Investigations
- Hypokalaemic alkalosis, in association with ↑ renin and aldosterone.
- Hypomagnesaemia.
- Hypocalciuria.

Treatment
- Potassium and magnesium replacement.
- Potassium-sparing diuretics may be required.
- See Table 3.5.

Table 3.5 Summary of features of renal tubular abnormalities

Syndrome*	BP	Renin	Aldosterone	Urinary calcium	Other
Bartter's	N	↑	↑	↑	
Gitelman's	N	↑	↑	↓	↓ Mg
Liddle's	↑	↓	↓	N	

* All three conditions have hypokalaemic alkalosis. N = normal.

Further reading

Amirlak I, Dawson KP (2000). Bartter's syndrome. *QJM* **93**, 207–15.

Furuhashi M, Kitamura K, Adachi M, *et al.* (2005). Liddle's syndrome caused by a novel mutation in the proline-rich PY motif of the epithelial sodium channel B-subunit. *J Clin Endocrinol Metab* **90**, 340–4.

Graziani G, Fedeli C, Moroni L *et al.* (2010) Gitelman syndrome: pathophysiological and clinical aspects. *QJM* **103**, 741–8.

Nakamura A, Shimizu C, Yoshida M *et al.* (2010) Problems in diagnosing atypical Gitelman's syndrome presenting with normomagnesaemia. *Clin Endocrinol* **72**, 272–6.

Mineralocorticoid deficiency

Epidemiology
Rare, apart from the hyporeninaemic hypoaldosteronism associated with diabetes mellitus.

Causes

Congenital
- Primary adrenal insufficiency due to:
    - *CAH*—certain types, most commonly 21-hydroxylase deficiency, are associated with MC deficiency; 📖 see p. 320.
    - *Congenital lipoid adrenal hyperplasia (CLAH)* caused by mutations in the genes encoding steroidogenic acute regulatory protein (StAR), responsible for rapid import of cholesterol into the mitochondrion, and the side chain cleavage protein (CYP11A1), responsible for the conversion of cholesterol to pregnenolone, i.e. the first step of steroidogenesis.
    - *Adrenal hypoplasia congenita (AHC)* caused by mutations in the genes encoding the transcription factors SF-1 (*NR5A1*) and DAX-1 (*NR0B1*) that play a crucial role in adrenal development.
    - *Adrenoleukodystrophy* affecting 1/20,000 ♂; very long chain fatty acids (VLCFA) cannot be oxidized in peroxisomes and accumulate in tissues and the circulation. CNS symptoms may be absent initially, in particular, in the milder form adrenomyeloneuropathy, but progressive demyelination can lead to hypertonic tetraparesis, dementia, epilepsy, coma, or death (in particular, in the early childhood onset variant adrenoleukodystrophy).
- Rare *inherited disorders* of aldosterone biosynthesis.
- *Pseudohypoaldosteronism*—inherited resistance to the action of aldosterone (📖 see p. 665). Autosomal dominant and recessive forms are described. Usually presents in infancy. Treated with sodium chloride.

Acquired
- All forms of non-congenital primary adrenal insufficiency—📖 see p. 266. In secondary adrenal insufficiency, the adrenals are anatomically intact, and thus regulation of mineralocorticoid secretion by the renin–angiotensin–aldosterone (RAA) system is intact.
- *Drugs*—heparin (heparin for >5 days may cause severe hyperkalaemia due to a toxic effect on the zona glomerulosa); ciclosporin.
- *Hyporeninaemic hypoaldosteronism*—interference with the renin–angiotensin system leads to mineralocorticoid deficiency and hyperkalaemic acidosis (type IV renal tubular acidosis), e.g. diabetic nephropathy. Treatment is fludrocortisone and potassium restriction. ACEI may produce a similar biochemical picture, but here the PRA will be elevated, as there is no angiotensin II feedback on renin.

Treatment
Fludrocortisone.

Adrenal insufficiency

Definition

Adrenal insufficiency is defined by the lack of cortisol, i.e. glucocorticoid deficiency, and may be due to destruction of the adrenal cortex (1°, Addison's disease and congenital adrenal hyperplasia (CAH); 📖 see p. 266) or due to disordered pituitary and hypothalamic function (2°).

Epidemiology

- Permanent adrenal insufficiency is found in 5 in 10,000 population.
- The most frequent cause is hypothalamic–pituitary damage, which is the cause of AI in 60% of affected patients.
- The remaining 40% of cases are due to primary failure of the adrenal to synthesize cortisol, with almost equal prevalence of Addison's disease (mostly of autoimmune origin, prevalence 0.9–1.4 in 10,000) and congenital adrenal hyperplasia (0.7–1.0 in 10,000).
- 2° adrenal insufficiency due to suppression of pituitary–hypothalamic function by exogenously administered, supraphysiological glucocorticoid doses for treatment of, for example, COPD or rheumatoid arthritis, is much more common (50–200 in 10,000 population). However, adrenal function in these patients can recover, following tapering and cessation of exogenous glucocorticoid administration.

Causes of secondary adrenal insufficiency

Lesions of the hypothalamus and/or pituitary gland

- Tumours—pituitary tumour, metastases, craniopharyngioma.
- Infection—tuberculosis.
- Inflammation—sarcoidosis, histiocytosis X, haemochromatosis, lymphocytic hypophysitis.
- Iatrogenic—surgery, radiotherapy.
- Other—isolated ACTH deficiency, trauma.

Suppression of the hypothalamo–pituitary–adrenal axis

- Glucocorticoid administration.
- Cushing's disease (after pituitary tumour removal).

Features of secondary adrenal insufficiency

As 1° (📖 see Clinical features, p. 123), except:
- Absence of pigmentation—skin is pale.
- Absence of mineralocorticoid deficiency.
- Associated features of underlying cause, e.g. visual field defects if pituitary tumour.
- Other endocrine deficiencies may manifest due to pituitary failure (📖 see p. 122).
- Acute onset may occur due to pituitary apoplexy.

Isolated **ACTH** deficiency

- Rare.
- Pathogenesis unclear—may be autoimmune (associated with other autoimmune conditions and antipituitary antibodies described in some patients); can be associated with autoimmune hypothyroidism.
- Absent ACTH response to CRH.
- POMC mutations and POMC processing abnormalities (e.g. proconvertase PC1).

Pathophysiology

Primary

- Adrenal gland destruction or dysfunction occurs due to a disease process which usually involves all three zones of the adrenal cortex, resulting in inadequate glucocorticoid, mineralocorticoid, and adrenal androgen precursor secretion. The manifestations of insufficiency do not usually appear until at least 90% of the gland has been destroyed and are usually gradual in onset, with partial adrenal insufficiency leading to an impaired cortisol response to stress and the features of complete insufficiency occurring later. Acute adrenal insufficiency may occur in the context of acute septicaemia (e.g. meningococcal or haemorrhage).
- Mineralocorticoid deficiency leads to reduced sodium retention and hyponatraemia and hypotension with ↓ intravascular volume, in addition to hyperkalaemia due to ↓ renal potassium and hydrogen ion excretion.
- Androgen deficiency presents in ♀ with reduced axillary and pubic hair and reduced libido. (Testicular production of androgens is more important in ♂.)
- Lack of cortisol −ve feedback increases CRH and ACTH secretion. Stimulation of skin melanocortin 1 receptors (MC1R) leads to skin pigmentation and other mucous membranes.

Secondary

- Inadequate ACTH results in deficient cortisol production (and ↓ androgens in ♀).
- There is no pigmentation because ACTH and POMC secretion is reduced. Mineralocorticoid secretion remains normal, as its primary regulator is the RAA system in kidney and adrenal gland which are intact. However, hyponatraemia may be present due to mild SIADH arising from the cortisol deficiency.
- The onset is usually gradual, with partial ACTH deficiency resulting in reduced response to stress. Prolonged ACTH deficiency leads to atrophy of the zona fasciculata and reduced ability to respond acutely to ACTH.
- Lack of stimulation of skin MC1R due to ACTH deficiency results in pale skin appearance.

Investigations

📖 see p. 125 for pituitary/hypothalamic disease and p. 268 for long-term endogenous or exogenous glucocorticoids.

Addison's disease

Causes of primary adrenal insufficiency

- Autoimmune—commonest cause in the developed world (approximately 70% cases).
- Autoimmune polyglandular deficiency—type 1 or 2 (see p. 270).
- *Malignancy*:
  - Metastatic (lung, breast, kidney—adrenal metastases found in ~50% of patients, but symptomatic adrenal insufficiency much less common and only observed with bilateral metastases).
  - Lymphoma (primary adrenal lymphoma, AI only if bilateral).
- Infiltration:
  - Amyloid.
  - Sarcoidosis.
  - Haemochromatosis.
- Infection:
  - Tuberculosis (medulla more frequently destroyed than cortex).
  - Fungal, e.g. histoplasmosis, cryptococcosis.
  - Opportunistic infections in, for example AIDS—CMV, *Mycobacterium intracellulare*, cryptococcus (up to 5% patients with AIDS develop 1° adrenal insufficiency in the late stages).
- Vascular haemorrhage:
  - Anticoagulants.
  - Waterhouse–Friderichsen syndrome in meningococcal septicaemia.
- *Infarction*—e.g. 2° to thrombosis in antiphospholipid syndrome.
- *Adrenoleukodystrophy*:
  - Inherited disorder caused by mutations in the X-linked ALD gene that encodes for the peroxisomal transporter protein ABCD1.
  - Diagnosed by measuring very long chain fatty acids.
  - Presents in childhood and adolescence.
  - Progresses in 50% to quadriparesis and dementia, in association with adrenal failure (= cerebral ALS); milder variant adrenomyeloneuropathy (AMN) causes spinal neurology only, and AI may precede manifestation of neurological symptoms; in 10–20%, AI is the sole manifestation of disease.
- Congenital adrenal hyperplasia—see p. 320.
- Adrenal hypoplasia congenita—very rare familial failure of adrenal cortical development due to mutations/deletion of the NR0B1 (DAX-1) or the NR5A1 (SF-1) genes.
- Congenital lipoid adrenal hyperplasia—very rare familial failure of adrenal steroidogenesis due to mutations in the genes encoding the steroidogenic acute regulatory protein (StAR; responsible for mitochondrial import of cholesterol) or the side chain cleavage enzyme CYP11A1 (responsible for conversion of cholesterol to pregnenolone, i.e. the first step of steroidogenesis).

- Familial glucocorticoid deficiency (FGD) due to mutations in genes encoding for proteins involved in the regulation of ACTH action, e.g. the ACTH receptor MC2R or the MC2R accessory protein MRAP that transfers MC2R to the adrenal cell membrane to facilitate ACTH binding.
- Triple A syndrome (*Achalasia, Addisonianism, Alacrimia*) (Allgrove syndrome):
  - Addison's due to ACTH resistance.
  - Autosomal recessive.
  - May get autonomic dysfunction, hypoglycaemia, and mental retardation.
  - Caused by mutations on the AAAS gene (12g13).
- Iatrogenic:
  - Bilateral adrenalectomy.
  - Drugs: ketoconazole, fluconazole, trilostane, abiraterone, etomidate, aminoglutethimide (inhibits cortisol synthesis), phenytoin, rifampicin (increases cortisol metabolism), mitotane (adrenolytic and increases cortisol metabolism).

Autoimmune adrenalitis

- Mediated by humoral and cell-mediated immune mechanisms. Autoimmune insufficiency associated with polyglandular autoimmune syndrome is more common in ♀ (70%).
- Adrenal cortex antibodies are present in the majority of patients at diagnosis, and although titres decline and eventually disappear, they are still found in approximately 70% of patients 10 years later. Up to 20% patients/year with +ve adrenal antibodies develop adrenal insufficiency. Antibodies to 21-hydroxylase are commonly found, although the exact nature of other antibodies that block the effect of ACTH, for example, is yet to be elucidated.
- Antiadrenal antibodies are found in <2% of patients with other autoimmune endocrine disease (Hashimoto's thyroiditis, diabetes mellitus, autoimmune hypothyroidism, hypoparathyroidism, pernicious anaemia). In addition, antibodies to other endocrine glands are commonly found in patients with autoimmune adrenal insufficiency (thyroid microsomal in 50%, gastric parietal cell, parathyroid, and ovary and testis). However, the presence of antibodies does not predict subsequent manifestation of organ-specific autoimmunity.
- Polyglandular autoimmune conditions (📖 see Autoimmune polyglandular syndrome (APS) type 1, p. 270; APS type 2, p. 271). The presence of 17-hydroxylase antibodies, in association with 21-hydroxylase antibodies, is a good marker of patients at risk of developing premature ovarian failure in association with 1° adrenal failure.
- Patients with type 1 diabetes mellitus and autoimmune thyroid disease only rarely develop autoimmune adrenal insufficiency. Approximately 60% of patients with Addison's disease have other autoimmune or endocrine disorders.

Clinical features

Chronic

- Anorexia and weight loss (>90%).
- Tiredness.
- Weakness—generalized, no particular muscle groups.
- Pigmentation—generalized but most common in skin areas exposed to friction or pressure (elbows and knees, and under bras and belts), mucosae, and scars acquired after onset of adrenal insufficiency. Look at palmar creases in Caucasians.
- Dizziness and postural hypotension.
- GI symptoms—nausea and vomiting, abdominal pain, diarrhoea.
- Arthralgia and myalgia.
- Symptomatic hypoglycaemia—rare in adults.
- ↓ axillary and pubic hair and reduced libido in ♀.
- Pyrexia of unknown origin—rarely.

Associated conditions

- Vitiligo.
- Features of other autoimmune endocrinopathies.

Laboratory investigations
- Hyponatraemia.
- Hyperkalaemia.
- Elevated urea.
- Anaemia (normocytic normochromic).
- Elevated ESR.
- Eosinophilia.
- Mild hypercalcaemia—↓ absorption, ↓ renal absorption of calcium.

Autoimmune polyglandular syndrome (APS) type 1

- Also known as autoimmune polyendocrinopathy, candidiasis, and ectodermal dystrophy (APECED).
- Autosomal recessive with childhood onset.
- Chronic mucocutaneous candidiasis.
- Hypoparathyroidism (90%), 1° adrenal insufficiency (60%).
- 1° gonadal failure (41%)—usually after Addison's diagnosis.
- 1° hypothyroidism.
- Rarely hypopituitarism, diabetes insipidus, type 1 diabetes mellitus.
- Associated chronic active hepatitis (20%), malabsorption (15%), alopecia (40%), pernicious anaemia, vitiligo.
- Mutations in the AIRE (autoimmune regulator) gene located on chromosome 21p22.3.

APS type 2

- Polygenic inheritance, association with HLADR3 and CTL4 regions, mixed penetrance.
- Adult onset.
- Adrenal insufficiency (100%).
- 1° autoimmune thyroid disease (70%), mostly hypothyroidism but also hyperthyroidism.
- Type 1 diabetes mellitus (5–20%)—often before Addison's diagnosis.
- 1° gonadal failure in affected women (5–20%).
- Rarely diabetes insipidus (<0.1%).
- Associated vitiligo, myasthenia gravis, alopecia, pernicious anaemia, immune thrombocytopenic purpura.

Eponymous syndromes

- Schmidt's syndrome:
    - Addison's disease, *and*
    - Autoimmune hypothyroidism.
- Carpenter syndrome:
    - Addison's disease, *and*
    - Autoimmune hypothyroidism, *and/or*
    - Type 1 diabetes mellitus.

Investigation of primary adrenal insufficiency

Electrolytes
• Hyponatraemia is present in 90% and hyperkalaemia in 65%.
• Elevated urea.

Serum cortisol and ACTH
• Undetectable serum cortisol is diagnostic of adrenal insufficiency, but the basal cortisol is often in the normal range. A cortisol >550nmol/L precludes the diagnosis. At times of acute stress, an inappropriately low cortisol is very suggestive of the diagnosis.
• Simultaneous 9 a.m. cortisol and ACTH will show an elevated ACTH for the level of cortisol. This is a very sensitive means of detecting Addison's disease but performs poorly in less clear-cut cases.
• NB Drugs causing ↑ cortisol-binding globulin (e.g. oestrogens) will result in higher total cortisol concentration measurements.

Response to ACTH
Short Synacthen® test
• Following basal cortisol measurement, 250 micrograms Synacthen® is administered IM and serum cortisol checked at 30 or 60min.
• Serum cortisol should rise to a peak of 550nmol/L (note that this cut-off may depend on local assay conditions).
• Failure to respond appropriately suggests adrenal failure.
  • A long Synacthen® test may be required to confirm 2° adrenal failure if ACTH is equivocal.
  • Recent onset of 2° adrenal failure (up to 4 weeks) may produce a normal response to a short Synacthen® test.

Long Synacthen® test
• Following basal cortisol level, depot Synacthen® 1mg IM is administered, and serum cortisol measured at 30, 60, 120min, and 4, 8, 12, and 24h. A normal response is an elevation in serum cortisol to >1,000nmol/L.
• Differentiation of 2° from 1° adrenal failure can be made more reliably following 3 days IM ACTH 1mg. This is because the test relies on the ability of the atrophic adrenal glands to respond to ACTH in 2° adrenocortical failure whereas, in 1° adrenal failure, the diseased gland is already maximally stimulated by elevated endogenous levels of ACTH and, therefore, unable to respond to further stimulation.
• Serum cortisol responses within the first 60min are superimposable with the short Synacthen® test.
• There is a progressive rise in cortisol secretion in 2° adrenal insufficiency but little or no response on 1° adrenal insufficiency.

Increased plasma renin activity (assessment of mineralocorticoid sufficiency)
This is one of the earliest abnormalities in developing 1° adrenal insufficiency.

Thyroid function tests
Reduced thyroid hormone levels and elevated TSH may be due to a direct effect of glucocorticoid deficiency (cortisol inhibits TRH) or due to associated autoimmune hypothyroidism; TSH is usually less than 10U/L in the former and above 10 in the latter. Re-evaluation is, therefore, required after adrenal insufficiency has been appropriately replaced for a few weeks. Initiation of thyroxine replacement prior to glucocorticoid replacement can trigger adrenal crisis, as thyroxine will speed up the inactivation of residual cortisol.

Establish cause of adrenal insufficiency
- *Adrenal autoantibodies* (detect antibodies to adrenal cortex and, more recently, specific antibodies to 21-hydroxylase, side chain cleavage enzyme, and 17-hydroxylase). 21-hydroxylase antibodies are the major component of adrenal cortex antibodies and are present in 80% of recent-onset autoimmune adrenalitis. Adrenal cortex antibodies (present in 80% patients of recent-onset autoimmune adrenalitis) are not detectable in non-autoimmune 1° adrenal failure.
- *Imaging*:
  - Adrenal enlargement, with or without calcification, may be seen on CT of the abdomen, suggesting tuberculosis, infiltration, or metastatic disease. The adrenals are small and atrophic in chronic autoimmune adrenalitis.
  - Percutaneous CT-guided adrenal biopsy is occasionally required.
- *Specific tests*—e.g. serological or microbiological investigations directed at particular infections, very long chain fatty acids (adrenoleukodystrophy) in ♂ and ♀ with antibody −ve isolated 1° adrenal insufficiency.

Acute adrenal insufficiency (risk higher in primary disease)
Clinical features
- Shock.
- Hypotension (often not responding to measures, such as inotropic support).
- Abdominal pain (may present as 'acute abdomen').
- Unexplained fever.
- Often precipitated by major stress, such as severe bacterial infection, major surgery, unabsorbed glucocorticoid medication due to vomiting.
- Occasionally occurs due to bilateral adrenal infarction.

Investigations
- As chronic.
- In the acute situation if the diagnosis is suspected, an inappropriately low cortisol (i.e. <600nmol/L) is often sufficient to make the diagnosis.

See Box 3.3 for emergency management.

Box 3.3 Emergency management of acute adrenal insufficiency

- This is a life-threatening emergency and should be treated if there is strong clinical suspicion rather than waiting for confirmatory test results.
- Blood should be taken for urgent analysis of electrolytes and glucose, in addition to cortisol and ACTH.

Fluids

Large volumes of 0.9% saline may be required to reverse the volume depletion and sodium deficiency. Several litres may be required in the first 24–48h, but caution should be exercised where there has been chronic hyponatraemia; in this circumstance, rapid correction of the deficit exposes the patient to risk of central pontine myelinolysis. If plasma sodium is <120mmol/L at presentation, aim to correct by no more than 10mmol/L in the first 24h.

Hydrocortisone

- A bolus dose of 100mg hydrocortisone is administered intravenously. Hydrocortisone 100mg IM is then continued 6-hourly for 24–48h or until the patient can take oral therapy. Double replacement dose hydrocortisone (20, 10, and 10mg orally) can then be instituted until well.
- This traditional regimen causes supraphysiological replacement, and some authors suggest lower doses, e.g. 150mg IV/24h.
- Specific mineralocorticoid replacement is not required, as the high-dose glucocorticoid has sufficient mineralocorticoid effects (40mg hydrocortisone equivalent to 100 micrograms fludrocortisone). Once the daily dose of glucocorticoid is reduced to less than 50mg after a couple of days and the patient is taking food and fluids by mouth, fludrocortisone 100 micrograms/day can be commenced.

Glucose supplementation

Occasionally required because of risk of hypoglycaemia (low glycogen stores in the liver as a result of glucocorticoid deficiency).

Investigate and treat precipitant

This is often infection.

Monitoring treatment

Electrolytes, glucose, and urea.

Treatment of primary adrenal insufficiency

Maintenance therapy

Glucocorticoid replacement

- Hydrocortisone is the treatment of choice for replacement therapy, as it is reliably and predictably absorbed and allows biochemical monitoring of levels.
- It is administered twice to thrice daily, e.g. 10mg immediately on waking, 5mg at midday, and 5mg at 4–5 p.m., or 15mg on waking and 5mg at midday.
- Longer-acting glucocorticoid preparations can be advantageous in patients with co-incident type 1 diabetes mellitus, e.g. 3mg prednisolone on waking and 1mg at 5pm.

Mineralocorticoid replacement

- Fludrocortisone (9-fluorohydrocortisone) is given at a dose of 100–150 micrograms daily; occasionally, lower (50 micrograms) or higher (200–250 micrograms) doses may be required. Aim to avoid significant postural fall in BP (>10mmHg).
- Plasma renin should be within the upper third of the normal reference range.
- 40mg hydrocortisone has the equivalent mineralocorticoid effect of 100 micrograms fludrocortisone.

DHEA replacement

- Dehydroepiandrosterone (DHEA) synthesis is also deficient in hypoadrenalism, resulting in reduced production of adrenal androgen precursors and thus invariably androgen deficiency in affected women.
- DHEA replacement (25–50mg/day) may improve mood and well-being as well as libido in women with AI.
- DHEA is not available as a UK-licensed preparation but is available from the USA as a dietary supplement.

Monitoring of therapy

Clinical

- For signs of glucocorticoid excess, e.g ↑ weight.
- BP (including postural change).
- Hypertension and oedema suggest excessive mineralocorticoid replacement whereas postural hypotension and salt craving suggest insufficient treatment.

Biochemical

- Serum electrolytes.
- Plasma renin (elevated if insufficient fludrocortisone replacement).
- Cortisol day curve to assess adequacy.

Intercurrent illness
- Cortisol requirements increase during severe illness or surgery.
- For moderate elective procedures or investigations, e.g. endoscopy or angiography, patients should receive a single dose of 100mg hydrocortisone before the procedure.
- For major surgery, patients should receive 100mg intravenously or intramuscularly with the premedication and receive:
  - 50–100mg IM hydrocortisone 6-hourly for the first 3 days, *or*
  - 100–150mg per 24h IV in 5% glucose before reverting rapidly to a maintenance dose.
- To cover severe illness, e.g. pneumonia, patients should receive 50–100mg IM hydrocortisone 6-hourly until resolution of the illness.
- See Box 3.4 for pregnancy.

Drug interactions
- Rifampicin:
  - Increases the clearance of cortisol.
  - Double usual dose of hydrocortisone.
- Mitotane:
  - Increases cortisol-binding globulin and induces CYP3A4, resulting in rapid inactivation of hydrocortisone.
  - Double usual dose of hydrocortisone, e.g. 20–10–10mg.
  - Topiramate—also induces CYP3A4 and accelerates clearance of glucocorticoids.

Box 3.4 Pregnancy
📖 also see Normal changes during pregnancy, p. 436.
- During normal pregnancy:
  - Cortisol-binding globulin gradually increases.
  - Free cortisol increases in the third trimester.
  - Progesterone increases, exerting an antimineralocorticoid effect.
  - Renin levels increase.
- In Addison's disease, therefore:
  - The usual glucocorticoid and mineralocorticoid replacement is continued initially.
  - Increase the hydrocortisone 25–50% in the third trimester.
  - Adjust mineralocorticoids to BP and serum potassium (not renin).
- Severe hyperemesis gravidarum during the first trimester may require temporary parenteral therapy, and patients should be warned about this to avoid precipitation of a crisis.
- During labour and for 24–48h:
  - Parenteral glucocorticoid therapy is administered (100mg IM every 6h), *or*
  - Hydrocortisone 100mg IV in 5% glucose per 24h.
  - Fluid replacement with IV 0.9% saline may be required.

Education of the patient

- Patient education is the key to successful management. Patients must be taught never to miss a dose. They should be encouraged to wear a MedicAlert/SOS bracelet or necklace and always to carry a steroid card.
- Every patient should know how to double the dose of glucocorticoid during febrile illness and to get medical attention if unable to take the tablets because of vomiting. They should have a vial of 100mg hydrocortisone, with syringe, diluent, and needle for times when parenteral treatment may be required (see Box 3.5).

Box 3.5 Emergency pack contents for Addison's patients

- 100mg vial hydrocortisone.
- Water for injection.
- 2mL syringe.
- 1 green needle.
- 1 blue needle.
- Cotton wool.
- Plaster.

NB Check expiry date of hydrocortisone.

Further reading

Arlt W (2009). The approach to the adult with newly diagnosed adrenal insufficiency. *J Clin Endocrinol Metab* **94**, 1059–67.

Arlt W, Allolio B (2003). Adrenal insufficiency. *Lancet* **361**, 1881–93.

Bornstein SR (2009). Predisposing factors for adrenal insufficiency. *N Engl J Med* **360**, 2328–39.

Lebbe M, Arlt W (2013). What is the best diagnostic and therapeutic management strategy for an Addison patient during pregnancy? *Clin Endocrinol (Oxf)* **78**, 497–502.

Mitchell AL, Pearce SH (2012). Autoimmune Addison disease: pathophysiology and genetic complexity. *Nat Rev Endocrinol* **8**, 306–16.

Wass JAH, Arlt W (2012). How to avoid precipitating an acute adrenal crisis. *BMJ* **345**, 6333.

Long-term glucocorticoid administration

Both exogenous glucocorticoid administration and endogenous excess glucocorticoids (Cushing's syndrome) lead to a −ve feedback effect on the hypothalamo–pituitary axis (HPA), leading to suppression of both CRH and ACTH secretion and atrophy of the zonae fasciculata and reticularis of the adrenal cortex. Administration (or endogenous over-production) of >50mg hydrocortisone equivalent per day will result in downregulation of mineralocorticoid production. However, the renin–angiotensin–aldosterone axis continues to function while the glucocorticoid excess ceases while the HPA axis will suffer from lasting suppression, with the time of recovery dependent on the duration of the preceding period of hypercortisolism. See Box 3.6 for steroid equivalents.

Short-term steroids

- Any patient who has received glucocorticoid treatment for <3 weeks is unlikely to have clinically significant adrenal suppression, and if the medical condition allows it, glucocorticoid treatment can be stopped acutely. A major stress within a week of stopping steroids should, however, be covered with glucocorticoids.
- Exceptions to this are patients who have other possible reasons for adrenocortical insufficiency, who have received >40mg prednisolone (or equivalent), where a short course has been prescribed within 1 year of cessation of long-term therapy, or evening doses (↑ HPA axis suppression).

Steroid cover

While receiving glucocorticoid treatment and within 1 year of steroid withdrawal, patients should receive standard steroid supplementation at times of stress, e.g. major trauma, surgery, and infection (📖 see p. 277).

Long-term steroids

- When patients are receiving supraphysiological doses (>5mg prednisolone or equivalent) of glucocorticoid, dose reduction depends on the activity of the underlying disease requiring glucocorticoid treatment.
- If the disease has resolved, the dose can be rapidly reduced to 5mg prednisolone by a reduction of 2.5mg every 3–5 days.
- Once the patient is established on 5mg prednisolone, consider changing to hydrocortisone (20mg in the morning), as this has a shorter half-life and will, therefore, lead to less prolonged suppression of ACTH.
- Daily hydrocortisone dose should be reduced by 2.5mg every 1–2 weeks, or as tolerated, until a dose of 10mg is reached. After 2–3 months, a short Synacthen® test should be performed. Once a short Synacthen® test demonstrates a normal response, hydrocortisone replacement can be stopped. Supplemental steroids during intercurrent illness are not required.

Cushing's syndrome

Patients with Cushing's syndrome on metyrapone or with recently treated disease, whatever the cause, may also have HPA axis suppression and may, therefore, need steroid replacement at times of stress.

Box 3.6 Steroid equivalents
- 1mg hydrocortisone.
- 1.5mg cortisone acetate.
- 0.20mg prednisolone.
- 0.0375mg dexamethasone.

4mg prednisolone ≡ 20mg hydrocortisone ≡ 0.75mg dexamethasone.

Adrenal incidentalomas

Definition and epidemiology

- An adrenal incidentaloma is an adrenal mass that is discovered incidentally upon imaging (e.g. CT chest or abdomen) carried out for reasons other than a suspected adrenal pathology.
- The incidental detection of an adrenal mass is becoming more common, as ↑ numbers of imaging procedures are performed and with technological improvements in imaging.
- Autopsy studies suggest incidence prevalence of adrenal masses of 1–6% in the general population.
- Imaging studies suggest that adrenal masses are present 2–3% in the general population. Incidence increases with ageing, and 8–10% of 70-year olds harbour an adrenal mass.

Importance

It is important to determine whether the incidentally discovered adrenal mass is:
- Malignant.
- Functioning and associated with excess hormonal secretion.

Differential diagnosis of an incidentally detected adrenal nodule

- Cortisol-secreting adrenal adenoma causing Cushing's syndrome or subclinical Cushing's syndrome (5%).
- Mineralocorticoid-secreting adrenal adenoma.
- CAH.
- Adrenocortical carcinoma (5–12%).
- Metastasis (2–10%; most prevalent breast, lung, kidney).
- Phaeochromocytoma (10–15%).
- Adrenal cysts (5%).
- Adrenal myelolipoma (5–10%).
- Haematoma.
- Ganglioneuroma (4%).

Investigations

- Clinical assessment for symptoms and signs of excess hormone secretion and signs of extra-adrenal carcinoma.
- Urinary free cortisol and overnight dexamethasone suppression test.
- Plasma free metanephrines (most sensitive and specific screening test; alternatively, urinary metanephrine—however, more cumbersome and less specific) (see p. 288).
- Aldosterone/renin ratio and serum potassium.
- A homogeneous mass with a low attenuation value prior to contrast administration (<10HU) on CT scan is likely to be a benign adenoma (low density = high fat content = benign) whereas a mass with high density (>20HU) has to be considered suspicious (differential diagnosis phaeochromocytoma/adrenocortical carcinoma/metastasis but also lipid-poor adenoma).

- Additional tests if adrenal carcinoma suspected:
  - 24h urinary excretion of corticosteroid metabolites.
  - DHEAS, 17α OH progesterone, progesterone.
  - 17α oestradiol (in ♂ only).
  - Androstenedione, testosterone.

Management

- Up to 20% of patients may develop hormonal excess during follow-up.
- Unlikely if tumour <3cm.
- Cortisol is the commonest excess hormone.
- Surgery if there is/are:
  - Evidence of a syndrome of hormonal excess attributable to the tumour.
  - Biochemical evidence of phaeochromocytoma.
  - Mass diameter >4cm (↑ likelihood of malignancy according to imaging or biochemistry (co-secretion of several corticosteroids indicative of malignancy) and definitely if >6cm in diameter).
  - Imaging features suggestive of malignancy (e.g. lack of clearly circumscribed margin, vascular invasion).
  - It should be noted that post-operative adrenal suppression may occur if, preoperatively, there is biochemical evidence of glucocorticoid excess and, therefore, glucorticoids may be necessary post-operatively.
- Non-surgical management:
  - Repeat biochemical screening annually.
  - In patients with tumours that remain stable on two imaging studies carried out at least 6 months apart or tumours that show clear criteria suggesting a benign adrenal mass (pre-contrast CT density <10HU) and do not exhibit hormonal hypersecretion over 3 years, further follow-up may not be warranted. As most adrenal incidentalomas are detected upon contrast CT, a follow-up investigation without contrast to determine pre-contrast tumour density is preferable; for larger nodules (>3cm), this might be combined with CT washout studies (<40% 15min after contrast indicative of malignancy).

Further reading

Mansmann G, Lau J, Balk E, et al. (2004). The clinically inapparent adrenal mass: update in diagnosis and management. Endocr Rev **25**, 309–40.

Turner HE, Moore NR, Byrne JV, et al. (1998). Pituitary, adrenal and thyroid incidentalomas. Endocr Rel Cancer **5**, 131–50.

Young WF Jr (2007). Clinical practice. The incidentally discovered adrenal mass. N Engl J Med **356**, 601–10.

Phaeochromocytomas and paragangliomas

Definition

- *Phaeochromocytomas* (aPCA) are chromaffin tumours arising from the adrenal medulla and secreting catecholamines.
- *Paragangliomas* are tumours arising from extra-adrenal sympathetic or parasympathetic nervous tissue.
- *Sympathetic paraganglia* occur as follows: in prevertebral, paravertebral, thoracoabdominal, in the pelvis area and close to reproductive organs, prostate, bladder, liver, and the organ of Zuckerkandl (at the bifurcation of the aorta). Tumours arising from this sympathetic tissue are termed extra-adrenal functional paraganglioma (eFPGL).

Parasympathetic paraganglia are located close to major arteries and nerves, e.g. carotid body, glomus jugulare, vagal, tympanic, pulmonary, and aorta. Tumours arising from the parasympathetic nervous system are referred to as head and neck paraganglioma (HNPGL), and only a minority of those shows endocrine activity (~25%).

Incidence

Rare tumours, accounting for <0.1% of causes of hypertension. However, it is a very important diagnosis due to:

- The development of potentially fatal hypertensive crises.
- The reversibility of all its manifestations after surgical removal of the tumour.
- The lack of long-term efficacy of medical treatment.
- The appreciable incidence of malignancy.
- The implications of the identification of an underlying genetic cause (>25% of cases, e.g. RET mutations and co-incident medullary carcinoma, VHL mutations and co-incident angiomas, or SDHB mutations and their potential for recurrent and malignant tumours).

Epidemiology

- Equal sex distribution, and most commonly present in the third and fourth decades. Up to 50% may be diagnosed post-mortem.
- Tumours may be bilateral, particularly where part of an inherited syndrome (see Table 3.6).
- 10% of aPCA/eFPGL occur in patients with a family history of phaeochromocytoma, and currently 25% of patients with apparently sporadic phaeochromocytoma are found to harbour a disease-causing mutation upon genetic analysis.

Multiple tumours, extra-adrenal location, or evidence of malignancy are indicators of a high likelihood of an underlying genetic cause. See Box 3.7 for who should be screened.

Table 3.6 Genetically caused syndromes associated with phaeochromocytomas

Familial phaeochromocytomas	Isolated autosomal dominant trait
MEN-2A and 2B (📖 see p. 592)	Mutation in RET proto-oncogene (chromosome 10)
	Primary hyperparathyroidism and medullary thyroid carcinoma associated with phaeochromocytoma (aPCA)
	MEN-2B also associated with marfanoid phenotype and mucosal neuromas (tongue) (📖 see p. 592)
von Hippel–Lindau syndrome (📖 see p. 580)	Mutation of VHL tumour suppressor gene (chromosome 3)
	Renal cell carcinoma, cerebellar haemangioblastoma, retinal angioma, renal and pancreatic cysts
	Phaeochromocytomas (aPCA/eFPGL) in 25%
Neurofibromatosis (📖 see p. 578)	Autosomal dominant condition caused by mutations of *NF1* gene on chromosome 17
	Phaeochromocytomas (aPCA/eFPGL) in 1.0% and mostly late presentation (>30 years)
Succinate dehydrogenase (SDH) mutations	SDHA: rare, autosomal dominant cause of aPCA, eFPGL, HNPGL
	SDHB: autosomal dominant cause of aPCA, eFPGL, HNPGL, and renal cell carcinoma. High frequency of malignancy and extra-adrenal tumours
	SDHC: autosomal dominant cause of HNPGL (rarely, also of aPCA, eFPGL)
	SDHD: autosomal dominant cause of HNPGL, aPCA, eFPGL (disease manifestation only in individuals with paternal inheritance of mutation)
TMEM127 (transmembrane encoding gene (chromosome 2q11))	Autosomal dominant cause of aPCA, eFPGL, HNPGL
MAX (MYC associated factor X, a tumour suppressor susceptibility gene)	Autosomal dominant cause of aPCA, higher incidence of bilateral and malignant tumours (as in SDHD parent-of-origin effect: disease manifestation only in individuals with paternal transmission of the mutation)

Box 3.7 Who should be screened for the presence of a phaeochromocytoma?
- Patients with a family history of MEN, VHL, neurofibromatosis, SDH, TMEM127, MAX gene mutations.
- Patients with paroxysmal symptoms.
- Young patients with hypertension.
- Patient developing hypertensive crisis during general anaesthesia/ surgery.
- Patients with unexplained heart failure.
- Patients with an adrenal incidentaloma.

Pathophysiology

Sporadic tumours are usually unilateral and <10cm in diameter. Tumours associated with familial syndromes are more likely to be bilateral and associated with pre-existing medullary hyperplasia.

Malignancy

- Approximately 15–20% are malignant, and these are characterized by local invasion or distant metastasis rather than capsular invasion.
- Differentiating benign and malignant tumours is difficult and mainly based on the presence of metastases, although chromosomal ploidy may be useful.
- Paragangliomas are more likely to be malignant and to recur.
- Typical sites for metastases are retroperitoneum, lymph nodes, bone, liver, and mediastinum.

Secretory products

- Catecholamine secretion is usually adrenaline or noradrenaline and may be constant or episodic.
- Phenylethanolamine-N-methyltransferase (PNMT) is necessary for methylation of noradrenaline to adrenaline and is cortisol-dependent.
- Paragangliomas (exception—organ of Zuckerkandl) secrete noradrenaline only, as they lack PNMT.
- Small adrenal tumours tend to produce more adrenaline whereas larger adrenal tumours produce more noradrenaline, as a proportion of their blood supply is direct, rather than corticomedullary, and therefore, lower in cortisol concentrations.
- Pure dopamine secretion is rare and may be associated with hypotension. These tumours are more likely to be malignant.
- Other non-catecholamine secretory products may also be produced, including VIP, neuropeptide Y, ACTH (associated with Cushing's syndrome), PTH, and PTHrP.

Clinical features

- Sustained or episodic *hypertension* often resistant to conventional therapy (BUT: more and more phaeochromocytomas are found incidentally following CT imaging, thus may not show any clinical signs and symptoms).
- The presence of palpitation, headaches, or sweating in a patient with hypertension should raise the diagnostic query of phaeochromocytoma.
- *General:*
  - Sweating and heat intolerance >80%.
  - Pallor or flushing.
  - Feeling of apprehension.
  - Pyrexia.
- *Neurological*—headache (throbbing or constant) (65%), paraesthesiae, visual disturbance, seizures.
- *Cardiovascular*—palpitations (65%), chest pain, dyspnoea, postural hypotension.
- *GI*—abdominal pain, constipation, nausea.
- *Skin*—livedo reticularis.
- *Endocrine*—paroxysmal thyroid swelling (noradrenaline-secreting).

Complications

- *Cardiovascular*—left ventricular failure, dilated cardiomyopathy (reversible), dysrhythmias.
- *Respiratory*—pulmonary oedema.
- *Metabolic*—carbohydrate intolerance, hypercalcaemia.
- *Neurological*—cerebrovascular, hypertensive encephalopathy.

Factors precipitating a crisis

- Straining.
- Exercise.
- Pressure on abdomen—tumour palpation, bending over.
- Surgery.
- Drugs:
  - Anaesthetics.
  - Unopposed β-blockade.
  - IV contrast agents.
  - Opiates.
  - Tricyclic antidepressants.
  - Phenothiazines.
  - Metoclopramide.
  - Glucagon.

Investigations of phaeochromocytomas and paragangliomas

Demonstrate catecholamine hypersecretion

24h urine collection is the standard test for screening for a phaeochromocytoma. In a patient with suggestive symptoms, this is usually sufficient to confirm or exclude the diagnosis. False −ves are more common when patients are asymptomatic and early in the disease. Particular care is needed in familial cases, incidentalomas, and in those in whom a general anaesthetic has precipitated a hypertensive episode. Metadrenalines (either urine or plasma) offer more specific diagnostic tools than measurement of unmetabolized catecholamines and provide the best biochemical tests for diagnosing phaeochromocytoma. See Table 3.8 for sensitivity and specificity of tests.

24h urine collection for catecholamines/metanephrines (see Tables 3.7 and 3.8)

- Urine is collected into bottles containing acid (warn patient).
- Because of the episodic nature of catecholamine secretion, at least 2× 24h collections should be performed. It is useful to perform a collection while a patient is having symptoms if episodic secretion is suspected.
- The sensitivity of urinary VMAs is less than free catecholamines or metadrenalines and also influenced by dietary intake and should not be used. Urinary metanephrines are of similar sensitivity but of superior specificity to urinary catecholamines.
- NB Tricyclic antidepressants and labetalol interfere with adrenaline measurements and should be stopped for 4 days (Box 3.8).
- For marginal elevation, urine collections should be repeated, avoiding nuts (walnuts), fruit (bananas and pineapple), potatoes, and beans.

Plasma metanephrine measurement

- Plasma metanephrines are the most sensitive test for detection of catecholamine excess and have only slightly lower specificity than urinary metanephrines (Table 3.8).
- If plasma metanephrines are borderline, urinary metanephrines may be used for confirmation.
- Routine measurement requires controlled conditions—supine and cannulated for 30min; however, false +ves are rare, thus screening can be carried out in the sitting position without 30min rest, and only borderline positive cases require repeat after 30min supine rest.
- Plasma catecholamines are elevated by renal failure, caffeine, nicotine, exercise, and some drugs.
- Catecholamine levels in asymptomatic individuals investigated for an adrenal incidentaloma or due to a familial condition are often diagnosed at an earlier stage and may, therefore, have lower catecholamines.

Table 3.7 Substances interfering with urinary catecholamine levels

Increased catecholamines	Decreased catecholamines	Variable effect
α-blockers	Monoamine oxidase inhibitors	Levodopa
β-blockers, e.g. phenoxybenzamine	Clonidine	Tricyclic antidepressants
Levodopa	Guanethidine and other adrenergic neurone blockers	Phenothiazines
Drugs containing catecholamines, e.g. decongestants		Calcium channel inhibitors
Metoclopramide		ACE inhibitors
Domperidone		Bromocriptine
Hydralazine		
Diazoxide		
Glyceryl trinitrate		
Sodium nitroprusside		
Nicotine		
Theophylline		
Caffeine		
Amphetamine		

Table 3.8 Sensitivity and specificity of tests

Test	Sensitivity (%)	Specificity (%)
Plasma metanephrines	97	92
Urinary metanephrines	85	95
Urinary catecholamines	88	78
Urinary VMA	65	88
Clonidine suppression test	97	
MRI	98	70
CT	93	70
MIBG	80	95

- Plasma and urinary methoxytyramine levels are indicators of malignancy and can show isolated increases in patients with 'biochemically negative' malignant phaeochromocytoma.

Clonidine suppression tests (📖 see Box 3.8, p. 291)

This test may be used to differentiate patients who have borderline catecholamine levels but may offer little advantage over the screening tests already described.

- Clonidine 300 micrograms orally—failure of suppression of plasma catecholamines into the normal range at 120 and 180min is suggestive of a tumour.

Provocative tests

These are not used routinely, as they do not enhance diagnostic accuracy and are potentially dangerous.

Localization of tumour

Imaging

- These are large tumours, in contrast to Conn's syndrome, and not easily missed with good quality imaging to the bifurcation of the aorta. Approximately 98% will be detected in the abdomen.
- <2% are in the chest, and 0.02% are in the head.
- Adrenal imaging with non-ionic contrast should be performed initially, then body imaging (ideally MRI) if tumour not localized in adrenal.
- *MRI.* Bright hyperintense image on T_2.
- *CT.* Less sensitive and specific—less good at distinguishing between different types of adrenal tumours.

^{123}I-MIBG scan (📖 see Box 3.9, p. 293)

- *Meta*-iodobenzylguanidine is a chromaffin-seeking analogue. Imaging using MIBG is +ve in 60–80% phaeochromocytomas and may locate tumours not visualized on MRI, e.g. multiple and extra-adrenal tumours and also metastases of the primary tumour.
- Specificity is nearly 100%.
- Performed preoperatively to exclude multiple tumours.
- NB Phenoxybenzamine may lead to false −ve MIBG imaging, so these scans should be performed before commencing this drug where possible.
- 18F fluorodopamine PET scanning is superior to MIBG in localizing metastatic disease. No K^+ iodide is necessary to block thyroid uptake.

Positron emission tomography
- [18F]fluorodeoxyglucose (FDG) and the norepinephrine analogue [11C]metahydroxyephedrine (mHED) have both been used as radionucleotides.
- Current data are insufficient to determine which radionucleotide has the greatest sensitivity and specificity.
- Sensitivity is better than MIBG and approaches 100%, but specificity is worse, with false +ves being reported.

Box 3.8 Test procedures
Clonidine suppression test
- Patient supine and cannulated for 30min.
- Clonidine 300 micrograms orally.
- Plasma catecholamines measured at time 0, 120, and 180min.
- Failure to suppress into the normal range is suggestive of a tumour.
- 1.5% false +ve rate in patients with essential hypertension.

Screening for associated conditions

Up to 24% of patients with apparently sporadic phaeochromocytomas may have a familial disorder, and high-risk patients should, therefore, be screened for the presence of associated conditions, even if asymptomatic. Screening can be performed either by looking for associated clinical manifestations or by genetic testing.

Genetic testing in non-syndromic phaeochromocytoma has shown a hereditary predisposition in 24%, of which 45% had germline mutations in VHL, 20% had mutations in RET, 18% mutations in SDHD, and 17% mutations in SDHB. See Box 3.8 for test procedures.

MEN 2 (📖 see p. 592)

- Serum calcium.
- Serum calcitonin (phaeochromocytomas precede medullary thyroid carcinoma in 10%).

VHL (📖 see p. 580)

- Ophthalmoscopy—retinal angiomas are usually the first manifestation.
- MRI—posterior fossa and spinal cord.
- US of kidneys—if not adequately imaged on MRI of adrenals.

NF1 (📖 see p. 578)

Clinical examination for *café-au-lait* spots and cutaneous neuromas.

Succinate dehydrogenase (subunits B, C, D)

- Reports of renal carcinomas: ensure adequate imaging of kidneys.
- The SDH enzyme consists of four subunits (A, B, C, and D). SDHC and SDHD anchor the two other components which form the catalytic core to the inner mitochondrial membrane. The enzyme is a component of Krebs' cycle and also regulates the downregulation of the transcription factor HIF1α.
- The succinate dehydrogenase D subunit gene is located on chromosome 11q21–23 and the B subunit on chromosome 1p35–6.
- Mutations in SDHB, SDHC, and SDHD may cause aPCA, eFPGL, and HNPGL.
- Mutations in SDHD have been associated with familial carotid body tumours.
- Germline SDHA mutations are associated with juvenile encephalopathy.
- SHD mutations show maternal imprinting so that only carriers who inherit the mutation paternally are at risk of developing a tumour.
- Rates of penetrance and malignancy vary: SDHB mutation may be associated with a more malignant phenotype.

Indications for screening for genetic conditions as a cause for phaeochromocytoma

- Bilateral tumours.
- Extra-adrenal tumour, including head and neck.
- Age of onset (<50 years 45% +ve, >40 years 7% +ve, >50 years 1% +ve).
- Malignancy.

Box 3.9 Drugs interfering with MIBG uptake in phaeochromocytoma*

- Opioids.
- Cocaine.
- Tramadol.
- Tricyclic antidepressants:
  - Amitriptyline, imipramine.
- Sympathomimetics:
  - Phenylpropanolamine, pseudoephedrine, amphetamine, dopamine, salbutamol.
- Antihypertensives/cardiovascular agents:
  - Labetalol, metoprolol, amiodarone, reserpine, guanethidine, calcium channel blockers—nifedipine and amlodipine, ACE inhibitors—captopril and enalapril.

* Should be discontinued 7–14 days prior to scan.

Management

Medical

- It is essential that any patient is fully prepared with α- and β-blockade before receiving IV contrast or undergoing a procedure, such as venous sampling or surgery.
- α-blockade must be commenced before β-blockade to avoid precipitating a hypertensive crisis due to unopposed α-adrenergic stimulation.
- *α-blockade*—commence phenoxybenzamine as soon as diagnosis made. Start at 10mg 2× day by mouth, and increase up to 20mg 4× day (doxazosin is an accepted alternative).
- *β-blockade*—use a β-blocker, such as propranolol 20–80mg 8-hourly by mouth, 48–72h after starting phenoxybenzamine and with evidence of adequate α-blockade (generally noted by a postural fall in BP).
- Treatment is commenced in hospital. Monitor BP, pulse, and haematocrit. The goal is a BP of 130/80 or less sitting and 100mg systolic standing, pulse 60–70 sitting and 70–80 standing. Reversal of α-mediated vasoconstriction may lead to haemodilution (check Hb preoperatively).
- To ensure complete blockade before surgery, IV *phenoxybenzamine* (1mg/kg over 4h in 100mL 5% glucose) can be administered on the 3 days before surgery. There is less experience with competitive α-adrenergic blockade, such as prazosin.
- See Table 3.9 for contraindicated drugs.

Surgical (also considered in 📖 see p. 610)

- Surgical resection is curative in the majority of patients, leading to normotension in at least 75%.
- Mortality from elective surgery is <2%. It is essential that the anaesthetic and surgical teams have expertise of management of phaeochromocytomas perioperatively.
- Surgery may be laparoscopic if the tumour is small and apparently benign. Careful perioperative anaesthetic management is essential, as tumour handling may lead to major changes in BP and also occasionally cardiac arrythmias. *Phentolamine*, *nitroprusside*, or *IV nicardipine* are useful to treat perioperative hypertension, and *esmolol* or *propranolol* for perioperative arrythmias. Hypotension (e.g. after tumour devascularization) usually responds to volume replacement but occasionally requires inotropic support.
- Risk factors for haemodynamic instability during surgery include a high noradrenaline concentration, large tumour size, postural drop after β-blockade, and a mean arterial pressure >100mmHg.

Table 3.9 Contraindicated drugs in phaeochromocytomas

Drug	Examples
β-blockers	Propranolol
D2 receptor antagonists	Metoclopramide Sulpiride Chlorpromazine
Tricyclic antidepressants	Imipramine Amitriptyline Paroxetine Fluoxetine
Monoamine oxidase inhibitors	
Sympathomimetics	Ephedrine Salbutamol Cocaine
Chemotherapeutic agents	
Opioid analgesics	
Neuromuscular blocking agents	Tubocurarine Suxamethonium
Peptide and corticosteroid hormones	Glucagon ACTH Dexamethasone

Follow-up

- Cure is assessed by 24h urinary free catecholamine measurement, but since catecholamines may remain elevated for up to 10 days following surgery, these should not be performed until 2 weeks post-operatively.
- Lifelong follow-up is essential to detect recurrence of a benign tumour or metastasis from a malignant tumour, as it is impossible to exclude malignancy on a histological specimen.
- Chromogranin A is also a useful marker (falsely elevated with proton pump therapy, steroids, liver and renal failure, essential hypertension, atrophic gastritis, prostatic carcinoma, and thyrotoxicosis).

Malignancy

- Malignant tumours require long-term α- and β-blockade. The tyrosine kinase inhibitor α-*methylparatyrosine* may help control symptoms.
- High-dose ^{131}I-MIBG can be used to treat metastatic disease.
- Chemotherapy, using *cyclophosphamide*, *vincristine*, *doxorubicin*, and *dacarbazine*, has been associated with symptomatic improvement.
- Radiotherapy can be useful palliation in patients with bony metastases.
- Novel treatment options for malignant phaeochromocytoma are urgently needed, and current studies explore VEGF inhibitors on the basis of the highly vascularized nature of the tumours.

Prognosis

- Hypertension may persist in 25% patients who have undergone successful tumour removal.
- 5-year survival for 'benign' tumours is 96%, and the recurrence rate is <10%.
- 5-year survival for malignant tumours is 44%.
- SHB gene mutation patients are associated with a shorter survival.

Further reading

Astuti D, Latif F, Dallol A, et al. (2001). Gene mutations in the succinate dehydrogenase subunit SDHB cause susceptibility to familial pheochromocytoma and to familial paraganglioma. *Am J Hum Genet* **69**, 49–54.

Ayala-Ramirez M, Chougnet CN, Habra MA, et al. (2012). Treatment with sunitinib for patients with progressive metastatic pheochromocytomas and sympathetic paragangliomas. *J Clin Endocrinol Metab* **97**, 4040–50.

Eisenhofer G, Lenders JW, Timmers H, et al. (2011). Measurements of plasma methoxytyramine, normetanephrine and metanephrine as discriminators of different hereditary forms of phaeochromocytoma. *Clin Chem* **57**, 411–20.

Erickson D, Kudva YC, Ebersold MJ, et al. (2001). Benign paragangliomas: clinical presentation and treatment outcomes in 236 patients. *J Clin Endocrinol Metab* **86**, 5210–16.

Gimm O, Armanios M, Dziema H, et al. (2000). Somatic and occult germ-line mutations in SDHD, a mitochondrial complex II gene, in nonfamilial phaeochromocytoma. *Cancer Res* **60**, 6822–5.

Ilias I, Yu J, Carrasquillo JA, et al. (2003). Superiority of 6-[18F]-fluorodopamine positron emission tomography versus [131I]-metaiodobenzylguanidine scintigraphy in the localization of metastatic pheochromocytoma. *J Clin Endocrinol Metab* **88**, 4083–7.

Jafri M, Maher ER (2012). The genetics of phaeochromocytoma: using clinical features to guide genetic testing. *Eur J Endocrinol* **166**,151–8.

Lenders JW, Eisenhofer G, Mannelli M, Pacak K (2005). Phaeochromocytoma. *Lancet* **366**, 665–75.

Neumann HP, Bausch B, McWhinney SR, et al. (2002). Germ-line mutations in nonsyndromic phaeochromocytoma. *N Engl J Med* **346**, 1459–66.

Reproductive endocrinology

Reproductive physiology

Anatomy

- Normal adult ♂ testicular volume 15–30mL.
- Normal adult ♀ ovarian volume 5–10mL.
- Two gonadotrophins LH and FSH address two gonadal cell types, with feedback from sex steroids and inhibin.
- Three important cells of the gonad:
  - *Interstitial cells.*♂ Leydig cells, ♀ theca cells—which are found in between the seminiferous tubules and follicles, respectively. Produce testosterone under LH drive.
  - *Cells supporting gametogenesis.* ♂ Sertoli cells, ♀ granulosa cells—secrete various hormones, including inhibin and Müllerian inhibitory factor (AMH) under FSH drive. The former inhibits FSH secretion from the pituitary gland, and the latter is responsible for suppressing ♀ sex organ development during sexual differentiation *in utero*. In adult ♀, AMH is produced in proportion to germ cell number and is, therefore, a marker of ovarian ageing.
  - *Germ cells.*♂ continue to make new germ cells throughout adult life in the basal membrane of tubules. ♀ cease to make new germ cells after birth and are, therefore, born with all of the 'eggs' that they will ever make.
- Functional units:
  - ♂ *seminiferous tubules.* Make up 90% of testicular volume. Spermatogenesis occurs here in the presence of high intratesticular concentrations of testosterone. Made up of germ cells and Sertoli cells through which spermatogonia mature to be released into the lumen of the tubule.
  - ♀ *Graafian follicle.* Primordial follicles are recruited in batches, mature over 2 months, with selection of a dominant follicle with single central oocyte surrounded by granulosa cells which convert theca-derived testosterone to oestradiol for ovulation. Follicles which do not proceed to ovulation become atretic.

See Fig. 4.6 for the sex steroid biosynthesis pathway.

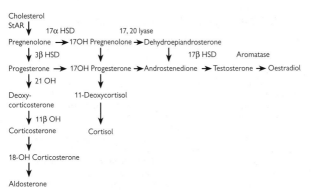

Fig. 4.6 Sex steroid biosynthesis pathway.

Regulation of gonadal function

(See Fig. 4.7 for normal menstrual cycle.)

Hypothalamus

- *Gonadotrophin-releasing hormone (GnRH)* is secreted by the hypothalamus in a pulsatile manner in response to stimuli from the cerebral cortex and limbic system via various neurotransmitters, e.g. leptin, kisspeptin, endorphins, catecholamines, and dopamine.
- GnRH release initially occurs during sleep in early puberty and then throughout the day in adulthood. It stimulates the secretion of *luteinizing hormone* (LH) and *follicle-stimulating hormone* (FSH) by the pituitary gland. The pattern of GnRH secretion is crucial for normal gonadotrophin secretion. Faster pulse frequencies are essential for LH secretion, whereas slower frequencies favour FSH secretion.
- Continuous administration of GnRH abolishes both LH and FSH secretion; therefore, superactive GnRH analogues (e.g. goserelin, triptorelin, leuprorelin) are used to suppress gonadal function.

Pituitary

- LH drives interstitial cell synthesis and secretion of testosterone in both sexes and triggers ovulation in ♀. Negative feedback by sex steroids.
- FSH in ♂ drives Sertoli cell-mediated sperm maturation and production of seminiferous tubule fluid as well as a number of substances thought to be important for spermatogenesis and inhibin. FSH in ♀ drives granulosa cell-mediated aromatization of androgens to oestradiol. Negative feedback mainly by inhibin.

Gonads

- Testosterone and small amounts of androstenedione (DHEA) and dihydrotestosterone (DHT) are produced by *Leydig cells.* ♂ testosterone has a circadian rhythm, with maximum secretion at around 8 a.m. and minimum around 9 p.m. ♀ testosterone production peaks at ovulation.
- Oestradiol production in ♂ mainly from peripheral conversion from androgens. In ♀, oestradiol rises with follicle maturation under FSH drive of granulosa cells. Oestradiol is also made by the placenta and corpus luteum.
- Progesterone secreted from *corpus luteum*, which is derived from granulosa cells, only after ovulation occurs. Peak production on day 21 of a 28-day cycle.

Regulation of gametogenesis

- Both FSH and LH are required for gametogenesis.
- LH ensures high intragonadal concentrations of testosterone (exogenous testosterone cannot substitute).
- FSH, through its action on Sertoli and granulosa cells, is vital for sperm and oocyte maturation.
- ♂. The whole process of spermatogenesis takes approximately 74 days, followed by another 12–21 days for sperm transport

through the epididymis. This means that events which may affect spermatogenesis may not be apparent for up to 3 months, and successful induction of spermatogenesis treatment may take 2 years.

- ♀. From primordial follicle to primary follicle, it takes about 180 days (a continuous process). It is then another 60 days to form a preantral follicle which then proceeds to ovulation three menstrual cycles later. Only the last 2–3 weeks of this process is under gonadotrophin drive, during which time the follicle grows from 2 to 20mm.

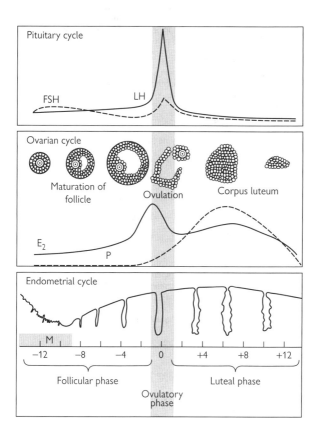

Fig. 4.7 The normal menstrual cycle.

Reproductive physiology

Sex steroid transport

Testosterone daily production rate in ♂ is 5–15mg; 2–4% of total testosterone circulates as free biologically active hormone. The rest is bound to proteins, particularly albumin and sex hormone-binding globulin (SHBG). Several equations are used to estimate free testosterone: free androgen index ((total testosterone/SHBG) × 100) is of limited value, and web-based calculators of bioactive testosterone have better validation.

Androstenedione is only about 6% SHBG-bound.

Oestradiol daily production rate in ♀ is 40–400 micrograms; 2–3% free oestradiol is biologically active; the rest is bound to SHBG.

Sex steroid metabolism

- Testosterone is converted in target tissues to the more potent androgen DHT in the presence of the enzyme 5α-reductase. There are multiple 5α-reductase isoenzymes; type 2 is the isoenzyme responsible for DHT synthesis in the genitalia, genital skin, and hair follicles. It is, therefore, essential for normal ♂ virilization and sexual development.
- Testosterone may alternatively be converted into oestradiol through the action of the aromatase enzyme, found in greatest quantities in testes and adipose tissue.
- Many effects previously attributed to testosterone are now known to be mediated by oestrogen—especially closure of epiphyses and maintenance of bone density.
- Testosterone and its metabolites are inactivated in the liver and excreted in the urine.
- Oestradiol is conjugated in the liver to sulphates and glucuronates and then extracted in the urine.

Androgen action

- Both testosterone and DHT exert their activity by binding to androgen receptors, the latter more avidly than testosterone.
- ♂ sexual differentiation during embryogenesis.
- Development and maintenance of ♂2° sex characteristics after puberty.
- Normal ♂ sexual function and behaviour.
- Spermatogenesis.
- Regulation of gonadotrophin secretion.

Oestrogen action

- Oestradiol binds to α (reproductive tissues) and β (bone, brain, heart, etc.) receptors.
- Development of ♀2° sex characteristics.
- Increase fat stores.
- Increase vaginal wall and uterine thickening.

Further reading

De Ronde W, Pols HAP, Van Leeuwen JPTM, *et al.* (2003). The importance of oestrogens in males. *Clin Endocrinol* **58**, 529–42.

Hirsutism

Definition

Hirsutism (not a diagnosis in itself) is the presence of excess hair growth in ♀ as a result of ↑ androgen production and ↑ skin sensitivity to androgens. See Table 4.1 for causes. See Box 4.1 for signs of virilization.

Physiology of hair growth

Before puberty, the body is covered by fine unpigmented hairs or vellus hairs. During adolescence, androgens convert vellus hairs into coarse, pigmented terminal hairs in androgen-dependent areas. The extent of terminal hair growth depends on the concentration and duration of androgen exposure as well as on the sensitivity of the individual hair follicle. Idiopathic hirsutism refers to those with normal investigations and presumably greater than average androgen receptor sensitivity.

The reason different body regions respond differently to the same androgen concentration is unknown but may be related to the number of androgen receptors in the hair follicle. Genetic factors play an important role in the individual susceptibility to circulating androgens, as evidenced by racial differences in hair growth.

Androgen production in women

In ♀, testosterone is secreted primarily by the ovaries and adrenal glands, although a significant amount is produced by the peripheral conversion of androstenedione and DHEA. Ovarian androgen production is regulated by luteinizing hormone, whereas adrenal production is ACTH-dependent. The predominant androgens produced by the ovaries are testosterone and androstenedione, and the adrenal glands are the main source of DHEA. Circulating testosterone is mainly bound to sex hormone-binding globulin (SHBG), and it is the free testosterone which is biologically active. Testosterone is converted to dihydrotestosterone in the skin by the enzyme 5α-reductase. Androstenedione and DHEA are not significantly protein-bound. See Fig. 4.1.

Table 4.1 Causes of hirsutism

Ovarian	PCOS	95%
	Androgen-secreting tumours	<1%
Adrenal	Congenital adrenal hyperplasia	1%
	Cushing's syndrome	<1%
	Androgen-secreting tumours	<1%
	Acromegaly	<1%
	Severe insulin resistance	<1%
Idiopathic	Normal US and endocrine profile	3%

Box 4.1 Signs of virilization
- Frontal balding.
- Deepening of voice.
- ↑ muscle size.
- Clitoromegaly.

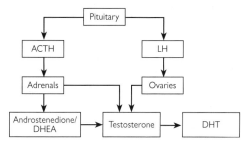

Fig. 4.1 Regulation of androgen production in ♀.

Evaluation of hirsutism

(See Box 4.2 for androgen-independent hair growth.)

Androgen-dependent hirsutism

Normally develops following puberty. Hairs are coarse and pigmented and typically grow in ♂ pattern. It is often accompanied by other evidence of androgen excess, such as acne, oily skin and hair, and male pattern alopecia.

History

- *Age and rate of onset of hirsutism.* Slowly progressive hirsutism following puberty suggests a benign cause, whereas rapidly progressive hirsutism of recent onset requires further immediate investigation to rule out an androgen-secreting neoplasm.
- *Menstrual history.* ?oligomenorrhoeic.
- Presence of other evidence of *hyperandrogenism*, e.g. acne or bitemporal hair recession.
- *Drug history.* Some progestins used in oral contraceptive preparations may be androgenic (e.g. norethisterone).
- Treatments are often based on subjective appearance, so be cautious if there is a great disparity between subjective and objective assessment. Consider psychological background.

Physical examination

- Distinguish between *androgen-dependent* and *androgen-independent* hair growth.
- Assess the *extent* and *severity* of hirsutism. The Ferriman–Gallwey score assesses the degree of hair growth in 11 regions of the body. This provides a semi-objective method of monitoring disease progression and treatment outcome but is mainly used in research rather than routine practice.
- *Virilization* should be looked for only in suspected cases of severe hyperandrogenism (see Box 4.1, p. 305).
- *Acanthosis nigricans* is indicative of insulin resistance and probable PCOS.
- *Rare causes* of hyperandrogenism, such as Cushing's syndrome and acromegaly, should be ruled out.

Box 4.2 Androgen-independent hair growth

Excess vellus hairs over face and trunk, including forehead. It does not respond to antiandrogen treatment.

  Causes of androgen-independent hair growth
- Drugs, e.g. phenytoin, ciclosporin, glucocorticoids.
- Anorexia nervosa.
- Hypothyroidism.
- Familial.

Laboratory investigation

Serum testosterone should be measured in all ♀ presenting with hirsutism. If this is <5nmol/L, then the risk of a sinister cause for her hirsutism is low. Further investigations and management of the individual disorders will be discussed in the following chapters.

Imaging

Pelvic ultrasound may be useful to diagnose PCOS. Idiopathic hirsutism refers to those with normal ovarian morphology, but this distinction is not clear-cut, as the level of detection of PCO morphology on US is operator-dependent.

Further reading

Koulori O, Conway G (2009). Management of hirsutism. *BMJ* **338**, 823–6.
Loriaux DL (2012). An approach to the patient with hirsutism. *JCEM* **97**, 2957–68.
Martin KA, Chang JR, Ehrmann DA, *et al.* (2008). Evaluation and treatment of hirsutism in premenopausal women: an Endocrine Society clinical practice guideline. *JCEM* **93**, 1105–20.

Polycystic ovary syndrome (PCOS)

Definition
- A heterogeneous clinical syndrome characterized by hyperandrogenism, mainly of ovarian origin, menstrual irregularity, and hyperinsulinaemia, in which other causes of androgen excess have been excluded (see Box 4.3).
- The diagnosis is further supported by the presence of characteristic ovarian morphology on US. Note the misnomer: the ovarian appearance refers to >12 *follicles*, i.e. polyfollicle syndrome.
- A distinction is made between polycystic ovary morphology on ultrasound (PCO which also occurs in congenital adrenal hyperplasia, acromegaly, Cushing's syndrome, and testosterone-secreting tumours) and PCOS—the syndrome. See Box 4.4 for secondary causes of PCOS.
- See Fig. 4.2 for abnormalities of hormone secretion.

Epidemiology
- PCOS is the most common endocrinopathy in ♀ of reproductive age; >95% of ♀ presenting to outpatients with hirsutism have PCOS.
- The estimated prevalence of PCOS ranges from 5 to 10% on clinical criteria. Polycystic ovaries on US alone are present in 20–25% of ♀ of reproductive age.
- First-degree ♂ relatives of women with PCOS have increased prevalence of metabolic syndrome and obesity than the general population.

Pathogenesis (📖 see Fig. 4.2, p. 309)
The fundamental pathophysiological defect is unknown, but both genetic and environmental factors are thought to play a role.

Genetic
- Familial aggregation of PCOS in 50% of ♀. A family history of type 2 diabetes mellitus is also more common in ♀ with PCOS.
- PCOS is probably a polygenic disorder.
- Implicated genes include those of the insulin pathway, testosterone biosynthesis enzymes, and obesity-related genes, including FTO gene.

Hyperandrogenism
- The main source of hyperandrogenaemia is the ovaries, although there may also be adrenal androgen hypersecretion which is poorly defined.
- The biochemical basis of ovarian dysfunction is unclear. Studies suggest an abnormality of cytochrome P450c17 activity, but this is unlikely to be the primary event but rather an index of ↑ steroidogenesis by ovarian theca cells.
- There is also an increase in the frequency and amplitude of GnRH pulses, resulting in the increase in LH concentration which is characteristic of the syndrome. This is probably due to anovulation and low progesterone levels.

Box 4.3 2003 Joint European Society of Human Reproduction and Embryology and American Society of Reproductive Medicine Consensus on the diagnosis criteria for PCOS (Rotterdam criteria)

At least two out of three of the following:
• Oligo-/amenorrhoea.
• Hyperandrogenism (clinical or biochemical).
• Polycystic ovaries on US and exclusion of other disorders.

Box 4.4 Secondary causes of polycystic ovary syndrome
• Congenital adrenal hyperplasia.
• Acromegaly.
• Cushing's syndrome.
• Testosterone-secreting tumours.

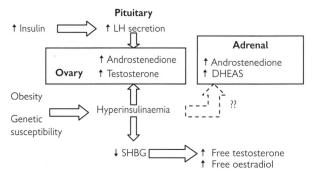

Fig. 4.2 Abnormalities of hormone secretion in PCOS.

Hyperinsulinaemia

- Approximately 70% of ♀ with PCOS are insulin-resistant, depending on the definition. The defect in insulin sensitivity appears to be selective, mainly affecting the metabolic effects of insulin (effects on muscle and liver) but sparing the ovaries where insulin acts as a co-gonadotrophin to amplify LH-mediated testosterone synthesis. Hyperinsulinaemia is exacerbated by obesity but can also be present in lean ♀ with PCOS.
- There is also evidence in a number of ♀ with PCOS of insufficient β-cell response to a glucose challenge, which is known to be a precursor to type 2 diabetes mellitus.
- Insulin also inhibits SHBG synthesis by the liver, with a consequent rise in free androgen levels.

Features

- *Onset of symptoms.* Symptoms often begin around puberty, after weight gain, or after stopping the oral contraceptive pill but can present at any time.
- *Oligo-/amenorrhoea* (70%). Due to anovulation. ♀ are usually well oestrogenized, so there is little risk of osteoporosis, unlike other causes of amenorrhoea.
- *Hirsutism* (66%):
  - 25% of ♀ also suffer from acne or male pattern alopecia. Virilization is not a feature of PCOS.
  - There is often a family history of hirsutism or irregular periods.
  - Slower onset of hirsutism makes a distinction from adrenal or ovarian tumours which are rapidly progressive and more likely to be associated with virilization and higher testosterone concentrations.
  - <1% of hirsute ♀ have non-classic congenital adrenal hyperplasia (⬚ see Clinical presentation, p. 321), and this should be excluded, particularly in ♀ with significantly raised serum testosterone levels.
- *Obesity* (50%). Symptoms worsen with obesity, as it is accompanied by ↑ testosterone concentrations as a result of hyperinsulinaemia. Acanthosis nigricans may be found in 1–3% of insulin-resistant ♀ with PCOS.
- *Infertility* (30%). PCOS accounts for 75% of cases of anovulatory infertility. The risk of spontaneous miscarriage is also thought to be higher than the general population, mainly because of obesity.

Rule out an androgen-secreting tumour

If there is:
- Evidence of virilization.
- Testosterone >5nmol/L (or >3nmol/L in post-menopausal ♀).
- Rapidly progressive hirsutism.
- *CT of adrenals or ultrasound of ovaries* will detect tumours >1cm.
- *Selective venous sampling* occasionally necessary to locate virilizing tumours undetected by imaging.
- *Ovarian suppression test* using GnRH analogues can establish ovarian origin of androgens.
- Adrenal tumours usually co-secrete cortisol as part of Cushing's syndrome.

Risks associated with PCOS

Type 2 diabetes mellitus

Type 2 diabetes mellitus is 2–4× more common in ♀ with PCOS. Impaired glucose tolerance affects 10–30% of ♀ with PCOS, and gestational diabetes is also more prevalent. The prevalence of diabetes mellitus is ↑ in ♀ with PCOS, independent of weight, but is highest in the obese group. Most important risk factor is family history of T2DM.

Dyslipidaemia

Several studies have shown an ↑ risk of hypercholesterolaemia, hypertriglyceridaemia, and low HDL cholesterol in ♀ with PCOS, but epidemiological studies of ♀ with PCOS have shown an ↑ mortality from ischaemic heart disease, despite their multiple cardiovascular risk factors.

Endometrial hyperplasia and carcinoma

In anovulatory ♀, endometrial stimulation by unopposed oestrogen results in endometrial hyperplasia. Several studies have also shown that this results in a 2–4-fold excess risk of endometrial carcinoma in ♀ with PCOS. The combination of obesity with adipose-derived oestrogen and oligomenorrhoea constitute the major risk group for uterine carcinoma.

Arterial disease

Meta-analyses suggest a 2-fold risk of arterial disease in women with PCOS relative to women without PCOS. This may not be entirely due to a high BMI.

Investigations of PCOS

The aims of investigations are mainly to exclude serious underlying disorders and to screen for complications, as the diagnosis is primarily clinical (see Box 4.3).

Confirmation of diagnosis

- Testosterone concentration:
  - Performed primarily as a screen for the presence of other causes of hyperandrogenism.
  - Often normal in ♀ with PCOS, and serum androgen concentrations do not reflect the degree of hirsutism because of variable androgen receptor sensitivity.
- LH concentration:
  - The higher the LH level, the more likely the risk of anovulation and infertility.
  - Cannot be used to diagnose PCOS, as it is normal in many affected ♀. Similarly, the traditional LH:FSH ratio is not a useful indicator.
- SHBG:
  - Low in 50% of ♀ with PCOS, owing to the hyperinsulinaemic state, with a consequent increase in circulating free androgens.
  - Useful indirect marker of insulin resistance.
- Free androgen index: FAI = 100 × (total testosterone/SHBG).
- Anti-Müllerian hormone (AMH) made by preantral follicles raised in PCOS but overlaps with normal range.
- Pelvic US of ovaries and endometrium:
  - Ultrasound criteria for PCO defined >12 follicles between 2–9mm in diameter or ovarian volume >10cm^3.
  - US is sensitive but not specific (occurs in CAH and Cushing's). Usually transvaginal but transabdominal possible in experienced hands.
  - False −ve results common in non-specialist scans.
  - Measurement of endometrial thickness is of major importance in the diagnosis of endometrial hyperplasia in the presence of anovulation. Endometrial hyperplasia is diagnosed if the endometrial thickness is >10mm.
  - Transvaginal US will also identify 90% of ovarian virilizing tumours.

Associated endocrinopathy

- *Serum prolactin.* In the presence of infertility or oligoamenorrhoea.
  - Mild hyperprolactinaemia (up to 2000mU/L) is present in up to 30% of ♀ with PCOS, and dopamine agonist treatment of this may be necessary if pregnancy is desired.
- 17OH progesterone (17OHP) level:
  - Used to exclude late-onset congenital adrenal hyperplasia.
  - Indicated in those with testosterone concentrations in excess of 5nmol/L or with evidence of virilization.
  - May also perform a Synacthen® test, looking for an exaggerated rise in 17OHP in response to ACTH in the presence of non-classic 21-hydroxylase deficiency (📖 see Clinical presentation, p. 321).
  - If the patient is ovulating, then all 17OHP measurements should be performed during the follicular phase of the cycle to avoid false +ves.
- DHEAS and androstenedione concentrations:
  - Both can be moderately raised in PCOS. DHEAS, although traditionally an adrenal marker, is probably of ovarian origin in most cases.
  - Do not need to measure routinely in ♀ with PCOS but indicated if serum testosterone >5nmol/L, in the presence of rapidly progressive hirsutism, or in the presence of virilization.
- Other:
  - Depending on clinical suspicion, e.g. urinary free cortisol or overnight dexamethasone suppression test if Cushing's syndrome is suspected, or IGF-1 if acromegaly suspected—but not routinely.

Screening for complications

- *Serum lipids and blood glucose.* All obese ♀ with PCOS should have an annual fasting glucose and fasting lipid profile. Consider OGTT in those with family history of T2DM.
- All ♀ with PCOS who fall pregnant should be screened for gestational diabetes.

Management of PCOS

(See Table 4.2.)

Weight loss

Studies have uniformly shown that weight reduction in obese ♀ with PCOS will improve insulin sensitivity and significantly reduce hyperandrogenaemia. Obese ♀ are less likely to respond to antiandrogens and infertility treatment. With a loss of 5%, ♀ with PCOS show improvement in hirsutism, restoration of menstrual regularity, and fertility.

Metformin

In obese and lean insulin-resistant ♀ with PCOS, metformin (1g–2.5g daily) improves insulin sensitivity, with a corresponding reduction in serum androgen and LH concentrations and an increase in SHBG levels. Metformin may regulate menstruation by improving ovulatory function but improved live birth rate not established. Metformin does not seem to improve response rates to ovulation induction using clomifene or gonadotrophins. Some benefits of metformin may be related to other lifestyle measures, such as diet and weight loss. Metformin is usually stopped at the diagnosis of pregnancy, as benefit in pregnancy is not proved outside of established GDM.

There have been few long-term studies looking at the effect of metformin on hirsutism, but it appears that its effects are modest at best, and most ♀ with significant hirsutism will require an antiandrogen.

♀ should be warned of its gastrointestinal side effects. In order to minimize these, they should be started on a low dose (500mg once daily) which may be ↑ gradually to a therapeutic dose over a number of weeks.

Hirsutism

Pharmacological treatment of hirsutism (see Table 4.2) is directed at slowing the growth of new hair. It can be combined with mechanical methods of hair removal, such as electrolysis and laser therapy. Therapy is most effective when started early. There is slow improvement over the first 6–12 months of treatment. Patients should be warned that facial hair is slow to respond, treatment is prolonged, and symptoms may recur after discontinuation of drugs. Adequate contraception is mandatory during pharmacological treatment of hirsutism because of possible teratogenicity.

Table 4.2 Pharmacological treatment of hirsutism

Ovarian androgen suppression	Combined oral contraceptive pill
	GnRH analogues (rarely)
Adrenal androgen suppression	Corticosteroids (rarely)
Androgen receptor antagonists	Spironolactone
	Cyproterone acetate
	Flutamide
Reductase inhibitor	Finasteride
Insulin sensitizers	Metformin
Topical inhibitors of hair follicle growth	Eflornithine

Ovarian androgen suppression

Combined oral contraceptive pill (COCP)

- The oestrogen component increases SHBG levels and thus reduces free androgen concentrations; the progestagen component inhibits LH secretion and thus ovarian androgen production.
- Dianette® (co-cyprindiol), which contains cyproterone acetate (2mg), or Yasmin®, which contains drospirenone, are preferred because the progestagens are antiandrogenic. Benefit of these brands over third generation COCP has not been established, so brands, such as Cilest®, Marvelon®, and Femodene®, make suitable alternatives.
- The effect of the COCP alone on hair growth is modest, so it may be combined with an antiandrogen.

GnRH analogues

- Suppress gonadotrophin secretion and thus ovarian androgen production.
- Rarely used. They cause oestrogen deficiency so have to be combined with 'add-back' oestrogen treatment. Also, they are expensive and need to be given parenterally.
- Use is confined to ♀ with severe hyperandrogenism in whom antiandrogens have been ineffective or not tolerated.

Androgen receptor blockers

These are most effective when combined with oral contraceptives. All are contraindicated in pregnancy. They act by competitively inhibiting the binding of testosterone and dihydrotestosterone to the androgen receptor.

Spironolactone

- Antiandrogen of choice, particularly in overweight ♀.
- *Dose.* 100–200mg a day.
- *Side effects.* Polymenorrhoea if not combined with the COCP. A fifth of ♀ complain of GI symptoms when on high doses of spironolactone. Potassium levels should be monitored, and other potassium-sparing drugs should be avoided.

Cyproterone acetate (CPA)
- *Dose.* 25–100mg, days 1–10 of the pill cycle, in combination with the COCP.
- *Side effects.* Amenorrhoea if given alone for prolonged periods or in higher doses. *Progesterone side effects.* Hepatic toxicity rare, but monitoring of liver function 6-monthly is recommended.
- A *washout period* of 3–4 months is recommended prior to attempting conception.

Flutamide
- A potent antiandrogen.
- *Dose.* 125–250mg a day; 1mg/kg daily may be effective and associated with a lower frequency of hepatic adverse effects.
- *Side effects.* Dry skin, nausea in 10%. However, there is a 0.4% risk of hepatic toxicity, and it should, therefore, be used with extreme caution.

5α-reductase inhibitors
Block the conversion of testosterone to the more potent androgen dihydrotestosterone.
- Finasteride:
  - *Dose.* 1–2.5mg a day. A weak antiandrogen.
  - *Side effects.* No significant adverse effects.
  - Can be used as monotherapy, or to combine with other antiandrogens or COCP.
  - Adequate contraceptive measures are mandatory because of its teratogenicity. In addition, pregnancy should not be attempted until at least 3 months after drug cessation.

Eflornithine 11.5%
- Irreversibly blocks the enzyme ornithine decarboxylase which is involved in growth of hair follicles.
- It is administered as a topical cream on the face to reduce new hair growth. Studies have shown its efficacy in the management of mild facial hirsutism, following at least 8 weeks of treatment. Treatment should be discontinued if there is no benefit at 4 months. It is not a depilatory cream and so must be combined with mechanical methods of hair removal.
- *Side effects.* Skin irritation with burning or pruritus, acne, hypersensitivity.

Amenorrhoea
- A minimum of a withdrawal bleed every 3 months minimizes the risk of endometrial hyperplasia.
- *Treatment:*
  - COCP.
  - Cyclical progestagen: Cerazette® (desogestrel) is a progesterone-only contraceptive pill with minimal androgenic properties. Medroxyprogesterone acetate 5–10mg bd for 12 days of each calendar month. Norethisterone should be avoided, as it is more androgenic.
  - Metformin (up to 1g bd) which also improves lipoprotein pattern.

Infertility

Ovulation induction regimens are indicated. Obesity adversely affects fertility outcome, with poorer pregnancy rates and higher rates of miscarriage, so weight reduction should be strongly encouraged.

Metformin

- Use remains controversial but probably does not improve pregnancy rates in insulin-resistant, particularly overweight, ♀ with PCOS. No reported teratogenic or neonatal complications.
- *Dose.* 500mg od after meals, to be ↑ gradually to 1g bd. If ovulation restored following 6 months of treatment, then continue for up to 1 year. If pregnancy does not occur, then consider other treatments.
- *Side effects.* Nausea, bloating, diarrhoea, vomiting.

Clomifene citrate

- Inhibits oestrogen negative feedback, ↑ FSH secretion and thus stimulating ovarian follicular growth.
- *Dose.* 25–150mg a day from day 2 of menstrual cycle for 5 days.
- *Response rates.* 80% ovulation rate, 67% pregnancy rate.
- *Complications.* 8% twins, 0.1% higher order multiple pregnancy. Risk of ovarian neoplasia following prolonged clomifene treatment remains unclear, so limit treatment to a maximum of six cycles.

Gonadotrophin preparations (hMG or FSH)

- Used in those unresponsive to clomifene. Low-dose regimes show better response rates and fewer complications, e.g. 75IU/day for 2 weeks, then increase by 37.5IU/day every 7 days, as required.
- 94% ovulation rate and 50% pregnancy rate.
- *Complications.* Hyperstimulation, multiple pregnancies.
- Close ultrasonic monitoring is essential.

Surgery

- Laparoscopic ovarian diathermy or laser drilling may restore ovulation in up to 90% of ♀, with cumulative pregnancy rates of 80% within 8 months of treatment. Particularly effective in slim ♀ with PCOS and high LH concentrations.
- *Complications.* Surgical adhesions although usually mild.

In vitro fertilization

- In ♀ who fail to respond to ovulation induction.
- 60–80% conception rate after six cycles.

Acne

Treatment for acne should be started as early as possible to prevent scarring. All treatments take up to 12 weeks before significant improvement is seen. All treatments, apart from benzoyl peroxide, are contraindicated in pregnancy.

Mild-to-moderate acne

Topical benzoyl peroxide 5%. Bactericidal properties. May use in conjunction with oral antibiotic therapy to reduce the risk of developing resistance to antibiotics. Side effects: skin irritation and dryness. Add oral antibiotics if no improvement after 2 months of treatment.

CHAPTER 4 **Reproductive endocrinology**

Moderate-to-severe acne

- *Topical retinoids*, e.g. tretinoin, isotretinoin. Useful alone in mild acne or in conjunction with antibiotics in moderately severe acne. Continue as maintenance therapy to prevent further acne outbreaks. Side effects: irritation, photosensitivity. Apply high factor sunscreen before sun exposure. Avoid in acne involving large areas of skin.
- *Oral antibiotics*, e.g. oxytetracycline 500mg bd, doxycycline 100mg od, or minocycline 100mg od. Response usually seen by 6 weeks and full efficacy by 3 months. Continue antibiotics for 2 months after control is achieved. Prescription usually given for a course of 3–6 months. Continue topical retinoids and/or benzoyl peroxide to prevent further outbreaks.
- *COCP and antiandrogens*. As for hirsutism.

Severe acne

Isotretinoin is very effective in ♀ with severe acne or acne which has not responded to other oral or topical treatments. Used early, it can minimize scarring in inflammatory acne. However, it is highly toxic and can only be prescribed by a consultant dermatologist. Also consider referring ♀ who develop acne in their 30s or 40s and ♀ with psychological problems as a result of acne.

Further reading

Diamanti-Kandarakis E, Dunaif A. (2012). Insulin resistance and the polycystic ovary syndrome revisited: an update on mechanisms and implications. *Endocr Rev* **33**, 981–1030.

Dunaif A (1997). Insulin resistance and polycystic ovary syndrome: mechanism and implications for pathogenesis. *Endoc Rev* **18**, 774–800.

Ehrmann DA (2005). Polycystic ovary syndrome. *N Engl J Med* **352**, 1223–36.

Ehrmann DA, Rychlik D (2003). Pharmacological treatment of polycystic ovary syndrome. *Semin Reprod Med* **21**, 277–83.

Ledger WL, Clark T (2003). Long term consequences of polycystic ovary syndrome. *Royal College of Obstetrics and Gynaecology* Guideline number 33. Royal College of Obstetrics and Gynaecology, London.

Lord JM, Flight IHK, Norman RJ (2003). Insulin sensitizing drugs for polycystic ovary syndrome. *Cochrane Database Syst review* 2003.

Neithardt AB, Barnes RB (2003). The diagnosis and management of hirsutism. *Semin Reprod Med* **21**,285–93.

Nestler JE (2008). Metformin for the treatment of the polycystic ovary syndrome. *N Engl J Med* **358**, 47–54.

Palomba S (2009). Evidence-based and potential benefits of metformin in the polycystic ovary syndrome: a comprehensive review. *Endocr Rev* **30**, 1–50.

Paradisi R (2010). Retrospective observational study on the effects and tolerability of flutamide in a large population of patients with various kinds of hirsutism over a 15-year period. *Eur J Endocrinol* **163**, 139–4.

Pierpoint T, McKeigue PM, Isaacs AJ, et al. (1998). Mortality of women with polycystic ovary syndrome at long term follow up. *J Clin Epidemiol* **51**, 581–6.

Randeva HS, et al. (2012). Cardiometabolic aspects of the polycystic ovary syndrome. *Endocr Rev* **33**, 812–41.

The Rotterdam ESHRE/ASRM-sponsored PCOS consensus workshop group (2004). Revised 2003 Consensus on diagnostic criteria and long-term health risks related to polycystic ovary syndrome. *Hum Reprod* **19**, 41–7.

Tsilchorozidou T, Overton C, Conway GS (2004). The pathophysiology of polycystic ovary syndrome. *Clin Endocrinol* **60**, 1–17.

Congenital adrenal hyperplasia (CAH) in adults

Definition
CAH is a group of inherited disorders characterized by a deficiency of one of the enzymes necessary for cortisol biosynthesis.
- >90% of cases are due to 21α-hydroxylase deficiency.
- Wide clinical spectrum, from presentation in neonatal period with salt wasting and virilization to non-classic CAH in adulthood.
- Autosomal recessive.
- Clinical presentation depends on severity of mutation.

Epidemiology
- Carrier frequency of classic CAH 1:60–1:100 in Caucasians.
- Carrier frequency of non-classic CAH 19% in Ashkenazi Jews, 13.5% in Hispanics, 6% in Italians, and 3% in other Caucasian populations.

Pathogenesis
Genetics
- *CYP21* encodes for the 21α-hydroxylase enzyme, located on the short arm of chromosome 6 (chromosome 6p21.3). In close proximity is the *CYP21* pseudogene, with 90% homology but no functional activity.
- 21α-hydroxylase deficiency results from gene mutations, partial gene deletions, or gene conversions in which sequences from the pseudogene are transferred to the active gene, rendering it inactive. There is a correlation between the severity of the molecular defect and the clinical severity of the disorder. Non-classic CAH is usually due to a point mutation (single base change); missense mutations result in simple virilizing disease, whereas a gene conversion or partial deletion usually results in presentation in infancy, with salt wasting or severe virilization.

Biochemistry
(See Fig. 4.3.)

21α-hydroxylase deficiency results in aldosterone and cortisol deficiency. Loss of −ve feedback from cortisol results in ACTH hypersecretion, and this causes adrenocortical hyperplasia and accumulation of steroid precursors 'above' the enzyme deficiency, including progesterone and 17-hydroxyprogesterone (17OHP). These are then shunted into androgen synthesis pathways, resulting in testosterone and androstenedione excess.

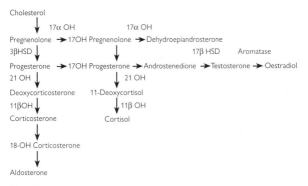

Fig. 4.3 Adrenal steroid biosynthesis pathway.

Clinical presentation

Classic CAH

- Most patients are diagnosed in infancy, and their clinical presentation is discussed elsewhere (📖 see Congenital adrenal hyperplasia, p. 320).
- *Problems persisting into adulthood.* Sexual dysfunction and subfertility in ♀, particularly in salt wasters. Reconstructive genital surgery is required in the majority of ♀ who were virilized at birth to create an adequate vaginal introitus. With improvement of medical care, normal pregnancy rates (90%) can be achieved.
- In ♂, high levels of adrenal androgens suppress gonadotrophins and thus testicular function. ↑ ACTH results in the development of testicular adrenal rest tissue (TARTs). These are always benign but may be misdiagnosed as testicular tumours. TARTs can be destructive, leading to testicular failure. Spermatogenesis is often low if CAH is poorly controlled.
- There is a significant risk of adrenal crises over lifetime.
- There is an impaired quality of life.

Non-classic CAH

- Due to partial deficiency of 21α-hydroxylase. Glucocorticoid and aldosterone production are normal, but there is overproduction of 17OHP and thus androgens.
- Present with hirsutism (60%), acne (33%), and oligomenorrhoea (54%), often around the onset of puberty. Only 13% of ♀ present with subfertility.
- Polycystic ovaries on US are common, and adrenal incidentalomas or hyperplasia are seen in 40%.
- Asymptomatic in ♂. The effect of non-classic CAH on ♂ fertility is unknown.

Investigations of CAH in adults

Because of the diurnal variation in adrenal hormonal secretion, all investigations should be performed at 9 a.m.

Diagnosis of non-classic CAH—17OHP measurement

Timing of measurement

- Screen in the follicular phase of the menstrual cycle. 17OHP is produced by the corpus luteum, so false +ve results may occur if measured in the luteal phase of the cycle.

Interpretation of result

- <5nmol/L—normal.
- >15nmol/L—CAH.
- 5–15nmol/L—proceed to ACTH stimulation test. A fifth will have non-classic CAH.

ACTH stimulation test

- Measure 17OHP 60min after ACTH administration.
- An exaggerated rise in 17OHP is seen in non-classic CAH.
- 17OHP level <30nmol/L post-ACTH excludes the diagnosis.
- Most patients have levels >45nmol/L.
- Levels of 30–45nmol/L suggest heterozygosity or non-classic CAH.
- Cortisol response to ACTH stimulation is usually low normal.

Other investigations

Androgens

- In poorly controlled classic CAH in ♀, testosterone and androstenedione levels may be in the adult ♂ range. Dehydroepiandrosterone sulphate levels are usually only mildly, and not consistently, elevated in CAH.
- Circulating testosterone, and particularly androstenedione, is elevated in non-classic CAH, but there is a large overlap with levels seen in PCOS, so serum androgen concentrations cannot be used to distinguish between the disorders.

Renin

- Plasma renin activity elevated due to aldosterone deficiency, indicating inadequate fludrocortisone dose if markedly raised.
- A proportion of ♀ with non-classic CAH may also have mildly elevated renin concentrations.

ACTH

- Greatly elevated in poorly controlled classic CAH.
- Usually normal levels in non-classic CAH.

See Table 4.3 for a list of enzyme deficiencies in CAH.

Table 4.3 Enzyme deficiencies in CAH

Enzyme deficiency	Incidence (per births)	Clinical features
Classic 21α-hydroxylase	1:10,000–1:15,000	Salt wasting, ambiguous genitalia in females, precocious pubarche in males
Non-classic 21α-hydroxylase (partial deficiency)	1:27–1:1,000	Hirsutism, oligomenorrhoea in pubertal girls, asymptomatic in boys
11β-hydroxylase	1:100,000	Ambiguous genitalia, virilization, hypertension
3β-hydroxylase	Rare	Mild virilization, salt wasting in severe cases
17α-hydroxylase	Rare	Delayed puberty in females, pseudohermaphroditism in males, hypertension, hypokalaemia

Management of CAH in adults

The aims of treatment of CAH in adulthood under specialist care are:
- To maintain normal energy levels and weight and avoid adrenal crises.
- To minimize hyperandrogenism and to restore regular menses and fertility in ♀.
- To avoid glucocorticoid over-replacement.
- To treat stress with adequate extra glucocorticoid.

Classic CAH

- *Prednisolone.* Total dose 5–7.5mg/day. Given in two divided doses, with one-third of the total dose given on waking (about 7 a.m.) and two-thirds of the dose on retiring. The aim is to suppress the early morning peak of ACTH and thus androgen secretion. The optimum dose is the minimum dose required to normalize serum androgens. Occasional patients who are not controlled on prednisolone may be optimally treated with nocturnal dexamethasone instead (0.25–0.5mg nocte).
- As with other forms of adrenal insufficiency, glucocorticoid doses should be doubled during illness. This is discussed in detail elsewhere (📖 see p. 274).
- Those with salt-losing form of CAH and who require mineralocorticoid replacement therapy with fludrocortisone in a dose of 50–200 micrograms/day is given as a single daily dose. The aim is to avoid suppression of plasma renin activity and risk of hypertension. Normal or slightly elevated levels are accepted.
- Bilateral adrenalectomy may, very occasionally, be considered for intractable infertility in females.
- *Pregnancy.* Patient and partners require prior CYP21 mutation analysis at the earliest opportunity to enable genetic counselling. If partner is a carrier, 50% risk of affected child (1 in 63 is a carrier of the 21 OH gene).

Non-classic CAH

- *Oligo-/amenorrhoea.* Prednisolone 2.5–5mg/day may be used but is often reserved to normalize ovulatory function.
- *Hirsutism and acne.* May alternatively, and more effectively, be treated as for PCOS (📖 see Management, p. 314). Spironolactone should be avoided because of the potential risk of salt wasting and thus hyperreninaemia.
- If plasma renin level is elevated, then fludrocortisone, given in a dose sufficient to normalize renin concentrations, may improve adrenal hyperandrogenism.
- ♂ may not require treatment. The occasional ♂ may need glucocorticoids to treat subfertility.

Management of pregnancy in CAH

- *Maternal classic CAH.* Screen patient/partner using basal ± ACTH-stimulated 17OHP levels (see Investigations, p. 322). If levels elevated, proceed to genotyping. If heterozygote, then preimplantation genetic diagnosis or prenatal treatment of fetus may be considered.
- Physiological prednisolone or hydrocortisone rarely needs adjusting in pregnancy. Routine biochemical markers cannot be used in pregnancy, so treat symptomatically.
- Adjust fludrocortisone against BP.
- Placental aromatase protects fetus from maternal androgens. >200 pregnancies reported to mothers with CAH—no case of fetal virilization recorded, so monitoring testosterone not required.
- >75% Caesarian section rate because of masculinized pelvis and surgical scarring following vaginoplasty.
- Routine glucocorticoid boost at delivery.

Prenatal treatment of pregnancies at risk of CAH

Aim of prenatal treatment is to prevent virilization of an affected ♀ fetus.

- Only to be considered if previous child from same partner with CAH or known mutations in both parents. Mutations must be identified well before trying to conceive (this cannot be done on the run).
- NOT for mothers with CAH, unless partner is a known carrier of a severe mutation.
- Only to be considered by experienced unit. Current guidelines consider this still in the realms of research, as long-term outcome of dexamethasone exposure to unaffected fetuses is unknown.

Treatment (commenced before 10 weeks' gestation)

Dexamethasone (20 micrograms/kg maternal body weight), in three divided doses a day, crosses the placenta and reduces fetal adrenal hyperandrogenism. Discontinue if ♂ fetus.

Outcome

50–75% of affected ♀ do not require reconstructive surgery.

Monitoring of treatment

Annual follow-up is usually adequate in adults.

- *Clinical assessment.* Measure BP and weight. Look for evidence of hyperandrogenism and glucocorticoid excess. Amenorrhoea in ♀ usually suggests inadequate therapy but may have to be accepted as can often not be achieved without excessive doses of glucocorticoid.
- Suppressed levels of 17OHP, testosterone (T), and renin are an indication for reduced dose of steroid. Normalizing will often result in complications from supraphysiological doses of glucocorticoids.
- Modestly raised or high normal levels of 17OHP, T, and renin are optimal.
- *Consider bone density which may be reduced by supraphysiological steroid doses.*
- Testicular function requires special attention. Low LH is a sign of raised adrenal androgens. Raised FSH may follow adrenal rests as a sign of testicular failure. US testis every 3–5 years. Consider sperm count/storage if adrenal rests are present.
- US ovaries not useful routinely, as PCO morphology is common.
- In men, testicular adrenal rest tumours may develop (up to 94%). Their detection may prevent infertility later. Ultrasound screening of the scrotum is suggested every 2 years.

Prognosis

Adults with treated CAH have a normal life expectancy. Improvement in medical and surgical care has also improved QoL for most sufferers. However, there are a few unresolved issues:

- *Height.* Despite optimal treatment in childhood, patients with CAH are, on average, significantly shorter than their predicted genetic height. Studies suggest that this may be due to overtreatment with glucocorticoids during infancy.
- *Fertility.* Mainly a problem in ♂ with poorly controlled classic CAH and adrenal rests.
- *Adrenal incidentalomas.* Benign adrenal adenomas have been reported in up to 50% of patients with classic CAH. ♂ with CAH may develop gonadal adrenocortical rests.
- *Psychosexual issues.* Gender dysphoria common in ♀. A significant number of ♀ with classic CAH, despite adequacy of vaginal reconstruction, are not sexually active.

Further reading

Arlt W, *et al.* (2010). Health status of adults with congenital adrenal hyperplasia: a cohort study of 203 patients. *J Clin Endocrinol Metab* **95**, 5110–21.

Aycan Z, Bas VN, Cetinkaya S, *et al.* (2013) Prevalence and long-term follow-up outcomes of testicular adrenal rest tumours in children and adolescent males with congenital adrenal hyperplasia. *Clin Endocrinol* **78**, 667–72.

Cabrera MS, Vogiatzi MG, New MI (2001). Long term outcome in adult males with classic congenital adrenal hyperplasia. *J Clin Endocrinol Metab* **86**, 3070–8.

Joint LWPES/ESPE CAH Working Group (2002). Consensus statement on 21-hydroxylase deficiency from the Lawson Wilkins Paediatric Endocrine Society and the European Society for Paediatric Endocrinology. *J Clin Endocrinol Metab* **87**, 4048–53.

Merke DP (2008). Approach to the adult with congenital adrenal hyperplasia due to 21-hydroxylase deficiency. *JCEM* **93**, 653–60.

New MI (2006). Extensive clinical experience: nonclassical 21-hydroxylase deficiency. *J Clin Endocrinol Metab* **91**, 205–14.

New MI, Carlson A, Obeid J, *et al.* (2001). Prenatal diagnosis for congenital adrenal hyperplasia in 532 pregnancies. *J Clin Endocrinol Metab* **86**, 5651–757.

Ogilvie CM, Crouch NS, Rumsby G, *et al.* (2006). Congenital adrenal hyperplasia in adults: a review of medical, surgical and psychological issues. *Clin Endocrinol* **64**, 2–11.

Premawaradhana LDKE, Hughes IA, Read GF, *et al.* (1997). Longer term outcome in females with congenital adrenal hyperplasia: the Cardiff experience. *Clin Endocrinol* **46**, 327–32.

Speiser PW, White PC (2003). Congenital adrenal hyperplasia. *N Engl J Med* **349**, 776–88.

Speiser PW, *et al.* (2010). Congenital adrenal hyperplasia due to steroid 21-hydroxylase deficiency: an Endocrine Society clinical practice guideline. *J Clin Endocrinol Metab* **95**, 4133–60.

Androgen-secreting tumours

Definition

Rare tumours of the ovary or adrenal gland which may be benign or malignant, which cause virilization in ♀ through androgen production.

Epidemiology and pathology

Androgen-secreting ovarian tumours

- 75% develop before the age of 40 years.
- Account for 0.4% of all ovarian tumours; 20% are malignant.
- Tumours are 5–25cm in size. The larger they are, the more likely they are to be malignant. They are rarely bilateral.
- Two major types:
  - Sex cord stromal cell tumours: often contain testicular cell types.
  - Adrenal-like tumours: often contain adrenocortical or Leydig cells.
- Other tumours, e.g. gonadoblastomas and teratomas, may also, on occasion, present with virilization.

Androgen-secreting adrenal tumours

- 50% develop before the age of 50 years.
- Larger tumours, particularly >6cm, are more likely to be malignant.
- Usually with concomitant cortisol secretion as a variant of Cushing's syndrome.

Clinical features

- *Onset of symptoms.* Usually recent onset of rapidly progressive symptoms.
- *Hyperandrogenism:*
  - Hirsutism of varying degree, often severe; male pattern balding and acne are also common.
  - Usually oligo-/amenorrhoea.
  - Infertility may be a presenting feature.
- *Virilization.* (🔲 see Box 4.1, p. 305.) Indicates severe hyperandrogenism, is associated with clitoromegaly, and is present in 98% of ♀ with androgen-producing tumours. Not usually a feature of PCOS.
- *Other:*
  - Abdominal pain.
  - Palpable abdominal mass.
  - Ascites.
  - Symptoms and signs of Cushing's syndrome are present in many of ♀ with adrenal tumours.

Investigations

See Fig. 4.4.

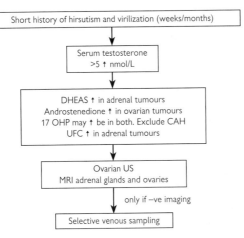

Fig. 4.4 Investigation of androgen-secreting tumours.

Management

Surgery
- Adrenalectomy or ovarian cystectomy/oophorectomy.
- Curative in benign lesions.

Adjunctive therapy
Malignant ovarian and adrenal androgen-secreting tumours are usually resistant to chemotherapy and radiotherapy.

Prognosis

Benign tumours
- Prognosis excellent.
- Hirsutism improves post-operatively, but clitoromegaly, male pattern balding, and deep voice may persist.

Malignant tumours
- *Adrenal tumours.* 20% 5-year survival. Most have metastatic disease at the time of surgery.
- *Ovarian tumours.* 30% disease-free survival and 40% overall survival at 5 years.

Further reading
Hamilton-Fairley D, Franks S (1997). Androgen-secreting tumours. In: Sheaves R, Jenkins PJ, Wass JAH (eds.) *Clinical endocrine oncology*, pp. 323–9. Blackwell Science, Oxford.
Rothman MS, Wierman ME (2011). How should postmenopausal androgen excess be evaluated? *Clin Endocrinol (Oxf)* **75**, 160–4.

Menstrual function disorder—assessment and investigation

Definitions

- *Oligomenorrhoea* is defined as the reduction in the frequency of menses to <9 periods a year.
- *1° amenorrhoea* is the failure of menarche by the age of 16 years. Prevalence ~0.3%
- *2° amenorrhoea* refers to the cessation of menses for >6 months in ♀ who had previously menstruated. Prevalence ~3%.
- See Table 4.4 for WHO categorization.

Aetiology

Although the list of causes is long (see Box 4.5 for causes), the majority of cases of secondary amenorrhoea can be accounted for by four conditions:
- Polycystic ovary syndrome.
- Hypothalamic amenorrhoea.
- Hyperprolactinaemia.
- Ovarian failure.

Table 4.4 WHO categorization of hypogonadism

WHO group	LH and FSH	Clinical
I	↓	Hypogonadotrophic hypogonadism
II	→	PCOS or mild hypothalamic amenorrhoea
III	↑	POF

Box 4.5 Causes of amenorrhoea

Physiological
- Pregnancy and lactation.
- Post-menopause.

Iatrogenic
- Depot medroxyprogesterone acetate.
- Levonorgestrel-releasing intrauterine device.
- Progesterone-only pill.

Pathological—1°
- Chromosomal abnormalities—50%:
  - Turner's syndrome.
  - Other X chromosomal disorders.
- 2° hypogonadism—25%:
  - Kallmann's syndrome.
  - Pituitary disease.
  - Hypothalamic amenorrhoea.
- Genitourinary malformations—15%:
  - Imperforate hymen.
  - Absence of uterus, cervix, or vagina, e.g. *Rokitansky syndrome*, *androgen insensitivity syndrome*.
- Other—10%:
  - CAH.
  - PCOS.

Most causes of 2° amenorrhoea can also cause 1° amenorrhoea.

Pathological—2°
- Ovarian—70%:
  - PCOS.
  - Premature ovarian failure.
- Hypothalamic—15%:
  - Hypogonadotrophic hypogonadism.
  - Hypothalamic amenorrhoea.
  - Weight loss.
  - Infiltrative lesions of the hypothalamus.
  - Drugs, e.g. opiates.
- Pituitary—5%:
  - Hyperprolactinaemia.
  - Hypopituitarism.
- Uterine—5%:
  - Intrauterine adhesions—*Asherman's syndrome*.
- Other endocrine disorders—5%:
  - Thyroid dysfunction.
  - Hyperandrogenism—Cushing's syndrome, CAH, tumour.

Menstrual function disorder—clinical evaluation

PCOS is the only common endocrine cause of amenorrhoea with normal oestrogenization—all other causes are oestrogen-deficient. Women with PCOS, therefore, are at risk of endometrial hyperplasia, and all others are at risk of osteoporosis.

History

- Oestrogen deficiency, e.g. hot flushes, reduced libido, and dyspareunia.
- Hypothalamic dysregulation, e.g. exercise and nutritional history, body weight changes, emotional stress, recent or chronic physical illness.
- In 1° amenorrhoea—history of breast development, history of cyclical pain, age of menarche of mother and sisters.
- In 2° amenorrhoea—duration and regularity of previous menses, family history of early menopause or familial autoimmune disorders, or galactosaemia.
- Anosmia may indicate Kallman's syndrome.
- Hirsutism or acne.
- Galactorrhoea.
- History suggestive of pituitary, thyroid, or adrenal dysfunction.
- Drug history—e.g. causes of hyperprolactinaemia, chemotherapy, hormonal contraception, recreational drug use.
- Obstetric and surgical history.

Physical examination

- Height, weight, BMI.
- Features of Turner's syndrome or other dysmorphic features.
- 2° sex characteristics.
- Galactorrhoea.
- Evidence of hyperandrogenism or virilization.
- Evidence of thyroid dysfunction.
- Anosmia, visual field defects.

Amenorrhoea with normal gonadotrophins—WHO group II

In routine practice, a common differential diagnosis is between mild version of PCOS and hypothalamic amenorrhoea (HA). The distinction between these conditions may require repeated testing, as a single snapshot may not discriminate. The reason to be precise is that PCOS is oestrogen-replete and will, therefore, respond to clomiphene citrate (an antioestrogen) for fertility. HA will be oestrogen-deficient and will need HRT and ovulation induction with pulsatile GnRH or hMG.

For comparison, see Table 4.5.

Table 4.5 Comparison of two common causes of amenorrhoea with normal gonadotrophins

	PCOS	Hypothalamic amenorrhoea
Exercise programme	Rare	Common
Androgen excess	Common	Rare
BMI usually	>21	<21
LH	↑ or →	↓ or →
Polycystic ovaries	90%	20%
Endometrial thickness	>4mm	<5mm

Menstrual function disorder—investigations

(See Fig. 4.5.)
- Is it 1° or 2° ovarian dysfunction?
  - FSH, LH, TFT, oestradiol, prolactin.
- Ultrasound:
  - Ovarian and uterine morphology—exclude anatomical abnormalities, PCOS, and Turner's syndrome.
  - Note that PCO morphology is present in 20% of all women, so their presence may be false +ve.
  - Endometrial thickness—to assess oestrogen status.
- Other tests, depending on clinical suspicion:
  - Induce withdrawal bleed with progesterone (e.g. 10mg medroxyprogesterone acetate bd for 7 days). If a bleed occurs, then there is adequate oestrogen priming and endometrial development. This test has poor specificity and sensitivity and has been abandoned in favour of ultrasound in many centres.
  - Serum testosterone in the presence of hyperandrogenism.
  - Karyotype in ovarian failure or disorder of sexual development suspects (absent uterus).
  - MRI of the pituitary fossa if FSH low or in the presence of hyperprolactinaemia.
  - Bone density if long-term oestrogen deficiency.

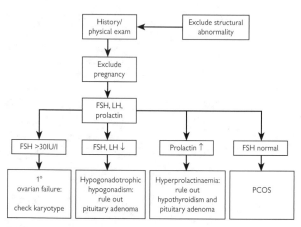

Fig. 4.5 Investigation of amenorrhoea.

Management of amenorrhoea

- Treat underlying disorder, for example:
  - Dopamine agonists for prolactinomas.
  - Pituitary surgery for pituitary tumours.
  - Eating disorder clinic in anorexia nervosa.
- Treat oestrogen deficiency—oestrogen/progestagen preparations.
- Treat infertility—📖 see p. 334.
- In PCOS with endometrial hyperplasia—progesterone withdrawal bleed, and consider hysteroscopy in resistant cases.
- See Box 4.6 for progesterone sensitivity.

Box 4.6 Progesterone sensitivity

- Skin condition occurs regularly premenstrually—settling with onset of menses.
- Dermatosis includes eczema, pompholyx, urticaria, and erythema multiforme.
- Autoantibodies present (+ve challenge test).

Further reading

Baird DT (1997). Amenorrhoea. *Lancet* **350**, 275–9.

Beswick SJ, Lewis HM, Stewart PM (2002). A recurrent rash treated by oophorectomy. *QJM* **95**, 636–7.

Hickey M, Balen A (2003). Menstrual disorders in adolescence: investigation and management. *Hum Reprod Update* **9**, 493–504.

Premature ovarian insufficiency (POI), including Turner's syndrome in adults

Definition

POI is a disorder characterized by amenorrhoea, oestrogen deficiency, and elevated gonadotrophins, developing in ♀ <40 years, as a result of loss of ovarian follicular function. See Box 4.7 for Turner's syndrome and Table 4.6 for correlation of karyotype with phenotype.

Epidemiology

- Incidence—0.1% of ♀ <30 years and 1% of those <40 years.
- Accounts for 10% of all cases of 2° amenorrhoea.
- 20% familial.
- 80% idiopathic.

Causes of POI

- Chromosomal abnormalities (5–10%):
  - Turner's syndrome.
  - Fragile X premutations.
  - Other X chromosomal abnormalities.
- Gene mutations:
  - Galactosaemia.
  - A variety of rare single gene defects that are not yet part of routine testing (e.g. NOBOX, FSHR, FOXL2).
- Autoimmune disease (20%).
- Iatrogenic:
  - Chemotherapy.
  - Radiotherapy.
  - Pelvic surgery.
- Other:
  - Enzyme deficiencies, e.g. 17-hydroxylase deficiency.
  - Infections, e.g. mumps, CMV.
- Idiopathic:
  - ? environmental toxin.

Pathogenesis

POI is the result of accelerated depletion of ovarian germ cells. Previously used term of 'resistant ovary syndrome' describes a mild form of POI that gradually progresses to amenorrhoea. Ovarian biopsy is no longer used, as this had no diagnostic value. Conversely, ovarian dysgenesis refers to early onset with primary amenorrhoea and describes the severe end of the condition.

POI is usually permanent and progressive, although a remitting course is also experienced and cannot be fully predicted, so all women must know that pregnancy is possible, even though fertility treatments are not effective (often a difficult paradox to describe). Spontaneous pregnancy has been reported in 5%.

Box 4.7 Turner's syndrome

(📖 also see Turner's syndrome, p. 336)
- Most common X chromosome abnormality in ♀, affecting 1:2,500 live ♀ births.
- Result of complete or partial absence of an X chromosome.
- *Clinical features.* Short stature and gonadal dysgenesis; 80% of affected ♀ have POI.
- *Characteristic phenotype.* Webbed neck, micrognathia, low-set ears, high arched palate, widely spaced nipples, and cubitus valgus.
- *Other associated abnormalities.* Aortic coarctation and other left-sided congenital heart defects, hypothyroidism, osteoporosis, skeletal abnormalities, lymphoedema, coeliac disease, congenital renal abnormalities, and ENT abnormalities.
- *Diagnosis.* Lymphocyte karyotype.
- *Management in adults:*
  - Sex hormone replacement therapy.
  - Treat complications.
- Follow-up:
  - Baseline renal US, thyroid autoantibodies.
  - Annual BMI, BP, TFT, lipids, fasting blood glucose, liver function.
  - 3–5-yearly echocardiogram and bone densitometry.
  - Hearing loss 5 years.

Table 4.6 Correlation of karyotype with phenotype

Karyotype	Phenotype
45, X (50%)	Most severe phenotype
	High incidence of cardiac and renal abnormalities
46, Xi(Xq) (20%)	↑ prevalence of thyroiditis, inflammatory bowel disease, and deafness
45, X/46, XX (10%)	Least severe phenotype
	↑ mean height
	Spontaneous puberty and menses in up to 40%
46, Xr(X) (10%)	Spontaneous menses in 33%
	Congenital abnormalities uncommon
	Cognitive dysfunction in those with a small ring chromosome
45, X/46, XY (6%)	↑ risk of gonadoblastoma (need gonadectomy)
Other (4%)	

Clinical presentation

- Amenorrhoea:
  - May be 1° or 2°.
- Symptoms of oestrogen deficiency:
  - Not present in those with 1° amenorrhoea.
  - 75% of ♀ who develop 2° amenorrhoea report hot flushes, night sweats, mood changes, fatigue, or dyspareunia; symptoms may precede the onset of menstrual disturbances.
- Autoimmune disease:
  - Screen for symptoms and signs of associated autoimmune disorders.
- Other:
  - Past history of radiotherapy, chemotherapy, or pelvic surgery.
  - +ve family history in 20% of patients; careful history is required to detect inheritance through father.
- With idiopathic POI, ovarian function can resume in most within a year of diagnosis. Spontaneous pregnancies have been recorded, so ultrasound assessment of follicles and measurement of inhibin B and oestradiol may be helpful.
- See Box 4.8 for autoimmune diseases.

Box 4.8 Autoimmune diseases and POI

- Responsible for 20% of cases of POI.
- A second autoimmune disorder is present in 10–40% of ♀ with autoimmune POI:
  - Autoimmune thyroid disease 25%.
  - Addison's disease 10%.
  - Type 1 diabetes mellitus 2%.
  - Myasthenia gravis 2%.
  - B12 deficiency.
  - SLE is also more common.
- Autoimmune endocrinopathies:
  - 60% of ♀ with autoimmune polyglandular syndrome type 1 (📖 see p. 270).
  - 25% of ♀ with autoimmune polyglandular syndrome type 2 (📖 see p. 271).
- Steroid cell antibodies are +ve in 60–100% of patients with Addison's disease in combination with POI. The presence of +ve steroid cell antibodies in ♀ with Addison's disease confers a 40% risk of ultimately developing POI. Other ovarian antibodies have little predictive value.

Investigation of POI

- *Serum gonadotrophins:*
  - Diagnosis is confirmed by serum FSH >40mIU/L on at least two occasions at least 1 month apart.
  - Disease may have a fluctuating course, with high FSH levels returning to normal and later regain of ovulatory function.
  - LH also elevated but FSH usually disproportionately higher than LH.
- *Serum oestradiol levels* are usually low.
- *Anti-Müllerian hormone*—only useful in early stages or at-risk groups, not in established cases.
- *Karyotype:*
  - All ♀ presenting with hypergonadotrophic amenorrhoea below age 40 should be karyotyped.
  - ♀ with Y chromosomal material should be referred for bilateral gonadectomy to prevent the development of gonadoblastoma.
- *Pelvic US*—to identify normal ovarian and uterine morphology.
- *Bone mineral density*—risk of osteoporosis.
- *Screen for autoimmune disease:*
  - Thyroid autoantibodies: if +ve, extend autoimmune screen to include adrenal, parietal cell, intrinsic factor.
  - Ovarian antibodies are rarely +ve—poor sensitivity.
  - TSH, vitamin B12.
  - Synacthen® test only if adrenal insufficiency is suspected clinically.
- *Ovarian biopsy*—not indicated.

Management of POI

Sex hormone replacement therapy

- Exogenous oestrogens (HRT) are required to alleviate symptoms and prevent the long-term complications of oestrogen deficiency—osteoporosis and possibly cardiovascular disease. Initial doses depend on the duration of amenorrhoea—if oestrogen-deficient for at least 12 months, then start on lowest doses of estradiol available to prevent side effects, but titrate up to full dose within 6 months. If recently amenorrhoeic, then full dose may be commenced immediately (see Table 4.7).
- Doses used in HRT are not contraceptive and do not suppress spontaneous ovarian follicular activity. Women who do not wish to conceive may use COCP instead of HRT—beware E2-deficient symptoms in pill-free week.
- HRT should be continued at least until the age of 50 years, the mean age of the natural menopause.
- In non-hysterectomized ♀, a progestagen should be added for 12–14 days a month to prevent endometrial hyperplasia.
- Low-dose androgen replacement therapy may improve persistent fatigue and poor libido, despite adequate oestrogen replacement.

Fertility

- A minority of ♀ with POI and a normal karyotype will recover spontaneously; 5% spontaneous fertility rate.
- Ovum donation is the only realistic chance of fertility. Pregnancy rate >50% per patient. Results are less good in ♀ if uterine damage after pelvic radiotherapy.
- Ovulation induction therapy has been tried, but the results have been poor.
- Glucocorticoid therapy has been used in autoimmune POI, but efficacy is poor.
- Recent improvements in methods of oocyte cryopreservation using rapid freezing in liquid nitrogen (vitrification) have allowed ♀ with high chance of POI (e.g. before chemo-/radiotherapy, Turner's syndrome mosaics with retained ovarian function) to store oocytes collected after superovulation.

Psychology

- Reduced self-esteem and sexual responsiveness.
- Reactive depression common at diagnosis and may return at critical times, such as pregnancy in a close friend.

For a full review of hormone replacement therapy, 📖 see Menopause, p. 342.

Table 4.7 Hormone replacement therapy in POI

Hormone replacement	Dose
Oestrogen	
Conjugated estrogens	0.625–1.25mg daily
Estradiol valerate	1–2mg daily
Transdermal estradiol	50–100 micrograms twice a week
Progestagen	12–14 days a month
Norethisterone	1mg
Medroxyprogesterone	10mg

Prognosis
- Mortality of ♀ with POI may be ↑ 2-fold.
- Oestrogen deficiency leads to:
  - ↑ risk of cardiovascular and cerebrovascular disease.
  - ↑ risk of osteoporosis. Up to two-thirds of ♀ with POI and a normal karyotype have ↓ BMD, with a Z score of −1 or less, despite at least intermittent hormone replacement therapy. This may be due to a combination of factors, including an initial delay in initiating ERT, poor compliance with ERT, and oestrogen 'underdosing'.

Further reading
Barlow DH (1996). Premature ovarian failure. *Baillière Clin Ob Gy* **10**, 361–84.

Davies MC, Cartwright B (2012). What is the best management strategy for a 20-year-old woman with premature ovarian failure? *Clin Endocrinol (Oxf)* **77**, 182–6.

Kalantaridou SN, Davis SR, Nelson LM (1998). Premature ovarian failure. *Endocrinol Metab Clin* **27**, 989–1006.

Nelson LM (2009). Clinical practice. Primary ovarian insufficiency. *N Engl J Med* **360**, 606–14.

Welte CK (2008). Primary ovarian insufficiency: a more accurate term for premature ovarian failure. *Clin End* **68**, 499–509.

Menopause

Definition

- The *menopause* is the permanent cessation of menstruation as a result of ovarian failure and is a retrospective diagnosis made after 12 months of amenorrhoea. The average age of ♀ at the time of the menopause is ~50 years, although smokers reach the menopause ~2 years earlier.
- The *perimenopause* encompasses the menopause transition and the first year following the last menstrual period.

Physiology

- Ovaries have a finite number of germ cells, with maximal numbers at 20 weeks of intrauterine life. Thereafter, there is a gradual reduction in the number of follicles until the perimenopause when there is an exponential loss of oocytes until the store is depleted at the time of the menopause.
- Inhibin B and anti-Müllerian hormone (AMH) are ovarian glycoproteins produced by follicles, as they develop from preantral to antral stages. Both may participate in ovarian paracrine regulation and, with other molecules, regulate the rate of attrition of follicles.
- Falling inhibin B levels result in fluctuating rise in FSH. Contrary to previous belief, average serum oestradiol levels may be high at the onset of the menopause transition as a result of FSH rise, falling only towards the end as the follicles are depleted.
- AMH is a useful early marker of ovarian ageing, being stable throughout the cycle and unaffected by COCP and without the marked fluctuations of FSH. AMH measurements, however, add nothing in routine practice or established menopause.
- See Table 4.8 for hormonal changes.

Long-term consequences

- *Osteoporosis.* During the perimenopausal period, there is an accelerated loss of bone mineral density (BMD), rendering post-menopausal ♀ more susceptible to osteoporotic fractures.
- *Ischaemic heart disease (IHD).* Post-menopausal ♀ are 2–3× more likely to develop IHD than premenopausal ♀, even after age adjustments. The menopause is associated with an increase in risk factors for atherosclerosis, including less favourable lipid profile, ↓ insulin sensitivity, and an ↑ thrombotic tendency.
- *Dementia.* ♀ are 2–3× more likely to develop Alzheimer's disease than ♂. It is suggested that oestrogen deficiency may play a role in the development of dementia.

Table 4.8 Hormonal changes during the menopausal transition

	Premenopause (from age 36 years)	Early perimenopause	Advanced perimenopause	Menopause
Menstrual cycle	Regular, ovulatory	Irregular, often short cycles, increasingly anovulatory	Oligomenorrhoea	Amenorrhoea
FSH	Rising but within normal range	Intermittently raised, especially in follicular phase	Persistently ↑	↑↑
AMH	Declining	Low	Low	Very low
E2	Normal	High normal	Normal/low	Low

Clinical presentation of menopause

There are marked cultural differences in the frequency of symptoms related to the menopause; in particular, vasomotor symptoms and mood disturbances are more commonly reported in western countries.

- *Menstrual disturbances* (90%). Cycles gradually become increasingly anovulatory and variable in length (often shorter) from about 4 years prior to the menopause. Oligomenorrhoea often precedes permanent amenorrhoea. In 10% of ♀, menses cease abruptly, with no preceding transitional period.
- *Hot flushes* (40%). Often associated with sweats and skin flushing. Highly variable and are thought to be related to fluctuations in oestrogen concentrations. Tend to resolve spontaneously within 5 years of the menopause.
- *Urinary symptoms* (50%). Atrophy of urethral and bladder mucosa after the menopause and ↓ sensitivity of α-adrenergic receptors of the bladder neck in the perimenopausal period. This may result in urinary incontinence and an ↑ risk of urinary tract infections.
- *Sexual dysfunction* (40%). Vaginal atrophy may result in dyspareunia and vaginal dryness. Additionally, falling androgen levels may reduce sexual arousal and libido.
- *Mood changes* (25–50%). Anxiety, forgetfulness, difficulty in concentration, and irritability have all been attributed to the menopause. ♀ with a history of affective disorders are at ↑ risk of mood disturbances in the perimenopausal period.

Evaluation of menopause (e.g. if HRT is being considered)

History
- Perimenopausal symptoms and their severity.
- Assess risk factors for cardiovascular disease and osteoporosis.
- Assess risk factors for breast cancer and thromboembolic disease.
- History of active liver disease.

Examination
- BP.
- Breasts.
- Consider pelvic examination for dyspareunia.

Investigations
- *FSH* levels fluctuate markedly in the perimenopausal period and correlate poorly with symptoms. Remember, a raised FSH in the perimenopausal period may not necessarily indicate infertility, so contraception, if desired, should continue until the menopause.
- *Mammography* indicated prior to starting oestrogen replacement therapy only in high-risk ♀; otherwise, mammography should be offered as per national screening programme.
- *Endometrial biopsy* does not need to be performed routinely but is essential in ♀ with abnormal uterine bleeding.

Hormone replacement therapy (HRT)

The aim of treatment of perimenopausal ♀ is to alleviate menopausal symptoms and optimize quality of life. The majority of women with mild symptoms require no HRT. See Table 4.9 for alternatives to HRT.

Benefits of HRT

Hot flushes

Respond well to oestrogen therapy in a dose-dependent manner. Start with a low dose, and increase gradually, as required, to control symptoms. High doses may be required initially, particularly in younger ♀ or in those whose symptoms develop abruptly (post-oophorectomy). In 75% of ♀, vasomotor symptoms settle within 5 years, so consider stopping HRT after 5 years of treatment. The dose of HRT should be gradually reduced over weeks, as sudden withdrawal of oestrogen may precipitate the return of vasomotor symptoms.

In ♀ with a contraindication to HRT or who are intolerant of it, non-hormonal therapies are summarized in Table 4.9.

Urinary symptoms

A trial of HRT, local or systemic, may improve stress and urge incontinence as well as the frequency of cystitis.

Vaginal atrophy

Systemic or local oestrogen therapy improves vaginal dryness and dyspareunia. A maximum of 6 months' use of vaginal cream is recommended, unless combined with a progestagen, as systemic absorption may increase the risk of endometrial hyperplasia. If oestrogens are not successful, then vaginal lubricants, e.g. Replens®, may help.

Osteoporosis

HRT has been shown to increase bone mineral density in the lumbar spine by 3–5% and at the femoral neck by about 2% by inhibiting bone resorption. The Women's Health Initiative (WHI) trial confirmed that HRT reduces the risk of both hip and vertebral fractures by 30%. HRT is not primarily used for bone protection, as other agents may have fewer side effects

Colorectal cancer

WHI showed a 20% reduction in the incidence of colon cancer in HRT users. However, HRT should currently not be prescribed solely to prevent colorectal cancer.

Risks of HRT

(Also see Box 4.9.)

Breast cancer

No personal or family history of breast cancer
There is an ↑ risk of breast cancer in HRT users which is related to the duration of use. The risk increases by 35%, following 5 years of use (over the age of 50), and falls to never-used risk 5 years after discontinuing HRT.

Table 4.9 Alternatives to HRT

Symptom	Management
Vasomotor symptoms	Venlafaxine (75mg od), paroxetine (20mg od), and fluoxetine (20mg od) have been shown to significantly reduce the frequency and severity of hot flushes with minimal side effects.
	Gabapentin (300mg tds) has also been shown to reduce the frequency and severity of hot flushes. Side effects include dizziness, somnolescence, and weight gain.
	Megestrol acetate in a dose of 20mg bd also reduces hot flushes by up to 70%, but its use is limited by side effects, particularly weight gain.
	Clonidine is less effective, reducing the occurrence of flushes by 20%, and is often associated with disabling side effects, such as dizziness, drowsiness, and a dry mouth.
	Citalopram (SSRI) 30mg may reduce hot flushes in 50% of patients.
Genitourinary symptoms	Vaginal lubricants, e.g. Replens®
Osteoporosis	Selective oestrogen receptor modulators (SERMs), e.g. raloxifene; however, these may exacerbate vasomotor symptoms, if present.Bisphosphonates, e.g. alendronic acid and risedronate

Box 4.9 A summary of contraindications to HRT

Absolute
- Undiagnosed vaginal bleeding.
- Pregnancy.
- Active DVT.
- Active endometrial cancer.
- Breast cancer.

Relative—seek advice
- Past history of endometrial cancer.
- Family or past history of thromboembolism.
- Ischaemic heart disease.
- Cerebrovascular disease.
- Active liver disease.
- Hypertriglyceridaemia

For ♀ aged 50 not using HRT, about 45 in every 1,000 will have cancer diagnosed over the following 20 years. This number increases to 47/1,000 ♀ using HRT for 5 years, 51/1,000 using HRT for 10 years, and 57/1,000 after 15 years of use. The risk is highest in ♀ on combined HRT compared with oestradiol alone. Mortality has not been shown to be ↑ in breast cancer developing in ♀ on HRT.

Family history of breast cancer
The risk of breast cancer may be ↑ 4-fold as a result of the family history, but there is little evidence that the risk is ↑ further by the use of HRT. HRT may be used in these ♀ if severe vasomotor symptoms are present after counselling regarding the above risks.

Past history of breast cancer
Avoid HRT in ♀ with a past history of breast cancer.

Venous thromboembolism (VTE)
Transdermal E2 is generally thought not to have an increased risk of VTE, which is why this group is favoured in most situations.

Oral HRT increases the risk approximately 3-fold, resulting in an extra two cases/10,000 woman-years. The risk is highest in the first year of use of HRT and has been shown to be halved by aspirin or statin therapy. This risk is markedly ↑ in ♀ who already have risk factors for DVT, including previous DVT, cardiovascular disease, and within 90 days of hospitalization.

Family history of DVT
If HRT is being considered because of severe vasomotor symptoms, then do a thrombophilia screen. If +ve, then avoid HRT. ♀ with a +ve family history of thromboembolism are still at a slightly ↑ risk themselves, even if the results of the thrombophilia screen are −ve, so consider transdermal route.

Past history of DVT/PE
Risk of recurrence is 5% per year, so avoid HRT unless on long-term warfarin therapy.

Cerebrovascular disease
HRT has been shown to increase the risk of ischaemic stroke in older ♀, particularly in the presence of atrial fibrillation. HRT should, therefore, not be used in ♀ with a history of cerebrovascular disease or atrial fibrillation, unless they are anticoagulated.

Endometrial cancer
No ↑ risk in ♀ taking continuous combined HRT preparations. ♀ using sequential combined preparations do not appear to have an ↑ risk of endometrial cancer initially, but the risk of endometrial hyperplasia does increase with long-term use (>5 years) despite regular withdrawal bleeds, so these ♀ need regular follow-up. ♀ with cured stage I tumours may safely take HRT.

Ovarian cancer
HRT may be associated with an ↑ risk of ovarian cancer, but the evidence is insufficient at present.

Gallstones
The risk of gallstones is ↑ 2-fold in HRT users.

Migraine
Migraines may increase in severity and frequency in HRT users. A trial of HRT is still worthwhile if indications are present, providing there are no focal neurological signs associated with the migraine. Modification in the dose of oestrogen or its preparation may improve symptoms. Avoid conjugated oestrogens, as these are most commonly associated with an increase in the frequency of migraines.

Endometriosis and uterine fibroids
The risk of recurrence of endometriosis or of growth of uterine fibroids is low on HRT.

Liver disease
Use parenteral or transcutaneous oestrogens to avoid hepatic metabolism, and monitor liver function in ♀ with impaired liver function tests. Do not use HRT in the presence of active liver disease or liver failure.

Areas of uncertainty with HRT

Cardiovascular disease (CVD)
Data from >30 observational studies suggest that HRT may reduce the risk of developing CVD by up to 50%. However, randomized placebo-controlled trials, e.g. the Heart and Oestrogen-Progestin Replacement Study (HERS) and the WHI trial, have failed to show that HRT protects against IHD. Currently, HRT should not be prescribed to prevent cardiovascular disease. However, it may be used cautiously in individual patients with CVD if QoL is significantly reduced from vasomotor symptoms.

Alzheimer's disease
Recent evidence suggests that the risk of developing Alzheimer's disease may be reduced by up to 50% in ♀ receiving HRT, particularly if started early in the menopause. However, in ♀ with established Alzheimer's disease, there is no evidence to suggest reversal of cognitive dysfunction following initiation of HRT. There is currently insufficient evidence to recommend the use of HRT to prevent Alzheimer's disease. In post-menopausal ♀ without dementia, HRT may improve certain aspects of cognitive function.

Mood disturbances
There has been a strongly held belief that HRT improves well-being and QoL in perimenopausal and post-menopausal ♀. However, in recent trials where QoL has been assessed, notably HERS and WHI, the improvement in QoL and improved sleep was only seen in ♀ with vasomotor symptoms.

Side effects commonly associated with HRT

- *Breast tenderness* usually subsides within 4–6 months of use. If troublesome, use lower oestrogen dose and increase gradually.
- *Mood changes* commonly associated with progestin therapy; manage by changing dose or preparation of progestin.
- *Irregular vaginal bleeding* may be a problem in ♀ on a continuous combined preparation; usually subsides after 6–12 months of treatment. Spotting persists in 10%—may change to a cyclic preparation. See Box 4.10.

Summary of WHI trial

(See Table 4.10.)

- Randomized controlled trial of the effects of continuous combined conjugated estrogens and medroxyprogesterone acetate on healthy asymptomatic post-menopausal ♀, mean follow-up 5.2 years.
- Mean age 63 years, with 66% of ♀ >60 years of age.
- 70% of participants were overweight or obese, and 50% were current or past smokers.
- Absolute risk was highest in the older age group (>65 years).
- Results of WHI cannot be extrapolated to younger HRT users (<55 years of age).
- It is unclear whether different HRT preparations or routes of administration would necessarily have the same benefit/risk profile.

Dietary phytoestrogens

Phytoestrogens are found in foods, such as soy beans, cereals, and seeds. Although they have oestrogen-like activity, data from clinical trials are conflicting. It appears that the effect of phytoestrogens on vasomotor symptoms is modest at best. Research does suggest that soy protein has a favourable effect on plasma lipid concentrations and may reduce the risk of cardiovascular disease. However, the actual daily dose required is unclear. Finally, data regarding the effect of phytoestrogens on bone loss and breast cancer risk are inconclusive. Phytoestrogen supplements cannot, therefore, be recommended for the prevention of chronic disease in peri- and post-menopausal ♀ until they are adequately evaluated in clinical trials.

Box 4.10 Who and how to investigate for irregular uterine bleeding

- *Sequential cyclical HRT.* Three or more cycles of bleeding before the ninth day of progestagen therapy, or change in the duration or intensity of uterine bleeding.
- *Continuous combined HRT.* In first 12 months if bleeding is heavy or extended, if it continues after 12 months of use, or if it starts after a period of amenorrhoea.
- *Endometrial assessment.* Vaginal US essential in ♀ with irregular uterine bleeding. Endometrial thickness of <5mm excludes disease in 96–99% of cases, a sensitivity similar to that of endometrial biopsy. However, specificity is poor, so if the endometrium is >5mm (as it will be in 50% of post-menopausal ♀ on HRT), endometrial biopsy will be required to rule out carcinoma.

Table 4.10 Risks and benefits per 10,000 ♀ treated with HRT per year (WHI trial)

Benefits	Number of patients
Hip fractures prevented	5
Colon cancer prevented	6
Adverse events:	
Coronary heart disease	7
Cerebrovascular events	8
Pulmonary embolism	5
Breast cancer (>5 years' use)	8

HRT regimens

Oestrogen preparations

See Table 4.11. In younger, symptomatic, often perimenopausal ♀, higher doses of oestrogen are often required initially, which can be reduced gradually to the lowest dose effective at controlling symptoms.

Older ♀ who have been amenorrhoeic for over a year should be started on the lowest possible dose of oestrogen.

Route of administration

- *Oral route* is the most popular. Disadvantages:
  - First pass hepatic metabolism results in increased thrombotic risk.
  - May be associated with nausea and may exacerbate liver disease.
  - Must be taken daily, so there is no breakthrough of symptoms.
- *Transdermal patches* avoid first pass effect and are thus ideal in ♀ with liver disease or hypertriglyceridaemia. Additionally, patches provide constant systemic hormone levels. However, 10% of ♀ develop skin reactions. Try to avoid moisture and to rotate patch sites to prevent this.
- *Gels* have the advantages of patches, but skin irritation is less common.
- *SC implants* have the advantage of good compliance. However, if side effects develop, implants are difficult to remove. Additionally, may release oestradiol for up to 3 years after insertion, and cyclical progestagens must be given until oestrogen levels are not detectable.

Progestagen preparations

See Table 4.12. Must be added in non-hysterectomized ♀ to avoid endometrial hyperplasia and subsequent carcinoma.

Sequential cyclical regimen

Give progestagen for a minimum of 10 days a month. Usually given for the first 12 days of each calendar month. Quarterly regimen available—progestagen given for 14 days 4× a year. However, the risk of endometrial hyperplasia on such a regimen is unknown.

99% of ♀ have a monthly withdrawal bleed. 10% may be amenorrhoeic, with no harmful consequences. Bleeding should start after the ninth day of progestagen therapy.

Continuous combined regimen

Lower doses of progestagen are given on a daily basis. Uterine bleeding is usually light in amount, but timing is unpredictable. Bleeding should stop in 90% of ♀ within 12 months, the majority in 6 months.

Ideal for older ♀ who do not want monthly withdrawal bleeds. Contraindicated in perimenopausal ♀, as irregular uterine bleeding is more likely and difficult to assess.

Tibolone (2.5mg a day)

A synthetic steroid with mixed oestrogenic, progestagenic, and weak androgenic activities. An alternative form of HRT, with little stimulation of the endometrium. It alleviates vasomotor symptoms, may improve mood and libido, and is protective against osteoporosis. Risks of VTE and breast cancer similar to oestrogen. 10% of ♀ may experience vaginal bleeding on tibolone.

Table 4.11 Oestrogen preparations

Preparation	Dose
Conjugated estrogens (PO)	0.625–1.25mg daily
Estradiol valerate (PO)	2mg daily
Estradiol transdermal patch	100 micrograms twice a week. New patch twice a week
Estradiol gel	1–1.5mg daily
Estradiol subcutaneous implant	25–100mg every 4–8 months. Check serum E2 prior to implant

Table 4.12 Progestagen preparations

Progestin	Cyclical dose (day 1–12)	Continuous daily dose
Dydrogesterone (least androgenic)	10mg	5mg
Medroxyprogesterone acetate	10mg	2.5–5mg (higher dose reduces bleeding)
Levonorgestrel	150 micrograms	Unknown
Norethisterone (most androgenic)	0.7–1mg	0.5–1mg

Androgen replacement therapy
(See Box 4.11.)
- The major androgens in premenopausal ♀ are androstenedione and testosterone, produced by both the ovaries and adrenal glands. Over 90% are bound to sex hormone-binding globulin and albumin. Androgens are thought to play a role in maintaining bone density and normal sexual and cognitive function in ♀.
- Total and free serum androstenedione and testosterone levels fall by up to 50% after the menopause as a result of both declining ovarian and adrenal androgen production.
- *Indications for androgen replacement therapy.* Poor well-being and libido, despite adequate oestrogen replacement therapy in ♀ with ovarian failure.
- *Mode of administration.* SC testosterone implants 50–100mg every 6–8 months. Testosterone patches (300 micrograms/24h) are also available. Always combine with oestrogen therapy.
- *Side effects and possible complications.* Hirsutism, acne, or virilization have been reported in approximately 20% of ♀. Adverse changes to lipid profile commonly occur. The effect on cardiovascular risk is unknown. The long-term effects of androgen therapy on the endometrium and breast tissue are unknown.

> **Box 4.11 Monitoring of women receiving androgen replacement therapy**
>
> **Clinical**
> - Exclude contraindications.
> - Polycythaemia.
> - Breast or endometrial cancer.
> - Assess efficacy.
> - Evaluate side effects.
>
> **Biochemical**
> - Lipid profile.
> - Liver function tests.
> - FBC (exclude polycythaemia).
> - Serum testosterone.

Further reading

Arlt W (2006). Androgen therapy in women. *Eur J Endocrinol* **154**, 1–11.

Davis SR, *et al.* (2008). Testosterone for low libido in postmenopausal women not taking estrogen. *N Engl J Med* **359**, 2005–17.

Humphries KH, Gill S (2003). Risks and benefits of hormone replacement therapy: the evidence speaks. *Can Med Assoc J* **168**, 1001–10.

Million Women Study Collaborators (2003). Breast cancer and hormone-replacement therapy in the Million women Study. *Lancet* **362**, 419–23.

Rymer J, Wilson R, Ballard K (2003). Making decisions about hormone replacement therapy. *BMJ* **326**, 322–6.

Writing Group for Women's Health Initiative Investigators (2002). Risks and benefits of estrogen plus progestin in healthy postmenopausal women: principal results from the Women's Health Initiative randomized controlled trial. *JAMA* **288**, 321–33.

Hormonal control of contraception

Formulations:
- Combined oral contraceptive pills.
- Transdermal and vaginal ethinylestradiol.
- Progesterone-only pills.
- Progesterone implants and injections.
- Intrauterine progesterone.
- Emergency contraception.

Combined oral contraceptive pills (COCP)

- Very effective contraception, with approximately 5 per 100 users falling pregnant per year.
- Good for cycle control and hyperandrogenic symptoms in young women, with low risk of thrombosis.
- *Oestrogens:*
  - Ethinylestradiol (EE2)—three doses: 20, 30, and 35 micrograms. Generally, the lowest effective dose is used, as risks thought to be dose-dependent—lowest doses less effective for menstrual control.
  - Estradiol—combined in one OCP with progestagens.
- *Progestagens:*
  - Second generation: *levonorgestrel* (150–250mg) and *norethisterone* (1mg)—though to have the lowest risk of thrombosis but more androgenic side effects.
  - Third generation: *norgestimate* and *desogestrel* are less androgenic but may be associated with an ↑ risk of thromboembolism.
  - Fourth generation: *drospirenone*—antiandrogenic properties.
  - Unclassified: *cyproterone acetate*—antiandrogenic, marketed for the treatment of acne rather than as COCP.

For a list of COCP preparations, see Box 4.12.
- Androgenicity: medroxyprogesterone < desogestrel < norethisterone.

COCP side effects
- Breakthrough bleeding.
- Low mood, reduced libido.
- Nausea.
- Fluid retention and weight gain.
- Breast tenderness and enlargement.
- Headache.
- Chloasma.

Benefits
- Ovarian cancer.
  - The risks of ovarian cancer are halved in ♀ who have been taking the COCP for 5 years or more. This risk reduction persists long after discontinuation of the COCP.
- Acne.
  - The COCP reduces free testosterone concentrations by suppressing ovarian production of androgens and by ↑ hepatic SHBG production. COCP with low androgenic progestagens often result in an improvement in acne.
- Menstrual disorders.
  - The COCP is associated with reduced menstrual flow and can, therefore, improve menorrhagia. The COCP can reduce dysmenorrhoea and premenstrual symptoms.

Risks
(See Table 4.13 for contraindications.)

Box 4.12 Examples of COCP preparations

First generation
- Norinyl-1®

Second generation
- BiNovum®
- Brevinor®
- Loestrin 20/30®
- Logynon®
- Microgynon 30/30 ED®

- Norimin®
- Ovranette®
- Ovysmen®
- Synphase®
- TriNovum®

Third generation
- Cilest®
- Femodene/ED®
- Femodette®
- Katya 30/75®

- Marvelon®
- Mercilon®
- Sunya 20/75®
- Triadene®

Fourth generation
- Yasmin®

Table 4.13 COCP contraindications

Absolute	Relative
History of heart disease—ischaemic or valvular	Migraine
Pulmonary hypertension	Sickle cell disease
History of arterial or venous thrombosis	Gallstones
History of cerebrovascular disease	Inflammatory bowel disease
High risk of thrombosis, e.g. factor V Leiden, antiphospholipid antibodies	Hypertension
Liver disease	Hyperlipidaemia
Migraine if severe or associated with focal aura	Diabetes mellitus
Breast or genital tract cancer	Obesity
Pregnancy	Smokers
Presence of two or more relative contraindications	
Age >35 years and a smoker	Otosclerosis
	Family history of thrombosis
	Family history of breast cancer

Consider using a progesterone-only pill in women with contraindications to the combined OCP.

Venous thromboembolism
- The risk of venous thromboembolism in non-pregnant ♀ (5 per 100,000 ♀/year) is ↑ 3-fold in ♀ on the COCP.
- The risk is highest in the first year of use, increases with age, and is ↑ in obese ♀.
- The risk of venous thromboembolism appears to be higher in ♀ taking COCPs containing desogestrel, gestodene, cyproterone acetate, or drospirenone, but absolute risk may be small in those with low risk and outweighed by benefits.
- ♀ with a family history of thromboembolism should undergo a thrombophilia screen before starting the COCP.

Arterial thrombosis
- There is a 10-fold excess risk of IHD in ♀ smokers over the age of 35 years who are on the COCP. The risk of IHD does not seem to be significantly ↑ in non-smokers who take low-dose COCP.
- The relative risk of ischaemic stroke is only slightly ↑ in ♀ taking low-dose COCP. The risk is ↑ in ♀ over the age of 35 years, smokers, or in ♀ with hypertension. The risk of haemorrhagic stroke does not seem to be ↑ by taking the COCP.
- Risk of either arterial or venous thrombosis returns to normal within 3 months of discontinuing the COCP.

Hypertension
May be caused by the COCP and, if already present, may be more resistant to treatment.

Hepatic disease
Raised hepatic enzymes may be seen in ♀ on the COCP. The incidence of benign hepatic tumours is also ↑.

Gallstones
The risk of developing gallstones is slightly ↑ by taking the COCP (RR = 1.2).

Breast cancer
- There may be a slightly ↑ risk of breast cancer in ♀ using the COCP (RR = 1.3), particularly in those who began taking the COCP in their teens.
- The risk does not seem to be related to the duration of exposure to the COCP nor to the EE2 dose.
- The relative risk of developing breast cancer returns to normal 10 years after discontinuing the COCP.

Cervical cancer
- The use of COCP appears to be associated with an excess risk of cervical cancer in ♀ who are HPV +ve. The risk increases with the duration of COCP use.
- It is not known whether the risk falls again following the discontinuation of COCP.

Thrombophilia screen
- Antithrombin III.
- Protein C.
- Protein S
- Factor V Leiden.

Practical issues

Age and the COCP
- ♀ with no risk factors for arterial or venous thrombosis may continue to use the combined COCP until the age of 50 years.
- Those with risk factors for thromboembolism and IHD should avoid COCP after the age of 35 years, particularly if they are smokers.
- Contraception after the menopause: assume fertile for the first year after last menstrual period if >50 years.

Breakthrough bleeding
Causes include:
- Genital tract disease.
- Insufficient oestrogen dose.
- Inappropriate progestagen.
- Missed pill.
- Taking two packets continuously.
- Gastroenteritis.
- Drug interactions, e.g. antibiotics, hepatic enzyme inducers.

Antibiotics and the COCP
Broad-spectrum antibiotics interfere with intestinal flora, thereby reducing bioavailability of the COCP. Additional methods of contraception should be used.

COCP and surgery
- Stop COCP at least 4 weeks before major surgery and any surgery to the legs. Do not restart until fully mobile for at least 2 weeks.
- If emergency surgery, then stop COCP and start antithrombotic prophylaxis.

Emergency contraception

Refers to contraception that a woman can use after unprotected sexual intercourse to prevent pregnancy.

- A single 1.5mg dose of the progestagen levonorgestrel is highly efficacious, with a pregnancy rate of 2–4% if taken within 72h of sexual intercourse. It is most effective the earlier it is taken. The dose is repeated if vomiting occurs within 3h of taking the pill.
- The *mechanism of action* is not clear but is thought to be due to inhibition of ovulation as well as a ↓ likelihood of endometrial implantation.
- *Side effects.* Nausea in up to 60% of ♀, vomiting in 10–20%. Consider antiemetic 1h before taking contraception. Other side effects—breast tenderness, fatigue, dizziness.
- *Contraindication*—pregnancy.
- ♀ should be advised to use barrier contraception until their next period.
- 98% of ♀ menstruate within 3–4 weeks of taking levonorgestrel. They should be encouraged to seek medical advice if they do not bleed in that time.
- If pregnancy does occur, levonorgestrel is not known to be teratogenic.

Further reading

Lidegaard O (2012). Thrombotic stroke and myocardial infarction with hormonal contraception. *N Engl J Med.* **366**, 2257–66.

Petitti DB (2003). Combination oestrogen-progestin oral contraceptives. *N Engl J Med* **349**, 1443–50.

Male hypogonadism

Definition
Failure of testes to produce adequate amounts of testosterone, spermatozoa, or both.

Epidemiology
- Klinefelter's syndrome (XXY) (□ see p. 370) is the most common congenital cause and is thought to occur with an incidence of 2:1,000 live births.
- Acquired hypogonadism is even more common, affecting 1:200 ♂.

Evaluation of male hypogonadism
Presentation
- Failure to progress through puberty.
- Sexual dysfunction.
- Infertility.
- Non-specific symptoms, e.g. lethargy, reduced libido, mood changes, weight gain.

The clinical presentation depends on:
- The age of onset (congenital vs acquired).
- The severity (complete vs partial).
- The duration (functional vs permanent).

Secondary hypogonadism

Definition
Hypogonadism as a result of hypothalamic or pituitary dysfunction.

Diagnosis
- Low 9 a.m. serum testosterone.
- Low normal or low LH and FSH, normal inhibin B and anti-Müllerian hormone.

Causes
(See Box 4.15.)

Kallmann's syndrome
A genetic disorder characterized by failure of episodic GnRH secretion ± anosmia. Results from disordered migration of GnRH-producing neurons into the hypothalamus.

Epidemiology
- Incidence of 1 in 10,000 ♂.
- ♂:♀ ratio = 4:1.

Diagnosis
- Anosmia in 75%.
- ↑ risk of cleft lip and palate, sensorineural deafness, cerebellar ataxia, and renal agenesis.
- Low testosterone, LH, and FSH levels.
- Rest of pituitary function normal.
- Normal MRI pituitary gland and hypothalamus; absent olfactory bulbs may be seen on MRI.
- Normalization of pituitary and gonadal function in response to physiological GnRH replacement.

Genetics
- Most commonly, a result of an isolated gene mutation.
- May be inherited in an X-linked (*KAL1*), autosomal dominant *FGFR1* mutation/*KAL2*, or recessive trait.
- *KAL1* gene mutation, responsible for some cases of X-linked Kallmann's syndrome, is located on Xp22.3. It has a more severe reproductive phenotype.
- Mutations of *FGFR1* (fibroblast growth factor receptor 1) gene, located on chromosome 8p11, is associated with the autosomal dominant form of Kallmann's syndrome. Affected ♂ have an ↑ likelihood of undescended testes at birth.
- 12–15% incidence of delayed puberty in families of subjects with Kallman's syndrome, compared with 1% in general population.
- ♂ with autosomal dominant form (*FGFR1* mutation)—50% transmitted to offspring who have increased likelihood of undescended testes at birth.

Management
- Androgen replacement therapy.
- When fertility is desired, testosterone is stopped and exogenous gonadotrophins are administered (see p. 408).

Box 4.15 Causes of secondary hypogonadism

- Idiopathic:
  - Kallmann's syndrome.
  - Other genetic causes, e.g. mutations of *GnRHR* or *GPR54* genes.
  - Idiopathic hypogonadotrophic hypogonadism (IHH).
  - Fertile eunuch syndrome.
  - Congenital adrenal hypoplasia (*DAX-1* gene mutation).
- Functional:
  - Exercise.
  - Weight changes.
  - Anabolic steroids.
  - Stress—physical/psychological.
  - Systemic illness.
  - Medication and recreational drugs.
- Structural:
  - Tumours, e.g. pituitary adenoma, craniopharyngioma, germinoma.
  - Infiltrative disorders, e.g. sarcoidosis, haemochromatosis.
  - Head trauma.
  - Radiotherapy.
  - Surgery to the pituitary gland or hypothalamus.
- Miscellaneous:
  - Haemochromatosis.
  - Prader–Willi syndrome.
  - Laurence–Moon–Biedl syndrome.

Idiopathic hypogonadotrophic hypogonadism (IHH)
- Congenital form is indistinguishable from Kallmann's syndrome, apart from the absence of anosmia. >90% of patients are ♂.
- GnRH receptor gene mutation is an uncommon cause of IHH.
- ♂ with acquired IHH may go through normal puberty and have normal testicular size but present with infertility or poor libido and potency. May be temporary, with normalization of gonadal function after stopping GnRH or testosterone therapy.

Fertile eunuch syndrome
- Incomplete GnRH deficiency. Enough to maintain normal spermatogenesis and testicular growth but insufficient for adequate virilization.
- May require testosterone/hCG for fertility.

Congenital adrenal hypoplasia
- Rare X-linked or autosomal recessive disease, caused by a mutation of the *DAX* gene which is located on the X chromosome.
- Presents with 1° adrenal failure in infancy.
- Hypothalamic hypogonadism is also present.

Structural
- Usually associated with other pituitary hormonal deficiencies.

- In children, craniopharyngiomas are the most common cause. Cranial irradiation for leukaemia or brain tumours may also result in 2° hypogonadism.
- The commonest lesions in adulthood are prolactinomas.

Systemic illness

Severe illness of any kind may cause hypogonadotrophic hypogonadism (see Box 4.14).

Drugs

- Anabolic steroids, cocaine, and narcotic drugs may all result in 2° hypogonadism.

All drugs causing hyperprolactinaemia (see Box 2.12, p. 141) will also cause hypogonadism.

Prader–Willi syndrome

A congenital syndrome, affecting 1:25,000 births, caused by loss of an imprinted gene on paternally derived chromosome 15q11–13.

It should be suspected in infancy in the presence of characteristic facial features (almond eyes, downturned mouth, strabismus, thin upper lip), severe hypotonia, poor feeding, and developmental delay. The child then develops hyperphagia due to hypothalamic dysfunction, resulting in severe obesity. Other characteristic features include short stature, small hands and feet, hypogonadotrophic hypogonadism, and learning disability.

- Type 2 diabetes occurs in 15–40% of adults.

Laurence–Moon–Biedl syndrome

Congenital syndrome characterized by severe obesity, gonadotrophin deficiency, retinal dystrophy, polydactyly, and learning disability.

Haemochromatosis

See Box 4.16.

Box 4.16 Haemochromatosis

Complications
- Central and primary hypogonadism.
- Diabetes mellitus.
- Liver cirrhosis.
- Addison's disease.

Diagnosed by genotyping.

Hypogonadotrophic hypogonadism (HH)

Definition
Hypogonadism as a result of gonadotrophin deficiency.

Diagnosis
- Low LH, FSH, oestradiol, testosterone.
- Rest of pituitary function normal.
- MRI: small pituitary gland, normal hypothalamus.
- Small gonads.
- Absent or delayed puberty, 1° amenorrhoea.
- Tall stature from delayed closure of epiphyses.
- Anosmia and absent olfactory bulbs on MRI in Kallmann's.

Causes
(See Box 4.13.)

Kallmann's syndrome
HH ± anosmia. Results from disordered migration of GnRH-producing neurons into the hypothalamus.

Epidemiology
- Incidence of 1 in 10,000 ♂.
- ♂:♀ ratio = 4:1.

Associated features
- Anosmia in 75%.
- Cleft lip and palate, sensorineural deafness, cerebellar ataxia, and renal agenesis.

Genetics
- Variable inheritance: X-linked (*KAL1*, Xp22.3), autosomal dominant *FGFR1* mutation (*KAL2*), or recessive trait.
- *KAL1* has a more severe reproductive phenotype.
- Mutations of fibroblast growth factor receptor 1 gene (*FGFR1*, 8p11) have an ↑ likelihood of undescended testes at birth.
- Variable penetrance: 12–15% incidence of delayed puberty in families of subjects with Kallmann's syndrome, compared with 1% in general population.

Idiopathic hypogonadotrophic hypogonadism (IHH)
- Congenital form is indistinguishable from Kallmann's syndrome, apart from the absence of anosmia.
- To date, ten single gene defects described, including *FGFR1*, *GnRH*, and *GnRHR* genes—none is available for routine screening at present.
- ♂ with acquired IHH may go through normal puberty and have normal testicular size but present with infertility or poor libido and potency.
- Spontaneous remission with normalization of gonadal function may occur at any age.
- *Fertile eunuch syndrome*. A mild form of IHH. Enough GnRH to maintain normal spermatogenesis and testicular growth but insufficient for adequate virilization.

Box 4.13 Causes of HH
- Single gene defects:
  - Kallmann's syndrome.
  - Idiopathic hypogonadotrophic hypogonadism (IHH).
- Functional:
  - Exercise, weight loss, stress, systemic illness.
  - Iatrogenic: anabolic steroids, opiates.
- Associated conditions:
  - Haemochromatosis.
  - CAH, especially ♂.
  - Pituitary disease.
- Syndromic:
  - Prader–Willi syndrome.
  - Laurence–Moon–Biedl syndrome.
  - CHARGE syndrome.
  - X-linked adrenal hypoplasia congenita.

Structural
- Usually associated with other pituitary hormonal deficiencies.
- In children, craniopharyngiomas are the most common cause. Cranial irradiation for leukaemia or brain tumours may also result in 2° hypogonadism.
- The commonest lesions in adulthood are prolactinomas.

Systemic illness
Severe illness of any kind may cause hypogonadotrophic hypogonadism (see Box 4.14).

Prader–Willi syndrome
A congenital syndrome affecting 1:25,000 births, caused by loss of an imprinted gene on paternally derived chromosome 15q11–13.

It should be suspected in infancy in the presence of characteristic facial features (almond eyes, downturned mouth, strabismus, thin upper lip), severe hypotonia, poor feeding, and developmental delay. The child then develops hyperphagia due to hypothalamic dysfunction, resulting in severe obesity. Other characteristic features include short stature, hypogonadotrophic hypogonadism, and learning disability.
- Type 2 diabetes occurs in 15–40% of adults.

Laurence–Moon–Biedl syndrome
Congenital syndrome characterized by severe obesity, gonadotrophin deficiency, retinal dystrophy, polydactyly, and learning disability.

CHARGE syndrome
The association of coloboma, heart anomaly, choanal atresia, retardation, genital and ear anomalies. A proportion also has HH.

> **Box 4.14 Systemic illness resulting in hypogonadism**
> - Any acute illness (e.g. myocardial infarction, sepsis, head injury).
> - Severe stress.
> - Haemochromatosis.
> - Endocrine disease (Cushing's syndrome, hyperprolactinaemia).
> - Liver cirrhosis.
> - Chronic renal failure.
> - Chronic anaemia (thalassaemia major, sickle cell disease).
> - GI disease (coeliac disease, Crohn's disease).
> - AIDS.
> - Rheumatological disease (rheumatoid arthritis).
> - Respiratory disease (e.g. chronic obstructive airways disease, cystic fibrosis).
> - Cardiac disease (e.g. congestive cardiac failure).

X-linked adrenal hypoplasia congenita

Rare X-linked or autosomal recessive disease, caused by a mutation of the *DAX* gene, which is located on the X chromosome.
- Presents with 1° adrenal failure in infancy.
- Hypothalamic hypogonadism is also present.

Management
- Androgen replacement therapy (📖 see p. 378).
- Oestrogen replacement therapy (📖 see p. 340).
- When fertility is desired, testosterone is stopped and exogenous gonadotrophins are administered (📖 see pp. 398, 408).

Primary hypogonadism

Due to testicular failure with normal hypothalamus and pituitary function. See Box 4.17 for clinical characteristics.

Diagnosis

- Low 9 a.m. serum testosterone.
- Elevated LH and FSH, low inhibin B, and anti-Müllerian hormone.

Causes

Genetic

Klinefelter's syndrome

The most common congenital form of 1° hypogonadism. It is thought that a significant number of men with Klinefelter's syndrome are not diagnosed.

Clinical manifestations will depend on the age of diagnosis. Patients with mosaicism tend to have less severe clinical features.

- Adolescence:
  - Small firm testes (mean 5mL).
  - Gynaecomastia.
  - Tall stature (↑ leg length).
  - Other features of hypogonadism.
  - Cognitive dysfunction.
- Adulthood:
  - Reduced libido and erectile dysfunction.
  - Gynaecomastia (50%).
  - Reduced facial hair.
  - Obesity.
  - Infertility.
- Risks:
  - Type 2 diabetes mellitus.
  - Osteoporosis.
  - Thromboembolism.
  - Malignancies, e.g. extragonadal germ cell tumours.
- Diagnosis:
  - Karyotyping: 47,XXY in 80%; higher grade chromosomal aneuploidies (e.g. 48,XXXY) or 46,XY/47,XXY mosaicism in the remainder.
  - Low testosterone, elevated FSH and LH.
  - Elevated SHBG and oestradiol.
  - Azoospermia.
- Management:
  - Lifelong androgen replacement.
  - May need surgical reduction of gynaecomastia.
  - Fertility: intracytoplasmic sperm injection (ICSI, 📖 see Management of male infertility, p. 409), using testicular spermatozoa from men with Klinefelter's syndrome, has resulted in successful pregnancies. However, couples should be counselled about the ↑ risk of chromosomal abnormalities in offspring.

Box 4.17 Testicular dysfunction—clinical characteristics of male hypogonadism

Testicular failure occurring before onset of puberty
- Testicular volume <5mL.
- Penis <5cm long.
- Lack of scrotal pigmentation and rugae.
- Gynaecomastia.
- High-pitched voice.
- Central fat distribution.
- Eunuchoidism:
  - Arm span 1cm greater than height.
  - Lower segment > upper segment.
- Delayed bone age.
- No ♂ escutcheon.
- ↓ body and facial hair.

Testicular failure occurring after puberty
- Testes soft, volume <15mL.
- Normal penile length.
- Normal skeletal proportions.
- Gynaecomastia.
- Normal ♂ hair distribution but reduced amount.
- Pale skin, fine wrinkles.
- Central fat distribution.
- Osteoporosis.
- Anaemia (mild).

Other chromosomal disorders
- XX males:
  - Due to an X to Y translocation, with only a part of the Y present in one of the X chromosomes.
  - Incidence 1:10,000 births.
  - Similar clinical and biochemical features to Klinefelter's syndrome. In addition, short stature and hypospadias may be present.
- XX/XO (mixed gonadal dysgenesis):
  - Occasionally, phenotypically ♂ with hypospadias and intra-abdominal dysgenetic gonads.
  - Bilateral gonadectomy is essential because of the risk of neoplasia, followed by androgen replacement therapy.
- XYY syndrome:
  - Taller than average but often have primary gonadal failure with impaired spermatogenesis.
- Y chromosome microdeletions:
  - Causes oligo-/azoospermia. Testosterone levels are not usually affected.
- Noonan's syndrome:
  - Autosomal dominant disorder, with an incidence of 1:1,000 to 1:2,500 live births.

- 46,XY karyotype and 2° external genitalia. However, several stigmata of Turner's syndrome (dysmorphic facial features, short stature, webbed neck, ptosis, low-set ears, lymphoedema) and ↑ risk of cardiac anomalies (valvular pulmonary stenosis and hypertrophic cardiomyopathy). Most have cryptorchidism and 1° testicular failure. May have a bleeding diathesis.

Cryptorchidism
- 10% of 2° neonates have undescended testes, but most of these will descend into the scrotum eventually so that the incidence of post-pubertal cryptorchidism is <0.5%.
- 15% of cases have bilateral cryptorchidism.

Consequences
- 75% of ♂ with bilateral cryptorchidism are infertile.
- 10% risk of testicular malignancy; highest risk in those with intra-abdominal testes.
- Low testosterone and raised gonadotrophins in bilateral cryptorchidism.

Treatment
- *Orchidopexy.* Best performed before 18 months, certainly before age 5 years, in order to reduce risk of later infertility.
- *Gonadectomy.* In patients with intra-abdominal testes, followed by androgen replacement.

Orchitis
- 25% of ♂ who develop mumps after puberty have associated orchitis, and 25–50% of these will develop 1° testicular failure.
- HIV infection may also be associated with orchitis.
- 1° testicular failure may occur as part of an autoimmune disease.

Chemotherapy and radiotherapy

- Cytotoxic drugs, particularly alkylating agents, are gonadotoxic. Infertility occurs in 50% of patients following chemotherapy for most malignancies, and a significant number of ♂ require androgen replacement therapy because of low testosterone levels.
- The testes are radiosensitive, so hypogonadism can occur as a result of scattered radiation during the treatment of Hodgkin's disease, for example.
- If fertility is desired, sperm should be cryopreserved prior to cancer therapy.

Other drugs

- Sulfasalazine, colchicines, and high-dose glucocorticoids may reversibly affect testicular function.
- Alcohol excess will also cause 1° testicular failure.

Chronic illness

Any chronic illness may affect testicular function, in particular chronic renal failure, liver cirrhosis, and haemochromatosis.

Testicular trauma

Testicular torsion is another common cause of loss of a testis, and it may also affect the function of the remaining testis.

Clinical assessment of hypogonadism

History

- *Developmental history.* Congenital urinary tract abnormalities, e.g. hypospadias, late testicular descent, or cryptorchidism.
- *Delayed or incomplete puberty.*
- *Infections,* e.g. mumps, orchitis.
- *Abdominal/genital trauma.*
- *Testicular torsion.*
- *Anosmia.*
- *Drug history,* e.g. sulfasalazine, antihypertensives, chemotherapy, cimetidine, radiotherapy; alcohol and recreational drugs also important.
- *General medical history.* Chronic illness, particularly respiratory, neurological, and cardiac.
- *Gynaecomastia.* Common (📖 see Gynaecomastia, pp. 382–3) during adolescence. Recent-onset gynaecomastia in adulthood—must rule out oestrogen-producing tumour.
- *Family history.* Young's syndrome (reduced fertility, bronchiectasis, and rhinosinusitis), cystic fibrosis, Kallmann's syndrome.
- *Sexual history.* Erectile function, frequency of intercourse, sexual techniques. Absence of morning erections suggests an organic cause of erectile dysfunction.

Physical examination

- Body hair distribution.
- Muscle mass and fat distribution.
- Eunuchoidism.
- Gynaecomastia.
- Genital examination:
  - *Pubic hair.* Normal ♂ escutcheon.
  - *Phallus.* Normal >5cm length and >3cm width.
  - *Testes.* Size (using Prader orchidometer) and consistency (normal >15m and firm).
  - Look for nodules or areas of tenderness.
- General examination: look for evidence of systemic disease.
  - Assess sense of smell and visual fields.
  - Reflexes.
  - Peripheral pulses.
  - Rectal examination.

Hormonal evaluation of testicular function

Serum testosterone

Diurnal variation in circulating testosterone, peak levels occurring in the early morning. 30% variation between highest and lowest testosterone levels, so 9 a.m. plasma testosterone essential. If level is low, this should be repeated.

Sex hormone-binding globulin (SHBG)
- Only 2–4% of circulating testosterone is unbound. 50% is bound to SHBG and the rest to albumin.
- Concentrations of SHBG should be taken into account when interpreting a serum testosterone result. SHBG levels may be affected by a variety of conditions (see Table 4.14).
- It is important to measure SBHG when testosterone values at 9 a.m. are under the normal range.

Gonadotrophins
Raised FSH and LH in 1° testicular failure and inappropriately low in pituitary or hypothalamic hypogonadism. Should always exclude hyperprolactinaemia in 2° hypogonadism.

Oestradiol
Results from the conversion of testosterone and androstenedione by aromatase. See Table 4.15 for causes of an elevated oestradiol. Request serum oestradiol level if gynaecomastia is present or a testicular tumour is suspected.

Table 4.14 Factors affecting SHBG concentrations

Raised SHBG	Low SHBG
Androgen deficiency	Hyperinsulinaemia
GH deficiency	Obesity
Ageing	Acromegaly
Thyrotoxicosis	Androgen treatment
Oestrogens	Hypothyroidism
Liver cirrhosis	Cushing's syndrome/glucocorticoid therapy
	Nephrotic syndrome

Table 4.15 Causes of raised oestrogens in ♂

Neoplasia:
Testicular
Adrenal
Hepatoma
Primary testicular failure
Liver disease
Thyrotoxicosis
Obesity
Androgen resistance syndromes
Antiandrogen therapy

Inhibin B and AMH

Gonadal glycoproteins secreted into the circulation. Useful markers of normal testicular functions; low if 1° testicular failure and normal if pituitary/hypothalamic dysfunction.

Other investigations

- Scrotal US (testicular volume/blood flow with Doppler/presence of hydrocele, etc.).
- Semen analysis (a normal semen analysis is indicative of gonadal health; ♂ with low sperm count should consider sperm cryopreservation to preserve fertility).

Dynamic tests

Of limited clinical value and are thus rarely performed routinely.

- hCG stimulation test:
  - Diagnostic test for examining Leydig cell function.
  - hCG 2000IU IM given on days 0 and 2; testosterone measured on days 0, 2, and 4.
  - In prepubertal boys with absent scrotal testes, a response to hCG indicates intra-abdominal testes. Failure of testosterone to rise after hCG suggests absence of functioning testicular tissue. An exaggerated response to hCG is seen in 2° hypogonadism.
- Clomifene stimulation test:
  - Used to assess the integrity of the hypothalamo–pituitary testicular axis.
  - A normal response to 3mg/kg (max 200mg) clomiphene daily for 7 days is a 2-fold increase in LH and FSH measured on days 0, 4, 7, and 10.
  - Subnormal response indicates hypothalamic or pituitary hypogonadism but does not differentiate between the two.

Further reading

AACE Hypogonadism Task Force (2002). American Association of Clinical Endocrinologists Medical Guidelines for clinical practice for the evaluation and treatment of hypogonadism in adult male patients–2002 Update. *Endoc Prac* **8**, 439–56.

Aksglaede L, Juul A (2013). Testicular function and fertility in men with Klinefelter syndrome: a review. *Eur J Endocrinol* **168**, R67–R76.

Lanfranco F, Kamischke A, Zitzmann M, *et al.* (2004). Klinefelter's syndrome. *Lancet* **364**, 273–83.

Miller JF (2012). Approach to the child with Prader-Willi syndrome. *J Clin Endocrinol Metab* **97**, 3837–44.

Semple RK, Topaloglu AK (2010). The recent genetics of hypogonadotrophic hypogonadism— novel insights and new questions. *Clin Endocrinol (Oxf)* **72**, 427–35.

Androgen replacement therapy

Treatment aims

- *Improve libido and sexual function.*
- *Improve mood and well-being.*
- *Improve muscle mass and strength.* Testosterone has direct anabolic effects on skeletal muscle and has been shown to increase muscle mass and strength when given to hypogonadal men. Lean body mass is also ↑ with a reduction in fat mass.
- *Prevent osteoporosis.* Hypogonadism is a risk factor for osteoporosis. Testosterone inhibits bone resorption, thereby reducing bone turnover. Its administration to hypogonadal ♂ has been shown to improve bone mineral density and reduce the risk of developing osteoporosis.

Androgen replacement therapy does not restore fertility—indeed, it suppresses normal spermatogenesis. ♂ with 2° hypogonadism who desire fertility may be treated with gonadotrophins to initiate and maintain spermatogenesis (📖 see p. 408). Prior testosterone therapy will not affect fertility prospects but should be stopped before initiating gonadotrophin treatment. ♂ with 1° hypogonadism will not respond to gonadotrophin therapy and may require donor insemination.

Indications for treatment

- In ♂ with established 1° or 2° hypogonadism of any cause.
- See Box 4.18 for contraindications.
- Treatment should be begun slowly with prolonged and/or severe hypogonadism.

NB Weight reduction is associated with a rise in testosterone.

Pretreatment evaluation

Clinical evaluation

History or symptoms of:
- Prostatic hypertrophy.
- Breast or prostate cancer.
- Cardiovascular disease.
- Sleep apnoea.

Examination

- Rectal examination of prostate.
- Breasts.

Laboratory evaluation

- Prostate-specific antigen (PSA) (NB PSA is often low in hypogonadal ♂, rising to normal age-matched levels with androgen replacement).
- Haemoglobin and haematocrit.
- Cholesterol profile.

See Box 4.19 for monitoring.

Box 4.18 Contraindications for androgen replacement therapy

Absolute
- Prostate cancer.
- Breast cancer.

Relative
- Benign prostate hyperplasia.
- Polycythaemia.
- Sleep apnoea.

Box 4.19 Monitoring of therapy

3 months after initiating therapy and then 6–12-monthly:
- Clinical evaluation—relief of symptoms of androgen deficiency and exclude side effects.
- Serum testosterone.
- Rectal examination of the prostate (if >45 years).
- PSA (if >45 years).
- Haemoglobin and haematocrit.
- Serum lipids.

Risks and side effects of androgen replacement therapy

(See Table 4.16 for testosterone preparations.)

Prostatic disease

- Androgens stimulate prostatic growth, and testosterone replacement therapy may therefore induce symptoms of bladder outflow obstruction in ♂ with prostatic hypertrophy.
- It is unlikely that testosterone increases the risk of developing prostate cancer, but it may promote the growth of an existing cancer.
- It may be possible to consider testosterone therapy after 4 years in low-risk patients with prostatic carcinoma after restaging and with careful PSA surveillance.

Polycythaemia

Testosterone stimulates erythropoiesis. Androgen replacement therapy may increase haemoglobin levels, particularly in older ♂. It may be necessary to reduce the dose of testosterone in ♂ with clinically significant polycythaemia.

Cardiovascular disease

Testosterone replacement therapy may cause a fall in both LDL and HDL cholesterol levels, the significance of which remains unclear. The effect of androgen replacement therapy on the risk of developing coronary heart disease is unknown.

Other

- *Acne.*
- *Gynaecomastia* is occasionally enhanced by testosterone therapy, particularly in peripubertal boys. This is the result of the conversion of testosterone to oestrogens.
- *Fluid retention* may result in worsening symptoms in those with underlying congestive cardiac failure or hepatic cirrhosis.
- *Obstructive sleep apnoea* may be exacerbated by testosterone therapy.
- *Hepatotoxicity* only with oral 17α alkylated testosterones.
- *Mood swings.*

Further reading

Bhasin S, *et al.* (2010). Testosterone therapy in men with androgen deficiency syndromes: an Endocrine Society clinical practice guideline. *J Clin Endocrinol Metab* **95**, 2536–59.

Handelsman DJ, Zajac JD (2004). Androgen deficiency and replacement therapy in men. *Med J Aust* **180**, 529–35.

Landau D, et al. (2012). Should testosterone replacement be offered to hypogonadal men treated previously for prostatic carcinoma? *Clin Endocrinol (Oxf)* **76**, 179–81.

Nieschlag E, Behre HM, Bouchard P, *et al.* (2004).Testosterone replacement therapy: current trends and future directions. *Hum Reprod Update* **10**, 409–19.

Rhoden EL, Morgentaler A (2004). Risks of testosterone replacement therapy and recommendations for monitoring. *N Engl J Med* **350**, 482–92.

Table 4.16 Testosterone preparations

Preparation	Dose	Advantages	Problems
IM testosterone esters	250mg every 2–3 weeks Monitor predose serum testosterone (should be above the lower limit of normal)	2–3 weekly dosage Effective, cheap	Painful IM injection Contraindicated in bleeding disorders Wide variations in serum testosterone levels between injections which may be associated with symptoms
'Nebido'®	1g 3-monthly (after loading dose)	Convenience of infrequent injections	
Testosterone implants	100–600mg every 3–6 months Monitor predose serum testosterone	Physiological testosterone levels achieved 3–6-monthly dosing	Minor surgical procedure Risk of infection and pellet extrusion (3–10%). Must remove pellet surgically if complications of androgen replacement therapy develop
Transdermal Gel (1%, 2%)	5–10g (1%), 2–4g (2%) gel daily	Physiological testosterone levels achieved Convenience	Skin reactions (rare) Possible person-to-person transfer through direct skin contact
Oral, e.g. testosterone undecanoate and mesterolone (analogue of DHT)	40mg tds, 25mg tds	Oral preparations	Highly variable efficacy and bioavailability Rarely achieves therapeutic efficacy Multiple daily dosing
Buccal testosterone	30mg bd	Physiological testosterone levels achieved	Local discomfort, gingivitis, bitter taste Twice daily dosing

Gynaecomastia

Definition

Enlargement of the ♂ breast, as a result of hyperplasia of the glandular tissue, to a diameter of >2cm (see Fig. 4.8). Common; present in up to one-third of ♂ <30 years and in up to 50% of ♂ >45 years.

See Box 4.20 for causes.

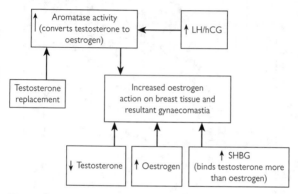

Fig. 4.8 Hormonal influences on gynaecomastia.

Box 4.20 Causes of gynaecomastia

See Fig. 4.8 for hormonal influences.
- Physiological:
  - Neonatal.
  - Puberty—about 50% of boys develop transient gynaecomastia.
  - Idiopathic—about 25% of all cases.
- Drugs (possible mechanisms: oestrogen-containing, androgen receptor blockers, inhibiting androgen production):
  - Oestrogens, antiandrogens, testosterone.
  - Spironolactone, ACE inhibitors, calcium antagonists, digoxin.
  - Alkylating agents.
  - Alcohol, marijuana, heroin, methadone.
  - Cimetidine.
  - Ketoconazole, metronidazole, antituberculous agents, tricyclic antidepressants, dopamine antagonists, opiates, benzodiazepines.
  - Antiretroviral drugs.
  - Imatinib (chronic myeloid leukaemia).
- Hypogonadism:
  - 1°.
  - 2°.
- Tumours:
  - Oestrogen- or androgen-producing testicular or adrenal tumours.
  - Human chorionic gonadotrophin-producing tumours, usually testicular, e.g. germinoma; occasionally ectopic, e.g. lung.
  - Aromatase-producing testicular or hepatic tumours.
- Endocrine:
  - Thyrotoxicosis.
  - Cushing's syndrome.
  - Acromegaly.
  - Androgen insensitivity syndromes.
- Systemic illness:
  - Liver cirrhosis.
  - Chronic renal failure.
  - HIV infection.
  - Malnutrition.

Evaluation of gynaecomastia

History
- Duration and progression of gynaecomastia.
- Further investigation warranted if:
  - Rapidly enlarging gynaecomastia.
  - Recent-onset gynaecomastia in a lean post-pubertal ♂.
  - Painful gynaecomastia.
- *Exclude underlying tumour,* e.g. testicular cancer.
- *Symptoms of hypogonadism.* Reduced libido, erectile dysfunction.
- *Symptoms of systemic disease,* e.g. hepatic, renal, and endocrine disease.
- *Drug history,* including recreational drugs, e.g. alcohol.

Physical examination
- *Breasts:*
  - Pinch breast tissue between thumb and forefinger—distinguish from fat.
  - Measure glandular tissue diameter. Gynaecomastia if >2cm.
  - If >5cm, hard, or irregular, investigate further to exclude breast cancer.
  - Look for galactorrhoea.
- *Testicular palpation:*
  - Exclude tumour.
  - Assess testicular size—? atrophy.
- *2° sex characteristics.*
- Look for evidence of *systemic disease,* e.g. chronic liver or renal disease, thyrotoxicosis, Cushing's syndrome, chronic cardiac or pulmonary disease.

Investigations
(See Fig. 4.9.)

Baseline investigations
- Serum testosterone.
- Serum oestradiol.
- LH and FSH.
- Prolactin.
- SHBG.
- hCG.
- Liver function tests.

Additional investigations
- If testicular tumour is suspected, e.g. raised oestradiol/hCG: testicular US.
- If adrenal tumour is suspected, e.g. markedly raised oestradiol: dehydroepiandrosterone sulphate; abdominal CT or MRI scan.
- If breast malignancy is suspected: mammography; FNAC/tissue biopsy.
- If lung cancer is suspected, e.g. raised hCG: chest radiograph.
- Other investigations, depending on clinical suspicion, e.g. renal or thyroid function.

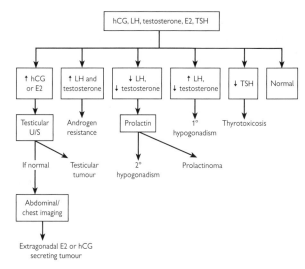

Fig. 4.9 Investigations of gynaecomastia.

Management of gynaecomastia

- Treat underlying disorder when present. Withdraw offending drugs where possible.
- Reassurance in the majority of idiopathic cases. Often resolves spontaneously.
- Treatment may be required for cosmetic reasons or to alleviate pain and tenderness.
- Drug treatment only partially effective. May be of benefit in treating gynaecomastia of recent onset.

Medical

See Table 4.17.

Surgical

Reduction mammoplasty may be required in ♂ with severe and persistent gynaecomastia.

Table 4.17 Medical treatment of gynaecomastia

Tamoxifen (10–30mg/day)	Antioestrogenic effects. Particularly effective in reducing pain and swelling if used in gynaecomastia of recent onset. A 3-month trial before referral for surgery may be of benefit.
Clomifene (50–100mg/day)	Antioestrogenic. May be effective in reducing breast size in pubertal gynaecomastia.
Danazol (300–600mg/day)	Non-aromatizable androgen. May also reduce breast size in adults. Its use is limited by side effects, particularly weight gain and acne.
Testolactone (450mg/day)	Aromatase inhibitor. May be effective in reducing pubertal gynaecomastia. However, tamoxifen appears to be more effective and better tolerated.
Anastrozole (1mg/day)	Another aromatase inhibitor. Clinical trials have failed to show a beneficial effect on gynaecomastia compared with placebo.

Further reading

Carlson HE (2011). Approach to the patient with gynecomastia. *J Clin Endocrinol Metab* **96**, 15-21.
Khan HN, Blarney RW (2003). Endocrine treatment of physiological gynaecomastia. *BMJ* **327**, 301–2.

Testicular tumours

Epidemiology
- 6/100,000 ♂ per year.
- Incidence rising, particularly in North West Europe.
  See Table 4.18 for classification.

Risk factors
- Cryptorchidism.
- Gonadal dysgenesis.
- Infertility/reduced spermatogenesis.

Prognosis
Seminomas
- 95% cure for early disease; 80% cure for stages II/IV.
- ↑ incidence of second tumours and leukaemias 20 years after therapy.

Non-seminoma germ cell tumours
- 90% cure in early disease, falling to 60% in metastatic disease.
- ↑ incidence of second tumours and leukaemias 20 years after therapy.

Stromal tumours
- Excellent prognosis for benign tumours.
- Malignant tumours are aggressive and are poorly responsive to treatment.

Table 4.18 Classification of testicular tumours

Tumours		Tumour markers
Germ cell tumours (95%)	Seminoma	None
	Non-seminoma	hCG, α-fetoprotein, CEA
	Mixed	
Stromal tumours (2%)	Leydig cell	
	Sertoli cell	
Gonadoblastoma (2%)		
Other (1%)	Lymphoma	
	Carcinoid	

Further reading
Griffin JE, Wilson JD (1998). Disorders of the testes and male reproductive tract. In: Wilson JD, Foster DW, Kronenberg HM, Larson PR (eds.) *Williams textbook of endocrinology*, 9th edn, pp. 819–76. WB Saunders, Philadelphia.

Erectile dysfunction

Definition

The consistent inability to achieve or maintain an erect penis sufficient for satisfactory sexual intercourse. Affects approximately 10% of ♂ and >50% of ♂ >70 years.

Physiology of male sexual function

- The erectile response is the result of the coordinated interaction of nerves, smooth muscle of the corpora cavernosa, pelvic muscles, and blood vessels.
- It is initiated by psychogenic stimuli from the brain or physical stimulation of the genitalia, which are modulated in the limbic system, transmitted down the spinal cord to the sympathetic and parasympathetic outflows of the penile tissue.
- Penile erectile tissue consists of paired corpora cavernosa on the dorsum of the penis and the corpus spongiosum. These are surrounded by fibrous tissue known as the tunica albuginea.
- In the flaccid state, the corporeal smooth muscle is contracted, minimizing corporeal blood flow and enhancing venous drainage.
- Activation of the erectile pathway results in penile smooth muscle relaxation and cavernosal arterial vasodilatation. As the corporeal sinuses fill with blood, the draining venules are compressed against the tunica albuginea, so venous outflow is impaired. This results in penile rigidity and an erection.
- Corporeal vasodilatation is mediated by parasympathetic neuronal activation, which induces nitric oxide release by the cavernosal nerves. This activates guanyl cyclase, thereby ↑ cGMP and causing smooth muscle relaxation.
- Detumescence occurs after the inactivation of cGMP by the enzyme phosphodiesterase, resulting in smooth muscle contraction and vasoconstriction.
- Ejaculation is mediated by the sympathetic nervous system.

Pathophysiology

Erectile dysfunction may thus occur as a result of several mechanisms:

- Neurological damage.
- Arterial insufficiency.
- Venous incompetence.
- Androgen deficiency.
- Penile abnormalities.

Evaluation of erectile dysfunction

History
Sexual history
- Extent of the dysfunction, its duration and progression.
- Presence of nocturnal or morning erections.
- Abrupt onset of erectile dysfunction which is intermittent is often psychogenic in origin.
- Progressive and persistent dysfunction indicates an organic cause.

Symptoms of hypogonadism
Reduced libido, muscle strength, and sense of well-being.

Full medical history
- For example, diabetes mellitus, liver cirrhosis, neurological, cardiovascular, or endocrine disease.
- Intermittent claudication suggests a vascular cause.
- A history of genitourinary trauma or surgery is also important.
- Recent change in bladder or bowel function may indicate neurological cause.
- Psychological history.

Drug history
Onset of impotence in relation to commencing a new medication.

Social history
- Stress.
- Relationship history.
- Smoking history.
- Recreational drugs, including alcohol.

Physical examination
- Evidence of 1° or 2° hypogonadism.
- Evidence of endocrine disorders:
  - Hyperprolactinaemia, thyroid dysfunction, hypopituitarism.
  - Other complications of diabetes mellitus, if present.
- Evidence of neurological disease:
  - Autonomic or peripheral neuropathy.
  - Spinal cord lesions.
- Evidence of systemic disease, for example:
  - Chronic liver disease.
  - Chronic cardiac disease.
  - Peripheral vascular disease.
- Genital examination:
  - Assess testicular size—? atrophy.
  - Penile abnormalities, e.g. Peyronie's disease.

See Box 4.21 for causes of erectile dysfunction.

Box 4.21 Causes of erectile dysfunction

- Psychological (20%):
  - Stress, anxiety.
  - Psychiatric illness.
- Drugs (25%):
  - Alcohol.
  - Antihypertensives, e.g. diuretics, β-blockers, methyldopa.
  - Cimetidine.
  - Marijuana, heroin, methadone.
  - Major tranquillizers.
  - Tricyclic antidepressants, benzodiazepines.
  - Digoxin.
  - Glucocorticoids, anabolic steroids.
  - Oestrogens, antiandrogens.
- Endocrine (20%):
  - Hypogonadism (1° or 2°).
  - Hyperprolactinaemia.
  - Diabetes mellitus (30–50% of ♂ with DM >6 years).
  - Thyroid dysfunction.
- Neurological:
  - Spinal cord disorders.
  - Peripheral and autonomic neuropathies.
  - Multiple sclerosis.
- Vascular:
  - Peripheral vascular disease.
  - Trauma.
  - Diabetes mellitus.
  - Venous incompetence.
- Other:
  - Haemochromatosis.
  - Debilitating diseases.
  - Penile abnormalities, e.g. priapism, Peyronie's disease.
  - Prostatectomy.

Investigation of erectile dysfunction

Baseline investigations

- Serum testosterone.
- Prolactin, LH, and FSH if serum testosterone low.
- Fasting blood glucose.
- Thyroid function tests.
- Liver function tests.
- Renal function.
- Serum lipids.
- Serum ferritin (haemochromatosis).

Additional investigations

Rarely required. To assess vascular causes of impotence if corrective surgery is contemplated:

- *Intracavernosal injection* of a vasodilator, e.g. alprostadil E1 or papaverine. A sustained erection excludes significant vascular insufficiency.
- *Penile Doppler ultrasonography*. Cavernous arterial flow and venous insufficiency are assessed.

Management of erectile dysfunction

Treat underlying disorder or withdraw offending drugs where possible.

Androgens

This should be first-line therapy in ♂ with hypogonadism (🕮 see p. 378). Hyperprolactinaemia, when present, should be treated with dopamine agonists and the underlying cause of hypogonadism treated.

Phosphodiesterase (PDE) inhibitors

(See Table 4.19 and Box 4.22.)

- Act by enhancing cGMP activity in erectile tissue by blocking the enzyme PDE-5, thereby amplifying the vasodilatory action of nitric oxide and thus the normal erectile response to sexual stimulation.
- Trials indicate a 50–80% success rate.

Alprostadil

- Alprostadil results in smooth muscle relaxation and vasodilatation.
- It is administered intraurethrally and is then absorbed into the erectile bodies.
- 60–66% success rate.
- *Side effects*. Local pain.

Intracavernous injection

- 70–100% success rate, highest in men with non-vasculogenic impotence.
- Alprostadil is a potent vasodilator. The dose should be titrated in 1 microgram increments until the desired effect is achieved in order to minimize side effects.
- Papaverine, a phosphodiesterase inhibitor, induces cavernosal vasodilatation and penile rigidity but causes more side effects.
- *Side effects:*
  - Priapism in 1–5%. Patients must seek urgent medical advice if an erection lasts >4h.
  - Fibrosis in the injection site in up to 5% of patients. Minimize risk by alternating sides of the penis for injection and injecting a maximum of twice a week.
  - Infection at injection site is rare.
- *Contraindication*. Sickle cell disease.
- *Injection technique*. Avoid the midline so as to avoid urethral and neurovascular damage. Clean the injection site; hold the penis under slight tension, and introduce the needle at 90°. Inject after the characteristic 'give' of piercing the fibrous capsule. Apply pressure to injection site after removing the needle to prevent bruising.

Vacuum device

Results are good, with 90% of ♂ achieving a satisfactory erection. The flaccid penis is put into the device and air is withdrawn, creating a vacuum which then allows blood to flow into the penis. A constriction band is then placed on to the base of the penis so that the erection is maintained. This should be removed within 30min.

- *Side effects*. Pain, haematoma.

Table 4.19 PDE-5 inhibitors

	Sildenafil	Vardenafil	Tadalafil
Dose (mg/day)	50–100	10–20	10–20
Recommended interval between drug administration and sexual activity	60min	30–60min	>30min
Half-life (h)	3–4	4–5	17
Adverse effects (%)			
Headaches	15–30	7–15	7–20
Facial flushing	10–25	10	1–5
Dyspepsia	2–15	0.5–6	1–15
Nasal congestion	1–10	3–7	4–6
Visual disturbance	1–10	0–2	0.1

Box 4.22 PDE-5 inhibitors—contraindications and cautions

Contraindications
- Recent myocardial infarction/stroke.
- Unstable angina.
- Current nitrate use, including isosorbide mononitrate/GTN.
- Hypotension (<90/50mmHg).
- Severe heart failure.
- Severe hepatic impairment.
- Retinitis pigmentosa.
- Ketoconazole or HIV protease inhibitors.

Cautions (reduce dose)
- Hypertension.
- Heart disease.
- Peyronie's disease.
- Sickle cell anaemia.
- Renal or hepatic impairment.
- Elderly.
- Leukaemia.
- Multiple myeloma.
- Bleeding disorders, e.g. active peptic ulcer disease.

Avoid concomitant opiates, including dihydrocodeine—may get prolonged erections (opiates increase cGMP in nerve endings).

Penile prosthesis
- Is usually tried in ♂ either reluctant to try other forms of therapy or when other treatments have failed. They may be semi-rigid or inflatable.
- *Complications.* Infection, mechanical failure.

Psychosexual counselling

Particularly for ♂ with psychogenic impotence and in ♂ who fail to improve with the above therapies.

Surgical
- Rarely indicated, as results are generally disappointing.
- Revascularization techniques may be available in specialist centres.
- Ligation of dorsal veins may restore erectile function temporarily in men with venous insufficiency, although rarely permanently.

Further reading

Beckman TJ, *et al.* (2006). Evaluation and medical management of erectile dysfunction. *Mayo Clinic Proc* **81**, 385–90.

Cohan P, Korenman SG (2001). Erectile dysfunction. *J Clin Endocrinol Metab* **86**, 2391–4.

Fazio L, Brick G (2004). Erectile dysfunction: management update. *Can Med Assoc J* **170**, 1429–37.

Shamloul R, Ghanem H (2013). Erectile dysfunction. *Lancet* **381**, 153–65.

Infertility

Definition

- Infertility, defined as failure of pregnancy after 1 year of unprotected regular (2× week) sexual intercourse, affects ~10% of all couples.
- Couples who fail to conceive after 1 year of regular unprotected sexual intercourse should be investigated.
- If there is a known predisposing factor or the ♀ partner is over 35 years of age, then investigation should be offered earlier.

Causes

(See Boxes 4.23 and 4.24.)
- ♀ factors (e.g. PCOS, tubal damage) 35%.
- ♂ factors (idiopathic gonadal failure in 60%) 25%.
- Combined factors 25%.
- Unexplained infertility 15%.

Box 4.23 Causes of female infertility

- Anovulation:
  - PCOS (80% of anovulatory disorders).
  - 2° hypogonadism.
  - Hyperprolactinaemia.
  - Thyroid dysfunction.
  - Hypothalamic disease.
  - Pituitary disease.
  - Systemic illness.
  - Drugs, e.g. anabolic steroids.
  - POF (5% of anovulatory disorders).
- Tubal disorders:
  - Infective, e.g. Chlamydia.
  - Endometriosis.
  - Surgery.
- Cervical mucus defects.
- Uterine abnormalities:
  - Congenital.
  - Intrauterine adhesions.
  - Uterine fibroids.

Box 4.24 Causes of male infertility

- Primary gonadal failure:
  - Genetic, e.g. Klinefelter's syndrome, Y chromosome microdeletions, immotile cilia/Kartagener's syndrome, cystic fibrosis.
  - Congenital cryptorchidism.
  - Orchitis.
  - Torsion or trauma.
  - Chemotherapy and radiotherapy.
  - Other toxins, e.g. alcohol, anabolic steroids.
  - Varicocele.
  - Idiopathic.
- 2° gonadal failure:
  - Hypogonadotrophic hypogonadism.
  - Structural hypothalamic/pituitary disease.
- Genital tract abnormalities:
  - Obstructive congenital, infective, post-surgical.
  - Sperm autoimmunity.
- Erectile dysfunction.
- Drugs, e.g. spironolactone, corticosteroids, sulfasalazine.
- Systemic disease, e.g. cystic fibrosis, Crohn's disease, and other chronic debilitating diseases.

Evaluation of female infertility

Sexual history
- *Frequency of intercourse*. Sexual intercourse every 2–3 days should be encouraged.
- *Use of lubricants*. Should be avoided because of the detrimental effect on semen quality.

Female factors
History
- *Age*. Fertility declines rapidly after the age of 36 years.
- *Menstrual history*:
  - Age at menarche.
  - Length of menstrual cycle and its regularity (e.g. oligo-/amenorrhoea).
  - Presence or absence of intermenstrual spotting.
- *Hot flushes* may be indicative of oestrogen deficiency.
- *Spontaneous galactorrhoea* may be caused by hyperprolactinaemia.
- *Hypothalamic hypogonadism*, suggested by excessive physical exercise (e.g. running >4 miles/day) or weight loss in excess of 10% in 1 year.
- *Drug history*:
  - Drugs which may cause hyperprolactinaemia (🕮 see Box 2.12, p. 141), including cocaine and marijuana.
  - Smoking is thought to have an adverse effect on fertility.
  - The use of anabolic steroids may cause 2° hypogonadism.
  - Cytotoxic chemotherapy or radiotherapy may cause ovarian failure.
- *Medical history*. Diabetes mellitus, thyroid or pituitary dysfunction, and other systemic illnesses.
- Exclude *tubal disease*:
  - Recurrent vaginal or urinary tract infections may predispose to pelvic inflammatory disease (PID).
  - Dyspareunia and dysmenorrhoea are often present.
  - Sexually transmitted disease and previous abdominal or gynaecological surgery all predispose to Fallopian tube obstruction.
- 2° *infertility*. Details of previous pregnancies, including abortions (spontaneous and therapeutic), and ectopic pregnancies should be ascertained.
- *Family history*. Suggestive of risk of POF, PCOS, endometriosis.

Physical examination
- *BMI*. The ideal BMI for fertility is 20–29.
- *2° sexual characteristics*. If absent, look for evidence of Turner's syndrome.
- *Hyperandrogenism*. PCOS.
- *Galactorrhoea*. Hyperprolactinaemia.
- *External genitalia and pelvic examination*.

Investigations
(See Fig. 4.10.)

- General assessment:
  - Measure TSH, free T4, and serum prolactin in ♀ with irregular menstrual cycles or who are not ovulating.
  - Serum testosterone, SHBG, 17OH progesterone if there is clinical evidence of hyperandrogenism, in the presence of irregular menstrual cycles, or if anovulation is confirmed.
  - *MRI of the pituitary fossa* in hyperprolactinaemia and hypogonadotrophic hypogonadism.
- Assess ovarian reserve:
  - Check serum FSH and LH. In ♀ who are not amenorrhoeic, this should be measured on days 2–6 of the menstrual cycle (day 1 = first day of menses). Follicular phase (FSH >10) is indicative of reduced ovarian reserve. Ovarian failure is diagnosed if FSH >30.
  - *Pelvic US.* Not only for uterine and ovarian anatomy but also for antral follicle count (number of small follicles as an estimate of ovarian ageing).
  - Consider AMH measurement.
- Assess ovulatory function:
  - Home ovulation kit testing of urinary LH reliable in regular cycles. Home temperature testing less reliable.
  - In ♀ with regular menstrual cycles—measure a midluteal progesterone (day 21 or approximately 7 days before expected onset of menses >30pmol/L consistent with ovulation).
  - Consider ovulation tracking by serial ultrasound if uncertain.
- *Exclude infection.* Send vaginal discharge for bacteriology, and do *Chlamydia trachomatis* serology.
- *Assess tubal patency* (refer to specialist multidisciplinary fertility clinic):
  - Hysterosalpingography (HSG) or laparoscopy and dye test (do in the early follicular phase of cycle to avoid doing during pregnancy).

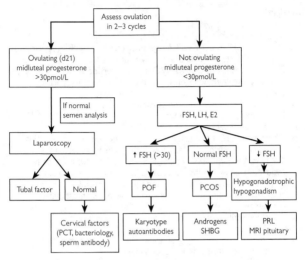

Fig. 4.10 Investigation of ♀ infertility.

Evaluation of male infertility

Male factors

History and physical examination

- Symptoms of androgen deficiency:
  - Reduced libido and potency.
  - Reduced frequency of shaving.
  - May be asymptomatic.
- *Drug history:*
  - Drug or alcohol abuse and the use of anabolic steroids may all contribute to hypogonadism.
  - Other drugs that may affect spermatogenesis, e.g. sulfasalazine, methotrexate.
  - Cytotoxic chemotherapy may cause 1° testicular failure.
- *History of infection,* e.g. mumps, orchitis, sexually transmitted disease, or epididymitis.
- *Bronchiectasis* may be associated with epididymal obstruction (Young's syndrome) or severe asthenospermia (immotile cilia syndrome).
- *Testicular injury or surgery* may cause disordered spermatogenesis.
- *2° sex characteristics* may be absent in congenital hypogonadism.
- *Anosmia.* Kallmann's syndrome.
- *Eunuchoid habitus* (📖 see Box 4.17, p. 371) suggestive of prepubertal hypogonadism.
- *Gynaecomastia* may suggest hypogonadism.
- *Testicular size* (using orchidometer):
  - Normal 15–25mL.
  - Reduced to <15mL in hypogonadism.
  - In Klinefelter's syndrome, they are often <5mL.
  - In patients with normal testicular size, suspect genital tract obstruction, e.g. congenital absence of vas deferens.
- Examine rest of *external genitalia.* Look for penile/urethral abnormalities and epididymal thickening.

Investigations

(See Fig. 4.11.)

Semen analysis

Essential in the diagnostic work-up of any infertile couple.
- If *normal* (see Table 4.20), then a ♂ cause is excluded.
- If *abnormal,* then repeat semen analysis approximately 6–12 weeks later.
- Semen collection should be performed after 3 days of sexual abstinence. See Table 4.20 for interpretation of results.
- If *azoospermia* is present, then rule out obstruction if FSH and testosterone concentrations are normal.
- *Asthenospermia,* or immotile sperm, is usually due to immunological infertility or infection, e.g. of the prostate (high semen viscosity and pH, and leukocytospermia).

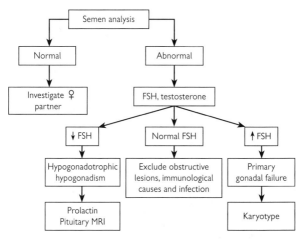

Fig. 4.11 Investigation of ♂ infertility.

Table 4.20 WHO criteria for normal semen analysis[1]

Test	Normal values (fertile)	Nomenclature for abnormal values
Volume	>2mL	Aspermia (no ejaculate)
pH	>7.2	
Total sperm number	>40 × 10⁶/ejaculate	Azoospermia (no sperm in ejaculate)
Sperm concentration	>48 × 10⁶/mL	Oligozoospermia
Motility	>63% progressive motility	Asthenospermia
Morphology	>12% normal forms	Teratospermia
Live sperm	>75%	Necrospermia
Leukocytes	<1 × 10⁶/mL	Leukocytospermia

[1] Reproduced with permission from Guzick DS, Overstreet JW, Factor-Litvak P, *et al.* (2001). Sperm morphology, motility, and concentration in fertile and infertile men. *New Engl J Med* **345**, 1388–93.

FSH, LH, testosterone, SHBG levels
- FSH may be elevated in the presence of normal LH and testosterone levels and oligospermia. This may be seen in ♂ who are normally virilized but infertile as a result of disordered spermatogenesis.
- Low FSH, LH, and testosterone concentrations suggest 2° hypogonadism. An MRI of the pituitary gland and hypothalamus is necessary to exclude organic disease.

Further investigations
- *Urinary bacteriology* should be performed in ♂ with leukocytospermia.
- *Scrotal US* may help in the diagnosis of chronic epididymitis. ♂ being investigated for infertility are at ↑ risk of testicular tumours.
- *Karyotyping* may be helpful in ♂ with 1° testicular failure. Klinefelter's syndrome (47,XXY) is a cause of infertility, and deletions on the long arm of the Y chromosome have been found in a significant proportion of azoospermic ♂.
- *Sperm antibodies* in semen should not be measured routinely, as specific treatment is rarely effective.
- *Testicular biopsy* is rarely diagnostic but may be used to retrieve sperm for assisted reproduction techniques in specialist fertility centres.
- *Sperm function tests* are not performed routinely.

Management of female infertility

Anovulation
- *Hypogonadotrophic (WHO class I):*
  - If hyperprolactinaemic, then dopamine agonists are usually effective.
  - Lifestyle changes if underweight/excessive exercise.
  - Otherwise, ovulation induction (📖 see Ovulation induction, p. 410).
- *Normogonadotrophic (WHO class II):*
  - Usually PCOS; weight reduction if obese.
  - Ovulation induction (📖 see Ovulation induction, p. 410).
- *Hypergonadotrophic (WHO class III):*
  - POF; ovum donation is only option.
  - Spontaneous transient remission possible in early POF.
  - If still cycling and FSH 15–25IU/L, ovarian hyperstimulation and IVF may be attempted but poor results.

Tubal infertility
- Surgical tubal reconstruction may be attempted in specialist centres.
- 50–60% 2-year cumulative pregnancy rate in patients with mild disease, but only 10% in more severe disease and high risk of ectopic pregnancy, so IVF may be more appropriate in ♀ with severe disease.
- Cumulative pregnancy rate at least 50% following IVF (20–35% per cycle), unless hydrosalpinx is present. ♀ with hydrosalpinx should be offered salpingectomy prior to IVF to improve success rates.

Endometriosis
- *Minimal/mild:*
  - GnRH agonists, danazol, and progestagens do not improve fertility.
  - Laparoscopic destruction of superficial disease improves pregnancy chances. Resection of ovarian endometriomas may improve ovarian folliculogenesis and thus fertility.
  - Assisted reproductive techniques (ART) (see Table 4.21) give pregnancy rate of 25–35% per cycle.
- *Moderate/severe:*
  - Surgery may improve fertility. However, ART often necessary.

Vaginal/cervical factors
- Each episode of acute PID causes infertility in 10–15% of cases.
- *Trachomatis* is responsible for half the cases of PID in developed countries. Treat both partners with antibiotics.

Uterine factors
- *Intracavity fibroids, polyps, uterine septum* can be resected hysteroscopically, with high chance of restoring fertility.
- *Intramural fibroids* may also reduce fertility and may require myomectomy.
- *Fibroid embolization* is not recommended for ♀ wishing fertility, as safety in pregnancy not established.

Table 4.21 Assisted reproductive techniques (ART)

Technique	Indications	Pregnancy rates	Notes
Intrauterine insemination (IUI) (usually offered up to six cycles)	Unexplained infertility Mild oligozoospermia ($>2 \times 10^6$ motile sperm) Mild endometriosis	<15% per cycle 15%	Washed and prepared motile spermatozoa are injected into the uterine cavity through a catheter just before ovulation. Superovulation may improve success rates but is associated with an increased risk of multiple pregnancy.
In vitro fertilization (IVF)	Most forms of infertility unless severe male factor	20–30% pregnancy rate per cycle 80–90% delivery rate after six cycles in women under the age of 35 years Success rates markedly reduced after 40 years of age Babies conceived by IVF have a 2× increased risk of low birthweight and preterm delivery	After superovulation, ovarian follicles are aspirated under ultrasonic guidance and are fertilized with prepared sperm in vitro. The embryos are then transferred back into the uterine cavity, usually 48h after insemination. Luteal support, using progesterone supplementation (pessaries or PO), is then provided until pregnancy is confirmed. May adopt a similar technique in women with premature ovarian failure using donated ova which are then fertilized in vitro with partner's sperm. Hormonal support will be required following embryo transfer.
Gamete intrafallopian transfer (GIFT)	Most forms of infertility unless severe male factor Do not use in women with tubal disease	Similar to IVF	Similar to IVF, except that retrieved follicles and sperm are injected laparoscopically into a Fallopian tube to fertilize naturally. Rarely performed in the UK, as it offers little advantage over IVF.
Intracytoplasmic sperm injection (ICSI)	Male infertility	20–30% per cycle if female partner under 40 years of age There is a small risk of sex chromosome abnormalities in males (1%) conceived following ICSI	Viable spermatozoa are injected directly into oocytes retrieved following superovulation. Embryos are then implanted into the uterus. Spermatozoa may be concentrated from an ejaculate or be aspirated from the epididymis or testis in men with obstructive azoospermia.

Management of male infertility

Hypogonadotrophic hypogonadism

- Gonadotrophins: chorionic gonadotrophin 1,500–2,000IU IM 2×
  week. Most also require FSH/hMG 150IU IM 3× week. Monitor serum
  testosterone and testicular size. Main side effect: gynaecomastia.

Or

- Pulsatile GnRH is not generally used in men.
  - Once testes are >8mL, semen analysis every 3–6 months. Takes
    at least 2 years to maximize spermatogenesis. Normalization of
    spermatogenesis in 80–90% of ♂.
  - Once spermatogenesis is induced, it may be maintained by hCG alone.

Idiopathic semen abnormalities

There is no evidence to suggest that the use of androgens, gonadotrophins, or antioestrogens help to improve fertility in ♂ with idiopathic
disorders of spermatogenesis.

Obstructive azoospermia

- Reversal of vasectomy will result in successful pregnancy in up to 50%
  of cases within 2 years.
- Microsurgery is possible for most other causes, with successful
  pregnancies in 25–35% of couples within 18 months of treatment.
  During surgery, sperm is often retrieved and stored for possible future
  intracytoplasmic sperm injection (ICSI).

Varicocele

Controversial association with ♂ subfertility. Surgical correction is currently not recommended for fertility treatment, as there is little evidence
that surgery improves pregnancy rates.

Unexplained infertility

Definition

Infertility despite normal sexual intercourse occurring at least twice weekly, normal semen analysis, documentation of ovulation in several cycles, and normal patent tubes (by laparoscopy).

Management

30–50% will become pregnant within 3 years of expectant management. If not pregnant by then, chances that spontaneous pregnancy will occur are greatly reduced, and ART should be considered. In ♀ >34 years of age, then expectant management is not an option, and up to six cycles of IUI or IVF should be considered.

Results

- Superovulation with IUI can achieve a pregnancy rate of 15% per cycle and cumulative delivery rate after several cycles of 50%.
- IVF offers a live birth rate per cycle of >30% in younger ♀ and a cumulative delivery rate approaching 80%.
- ICSI allows IVF to be offered in severe oligospermia, with pregnancy rates equivalent to standard IVF. Slight increase in congenital malformations after ICSI. Significant risk of multiple pregnancies with any form of ART.

Ovulation induction

Indications
- Anovulation due to:
  - PCOS.
  - Hypopituitarism.
  - Hypogonadotrophic hypogonadism.
- Controlled ovarian hyperstimulation for IVF.

Pretreatment assessment
- Exclude thyroid dysfunction and hyperprolactinaemia.
- Check rubella serology.
- Confirm normal semen analysis.
- Confirm tubal patency (laparoscopy, hysterosalpingogram (HSG), or hysterosalpingo-contrast-sonography (HyCoSy)) prior to gonadotrophin use and/or after failed clomiphene use.
- Optimize lifestyle: maintain satisfactory BMI, exercise in moderation, reduce alcohol intake, and stop smoking.
- Baseline pelvic US is essential to exclude ovarian masses and uterine abnormalities prior to treatment.

Clomifene citrate
- *Mode of action:*
  - Antioestrogen blocking normal –ve feedback, thereby ↑ pulse frequency of GnRH. This stimulates FSH and LH release, thereby stimulating the production of one or more dominant ovarian follicles.
  - Antioestrogen effect on endometrium, cervix, and vagina.
- *Indications.* Eugonadotrophic anovulation, e.g. PCOS. May also be used in unexplained infertility. Requires normal hypothalamo–pituitary–ovarian axis to work, therefore ineffective in hypogonadotrophic hypogonadism.
- *Administration.* Start on days 2–5 of menstrual cycle (may have to induce bleed by giving a progestagen for 10 days), and take for a total of 5 days.
- *Dose:*
  - Most require 50–100mg/day for 5 days.
  - Should be used with ovulation tracking by ultrasound to avoid multiple pregnancies and to confirm effectiveness.
  - Spontaneous ovulation should occur 5–10 days after last day of medication.
  - Remain on optimum dose for 6–12 months.
- *Efficacy:*
  - 80–90% ovulate, with conception rates of 50–60% in first six ovulatory cycles. May enhance chances of ovulation in non-responders by the administration of 10,000IU of hCG midcycle (use US guidance; administer hCG when leading follicle is at least 20mm).
- *Side effects:*
  - Hot flushes in 10%, mood swings, depression and headaches in 1%, pelvic pain in 5%, nausea in 2%, breast tenderness in 5%, hair loss in 0.3%, visual disturbances in 1.5%.

- • Ovarian hyperstimulation syndrome (OHSS) in 1%.
    - • Multiple pregnancies in 7–10%.
- • *Risk of ovarian cancer.* Unknown. Infertility is associated with an ↑ risk of ovarian cancer. Additionally, one study suggests a 2-fold ↑ risk of low-grade ovarian cancer, following long-term clomifene use. Further studies necessary, but currently recommended maximum treatment duration is 6–12 months.
- • *Tamoxifen* is also an antioestrogen which has similar properties to clomifene. It can be used to induce ovulation, with results comparable to clomifene. The dose used is 20–40mg od for 5–7 days, starting on days 2–5 of menstrual cycle. Letrozole 5mg also used in some countries—similar effectiveness.

Ovarian diathermy

- • Laparoscopic ovarian diathermy in 4–10 points on the surface of the ovaries may be used in ♀ with PCOS who have failed to conceive on clomiphene.
- • Its ovulation rate of >80% and pregnancy rate of >60% are comparable to gonadotrophin therapy without the risk of multiple pregnancies or OHSS. It is most effective in slim ♀ with PCOS with a high LH.
- • There is a low risk of pelvic adhesions following ovarian diathermy and a theoretical risk of premature ovarian failure.

Gonadotrophins

- • *Indications:*
    - • Hypogonadotrophic hypogonadism.
    - • ♀ with PCOS who are clomiphene-resistant.
    - • For superovulation, as part of ART.
- • *Dose and administration.* Several regimens available; all require close monitoring with vaginal US.
- • One suggested regime (low-dose step-up approach):
    - • Start at 50–75IU/day hMG (or FSH) on days 2–4 of the menstrual cycle. Titrate the dose up at approximately weekly intervals, according to follicle development to achieve up to three follicles over 14mm.
    - • If >3 mature follicles (>14mm) develop or E2 >3,000pmol/L, then abandon cycle and restart on half-dose hMG/FSH because of risk of OHSS.
    - • Otherwise, give hCG at a dose of 5,000IU to trigger ovulation when follicle >18mm diameter. May increase to 10,000IU in subsequent cycle if ovulation does not occur.
    - • May use gonadotrophins for a total of six cycles. If unsuccessful, then consider IVF.
- • *Efficacy.* 80–85% pregnancy rate after six cycles.
- • *Side effects:*
    - • Multiple pregnancies (20%).
- • *OHSS:*
    - • A potentially fatal syndrome of ovarian enlargement and ↑ vascular permeability, with accumulation of fluid in the peritoneal, pleural, and pericardial cavities. Occurs after hCG stimulation and is more severe if pregnancy occurs due to endogenous hCG production. Withhold hCG in at-risk cycles.

- Mild OHSS occurs in up to 25% of stimulated cycles and results in abdominal bloating and nausea. It resolves with bed rest and fluid replacement. Severe OHSS, associated with hypotension, markedly enlarged ovaries, ascites, and pleural and pericardial effusions, occurs in <0.1%. ♀ need to be hospitalized and resuscitated, as there is an ↑ mortality from disseminated intravascular coagulation and pulmonary emboli. Management should be led by an expert reproductive endocrinologist.
- Risk factors for OHSS are multiple follicles, young age, PCOS, and previous OHSS.
- IVF superovulation should be accompanied by use of a GnRH agonist, starting from midluteal phase of the preceding cycle (long protocol) or a GnRH antagonist starting in the midfollicular phase of the stimulation cycle (antagonist protocol). These strategies prevent premature ovulation before eggs can be collected and significantly improve pregnancy rates.

Pulsatile GnRH

- *Indications.* Hypothalamic hypogonadism with normal pituitary function.
- *Dose and administration.* Pulsatile GnRH using an infusion pump which is worn continuously. This delivers a dose of GnRH every 90min, delivered subcutaneously (15–20 micrograms/90min).
- This treatment is favoured over hMG because of lower risk of OHSS or multiple pregnancies.
- *Side effects.* Allergic reaction.
- *Efficacy.* Cumulative pregnancy rate of 70–90%.

Cryopreservation, fertility, and cancer treatment

- Chemotherapy and/or radiotherapy for some cancers can adversely affect ♂ and ♀ fertility, resulting in gonadal failure.
- ♂ patients should be offered the chance of sperm cryopreservation and storage prior to commencing cancer treatment so that future fertility may be an option.
- ♀ cancer patients may consider either superovulation with oocyte cryopreservation or IVF with embryo freezing if with established partner. Requires a 3–6 weeks' delay in initiation of chemo-/radiotherapy which must be sanctioned by oncologist.

Human Fertilisation and Embryology Act (UK)

- The Human Fertilisation and Embryology Authority (HFEA) is a statutory body set up to inspect, monitor, and license fertility centres offering IUI, IVF, ICSI, and/or donor sperm or egg insemination and to regulate all research involving human embryos. It is also required to keep a register of all IVF treatment cycles and of all children born as a result of IVF or donor sperm or oocytes. The HFEA also provides information to couples seeking fertility treatment or potential donors.
- The HFEA is accountable to the Secretary of State for Health and advises government ministers, as required, particularly regarding new developments in fertility technology or research.

Further reading

Braude P, Muhammed S (2003). Assisted conception and the law in the United Kingdom. *BMJ* **327**, 978–81.

Farhat R, et al. (2010). Outcome of gonadotropin therapy for male infertility due to hypogonado-trophic hypogonadism. *Pituitary* **13**, 105–10.

Hamilton-Fairley D, Taylor A (2003). Anovulation. *BMJ* **327**, 546–9.

Hirsh A (2003). Male subfertility. *BMJ* **327**, 669–72.

Royal College of Obstetrics and Gynaecology (2004). Fertility assessment and treatment for people with fertility problems. RCOG, pp.1–208. Royal College of Obstetrics and Gynaecology, London.

Disorders of sexual differentiation

Definition
Discordance between three elements of sexual development: genetic sex, gonadal structure, or genital appearance.

Clinical presentation
- *Infancy.* Ambiguous genitalia (see evaluation discussed in Assessment of ambiguous genitalia, p. 545).
- *Puberty:*
  - Failure to progress through puberty (♂ or ♀ phenotype).
  - 1° amenorrhoea in a ♀ phenotype.
  - Virilization of a ♀ phenotype.
- *Adulthood:*
  - Hypogonadism.
  - Infertility.

Evaluation
- *Karyotype.* 46,XX vs 46,XY ♂ or ♀.
- Imaging:
  - Look for presence of testes or ovaries and uterus.
  - Most easily performed using pelvic US, but MRI may be more sensitive in identifying internal genitalia and abnormally sited gonads in cryptorchidism.

Hormonal evaluation
- LH, FSH, testosterone, oestradiol, SHBG.
- hCG stimulation test (see Clinical assessment, p. 119)—to assess the presence of functioning testicular material. Measure testosterone, androstenedione, DHT, and SHBG post-stimulation.
- Others, depending on clinical suspicion, for example:
  - 5α-reductase deficiency—check DHT levels before and after hCG stimulation.
  - 21-hydroxylase deficiency—17-hydroxyprogesterone ± ACTH stimulation (see Investigations, p. 322).
  - Urinary steroid profile—mass spectrometry and gas chromatography as screen for some enzyme defects.

See Box 4.25 for causes.

Box 4.25 Causes of disorders of sexual differentiation

(📖 see also Assessment of ambiguous genitalia, p. 545.)

46,XY DSD

- XY gonadal dysgenesis (Swyer syndrome):
  - Cause unknown in the majority.
  - 20% SRY gene mutation.
- Leydig cell hypoplasia:
  - LH receptor gene mutation.
- Biochemical defects of androgen synthesis, for example:
  - 3β-HSD, 17α-hydroxylase/17,20-desmolase or 17β-HSD deficiencies.
- Androgen receptor defects:
  - Androgen insensitivity syndrome (📖 see pp. 416, 546).
- 5α-reductase deficiency:
  - Mutation of 5α-reductase type 2 gene.
  - Autosomal recessive inheritance.
  - High testosterone but low DHT concentrations.
  - Phenotype can range from ♀ external genitalia to ♂ with hypospadias. Characteristically virilize after puberty.
- Persistent Müllerian duct syndrome:
  - Müllerian inhibitory substance (MIS), also called anti-Müllerian hormone (AMH), or MIS receptor gene mutation.
- Ovotesticular DSD.

46,XX DSD

- Excess fetal androgens—CAH:
  - 21-OH deficiency (90%).
  - 11B-OH deficiency.
- Excess maternal androgens:
  - Drugs.
  - Virilizing tumours.
- Placental aromatase deficiency.
- 46,XX ♂
  - Due to a Y to X translocation so that the SRY gene is present.
  - Phenotype similar to Klinefelter's syndrome.
- Ovotesticular DSD.

Androgen insensitivity syndrome

Pathogenesis

- Results from a mutation in androgen receptor gene (Xq11–12). Inherited in an X-linked recessive fashion, but approximately 40% of patients have a –ve family history, i.e. *de novo* mutations.
  - Severity of mutation variable—results in phenotype spectrum from normal female, through partially virilized XY DSD, to infertile male: Reifenstein's syndrome (undervirilized ♂ with gynaecomastia and hypospadias).
- Incidence 1:20,000–1:64,000.

Clinical features

- *Complete androgen insensitivity* results in normal ♀ external genitalia. However, the vagina is often shorter than normal and may rarely be absent. Testes are usually located in the abdomen or in the inguinal canal. There is no spermatogenesis.
- Presents in childhood with inguinal testicular hernia or 1° amenorrhoea at puberty. Pubertal development is normal, apart from little or no pubic and axillary hair. Body habitus, gender identity, and psychological development are ♀.
- *Partial androgen insensitivity* has a wide phenotypic spectrum, ranging from ambiguous genitalia to a normal ♂ phenotype, presenting with infertility.

Evaluation

- Key features are raised LH, normal FSH, and testosterone levels normal or slightly raised (♂ range). hCG stimulation results in a further rise in testosterone, with little increase in SHBG.
- Androgen receptor mutation screening if possible female carriers exist in pedigree.

Management

- Orchidectomy to prevent malignancy. Exact timing of surgery is controversial, but it is usually performed in adolescence after attaining puberty. In phenotypic ♀ with partial androgen insensitivity, gonadectomy may be performed before puberty to avoid virilization.
- Oestrogen replacement therapy in phenotypic ♀.
- High-dose androgen therapy in ♂ with Reifenstein's syndrome may improve virilization.

Ovotesticular DSD

Pathogenesis
- Unknown. May be familial.
- Previously known as true hermaphroditism.
- Affected individuals have both ovarian and testicular tissue, either in the same gonad (ovotestis) or an ovary on one side and a testis on the other. A uterus and a Fallopian tube are usually present, the latter on the side of the ovary or ovotestis. Wolffian structures may be present in a third of individuals on the side of the testis. The testicular tissue is usually dysgenetic, although the ovarian tissue may be normal.

Clinical features
- Most individuals have ambiguous genitalia and are raised as ♂, but just under 10% have normal ♀ external genitalia.
- At puberty, 50% of individuals menstruate, which may present as cyclic haematuria in ♂, and most develop breasts.
- Feminization and virilization vary widely. Most are infertile, but fertility has been reported.
- 2% risk of gonadal malignancy, higher in 46,XY individuals.

Evaluation
- 46,XX in 70%, 46,XX/46,XY in 20%, and 46,XY in 10%.
- Hypergonadotrophic hypogonadism is usual.
- Diagnosis can only be made on gonadal biopsy.

General principles of management

Assignment of gender and reconstructive surgery

Virilized females
- The majority are brought up as ♀.
- The timing of feminizing surgery remains controversial but is usually deferred until adolescence. The decision should be made on an individual basis by a multidisciplinary specialist team, the parents, and ideally the patient. It appears that a significant number of children who have surgery performed during infancy will require further surgery in their teens. The results of feminizing genitoplasty, which involves clitoral reduction and vaginoplasty, with regard to sexual function are unclear.

Undervirilized males
- The decision regarding gender reassignment is complex and depends on the degree of sexual ambiguity, aetiology, the potential for normal sexual function and fertility, and social circumstances.
- Individuals with complete androgen insensitivity are assigned a ♀ sex, as they are resistant to testosterone therapy, develop ♀ sexual characteristics, and have a ♀ gender identity.
- Sex assignment of other forms depends on phallic size. A trial of 3 months of testosterone may be used to enhance phallic growth.
- Penile reconstruction and orchidopexy by an experienced urologist may be considered in some patients. Testicular prostheses may be required if orchidopexy is not possible. The optimal procedure and timing of surgery remain controversial, and the decision should ideally be made involving the patient when he is old enough to give informed consent. Results of surgery on sexual function are mixed.

Gonadectomy
- ↑ risk of gonadoblastoma in most individuals with abdominal testes. Risk is highest in those with dysgenetic gonads and Y chromosome material. Bilateral gonadectomy should, therefore, be performed (usually laparascopically).
- Optimal timing of the gonadectomy is unknown. In androgen insensitivity, the risk of gonadoblastoma appears to rise only after the age of 20 years, so orchidectomy is recommended in adolescence after attaining puberty. In most other disorders, gonadectomy prior to puberty is recommended.
- Early bilateral orchidectomy should also be performed in 46,XY subjects with 5α-reductase deficiency or 17β-HSD deficiency who are being raised as ♀ to prevent virilization at puberty.

Hormone replacement therapy

- Patients with disorders of adrenal biosynthesis, e.g. CAH, require lifelong glucocorticoid and usually mineralocorticoid replacement therapy.
- Gender-assigned ♂ require long-term testosterone replacement therapy.
- Individuals with 5α-reductase deficiency usually receive supraphysiological doses of testosterone in order to achieve satisfactory DHT levels.
- Gender-assigned ♀ should receive oestrogen replacement therapy to induce puberty, and this should be continued until about the age of 50.

Psychological support

- Disorders relating to sexual identity and function require expert counselling.
- Patient support groups are often helpful.

Further reading

Creighton S, Minto C (2001). Managing intersex. *BMJ* **323**, 1264–5.
MacLaughlin DT, Donahoe PK (2004). Sex determination and differentiation. *N Engl J Med* **350**, 367–78.
Vogiatzi MG, New MI (1998). Differential diagnosis and therapeutic options for ambiguous genitalia. *Curr Opin Endocrinol Diabet* **5**, 3–10.
Warne GL, Zajac JD (1998). Disorders of sexual differentiation. *Endocrinol Metab Clin North Am* **27**, 945–67.

Transsexualism

Definition

A condition in which an apparently anatomically and genetically normal person feels that he or she is a member of the opposite sex. *Gender dysphoria* is an irreversible discomfort with the anatomical gender, which may be severe, often developing in childhood.

Epidemiology

- More common in ♂.
- Estimated prevalence of 1:13,000 ♂ and 1:30,000 ♀.

Aetiology

- Unknown and controversial.
- Some evidence that it may have a neurobiological basis. There appear to be sex differences in the size and shape of certain nuclei in the hypothalamus. ♂ to ♀ transsexuals have been found to have ♀ differentiation of one of these nuclei, whereas ♀ to ♂ transsexuals have been found to have a ♂ pattern of differentiation.

Management

Standards of care

- Multidisciplinary approach between psychiatrists, endocrinologists, and surgeons. Patient should be counselled about the treatment options, risks, and implications, and realistic expectations should be discussed.
- Endocrine disorders should be excluded prior to entry into the gender reassignment programme, i.e. ensure normal internal and external genitalia, karyotype, gonadotrophins, and testosterone/oestradiol.
- Psychiatric assessment and follow-up is essential before definitive therapy. The transsexual identity should be shown to have been persistently present for at least 2 years to ensure a permanent diagnosis.
- Following this period, the subject should dress and live as a member of the desired sex under the supervision of a psychiatrist. This should continue for at least 3 months before hormonal treatment and 1 year before surgery.
- Psychological follow-up and expert counselling should be available, if required, throughout the programme, including after surgery.
- In adolescents, puberty can be reversibly halted by GnRH analogue therapy to prevent irreversible changes in the wrong gender until a permanent diagnosis is made.
- See Box 4.27 for monitoring of therapy.

Box 4.26 Contraindications to hormone manipulation

Feminization
- Prolactinoma.
- Family history of breast cancer.
- Risk of thromboembolism.
- Active liver disease.
- Cardiovascular or cerebrovascular disease.
- Other contraindication to oestrogen therapy (📖 see p. 347).

Masculinization
- Cardiovascular disease.
- Active liver disease.
- Polycythaemia.
- Cerebrovascular disease.

Box 4.27 Monitoring of therapy
- Every 3 months for first year, then every 6 months.
- Hormonal therapy is lifelong, and so patients should be followed up indefinitely.

Male to female
- Physical examination.
- Liver function tests.
- Serum lipids and glucose.
- LH, oestradiol, prolactin.
- PSA (>50 years).
- ? mammogram (>50 years).
- Bone densitometry.

Female to male
- Physical examination.
- Liver function tests.
- Serum lipids and blood glucose.
- LH, testosterone.
- FBC (exclude polycythaemia).
- Bone densitometry.

Hormonal manipulation

See Box 4.26 for contraindications.

Male to female transsexuals

- Suppress ♂ 2° sex characteristics: cyproterone acetate (CPA) (100mg/day).
- Induce ♀ 2° sex characteristics:
  - Ethinylestradiol 100 micrograms/day or estradiol valerate 2mg bd/ tds or estradiol patch 100 micrograms 2×/week (stop smoking).
  - Medroxyprogesterone acetate 10mg od.
- *Aims:*
  - Breast development—maximum after 2 years of treatment.
  - Development of ♀ fat distribution.
  - ↓ body hair and smoother skin. However, facial hair is often resistant to treatment.
  - ↓ muscle bulk and strength.
  - Reduction in testicular size.
  - Hormonal manipulation has little effect on voice.

- Reduce dose of CPA following gender reassignment surgery, and discontinue, if possible. However, some subjects will require an antiandrogen in order to keep oestradiol doses to a minimum (see Table 4.22).
- The dose of oestrogen may be reduced after gender reassignment surgery (see Table 4.22).
- Change to transdermal oestrogens if >40 years old. Change to HRT doses once >50 years old.
- Adjust oestrogen dose, depending on plasma LH and oestradiol levels.
- *Side effects* (particularly while on high-dose EE2 + CPA therapy):
  - Hyperprolactinaemia.
  - Venous thromboembolism.
  - Abnormal liver enzymes.
  - Depression.
  - ? ↑ risk of breast cancer.

Female to male transsexuals
- Induce ♂ 2° sex characteristics and suppress ♀2° sex characteristics: parenteral testosterone (see Table 4.22).
- *Aims:*
  - Cessation of menstrual bleeding.
  - Atrophy of uterus and breasts.
  - Increase muscle bulk and strength.
  - Deepening of voice (after 6–10 weeks).
  - Hirsutism.
  - ♂ body fat distribution.
  - Increase in libido.
- Once sexual characteristics are stable (after approximately 1 year of treatment) and following surgery, reduce testosterone dose, based on serum testosterone and LH levels.
- *Side effects:*
  - Acne (in 40%).
  - Weight gain.
  - Abnormal liver function.
  - Adverse lipid profile.

Gender reassignment surgery
- Performed at least 6–9 months after starting sex hormone therapy.
- A second psychiatric opinion should be sought prior to referral for surgery.
- Usually performed in several stages.

Male to female transsexuals
- Bilateral orchidectomy and resection of the penis.
- Construction of a vagina and labia minora.
- Clitoroplasty.
- Breast augmentation.

Table 4.22 Maintenance hormone regimens in the treatment of transsexualism

Feminization (post-surgery)	Masculinization (pre- and post-surgery)
<40 years: Ethinylestradiol 30–50 micrograms od Estradiol valerate (oral) 2–4mg od Estradiol valerate (transdermal) 50 micrograms 2×/week Conjugated estrogens 1.25mg od	Testosterone 250mg IM every 2 weeks Transdermal testosterone (gel or patch) 5mg od
>40 years: Transdermal estradiol 50 micrograms 2×/week May need to continue cyproterone acetate 50mg od or add spironolactone 100–200mg od Role of progestin not established	

Female to male transsexuals
- Bilateral mastectomy.
- Hysterectomy and salpingo-oophorectomy.
- Phalloplasty and testicular prostheses.

Prognosis
- Significantly ↑ morbidity in ♂ to ♀ transsexuals from thromboembolism.
- Hyperprolactinaemia and elevation in liver enzymes are self-limiting in the majority of cases.
- The risk of osteoporosis is not thought to be ↑ in transsexuals.
- There may be a slightly ↑ risk of breast cancer in ♂ to ♀ transsexuals.
- Results from reconstructive surgery, particularly in ♀ to ♂ transsexuals, remain suboptimal.
- There is an ↑ risk of depressive illness and suicide in transsexual individuals.

Further reading

Gooren LJ (2011). Clinical practice. Care of transsexual persons. *N Engl J Med* **364**, 1251–7.
Gooren LJ, Giltay EJ, Brunck MC (2008). Long-term treatment of transsexuals with cross-sex hormones: extensive personal experience. *J Clin Endocrinol Metab* **93**, 19–25.
Levy A, Crown A, Reid R (2003). Endocrine intervention for transsexuals. *Clin Endocrinol* **59**, 409–18.
Moore E, Wisniewski A, Dobs A (2003). Endocrine treatment of transsexual people: a review of treatment regimens, outcomes and adverse effects. *J Clin Endocrinol Metab* **88**, 3467–73.
Schlatterer K, von Werder K, Stalla GK (1996). Multistep treatment concept of transsexual patients. *Exp Clin Endocrinol Diabet* **104**, 413–19.

Endocrinology in pregnancy

Thyroid and parathyroid disorders

Normal physiology

Effect of pregnancy on thyroid function

- *Iodine stores.* Fall due to ↑ renal clearance and transplacental transfer to fetus.
- *Thyroid size.* Increase in thyroid volume by 10–20% due to hCG stimulation and relative iodine deficiency.
- *Thyroglobulin.* Rise corresponds to rise in thyroid size.
- *Thyroid-binding globulin (TBG).* Twofold ↑ in concentration as a result of reduced hepatic clearance, and ↑ synthesis stimulated by oestrogen. Concentration plateaus at 20 weeks' gestation and falls again post-partum.
- *Total T_4 and T_3.*↑ concentrations, corresponding to rise in TBG.
- *Free T_4 and T_3.* There may be a small rise in concentration in first trimester due to hCG stimulation, then fall into normal range. During second and third trimester, FT_4 concentration is often just below the normal reference range.
- *Thyroid-stimulating hormone (TSH).* Within normal limits in pregnancy. However, suppressed in 13.5% in first trimester, 4.5% in second trimester, and 1.2% in third trimester due to hCG thyrotropic effect. +ve correlation between free T_4 and hCG levels, and –ve correlation between TSH and hCG levels in first half of pregnancy. Upper limit of normal range is higher in pregnancy.
- *Thyrotropin-releasing hormone (TRH).* Normal.
- *TSH receptor antibodies.* When present in high concentrations in maternal serum, may cross the placenta. Antibody titre decreases with progression of pregnancy.

Fetal thyroid function

- TRH and TSH synthesis occurs by 8–10 weeks' gestation, and thyroid hormone synthesis occurs by 10–12 weeks' gestation.
- TSH, total and free T_4 and T_3, and TBG concentrations increase progressively throughout gestation.
- Maternal TSH does not cross the placenta, and although TRH crosses the placenta, it does not regulate fetal thyroid function. Iodine crosses the placenta, and excessive quantities may induce fetal hypothyroidism. Maternal T_4 and T_3 cross the placenta in small quantities and are important for fetal brain development in the first half of gestation.

Maternal hyperthyroidism

(📖 see Thyrotoxicosis in pregnancy, p. 44.)

Incidence
- Affects 0.2% of pregnant women.
- Most are diagnosed before pregnancy or in the first trimester of pregnancy.
- In women with Graves's disease in remission, exacerbation may occur in first trimester of pregnancy.

Graves's disease
- The commonest scenario is pregnancy in a patient with pre-existing Graves's disease on treatment, as fertility is low in patients with untreated thyrotoxicosis. Newly diagnosed Graves's disease in pregnancy is unusual.
- Aggravation of disease in first trimester, with amelioration in second half of pregnancy because of a decrease in maternal immunological activity at that time.
- Symptoms of thyrotoxicosis are difficult to differentiate from normal pregnancy. The most sensitive symptoms are weight loss and tachycardia. Goitre is found in most patients.

Management
- Risks of uncontrolled hyperthyroidism to mother: heart failure/arrhythmias.
- Antithyroid drugs (ATDs) are the treatment of choice but cross the placenta.
- Propylthiouracil (PTU) should be used in the first trimester in case of teratogenic effects of carbimazole (check liver function monthly). Thereafter, carbimazole is recommended.
- Carbimazole use in pregnancy was discouraged, as it was thought to be associated with aplasia cutis, a rare scalp defect, though recent studies have shown no increase in rate. Studies have shown that carbimazole may be associated with choanal and oesophageal atresia, but the maternal hyperthyroidism may be a factor in this.
- Propylthiouracil may rarely be associated with hepatocellular inflammation, which, in severe cases, can lead to liver failure and death. A recent study also showed that PTU was associated with low birthweight infants.
- A short course of 40mg of propranolol tds can be used initially for 2–3 weeks while antithyroid drugs take affect.
- Most patients will be on a maintenance dose of ATD. A high dose of ATD may be necessary initially to achieve euthyroidism as quickly as possible (carbimazole 20–40mg/day or propylthiouracil 200–400mg/day) in newly diagnosed patients, then use the minimal dose of ATD to maintain euthyroidism.
- Do not use block and replace regime as higher doses of ATDs required, and there is minimal transplacental transfer of T_4, thereby risking fetal hypothyroidism.
- Monitor TFTs every 4–6 weeks.

- Aim to keep FT$_4$ at upper limit of normal and TSH low normal (<2.5mU/L—first trimester, <3.0mU/L—second trimester, <3.5mU/L—third trimester).
- In ~30% of women, ATD may be discontinued at 32–36 weeks' gestation. Consider if euthyroid for at least 4 weeks on lowest dose of ATD, but continue to monitor TFTs frequently. The presence of a large goitre or ophthalmopathy suggests severe disease and the chances of remission are low, so do not stop ATD. Graves's disease can flare in the post-natal period due to increase in the maternal antibody levels, so patients should be monitored closely in the post-partum period.
- Risks of neonatal hypothyroidism and goitre are reduced if woman on carbimazole 20mg or less (200mg propylthiouracil or less) in last few weeks of gestation.
- Breastfeeding is safe at doses of less than 150mg of PTU and 15mg carbimazole, as only small amounts pass into the breast milk (<0.7% PTU and 0.5% carbimazole).
- If higher doses are given, we recommend breastfeeding prior to taking medication, and the dose can be divided throughout the day. Neonatal thyroid function needs to be monitored.
- Surgical management of thyrotoxicosis is rarely necessary in pregnancy. Only indication: serious ATD complication (e.g. agranulocytosis) or drug resistance. There is a possible ↑ risk of spontaneous abortion or preterm delivery associated with surgery during pregnancy. The second trimester is the optimal time for surgery, as organogenesis is complete and less chance of anaesthesia and surgery inducing labour.
- Radioiodine therapy is contraindicated in pregnancy, during breastfeeding, and for 4 months prior to conception.

Infants born to mothers with Graves's disease
- Risks to fetus of uncontrolled thyrotoxicosis:
  - ↑ risk of spontaneous miscarriage and stillbirth.
  - Intrauterine growth restriction (IUGR).
  - Preterm labour.
  - Fetal or neonatal hyperthyroidism.
- Follow-up of babies born to mothers on ATDs show normal weight, height, and intellectual function.
- *Fetal hypothyroidism.* May occur following treatment of mother with high doses of ATDs (>200mg PTU/day; >20mg carbimazole), particularly in the latter half of pregnancy. This is rare and may be diagnosed by demonstrating a large fetal goitre on fetal US in the presence of fetal bradycardia.
- *Fetal hyperthyroidism.* May occur after week 25 of gestation. It results in IUGR, fetal goitre, and tachycardia (fetal heart rate >160bpm) and has high mortality if not treated. It may develop if the mother has high titres of TSH-stimulating antibodies (TSAb) which can cross the placenta. Treat by giving mother ATD, and monitor fetal heart rate (aim <140bpm), growth, and goitre size. It is important to remember women with Graves's disease who have been treated with radioiodine or surgery can still have high antibody titres and therefore need monitoring.

- *Neonatal thyrotoxicosis.* Develops in 1% of infants born to thyrotoxic mothers. Transient, usually subsides by 6 months, but up to 30% mortality if untreated. Treat with ATD and β-blockers.

Hyperemesis gravidarum (gestational hyperthyroidism)
- Characterized by severe vomiting and weight loss. Cause unknown.
- Begins in early pregnancy (weeks 6–9 of gestation) and tends to resolve spontaneously by week 20 of gestation.
- Biochemical hyperthyroidism in two-thirds of affected women, but T_3 is less commonly elevated. Mechanism: hCG has TSH-like effect, thus stimulating the thyroid gland and suppressing TSH secretion.
- Degree of thyroid stimulation correlates with severity of vomiting.
- No other evidence of thyroid disease, i.e. no goitre, no history of thyroid disease, no ophthalmopathy, and –ve thyroid autoantibodies (10% population is +ve for thyroid antibodies).
- Antithyroid drugs not required and do not improve symptoms of hyperemesis.

Causes of maternal hyperthyroidism
- Graves's disease (85% of cases).
- Toxic nodule.
- Toxic multinodular goitre.
- Hydatidiform mole.

Maternal hypothyroidism

Prevalence
- 2.5% subclinical hypothyroidism.
- 1–2% overt hypothyroidism.

Risks of suboptimal treatment during pregnancy
- *Spontaneous miscarriage.* Twofold ↑ risk.
- *Pre-eclampsia.* 21% of suboptimally treated mothers have pregnancy-induced hypertension (PIH).
- Also ↑ risk of anaemia during pregnancy and post-partum haemorrhage.
- The fetus is dependent on maternal thyroxine until fetal production starts at 12 weeks.
- Risk of impaired fetal intellectual and cognitive development.
- ↑ risk of perinatal death.
- Other risks to fetus are those associated with PIH (IUGR, preterm delivery, etc.).
- The risk of congenital malformations is not thought to be ↑.

Management
- Spontaneous pregnancy in overtly hypothyroid women is unusual, as hypothyroid women are likely to have anovulatory menstrual cycles.
- *Levothyroxine therapy.* Start on 100 micrograms. Measure TSH and free T_4 4 weeks later.
- For women on thyroxine, optimize therapy prior to pregnancy.
- If already on T_4 before pregnancy, on confirmation of pregnancy, increase dose by 30% (25–50 micrograms) because of increased TBG and thyroid hormone requirements.
- *Aim.* TSH—lower part of normal range; FT_4—upper end of normal.
- Many women are suboptimally replaced prior to pregnancy, so their dose needs to be increased in response to abnormal TFTs. After delivery, they should continue on this increased dose, with monitoring of biochemistry.
- NB Do not give $FeSO_4$ simultaneously with T_4—reduces its efficacy. Separate times for drug ingestion by at least 2h.

Causes of maternal hypothyroidism
- Hashimoto's thyroiditis (most common cause).
- Previous radioiodine therapy or thyroidectomy.
- Previous post-partum thyroiditis.
- Hypopituitarism.

Positive thyroid antibodies but euthyroid
- Twofold excess risk of spontaneous miscarriage.
- No other complications.
- No risk of neonatal hypothyroidism.
- Risk of PIH not ↑.
- The occasional mother will develop hypothyroidism towards the end of the pregnancy, so check TFTs between weeks 28–32 of gestation.
- ↑ risk of post-partum thyroiditis, so check TSH at 3 months post-partum.

Post-partum thyroid dysfunction

Prevalence
- 5–10% of women within 1 year of delivery or miscarriage.
- 3× more common in women with type 1 diabetes mellitus.

Aetiology
- Chronic autoimmune thyroiditis (🕮 see Other types of thyroiditis, p. 72).

Clinical presentation
- *Hyperthyroidism (32%):*
  - Within 4 months of delivery.
  - The most common symptom is fatigue.
  - Usually resolves spontaneously in 2–3 months.
- *Hypothyroidism (43%):*
  - Develops 4–6 months after delivery.
  - Symptoms may be mild and non-specific.
  - There may be an ↑ risk of post-partum depression.
- *Hyperthyroidism followed by hypothyroidism (25%).*
- *Spontaneous recovery* in 80% within 6–12 months of delivery.

Differential diagnosis
- Graves's disease may relapse in the post-partum period. This is differentiated from post-partum thyroiditis by a high uptake on radioiodine scanning.
- Lymphocytic hypophysitis may cause hypothyroidism. However, serum TSH concentrations are inappropriately low.

Investigation
- Thyroid peroxidase antibodies are +ve in 80%.
- Radionuclide uptake scans are rarely necessary. However, there is low uptake during the thyrotoxic phase, differentiating it from Graves's disease where uptake is ↑.

Management
- β-blockers if thyrotoxic and symptomatic until TFTs normalize. Antithyroid medication is unnecessary.
- Levothyroxine if TSH >10 or if TSH between 4–10 and symptomatic.
- No consensus as to how long to treat with thyroxine. Two options:
  - Halve dose at about 12 months post-natal, and check TFTs 6 weeks later. If normal, then withdraw T_4, and check TFTs 6 weeks later.
  - Withdraw treatment 1 year after completion of family.

Prognosis
- Recurrence in future pregnancies in 25% of women.
- Permanent hypothyroidism develops in up to 30% of women within 10 years. If treatment is withdrawn, then annual TSH measurements are essential.

Thyroid cancer in pregnancy

(🕮 see Thyroid cancer and pregnancy, p. 102.)

Parathyroid disorders

Calcium metabolism in pregnancy

- There are increased calcium requirements in pregnancy; 25–30g is transferred to the baby.
- There is increased maternal intestinal absorption of calcium.
- Due to increased renal blood flow, there is increase in the renal excretion of calcium.

Primary hyperparathyroidism in pregnancy

- Rare—8 cases in 100,000 in women of childbearing age.
- In pregnancy, the hypercalcaemia may improve due to the fetal transfer of calcium.
- Diagnosis is made by finding a raised PTH in the presence of a raised calcium.
- Ultrasound can be used to locate the adenoma.
- Can cause serious maternal morbidity which includes hyperemesis, nephrolithiasis, peptic ulcers, and pancreatitis. It is also associated with pre-eclampsia, recurrent miscarriage, preterm labour.
- Fetal complications include IUGR and neonatal death. The high circulating maternal calcium can lead to suppression of fetal parathyroid development, leading to hypocalcaemia of the fetus after delivery. Neonates normally present at days 5–14 with poor feeding, tetany, and convulsions.

Management

- Hypercalcaemia is treated with IV fluids.
- If mild, women can be advised to increase their fluid intake. Calcium levels should be monitored throughout pregnancy, with surgery arranged post-partum.
- If calcium remains persistently high (>2.85mmol/L), then parathyroidectomy can be arranged in the second or early third trimester.

Hypoparathyroidism

- Pregnancy increases the demand for vitamin D. Therefore, replacement doses will need to be increased in pregnancy.
- Maternal levels of corrected calcium and vitamin D should be checked monthly.
- Untreated hypoparathyroidism leads to miscarriage, fetal hypocalcaemia, and neonatal rickets.

Further reading

Abalovich M, Amino N, Barbour LA, *et al.* (2007). Management of thyroid dysfunction during pregnancy and post-partum: an Endocrine Society clinical practice guideline. *J Clin Endocrinol Metab* **92**(8 Suppl), S1–47.

Alexander EK, Marqusee E, Lawrence J, *et al.* (2004). Timing and magnitude of increases in levothyroxine requirements during pregnancy in women with hypothyroidism. *N Engl J Med* **351**, 241–9.

Azizi F, Amouzegar A (2011). Management of hyperthyroidism during pregnancy. *Eur J Endocrinol* **164**, 871–6.

Chen C, Xirasager S, *et al.* (2011). Risk of adverse perinatal outcomes with antithyroid treatement during pregnancy: a national population based study. *BJOG* **118**, 1365–73.

Cooper S, Rivkees S (2009). Putting propylthiouracil in perspective. *J Clin Endocrinol Metab* **94**, 1881–2.

De Groot L, *et al.* (2012). Management of thyroid dysfunction during pregnancy and post-partum: an Endocrine Society clinical practice guideline. *J Clin Endocrinol Metab* **97**, 2543–65.

Lazarus JH. (2011).Thyroid function in pregnancy. *Br Med Bull* **97**, 137–48.

LeBeau SO, Mandell SJ (2006). Thyroid disorders during pregnancy. *Endocrinol Metab Clin North Am* **35**, 117–36.

Norman J, *et al.* (2009). Hyperparathyroidism during pregnancy and the effect of rising calcium on pregnancy loss: a call for earlier intervention. *Clin Endocrinol (Oxf)* **71**, 104–9.

Poppe K, Glinoer D (2003). Thyroid autoimmunity and hypothyroidism before and during pregnancy. *Hum Reprod Update* **9**, 149–61.

Sato K (2008). Hypercalcemia during pregnancy, puerperium and lactation: Review and a case report of hypercalcemic crisis after delivery due to excessive productin of PTH-related protein (PTHrP) without malignancy (humoral hypercalcemia of pregnancy). *Endocrin J* **55**, 959–66.

Stagnaro-Green A (2002). Post-partum thyroiditis. *J Clin Endocrinol Metab* **87**, 4042–7.

Pituitary disorders

Normal anatomical changes during pregnancy

- *Prolactin (PRL)-secreting cells.* Marked lactotroph hyperplasia during pregnancy.
- *Gonadotrophin-secreting cells.* Marked reduction in size and number.
- *TSH and ACTH-secreting cells.* No change in size or number.
- *Anterior pituitary.* Size increases by up to 70% during pregnancy. May take 1 year to shrink to near pre-pregnancy size in non-lactating women. Gradual slight increase in size with each pregnancy.
- *MRI.* Enlarged anterior pituitary gland, but stalk is midline. Posterior pituitary gland may not be seen in late pregnancy.

Normal physiology during pregnancy

- *Serum PRL.* Concentrations increase markedly during pregnancy and fall again to pre-pregnancy levels approximately 2 weeks post-partum in non-lactating women.
- *Serum LH and FSH.* Undetectable levels in pregnancy and blunted response to GnRH because of −ve feedback inhibition from high levels of sex hormones and PRL.
- *Serum TSH, T_4, and T_3.* TSH may be suppressed in the first trimester of pregnancy. Free thyroid hormones usually at the lower end of the normal range.
- *Growth hormone (GH) and IGF-I.* Low maternal GH levels and blunted response to hypoglycaemia due to placental production of GH-like substance. IGF-I levels are normal or high in pregnancy.
- *ACTH and cortisol.* CRH, ACTH, and cortisol levels are high in pregnancy, as both CRH and ACTH are produced by the placenta. In addition, oestrogen-induced increase in cortisol-binding globulin (CBG) synthesis during pregnancy will further increase maternal plasma cortisol concentrations. During the latter half of pregnancy, there is a progressive increase of ACTH and cortisol levels, peaking during labour. Incomplete suppression of cortisol, following dexamethasone suppression test, and exaggerated response of cortisol to CRH stimulation. However, normal diurnal variation persists.

Prolactinoma in pregnancy

Effect of pregnancy on tumour size

Risk of significant tumour enlargement (i.e. resulting in visual field disturbances or headaches):
- Microadenoma 1–2%.
- Macroadenoma 15–35%.
- Macroadenoma treated with surgery and/or radiotherapy before pregnancy 4–7%.

Effect of dopamine agonists on the fetus

Bromocriptine

Over 6,000 pregnancies have occurred in women receiving bromocriptine in early pregnancy, and the incidence of complications in these pregnancies with regard to fetal outcome is similar to that of the normal population, indicating that bromocriptine is probably safe in early pregnancy. Data are available on children whose mothers received bromocriptine throughout pregnancy, and again the incidence of congenital abnormalities is negligible. Children who are exposed to bromocriptine *in utero* have normal psychological development in follow-up.

The FDA has withdrawn the licence for use of bromocriptine post-partum to suppress lactation, as there was an increased incidence of adverse incidents which included myocardial infarction and stroke. We would advise caution, particularly in women with pre-eclampsia.

Cabergoline

Also probably safe in early pregnancy and has been used in >380 pregnancies, with no ↑ risk of fetal loss or congenital abnormalities, but fewer data are available. There are more data on the long-term safety of bromocriptine, but cabergoline is being used increasingly as it is better tolerated.

Quinagolide

It has been used in >176 pregnancies, with a slightly higher rate of congenital abnormalities compared to the background rate.

Recent controversy

The Medicine and Health Regulatory Authority issued guidance on the use of cabergoline in pregnancy, stating it should be stopped 1 month pre-pregnancy. This recommendation is based on data in Parkinson's patients where high doses are used and an increased rate of cardiac and pulmonary fibrosis has been reported. There are no published data on similar conditions occurring in the fetus. Current practice is to use bromocriptine first-line in women hoping to conceive, and cabergoline if they cannot tolerate bromocriptine. Quinagolide is reserved for patients who are unable to tolerate the other dopamine agonists.

Management of prolactinoma

Microprolactinoma

- After recent MRI, initiate dopamine agonist therapy to induce normal ovulatory cycles and fertility.
- Stop bromocriptine as soon as pregnancy is confirmed.
- Assess for visual symptoms and headache at each trimester, although the risk of complications is low (<5%). Serum PRL levels are difficult to interpret during pregnancy, as they are normally elevated; therefore, they are not measured.
- MRI is indicated in the occasional patient who becomes symptomatic.
- In the post-partum period, recheck serum PRL level 2 months after cessation of breastfeeding. Reassess size of microprolactinoma by MRI only if serum PRL level is higher than pre-pregnancy concentrations.
- 40–60% chance of remission of microprolactinoma following pregnancy.

Macroprolactinoma

Management is controversial and must, therefore, be individualized. Three possible approaches:

- Bromocriptine (because cabergoline does not have a licence in pregnancy) may be used throughout pregnancy to reduce the risk of tumour growth. The patient is monitored by visual fields at each trimester or more frequently if symptoms of tumour enlargement develop. This is probably the safest, and thus preferred, approach.
- May use bromocriptine or cabergoline to induce ovulation, and then stop it after conception. However, patient must be monitored very carefully during pregnancy with monthly visual field testing.
- If symptoms of tumour enlargement develop or there is deterioration in visual fields, then MRI should be performed to assess tumour growth. If significant tumour enlargement develops, then bromocriptine therapy should be initiated.
- Alternatively, the patient may undergo surgical debulking of the tumour and/or radiotherapy before seeking fertility. This will significantly reduce the risk of complications associated with tumour growth. However, this approach may render them gonadotrophin-deficient. These patients should again be monitored during pregnancy, using regular visual fields.

MRI should be performed in the post-partum period in women with macroprolactinomas to look for tumour growth.

Breastfeeding

- There is no contraindication to breastfeeding.
- If the mother would like to breastfeed, dopamine receptor agonists will have to be discontinued prior to birth, as they inhibit lactation. The decision to discontinue medication should be assessed on a case-by-case basis, dependent upon the potential risk of optic nerve/chiasm compression.

Cushing's syndrome

- Pregnancy is rare in women with untreated Cushing's syndrome, as 75% of them will experience oligo- or amenorrhoea.
- Adrenal disease is the most common cause of Cushing's syndrome developing in pregnancy, responsible for over 50% of reported cases.
- The diagnosis of Cushing's syndrome is difficult to establish during pregnancy. However, the presence of purple striae and proximal myopathy should alert the physician to the diagnosis of Cushing's syndrome.
- If suspected, the investigation of Cushing's syndrome should be carried out as in the non-pregnant state.
- The circulating levels of cortisol rise during normal pregnancy. This is due to a combination of the increased levels of cortisol-binding globulin, stimulated by the raised oestrogen, and the placental CRH production which is biologically active.
- 24h urinary free cortisol measurements remain normal in the first trimester but can increase by 3× by term in a normal pregnancy.
- Non-suppression of cortisol production on a low-dose dexamethasone suppression test may be a feature of a normal pregnancy. There are no internationally agreed normal values in pregnancy, so interpretation of dynamic testing is difficult.
- The diurnal variation of cortisol secretion is, however, preserved in normal pregnancy.
- Diagnosis is important, as pregnancy in Cushing's syndrome is associated with a high risk of maternal and fetal complications (see Table 5.1).

Management of Cushing's syndrome

- *First trimester:*
  - Offer termination of pregnancy and instigate treatment, particularly if adrenal carcinoma.
  - Alternatively, surgical treatment early in the second trimester.
- *Second trimester:*
  - Surgery, e.g. adrenalectomy or pituitary adenomectomy. Minimal risk to fetus.
- *Third trimester:*
  - ↑ risk of diabetes mellitus.
  - Deliver baby as soon as possible (preferably by vaginal delivery to minimize the risk of poor wound healing following a Caesarean section), and instigate treatment.
- Metyrapone used in doses of <2g/day generally well tolerated in pregnancy. It can cause hypertension and has been associated with development of pre-eclampsia and fetal hypoadrenalism.
- Ketoconazole has been used successfully in a few pregnancies; it is antiandrogenic in rats, so caution should be used if the infant is male.
- Aminoglutethimide causes fetal masculinization so is not recommended.
- Post-operative glucocorticoid replacement therapy will be required.
- Treatment of Cushing's syndrome in pregnancy may reduce maternal and fetal morbidity and mortality.
- See Table 5.1 for complications.

Table 5.1 Complications of Cushing's syndrome in pregnancy

Maternal complications	Incidence (%)	Fetal complications	Incidence (%)
Hypertension	70	Spontaneous abortion	12
Diabetes mellitus	27	Perinatal death	18
Congestive cardiac failure	7	Prematurity	60
Poor wound healing	6	Congenital malformations	Low risk; no risk of virilization
Death	4		

Acromegaly

- Fertility in acromegaly is reduced, partly due to hyperprolactinaemia (if present), in addition to secondary hypogonadism. However, there have been several reported cases of pregnancy in acromegaly.
- Diagnosis in pregnancy is difficult, as the placenta secretes growth hormone and, though different from maternal GH, assays may not be able to detect this. IGF-1 also increases in normal pregnancy.
- Acromegaly increases the risk of gestational diabetes and hypertension, so women should be screened.
- However, in the absence of diabetes mellitus, there does not appear to be an excess of perinatal morbidity or mortality in babies born to women with acromegaly.
- Significant tumour enlargement occasionally occurs, together with enlargement of the normal pituitary lactotrophs, so monthly visual field testing is recommended.
- Bromocriptine can be used in pregnancy, but there is less response compared to prolactinomas.
- There are limited reports of somatostatin analogues and somatostatin receptor agonists use in pregnancy, with no apparent adverse events. They do cross the placenta. We would not advocate their use until more data are available on their safety in pregnancy. Women are generally advised to stop medication on conception.
- Headaches may be helped with both somatostatin analogues and bromocriptine.
- Treatment may be deferred until after delivery in the majority of patients.

Non-functioning pituitary tumours

- These tumours are the second commonest pituitary tumours, but there is little reported about the incidence in pregnancy. Women may present with compression effects due to tumour enlargement.
- If diagnosed pre-pregnancy, then visual field assessment in each trimester is sufficient.
- If field defects develop during pregnancy, bromocriptine may be used which will decrease the size of the normal lactotrophs and thereby improving field defects.

Hypopituitarism in pregnancy

Pre-existing hypopituitarism
- Most commonly due to surgical treatment of and/or radiotherapy for a pituitary adenoma.
- May require ovulation induction and thus conception by gonadotrophin stimulation.

Lymphocytic hypophysitis
(📖 see also Lymphocytic hypophysitis, p. 194.)
- Rare disorder thought to be autoimmune in origin.
- Characterized by pituitary enlargement on imaging and variable loss of pituitary function.
- Most commonly seen in women in late pregnancy or in the first year post-partum.
- Symptoms are due to pressure effects, e.g. visual field defects and headaches, or due to hormonal deficiency.
- Most common hormonal deficiencies:
  - ACTH and vasopressin deficiency.
  - TSH deficiency may also exist.
  - Gonadotrophins and GH levels are usually normal.
  - PRL levels may be mildly elevated in a third, and low in a third.
- *Differential diagnosis:*
  - Pituitary adenoma.
  - Sheehan's syndrome.
- MRI often reveals diffuse homogeneous contrast enhancement of the pituitary gland. However, the diagnosis is often only made definitively by pituitary biopsy.
- There is an association with other autoimmune diseases, particularly Hashimoto's thyroiditis.
- Course variable. Pituitary function may deteriorate or improve with time.

Management
- Pituitary hormone replacement therapy, as required.
- Surgical decompression if pressure symptoms persist.
- A course of high-dose steroid therapy is controversial, with mixed results.

Causes of hypopituitarism during pregnancy
- Pre-existing hypopituitarism.
- Pituitary adenoma.
- Lymphocytic hypophysitis.
- Sheehan's syndrome.

Management of pre-existing hypopituitarism during pregnancy
- *Hydrocortisone.* Dose may need to be ↑ in the third trimester of pregnancy by 10mg a day, as the increase in CBG will reduce the bioavailability of hydrocortisone. Parenteral hydrocortisone in a dose of 100mg IM every 6h should be given during labour and the dose reduced back to maintenance levels in the post-partum period (24–72h).

- *Thyroxine.* Requirements may increase, as pregnancy progresses. Monitor free T_4 each trimester, and increase T_4 dose accordingly.
- *GH.* There are little data on the effects of GH on pregnancy, but case reports do not suggest a detrimental effect on fetal outcome. However, until more data accrue, GH should be stopped prior to pregnancy. Moreover, as the placenta synthesizes a GH variant, GH therapy is unnecessary.
- *Vasopressin.* The placenta synthesizes vasopressinase, which breaks down vasopressin but not desmopressin. Women with partial diabetes insipidus may, therefore, require desmopressin treatment during pregnancy. Those already receiving desmopressin may require a dose increment during pregnancy. Vasopressinase levels fall rapidly after delivery.

Sheehan's syndrome

Post-partum pituitary infarction/haemorrhage, resulting in hypopituitarism. Increasingly uncommon in developed countries with improvements in obstetric care and management of post-partum haemorrhage.

Pathogenesis
- The enlarged pituitary gland of pregnancy is susceptible to any compromise to its blood supply.
- Investigations will confirm hypopituitarism.

Risk factors
- Post-partum haemorrhage.
- Type 1 diabetes mellitus.
- Sickle cell disease.

Clinical features
- Failure of lactation.
- Involution of breasts.
- Fatigue, lethargy, and dizziness.
- Amenorrhoea.
- Loss of axillary and pubic hair.
- Symptoms of hypothyroidism.
- Diabetes insipidus is rare.

Management
Pituitary hormone replacement therapy (📖 see Background, p. 127).

Further reading

Caron P, *et al.* (2010). Acromegaly and pregnancy: a retrospective multicenter study of 59 pregnancies in 46 women. *J Clin Endocrinol Metab* **95**, 4680–7.

Karaca Z, *et al.* (2010). Pregnancy and pituitary disorders. *Eur J Endocrinol* **162**, 453–75.

Kovacs K (2003). Sheehan syndrome. *Lancet* **361**, 520–2.

Lindsay JR, *et al.* (2005). Cushing's syndrome during pregnancy: personal experience and review of the literature. *J Clin Endocrinol Metab* **90**, 3077–83.

Medicines and Healthcare Products Regulatory Agency (2008). *Drug safety update* **2**(3).

Molitch M (2006). Pituitary disorders in pregnancy. *Endocrinol Metab Clin North Am* **35**, 99–116.

Molitch ME (2011). Prolactinoma in pregnancy. *Best Pract Res Clin Endocrinol Metab* **25**, 885–96.

Sam S, Molitch M (2003). Timing and special concerns regarding endocrine surgery during pregnancy. *Endocrinol Metab Clin North Am* **32**, 337–54.

Webster J (1996). A comparative review of the tolerability profiles of dopamine agonists in the treatment of hyperprolactinaemia and inhibition of lactation. *Drug Saf* **14**, 228–38.

Adrenal disorders

Normal changes during pregnancy

Changes in maternal adrenocortical function
Markedly ↑ concentrations of all adrenal steroids due to ↑ synthesis and ↓ catabolism.

Feto-placental unit
- *Fetal adrenal gland.* DHEAS is produced in vast quantities by the fetal adrenal gland. This is the major precursor for oestrogen synthesis by the placenta. The fetal adrenal gland has a large capacity for steroidogenesis. Stimulus for fetal adrenal gland unknown—possibly hCG or PRL.
- *Placenta:*
  - Maternal glucocorticoids are largely inactivated in the placenta by 11β-HSD. Maternal androgens are converted to oestrogens by placental aromatase, thus protecting ♀ fetus from virilization.
  - Maternal catecholamines are broken down by placental catechol-O-methyl transferase and monoamine oxidase activity.

Addison's disease in pregnancy

- No associated fetal morbidity in women who have pre-existing primary adrenal insufficiency, as fetus produces and regulates its own adrenal steroids.
- Management of Addison's disease does not differ in pregnancy.
- Glucocorticoids which are metabolized by placental 11β-HSD preferred (i.e. prednisolone or hydrocortisone) to avoid fetal adrenal suppression.
- Increase hydrocortisone dose by about 10mg during the third trimester of pregnancy and at any time in case of intercurrent illness.
- High-dose intramuscular hydrocortisone should be given at the time of delivery to cover the stress of labour.
- Doses may be tapered to normal maintenance doses in the post-partum period (see Box 5.1).
- Addison's disease developing in pregnancy may result in an adrenal crisis, particularly at the time of delivery, because of a delay in diagnosis.
- In early pregnancy, vomiting, fatigue, hyperpigmentation, and low BP may be wrongly attributed to pregnancy. However, persisting symptoms should alert the clinician.
- If suspected, the diagnosis is confirmed by the presence of low serum cortisol concentrations, with failure to rise following ACTH stimulation, and high ACTH levels. However, the normal ranges for serum ACTH and cortisol concentrations have not been established in pregnancy. One review suggests a value of <828nmol/L 30min after short Synacthen® test would be diagnostic in pregnancy, but this has yet to be agreed internationally.
- Chronic maternal adrenal insufficiency may be associated with intrauterine fetal growth restriction.
- There is no ↑ risk of developing Addison's disease in the immediate post-partum period.

Box 5.1 Management of adrenal insufficiency during pregnancy

- Hydrocortisone 20–30mg PO in divided doses, as per pre-pregnancy dose. Increase in third trimester.
- Fludrocortisone 50–200 micrograms PO, as per pre-pregnancy dose, but requirements may increase. As renin goes up during pregnancy, this is monitored by BP and K.

During uncomplicated labour

- Hydrocortisone 100mg IM 6-hourly for 24h, then reduce to maintenance dose over 72h.
- Keep well hydrated.
- Fludrocortisone may be discontinued while on high doses of hydrocortisone.

Congenital adrenal hyperplasia

- Fertility is reduced, particularly women with the salt-wasting form of CAH.
- Reasons:
  - Inadequate vaginal introitus despite reconstructive surgery.
  - Anovulation as a result of hyperandrogenaemia.
  - Adverse effects of elevated progestagen levels on endometrium.
- 60–80% of women with CAH and an adequate vaginal introitus are fertile.
- Fertility may be maximized by optimal suppression of hyperandrogenism by glucocorticoid therapy (📖 see Management, p. 324).
- No major complications in pregnancy are known in women with CAH, apart from a possibly ↑ incidence of pre-eclampsia.
- However, women are more likely to require Caesarean section for cephalopelvic disproportion.
- Management is the same as in the non-pregnant woman, and steroids are ↑ at the time of delivery as for Addison's disease (📖 see p. 266).
- Monitor serum testosterone and electrolytes every 6–8 weeks; if levels increase, then increase dose of corticosteroids.
- Risk to fetus:
  - No risk of virilization from maternal hyperandrogenism, as placenta will aromatize androgens to oestrogens.
  - Glucocorticoids do not increase the risk of congenital abnormalities.
  - If partner is a heterozygote or homozygote for CAH, then the fetus has a 50% risk of CAH. Prenatal treatment with dexamethasone will then be necessary to avoid virilization of a ♀ fetus (📖 see Management of pregnancy in CAH, p. 325).

Phaeochromocytoma

- Rare but potentially lethal in pregnancy. Maternal mortality may still be as high as 17% and fetal mortality as high as 30% if not treated promptly.
- Maternal death can be due to stroke, pulmonary oedema, arrhythmia, and myocardial infarction, with the greatest risk during labour. Placental vasoconstriction can lead to spontaneous fetal death, intrauterine growth restriction, and fetal hypoxia.
- Hypertensive crisis can be precipitated by labour, delivery, opiates, metoclopramide, and general anaesthesia.
- Women can present with palpitations, sweating, headache, anxiety, dyspnoea, vomiting, and hyperglycaemia.
- Phaeochromocytoma needs to be differentiated from women with pre-eclampsia, so suspect in women with hypertension, persistent or intermittent, especially in:
  - The absence of proteinuria or oedema, or presence of other features.
  - Hypertension developing before 20 weeks' gestation, or
  - Persistent glycosuria.
- Prenatal screening in high-risk women, e.g. those with a history or family history of MEN-2 or von Hippel–Lindau syndrome.
- Diagnose by 24h urinary catecholamine collection (normal ranges are unaltered in pregnancy) or raised plasma catecholamines.
- Labetalol and methyldopa can give false +ves.
- Tumour localization is important—MRI is the imaging of choice in pregnancy.

Management of phaeochromocytoma

- *α-blockade: phenoxybenzamine*. Reduces fetal and maternal morbidity and mortality. Appears to be safe in pregnancy. The starting dose is 10mg 12-hourly and is built up gradually to a maximum of 20mg every 8h. Oral prazosin and IV phentolamine can also be used.
- *β-blockade: propranolol*. Only after adequate α-blockade. May increase the risk of intrauterine fetal growth restriction if started in the first trimester, but benefits outweigh risks. Give in a dose of 40mg 8-hourly.
- *Surgery*. Timing is controversial. Some recommend, before 24 weeks' gestation, surgical removal of phaeochromocytoma (relatively safe following α- and β-blockade). After 24 weeks' gestation, surgery should be deferred until fetal maturity. The preferred method of delivery is usually elective Caesarean section. Ensure adequate adrenergic blockade before surgery. Surgery can be delayed until after delivery.

Conn's syndrome

- Rare in pregnancy, with <50 cases reported.
- Diagnosed with hypertension and hypokalaemia.
- Has been associated with placental abruption.
- Maternal mortality has been reported.

Diagnosis

- A suppressed renin and raised aldosterone (compared to normal pregnancy ranges) confirm the diagnosis.
- US or MRI can be used to localize tumour.

Management

- Standard treatment for hypertension in pregnancy.
- Amiloride can be used in pregnancy.
- Spironolactone should be avoided, as associated with ambiguous sexual genitalia in male rats.

Further reading

Ahlawat SK, Jain S, Kumaro S, Varma S, Sharma BK (1999). Phaeochromocytoma associated with pregnancy: case report and review of the literature. *Obstet Gynecol Surv* **54**, 728–37.

Hadden DR (1995). Adrenal disorders of pregnancy. *Endocrinol Metab Clin North Am* **24**, 139–51.

Lindsay JR, Nieman LK (2006). Adrenal disorders in pregnancy. *Endocrinol Metab Clin North Am* **35**, 1–20.

Robar C, Porremba J, Pelton J, Hudson L, Higby K (1998). Current diagnosis and management of aldosterone-producing adenomas during pregnancy. *Endocrinologist* **8**, 403–8.

Sam S, Molitch M (2003). Timing and special concerns regarding endocrine surgery during pregnancy. *Endocrinol Metab Clin North Am* **32**, 337–54.

Calcium and bone metabolism

Calcium and bone physiology

Bone turnover

In order to ensure that bone can undertake its mechanical and metabolic functions, it is in a constant state of turnover (see Fig. 6.1).

- *Osteoclasts*—derived from the monocytic cells; resorb bone.
- *Osteoblasts*—derived from the fibroblast-like cells; make bone.
- *Osteocytes*—buried osteoblasts; sense mechanical strain in bone.

Bone mass during life

(see Fig. 6.2)

Bone is laid down rapidly during skeletal growth at puberty. Following this, there is a period of stabilization of bone mass in early adult life. After the age of ~40, there is a gradual loss of bone in both sexes. This occurs at the rate of approximately 0.5% annually. However, in ♀ after the menopause, there is a period of rapid bone loss. The accelerated loss is maximal in the first 2–5 years after the cessation of ovarian function and then gradually declines until the previous gradual rate of loss is once again established. The excess bone loss associated with the menopause is of the order of 10% of skeletal mass. This menopause-associated loss, coupled with higher peak bone mass acquisition in ♂, largely explains why osteoporosis and its associated fractures are more common in ♀.

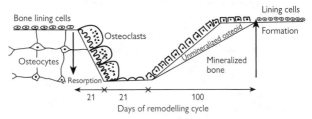

Fig. 6.1 Bone turnover during remodelling cycle.

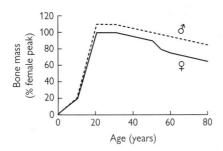

Fig. 6.2 Bone mass and age.

Calcium

Roles of calcium
- Skeletal strength.
- Neuromuscular conduction.
- Stimulus secretion coupling (e.g. chromaffin cells).

Calcium in the circulation
Circulating calcium exists in several forms (see Fig. 6.3).
- Ionized—biologically active.
- Complexed to citrate, phosphate, etc.—biologically active.
- Bound to protein, mainly albumin—inactive.

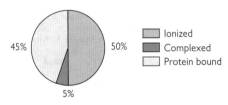

Fig. 6.3 Forms of circulating calcium.

Investigation of bone

Bone turnover markers

Used in some centres.

May be useful in:
- Assessing overall risk of osteoporotic fracture.
- Judging response to treatments for osteoporosis.

Resorption markers
- *Collagen crosslinks.* These are products of collagen degradation. The small fragments of the ends of the collagen molecule are known as *telopeptides* (NTX and CTX), and the measurement of these in blood is the preferred biochemical measure of bone resorption.

Formation markers
- *Total alkaline phosphatase* is not specific to bone and is also found in liver, intestine, and placenta. It is also insensitive to small changes in bone turnover and is only of general use in monitoring the activity of Paget's disease.
- *Bone-specific alkaline phosphatase* is a more specific and reliable measure of bone formation.
- *Osteocalcin* is a component of bone matrix, and the serum level of osteocalcin reflects osteoblast activity.
- *P1NP* is a procollagen fragment released from the N terminal as type 1 collagen is laid down. When measured in serum, it is the most sensitive and specific marker of bone formation.

The clinical utility of routine measurements of bone turnover markers is not yet established.

Bone imaging

Skeletal radiology

- Useful for:
  - Diagnosis of fracture.
  - Diagnosis of specific diseases (e.g. Paget's disease and osteomalacia).
  - Identification of bone dysplasia.
- Not useful for assessing bone density.

Isotope bone scanning

Bone-seeking isotopes, particularly ^{99m}technetium-labelled bisphosphonates, are concentrated in areas of localized ↑ bone cell activity. Isotope bone scans are useful for identifying localized areas of bone disease, such as fracture, metastases, or Paget's disease. However, isotope uptake is not selective, and so ↑ activity on a scan does not indicate the nature of the underlying bone disease. Hence, subsequent radiology of affected regions is needed to establish the diagnosis.

Isotope bone scans are particularly useful in Paget's disease to establish the extent and sites of skeletal involvement and the underlying disease activity.

Bone mass measurements

(See Table 6.1.)

Interpretation of results

- Bone mass is quoted in terms of the number of standard deviations (SD) from an expected mean. The most useful way of expressing this is as T scores. T scores represent observed bone mass in comparison to a sex-matched young, healthy population. Z scores are sometimes quoted and relate to bone density, according to a sex- and an age-matched group.
- A reduction of one SD in bone density will approximately double the risk of fracture.
- WHO has established criteria for the diagnosis of osteoporosis in post-menopausal ♀ (see 📖 p. 493).
- No similar criteria have been set in ♂, but the same thresholds are generally accepted.
- For some 2° causes of osteoporosis, particularly glucocorticoid use, a less stringent criterion of T score <−1.5 should be used as a bone density-determined treatment intervention threshold.

Table 6.1 Measurement of bone density

Technique	Site	Measures	Radiation	Reproducibility
Dual-energy absorptiometry (DXA)	Spine* Femur* Whole body Forearm	Bone mineral per unit area (g/cm²)	~1µSv per site	<1% at spine <2% at femur
Quantitative computed tomography (QCT)	Spine Forearm	True bone mineral density (BMD) (g/cm³)	~50µSv at spine	~1%

* Accepted as 'gold standard' measurement.

Bone biopsy

Bone biopsy is occasionally necessary for the diagnosis of patients with complex metabolic bone diseases. This is usually in the context of suspected osteomalacia. Bone biopsy is not indicated for the routine diagnosis of osteoporosis. *It should only be undertaken in highly specialist centres with appropriate expertise.*

Investigation of calcium, phosphate, and magnesium

Blood concentration

Calcium

Measurement of serum calcium does not require patients to be fasted. Blood for parathyroid hormone (PTH) and phosphate level measurements should, however, ideally be collected after an overnight fast.

In most clinical situations, direct measurement of ionized calcium concentration is unnecessary. However, it is important to adjust the measured calcium concentration for the prevailing serum albumin concentration (see Box 6.1).

Phosphate and magnesium

Measurements of plasma phosphate and magnesium are not conventionally adjusted for plasma protein concentrations.

Box 6.1 Adjustment of measured calcium concentration

Adjusted Ca = measured Ca + 0.02 × (40 − albumin)

(Where calcium is in mmol/L and albumin in g/L.)

Urine excretion

Calcium

Measurement of 24h urinary excretion of calcium provides a measure of risk of renal stone formation or nephrocalcinosis in states of chronic hypercalcaemia. In other circumstances, particularly in the assessment of the cause of hypercalcaemia (1° hyperparathyroidism versus familial hypocalciuric hypercalcaemia), an estimate of the renal handling of calcium is more useful. This is most commonly estimated from the ratio of the renal clearance of calcium to that of creatinine in the fasting state (see Box 6.2). If all values are in mmol/L, the ratio is typically >0.02 in 1° hyperparathyroidism; values <0.01 are suggestive of hypocalciuric hypercalcaemia. (Exclude other causes of hypocalciuria, including renal insufficiency, vitamin D deficiency.)

Phosphate

A 24h measurement of phosphate excretion largely reflects dietary phosphate intake and has little clinical utility.

Box 6.2 Calculation of calcium/creatinine excretion ratio

CaE = [Urine calcium (mmol)/urine creatinine (mmol)]
$\times$ [(plasma creatinine (micromol)/1000)/plasma calcium (mmol)]

= <0.01 in FHH

= >0.02 in primary hyperparathyroidism

Calcium-regulating hormones

Parathyroid hormone

Careful attention should be paid to local requirements for collecting blood for PTH measurement. Since PTH secretion is suppressed by calcium ingestion, it should be measured in the fasting state. The reference range depends on the precise assay employed, but typical values are 10–60pg/mL (1–6pmol/L).

Vitamin D and its metabolites

25OH vitamin D (25OHD)

This is the main storage form of vitamin D, and the measurement of 'total vitamin D' is the most clinically useful measure of vitamin D status.

Internationally, there remains controversy around a 'normal' or 'optimal' concentration of vitamin D. Levels over 50nmol/L are generally accepted as satisfactory and values <25nmol/L representing deficiency. True osteomalacia occurs with vitamin D values <15nmol/L.

Low levels of 25OHD can result from a variety of causes (see Vitamin D deficiency, p. 484). It is unlikely that serious intoxication will occur with 25OHD concentrations of <125nmol/L.

1,25(OH)$_2$ vitamin D (1,25(OH)$_2$D)

Although this is the active form of vitamin D, measurement of its concentration is rarely indicated. It is sometimes useful diagnostically in conditions of extrarenal synthesis of 1,25(OH)$_2$D, such as in sarcoidosis.

Parathyroid hormone-related peptide (PTHrP)

It is possible to measure the level of this oncofetoprotein in serum, but this is very rarely indicated. Sample collection involves specific requirements.

Calcitonin

Calcitonin assays are available, but their utility is confined to the diagnosis and monitoring of medullary carcinoma of the thyroid. There is no role for calcitonin measurements in the routine investigation of calcium and bone metabolism.

Hypercalcaemia

Epidemiology

Hypercalcaemia is found in 5% of hospital patients and in 0.5% of the general population.

Causes

Many different disease states can lead to hypercalcaemia. These are listed by order of importance in hospital practice in Box 6.3. In asymptomatic community-dwelling subjects, the vast majority of hypercalcaemia is the result of hyperparathyroidism.

Clinical features

Notwithstanding the underlying cause of hypercalcaemia, the clinical features are similar. With adjusted serum calcium levels <3.0mmol/L, significant related symptoms are unlikely. With progressive increases in calcium concentration, the likelihood of symptoms increases rapidly.

The clinical features of hypercalcaemia are well recognized (see Box 6.4); unfortunately, they are non-specific and may relate to underlying illness.

Clinical signs of hypercalcaemia are rare. With the exception of band keratopathy, these are not specific. It is important to seek clinical evidence of underlying causes of hypercalcaemia, particularly malignant disease.

In addition to specific symptoms of hypercalcaemia, symptoms of long-term consequences of hypercalcaemia should be sought. These include the presence of bone pain or fracture and renal stones. These indicate the presence of chronic hypercalcaemia.

Investigation of hypercalcaemia

Confirm the diagnosis

Serum calcium (adjusted for albumin).

Determine the mechanism

- ↑ *PTH.* Parathyroid overactivity (1° or tertiary hyperparathyroidism can also occur in familial hypocalciuric hypercalcaemia and in lithium therapy due to faulty calcium-sensing).
- ↓ *PTH.* Parathyroid-independent cause.
- *Normal PTH:*
  - May imply parathyroid overactivity—incomplete suppression.
  - May imply altered calcium sensor—familial hypocalciuric hypercalcaemia—calcium/creatinine excretion ratio will be low.
- Urine calcium to determine calcium/creatinine excretion ratio (not correlated with the risk of stones).

Seek underlying illness (where indicated)

- History and examination.
- Chest X-ray.
- FBC and ESR.
- Biochemical profile (renal and liver function).
- Thyroid function tests (exclude thyrotoxicosis).

- 25OHD (rarely 1,25(OH)$_2$D).
- Plasma and urine protein electrophoresis (exclude myeloma).
- Serum cortisol (short Synacthen® test (exclude Addison's disease)).

To determine end-organ damage
- 24h urine calcium (± urine creatinine for reproducibility).
- Renal tract ultrasound (calculi, nephrocalcinosis).
- Skeletal radiographs (lateral thoracolumbar spine, hands).
- BMD by DXA.
- (Bone turnover markers.)

Box 6.3 Causes of hypercalcaemia

Common
- Hyperparathyroidism:
  - 1°.
  - Tertiary.
- Malignancy:
  - Humoral hypercalcaemia.
  - Multiple myeloma.
  - Bony metastases.

Uncommon
- Vitamin D intoxication.
- Familial hypocalciuric hypercalcaemia.
- Sarcoidosis and other granulomatous diseases.
- Thiazide diuretics.
- Lithium.
- Immobilization.
- Hyperthyroidism.
- Renal failure.
- Addison's disease.
- Vitamin A intoxication.

Box 6.4 Clinical features of hypercalcaemia

Renal	Gastrointestinal	CNS	Other
• Polyuria.	• Anorexia.	• Confusion.	• Pruritus.
• Polydipsia.	• Vomiting.	• Lethargy.	• Sore eyes.
	• Constipation.	• Depression.	
	• Abdominal pain.		

Primary hyperparathyroidism

Present in up to 1 in 500 of the general population where it is predominantly a disease of post-menopausal ♀ (14/100,000 ♂, 28/100,000 ♀).

The normal physiological response to hypocalcaemia is an increase in PTH secretion. This is termed 2° *hyperparathyroidism* and is not pathological in as much as the PTH secretion remains under feedback control. Continued stimulation of the parathyroid glands can lead to autonomous production of PTH. This, in turn, causes hypercalcaemia which is termed *tertiary hyperparathyroidism*. This is usually seen in the context of renal disease but can occur in any state of chronic hypocalcaemia, such as vitamin D deficiency or malabsorption.

Pathology
- 85% single adenoma.
- 14% hyperplasia (may be associated with other endocrine abnormalities, particularly multiple endocrine neoplasia (MEN) types 1 and 2 (📖 see MEN type 1, pp. 586–7; MEN type 2, pp. 592–3).
- <1% carcinoma (express the lectin galectin-3).

Clinical features
- Majority of patients are asymptomatic.
- Features of hypercalcaemia.
- End-organ damage—see Box 6.5.

Natural history
- In majority of patients without end-organ damage, disease is benign and stable.
- A significant minority (2–3% per annum) will develop new indications for surgery.
- Excess deaths probably linked to cardiovascular diseases and possibly malignancy.

Investigation
(See Box 6.6.) Potential diagnostic pitfalls:
- FHH—differentiate with calcium/creatinine excretion ratio (📖 see Familial hypocalciuric hypercalcaemia (FHH), pp. 457, 470) (<0.01 in FHH; >0.02 in hyperparathyroidism).
- Long-standing vitamin D deficiency where the concomitant osteomalacia and calcium malabsorption can mask hypercalcaemia which becomes apparent only after vitamin D repletion. Consider other causes of a raised PTH (see Box 6.7).
- Drugs associated with hypercalcaemia (e.g. thiazides and lithium).

Investigation is, therefore, primarily aimed at determining the presence of end-organ damage from hypercalcaemia in order to determine whether operative intervention is indicated.

Box 6.5 End-organ damage in hyperparathyroidism

Bone
- Osteoporosis:
  - Common.
  - Affects all sites, but predominant loss is in peripheral cortical bone.
- Radiographic changes:
  - Uncommon.
  - Include subperiosteal resorption, abnormal skull vault, eroded lamina dura (around teeth), and bone cysts.
- Osteitis fibrosa cystica:
  - Rare.
  - Usually with tertiary hyperparathyroidism.

Kidneys
- Renal calculi.
- Nephrocalcinosis.
- Renal impairment.

Joints
- Chondrocalcinosis.
- Pseudogout.

Pancreatitis

Box 6.6 Diagnosis of primary hyperparathyroidism

- Ca > NR (2.60mmol (adjusted) × 2).
- U&E normal.
- Not on lithium or thiazide diuretic.
- PTH >3.0pmol (20% patients have PTH within upper part NR).
- Urine Ca >2.5mmol/day.

Box 6.7 Other causes of raised PTH

- Renal insufficiency.
- Vitamin D deficiency.
- Renal hypercalciuria.
- Drugs (e.g. lithium, thiazides).

Exclusion of underlying condition

- 1° hyperparathyroidism (PHP) can be associated with genetic abnormalities, especially MEN-1 and 2, as well as familial hyperparathyroidism.
- These conditions should be sought in patients presenting with PHP and a family history in ≥1 first-degree relatives or at a young age (<40 years).

Localization of abnormal parathyroid glands

This should only form part of a preoperative assessment and is not indicated in the initial diagnosis of hyperparathyroidism.

- Localization with two separate techniques (usually US and ^{99m}Tc-sestamibi) is imperative before minimally invasive parathyroidectomy.
- Otherwise, open bilateral neck exploration by an experienced surgeon is optimal in the first instance.
- After failed neck exploration, other localizing techniques are required, which include:
  - ^{99m}Tc-sestamibi.
  - Thallium/technetium subtraction scanning (less sensitive).
  - CT.
  - US.
- Angiography with selective venous sampling may be employed in difficult cases but should be confined to specialist centres with experience in this technique.

Treatment of hyperparathyroidism

Parathyroid surgery

(Aspects of parathyroid surgery also covered on 🕮 see p. 608.)

- For indications, see Table 6.2.
- Only by experienced surgeon (>20 procedures per year):
  - *Adenoma.* Remove affected gland—often by minimally invasive surgery.
  - *Hyperplasia.* Partial parathyroidectomy (perhaps with reimplantation of tissue in more accessible site).

Observation

- Suitable for patients with mild disease with no evidence of end-organ damage.
- Most such patients have stable disease over many years but do require monitoring:
  - *Annual* serum calcium and renal function, BP.
  - *Every 2–3 years*—BMD, renal US.
- Any significant deterioration is an indication for surgery.

Medical management

Only indicated if patient not suitable for surgery.

- Hormone replacement therapy:
  - Preserves bone mass.
  - Consider long-term risks (breast cancer, venous thrombosis, heart disease, and stroke).
- Bisphosphonates:
  - Clinically inconsequential effect on plasma and urine calcium.
  - Preserve bone mass.
- Calcium-sensing receptor agonists:
  - Cinacalcet (30mg twice daily) reduces serum but not urinary calcium concentration. It increases sensitivity of calcium-sensing receptor, decreasing PTH secretion. It is licensed for patients with severe 2° hyperparathyroidism on dialysis, parathyroid carcinoma, and patients with PHP in whom parathyroid surgery is contraindicated or clinically inappropriate. It may also be used if the neck has been explored and the parathyroid adenoma has not been found.

Indications for surgery in primary hyperparathyroidism

It is generally accepted that all patients with symptomatic hyperparathyroidism or evidence of end-organ damage should be considered for parathyroidectomy. This would include:

- Definite symptoms of hypercalcaemia. There is less good evidence that non-specific symptoms, such as abdominal pain, tiredness, or mild cognitive impairment, benefit from surgery.
- Impaired renal function.
- Renal stones (symptomatic or on radiograph).
- Parathyroid bone disease, especially osteitis fibrosis cystica.
- Pancreatitis.

Guidelines for the management of asymptomatic hyperparathyroidism have been produced on the basis of a consensus development conference in the USA[1] and following review of evidence in the UK.[2] Although there are some differences between these approaches, there is also considerable similarity.

Conservative management

- Patients not managed with surgery require regular follow-up.
- Again, there is some difference between recommendations in the UK and USA (see Table 6.3).

Table 6.2 Table comparing indications for parathyroidectomy in asymptomatic patients in the USA compared with the UK

	UK	USA
Serum calcium	3.00mmol/L	~2.85mmol/L
Urine calcium	10mmol/day (perhaps)	Test not indicated
Creatinine clearance	No guidance	<60mL/min
BMD	T score <−2.5	T score <−2.5 or previous fragility fracture
Age	<50	<50

Table 6.3 Table comparing management recommendations for patients in the USA compared with the UK

	UK	USA
Serum calcium	6 months	12 months
Serum creatinine	6 months	12 months
BP	6 months	No recommendation
PTH	12 months	No recommendation
Urine calcium	12 months	Not indicated
Urine creatinine	12 months	Not indicated
BMD	24–36 months	12–24 months
Abdominal X-ray/US	36 months	Not indicated

References

1. Bilezikian JP, Khan AA, Potts JT Jr, et al. (2009). Guidelines for the management of asymptomatic primary hyperparathyroidism: Summary Statement from the Third International Workshop. *J Clin Endocrinol Metab* **94**, 335–9.
2. Davies M, Fraser WD, Hoskin DJ (2002). The management of primary hyperparathyroidism. *Clin Endocrinol (Oxf)* **57**, 145–55.

Complications of parathyroidectomy

Mechanical
- Vocal cord paresis:
  - May be permanent, particularly with repeated surgery.
- Tracheal compression from haematoma.

Metabolic (hypocalcaemia)
- Transient:
  - Due to suppression of remaining glands.
  - May sometimes require oral therapy with calcium ± vitamin D metabolites.
- Severe:
  - Due to hungry bones—rare. Treatment with calcitriol 1 microgram/day (sometimes higher dose required) and oral calcium, 3× daily, may be required for several weeks.
  - Occurs in patients with pre-existing bone disease.
  - Minimize risk by pretreatment of any vitamin D deficiency for several weeks. Risk of significant worsening of hypercalcaemia is low, but monitoring of serum calcium is recommended.
  - Acute severe hypocalcaemia requires initial IV calcium to stabilize metabolic status.

Outcome after surgery
- <5% fail to become normocalcaemic, and these should be considered for a second operation.
- All patients with hyperplasia (including MEN) identified on histopathology should have long-term monitoring of serum calcium to detect recurrent primary hyperparathyroidism.
- Patients rendered permanently hypoparathyroid by surgery require lifelong supplements of active metabolites of vitamin D with calcium. This can lead to hypercalciuria, and the risk of stone formation may still be present in these patients. Target serum calcium in these patients should be towards the low end of the reference range to minimize hypercalciuria.

Other causes of hypercalcaemia

Hypercalcaemia of malignancy

Mechanism
See Table 6.4.

Clinical features
Hypercalcaemia is usually a late manifestation of malignant disease, and the primary lesion is usually evident by the time hypercalcaemia is expressed (50% of patients die within 30 days). One exception to this is in small endocrine tumours, such as carcinoids and islet cell tumours, which can produce humoral mediators of hypercalcaemia (PTHrP) in the absence of significant spread. Symptoms of hypercalcaemia are non-specific and frequently difficult to distinguish from those of the underlying disease.

Investigation
See investigation of hypercalcaemia in 🕮 Clinical features, p. 460.
Factors suggesting hypercalcaemia of malignancy include:
- ↑ calcium.
- ↓ PTH.
- Other features of malignant disease.
- ↑ PTHrP—not usually measured in clinical practice.

Steroid suppression tests are rarely indicated. May suppress with malignancy but not with primary hyperparathyroidism.

Treatment
Frequently, patients requiring treatment will have severe symptomatic hypercalcaemia. Often, emergency treatment is necessary to stabilize the patient. In such circumstances, the principles of management are the same as those of severe hypercalcaemia from any cause (🕮 see Box 6.8, p. 470).

Table 6.4 Types of hypercalcaemia associated with cancer

Type	Frequency (%)	Bone metastases	Causal agent	Tumour type
Local osteolysis	20	Common Extensive	Cytokines Chemokines PTHrP	Breast Myeloma Lymphoma
Humoral	80	Minimal	PTHrP	Squamous carcinoma Renal Ovarian Endometrial Breast HTLV Lymphoma
1,25OH vit D	<1	Variable	1,25(OH)$_2$D	Lymphoma
Ectopic PTH	<1	Variable	PTH	Variable

Box 6.8 Management of severe hypercalcaemia
- Vigorous rehydration 200–500mL/h.
- Disodium pamidronate 60–90mg or zoledronic acid 5mg IV.
- Calcium falls within 12h, nadir 4–7 days.
- Duration of effect is variable but usually 1–6 weeks.

1. Stabilize the level of hypercalcaemia, and prevent any further decline in renal function. This requires the IV infusion of large quantities of 0.9% saline, frequently 3–6L over the first 24h. If there is a danger of salt and water retention, a loop diuretic may be added. This is the only role of diuretics in the management of hypercalcaemia and is not routine practice, contrary to previous historical texts. Loop diuretics can precipitate intravascular volume depletion and worsening hypercalcaemia. In severe renal impairment, dialysis may be of value.

2. Once the patient is volume-replete, it is necessary to treat the cause of the hypercalcaemia. The most effective therapy available for this is IV bisphosphonate—pamidronate (60–90mg) or zoledronic acid (5mg) are the most frequently used. Repeat doses may be required. Even patients who are acutely hypercalcaemic can rarely develop hypocalcaemia following IV bisphosphonate therapy, especially if they are vitamin D-deficient.

3. Calcitonin and glucocorticoids are rarely used in the acute management of hypercalcaemia nowadays.

Familial hypocalciuric hypercalcaemia (FHH)

FHH—also known as familial benign hypercalcaemia. Three types exist: FHH 1–3 (see Table 6.5).

- Very rare cause of hypercalcaemia.
- Autosomal dominant, with virtually complete penetrance, but may also be autosomal recessive.
- Mutation in the calcium-sensing receptor which reduces its sensitivity such that the body behaves as if it were experiencing normocalcaemia, even though the serum calcium level is elevated.
- Generally benign and is not usually associated with symptoms or adverse effects, such as renal stones or bone disease.
- Does not usually show any sustained benefit from parathyroidectomy.
- The homozygous state produces severe life-threatening hypercalcaemia soon after birth (neonatal severe hyperparathyroidism). In such cases, total parathyroidectomy is lifesaving.
- See Box 6.8 for management of hypercalcaemia.

Patients have low urine calcium excretion (24h <2.5mmol, fasting calcium/creatinine excretion ratio <0.01 (Box 6.2, p. 457)).

Table 6.5 Three types of FHH

FHH 1 60%	FHH 2	FHH 3 20%
Autosomal dominant	Autosomal dominant	Autosomal dominant
Disorder of extracellular calcium homeostasis ↑ Ca in serum ↓ Ca in urine (Ca/Cr ratio <0.01)		
Chromosome 3q 21.1	19p	13q 133
Normal PTH Mild ↑ Mg		↑ PTH ↓ PO$_4$ Osteomalacia
Asymptomatic Occasional pancreatitis Chondrocalcinosis 1° hyperparathyroidism Osteoporosis Kidney stones		

Further reading

Lietman SA, et al. (2009). A novel loss-of-function mutation, Gln459Arg, of the calcium-sensing receptor gene associated with apparent autosomal recessive inheritance of familial hypocalciuric hypercalcemia. *J Clin Endocrinol Metab* **94**, 4372–9.

Nesbit MA, et al. (2013). Mutations in AP2S1 cause familial hypocalciuric hypercalcemia type 3. *Nat Genet* **45**, 93–7.

Nesbit MA, Hannan FM, Howles SA, et al. (2013). Mutations affecting G-protein subunit α11 in hypercalcemia and hypocalcemia. *N Engl J Med* **368**(26):2476–86.

Pallais JC, Kifor O, Chen YB, et al. (2004). Acquired hypocalciuric hypercalcemia due to autoantibodies against the calcium-sensing receptor. *N Engl J Med* **351**, 362–9.

Vitamin D intoxication

- The diagnosis is established by the presence of greatly elevated concentrations of 25OHD (>125nmol/L) and 1,25(OH)$_2$D, together with suppressed PTH. If calcitriol or alfacalcidol is the offending compound, then 25OHD levels will not be elevated.
- In mild cases, particularly when the active vitamin D metabolites are involved, the only treatment necessary is to withdraw the offending treatment and let the calcium settle. If the longer-acting vitamin D metabolites are involved, then active treatment may be necessary.
  - Patients should first be stabilized with a saline infusion (see Box 6.8).

Following this, the traditional management has been to give high-dose oral glucocorticoid, such as prednisolone 40mg daily, although IV bisphosphonates should also be considered in the acute setting.

Sarcoidosis

- Together with other granulomatous disorders, sarcoidosis causes hypercalcaemia by extrarenal production of 1,25(OH)$_2$D in granulomata. This process is not under feedback inhibition but is substrate-regulated. The hypercalcaemia is, therefore, dependent on vitamin D supply. Patients may present with hypercalcaemia in summer or following foreign holidays when the endogenous production of vitamin D is maximal.
- The biochemical picture is of normal 25OHD, raised 1,25(OH)$_2$D, and suppressed PTH. In addition, other markers of sarcoid activity, such as raised angiotensin-converting enzyme (ACE) activity, are frequently present.
- Treatment with high-dose glucocorticoids is recommended to control sarcoid activity and to minimize the GI effects of the excess 1,25(OH)$_2$D.

Further reading

Bilezikian JP, Watts JT Jr, Fuleihan Gel-H, et al. (2002). Summary statement from a workshop on asymptomatic primary hyperparathyroidism: a perspective for the 21st century. *J Clin Endocrinol Metab* **87**, 5353–61.

Marcocci C, et al. (2011). Primary hyperparathyroidism. *N Engl J Med* **365**, 2389–97.

Palazzo FF, Sadler GP (2004). Minimally invasive parathyroidectomy. *BMJ* **328**, 849–50.

Peacock M, Bilezikian JP, Klassen PS, et al. (2005). Cinacalcet hydrochloride maintains long-term normocalcemia in patients with primary hyperthyroidism. *J Clin Endocrinol Metab* **90**, 135-41.

Stewart AF (2005). Clinical practice. Hypercalcemia associated with cancer. *N Engl J Med* **352**, 373–9.

Yu N, et al. (2011). A record linkage study of outcomes in patients with mild primary hyperparathyroidism: the Parathyroid Epidemiology and Audit Research Study (PEARS). *Clin Endocrinol (Oxf)* **75**,169–76.

Hypocalcaemia

Causes

Although hypocalcaemia can result from failure of any of the mechanisms by which serum calcium concentration is maintained, it is usually the result of either failure of PTH secretion or because of the inability to release calcium from bone. These causes are summarized in Box 6.9.

Clinical features

The clinical features of hypocalcaemia are largely as a result of ↑ neuro-muscular excitability. In order of ↑ severity, these include:
- Tingling—especially of fingers, toes, or lips.
- Numbness—especially of fingers, toes, or lips.
- Cramps.
- Carpopedal spasm.
- Stridor due to laryngospasm.
- Seizures.

The symptoms of hypocalcaemia tend to reflect the severity and rapidity of onset of the metabolic abnormality.

Clinical signs of hypocalcaemia depend upon the demonstration of neuro-muscular irritability before this necessarily causes symptoms:
- *Chvostek's sign* is elicited by tapping the facial nerve in front of the ear. A +ve result is indicated by twitching of the corner of the mouth. Slight twitching is seen in up to 15% of normal ♀, but more major involvement of the facial muscles is indicative of hypocalcaemia or hypomagnesaemia.
- *Trousseau's sign* is produced by occlusion of the blood supply to the arm by inflation of a sphygmomanometer cuff above arterial pressure for 3min. If +ve, there will be carpopedal spasm which may be accompanied by painful paraesthesiae.

In addition, there may be clinical signs and symptoms associated with the underlying condition:
- *Vitamin D deficiency* may be associated with generalized bone pain, fractures, or proximal myopathy (📖 see p. 484).
- *Hypoparathyroidism* can be accompanied by mental slowing and personality disturbances as well as extrapyramidal signs, cataracts, and papilloedema.
- If *hypocalcaemia* is present during the development of permanent teeth, these may show areas of enamel hypoplasia. This can be a useful physical sign, indicating that the hypocalcaemia is long-standing.

Box 6.9 Causes of hypocalcaemia

Hypoparathyroidism
- Destruction of parathyroid glands:
  - Surgical.
  - Autoimmune.
  - Radiation.
  - Infiltration.
- Failure of parathyroid development:
  - Isolated, e.g. X-linked.
  - With other abnormalities, e.g. di George syndrome (with thymic aplasia, immunodeficiency, and cardiac anomalies).
- Failure of PTH secretion:
  - Magnesium deficiency.
  - Overactivity of calcium-sensing receptor.
- Failure of PTH action:
  - Pseudohypoparathyroidism—due to G protein abnormality.

Failure of release of calcium from bone
- Osteomalacia:
  - Vitamin D deficiency.
  - Vitamin D resistance.
  - Renal failure.
- Inhibition of bone resorption:
  - Hypocalcaemic drugs, e.g. cisplatin, calcitonin, oral phosphate.
- ↑ uptake of calcium into bone:
  - Osteoblastic metastases (e.g. prostate).
  - Hungry bone syndrome.

Complexing of calcium from the circulation
- ↑ albumin-binding in alkalosis.
- Acute pancreatitis:
  - Formation of calcium soaps from autodigestion of fat.
  - Abnormal PTH and vitamin D metabolism.
  - Phosphate infusion.
- Multiple blood transfusions—complexing by citrate.

Pseudohypoparathyroidism
- Resistance to parathyroid hormone action.
- Due to defective signalling of PTH action via cell membrane receptor.
- Also affects TSH, LH, FSH, and GH signalling.
- Most commonly caused by autosomal dominant mutation of *GNAS1* gene.
- Significant imprinting:
  - Maternal transmission leads to full blown syndrome of hormone resistance.
  - Paternal transmission causes only phenotypic features of Albright's hereditary osteodystrophy.

Albright's hereditary osteodystrophy

Patients with the most common type of pseudohypoparathyroidism (type Ia) have a characteristic set of skeletal abnormalities, known as Albright's hereditary osteodystrophy. This comprises:

- Short stature.
- Obesity.
- Round face.
- Short metacarpals.

Some individuals with Albright's hereditary osteodystrophy do not appear to have a disorder of calcium metabolism. In the past, the term *pseudopseudohypoparathyroidism* has been used to describe these. However, it is now clear that these reflect different manifestations of the same underlying genetic defect as a result of imprinting. In the light of the same underlying aetiology, there has been a tendency to avoid the more cumbersome designations and to refer to all such patients as having Albright's hereditary osteodystrophy.

Investigation

- Serum calcium.
- PTH—the presence of a low, or even normal, PTH concentration implies failure of PTH secretion in the presence of hypocalcaemia.
- Total vitamin D.
- Magnesium.
- Ellsworth–Howard test can be performed if pseudohypoparathyroidism suspected (measurement of serum and urinary phosphorous after IV administration of parathyroid hormone).

Treatment of hypocalcaemia

- *Acute symptomatic hypocalcaemia* is a medical emergency and demands urgent treatment whatever the cause (see Box 6.10).
- Treatment of *chronic hypocalcaemia* is more dependent on the cause.

Chronic hypocalcaemia

Hypoparathyroidism

- In hypoparathyroidism, the target serum calcium should be at the low end of the reference range. The reason for this is that the renal retention of calcium brought about by PTH has been lost. Thus, any attempt to raise the plasma calcium well into the normal range is likely to result in unacceptable hypercalciuria, with the risk of nephrocalcinosis and renal stones.
- In patients with mild parathyroid dysfunction, it may be possible to achieve acceptable calcium concentrations by using calcium supplements alone. If used in this way, these need to be given in large doses, perhaps as much as 1g elemental calcium 3× daily.
- The majority of patients will not achieve adequate control with such treatment. In those cases, it is necessary to use vitamin D or its metabolites in pharmacological doses to maintain plasma calcium. The more potent analogues of vitamin D, such as *calcitriol* or *alfacalcidol*, have the advantage over high-dose calciferol that it is easier to make changes in therapy in response to plasma calcium levels. If hypercalcaemia does occur, it settles much more quickly following withdrawal of these compounds than calciferol. The dose of vitamin D metabolite is determined by the clinical response but usually lies in the range of 0.5–2 micrograms daily of one of the potent activated vitamin D analogues. Serum calcium must be checked on an ongoing basis, and close monitoring should occur around times of dose adjustments.
- It is essential to ensure an adequate intake of calcium as well as appropriate doses of activated vitamin D analogues. In some patients, it is necessary to give calcium supplementation, particularly in the young.
- PTH (1-84) is a not yet approved therapy but may improve quality of life.

Pseudohypoparathyroidism

- The principles underlying the treatment of pseudohypoparathyroidism are the same as those underlying hypoparathyroidism.
- Patients with the most common form of pseudohypoparathyroidism may have resistance to the action of other hormones which rely on G protein signalling. They, therefore, need to be assessed for thyroid and gonadal dysfunction (because of defective TSH or gonadotrophin action). If these deficiencies are present, they need to be treated in the conventional manner.

Vitamin D deficiency

Treatment of osteomalacia and vitamin D deficiency is described on see p. 484.

Box 6.10 Treatment of acute hypocalcaemia
- Patients with tetany or seizures require urgent IV treatment with calcium gluconate (less irritant than calcium chloride).
  - This is a 10% w/v solution (10mL = 2.25mmol elemental calcium).
  - The solution should always be further diluted to minimize the risk of phlebitis or tissue damage if extravasation occurs.
- Initially, 20mL of 10% calcium gluconate should be diluted in 100–200mL of 0.9% saline or 5% glucose and infused over about 10min.
- Repeat if symptoms not resolved.
- Care must be taken if the patient has heart disease, especially if taking digoxin, as too rapid elevation of the plasma calcium can cause arrhythmias. Cardiac monitoring is advisable.
- In order to maintain the plasma calcium, a calcium infusion is required. 40mL of 10% calcium gluconate should be added to 1L of saline or glucose solution and infused over 24h.
- The plasma calcium should be checked regularly (not less than 6-hourly) and the infusion rate adjusted in response to the change in concentration.
- Failure of the plasma calcium to respond to infused calcium should raise the possibility of underlying hypomagnesaemia. This can be rapidly ascertained by plasma magnesium estimation and, if appropriate, a magnesium infusion commenced (📖 see Treatment, p. 488).
- In circumstances where hypoparathyroidism could be predicted (such as block dissection of the neck), infusion of calcium gluconate in an initial dose of 50mL 10% solution (~11mmol Ca) diluted in normal saline over 24h should be given to avoid post-operative hypocalcaemia. This dose should be adjusted in the light of regular calcium estimations.
- Once oral or NG tube intake is possible, calcium and active vitamin D metabolites should be substituted as above.

Overactivity of calcium-sensing receptor

This leads to a condition known as autosomal dominant hypocalcaemia. It is a benign condition in which the hypocalcaemia is usually asymptomatic. Treatment should be avoided in the absence of symptoms, as elevation of calcium levels, even to within the normal range, may cause renal impairment.

Further reading

Bilezikian JP, *et al.* (2011). Hypoparathyroidism in the adult: epidemiology, diagnosis, pathophysiology, target-organ involvement, treatment, and challenges for future research. *J Bone Miner Res* **26**, 2317–37.

Cooper MS, Gittoes NJ (2008). Diagnosis and management of hypocalcaemia. *BMJ* **336**, 1298–302.

Shoback D (2008). Hypoparathyroidism *N Engl J Med* **359**, 391–403.

Rickets and osteomalacia and hypophosphataemia

Definitions

Osteomalacia occurs when there is inadequate mineralization of mature bone. *Rickets* is a disorder of the growing skeleton where there is inadequate mineralization of bone as it is laid down at the epiphysis. In most instances, osteomalacia leads to build-up of excessive unmineralized osteoid within the skeleton. In rickets, there is build-up of unmineralized osteoid in the growth plate. This leads to the characteristic radiological appearance of rickets, with widening of the growth plate and loss of definition of the ossification centres. These two related conditions may coexist. See Box 6.11 for vitamin D resistance and Box 6.12 for abnormal vitamin D metabolism.

Clinical features

Osteomalacia

- Bone pain.
- Deformity.
- Fracture.
- Proximal myopathy.
- Hypocalcaemia (in vitamin D deficiency).

Rickets

- Growth retardation.
- Bone pain and fracture.
- Skeletal deformity:
  - Bowing of the long bones.
  - Widening of the growth plates, widening of the wrists, 'rickety rosary' (costochondral junctions enlarged).

Diagnosis

- The diagnosis of osteomalacia is usually based on the appropriate biochemical findings (see Table 6.6).
- The majority of patients with osteomalacia will show no specific radiological abnormalities.
- The most characteristic abnormality is the *Looser's zone* or pseudofracture. If these are present, they are virtually pathognomonic of osteomalacia.
- In clinical practice, bone biopsy is rarely indicated.

Box 6.11 Vitamin D resistance

Several different kindreds have been shown to have a defective vitamin D receptor. This condition is inherited as an autosomal recessive condition. It produces hypocalcaemia and osteomalacia, with elevated serum levels of $1,25(OH)_2D$. Approximately two-thirds of affected individuals have total alopecia. This condition is known as vitamin D-dependent rickets type II. If alopecia is present, it is often termed type IIA in contrast to type IIB where hair growth is normal.

Treatment usually requires administration of large doses of active vitamin D metabolites, sometimes reaching doses of 60 micrograms of calcitriol daily.

Box 6.12 Abnormal vitamin D metabolism

The most common cause of failure of 1α-hydroxylase is renal failure. Congenital absence of this enzyme leads to a condition known as vitamin D-dependent rickets type I. This is inherited in an autosomal recessive fashion. It leads to profound rickets, with myopathy and enamel hypoplasia. Very large doses of calciferol are needed to heal the bone lesions which, in contrast, will respond to physiological doses of alfacalcidol or calcitriol.

In practice, liver disease seldom results in clinical problems of vitamin D metabolism.

Table 6.6 Biochemical findings and causes of rickets and osteomalacia

	Ca	PO$_4$	Alkaline phosphatase	25OHD	1,25(OH)$_2$D	PTH	Other
Vitamin D deficiency	↓	↓	↑	↓	↓	↑	
Renal failure	↓	↑	↑	N	↓	↑	↓ GFR
VDDR type I (deficient 1α-hydroxylase)	↓	↓	↑	N	↓	↑	
VDDR type II (deficient vitamin D receptor)	↓	↓	↑	N	↑	↑	
X-linked hypophosphataemia (vitamin D-resistant rickets)	N	↓	↑	N	N	N or ↑	
Oncogenic	N or ↓	↓	↑	N	↓	N	May have aminoaciduria, proteinuria
Phosphate depletion	N	↓	↑	N	↑	N	↑ urine Ca
Fanconi syndrome	↓ or N	↓	↑	N	↑	N	Acidosis, aminoaciduria, glycosuria
Renal tubular acidosis	↓ or N	↓	↑	N	N or ↓	N	Acidosis
Toxic (etidronate, fluoride)	N	N	N	N	N	N	Diagnosed on biopsy

Vitamin D deficiency

Causes
- Poor sunlight exposure:
  - Elderly housebound.
  - Extensive skin coverage with clothes.
- Poor diet (especially vegetarians):
  - Malabsorption.
  - ↑ catabolism of vitamin D.
- 2° hyperparathyroidism:
  - Malabsorption.
  - Post-gastrectomy.
  - Enzyme-inducing drugs, e.g. phenytoin.

Investigation
The diagnosis of vitamin D deficiency is based on the characteristic biochemical abnormalities (see Table 6.6). Frank osteomalacia is usually associated with very low levels of 25OHD (<15nmol/L), but the associated 2° hyperparathyroidism frequently results in normal, or even elevated, concentrations of $1,25(OH)_2D$.

Treatment
- Treatment is best given in the form of calciferol to restore body stores, correct biochemical abnormalities, and heal bony abnormalities. Although the use of the active metabolites of vitamin D will heal the bony abnormalities, it will not correct the underlying biochemical problem and is associated with ↑ risk of hypercalcaemia.
- In adults, treatment can be given as a daily dose of calciferol (800–1,000IU) which is often most easily administered in combination with a calcium supplement. An alternative, which is particularly helpful if poor compliance is suspected, is to give a single large dose of 150,000–300,000IU. This is most effectively given as a single oral dose (3–6 × 1.25mg tablets of ergocalciferol) which can be supervised in clinic. It is possible to give a similar dose by IM injection, but the absorption from this route is variable.
- Following treatment, there is usually a rapid improvement of myopathy and symptoms of hypocalcaemia. Bone pain frequently persists longer, and biochemical abnormalities may not settle for several months. Indeed, following the onset of therapy, markers of bone turnover, such as alkaline phosphatase, might even show a transient increase, as the osteoid is mineralized and remodelled.

X-linked hypophosphataemia
- X-linked dominant genetic disorder.
- Severe rickets and osteomalacia.
- Mutation of an endopeptidase gene (*PHEX*).

Clinical features
- The abnormal phosphate levels are often detected early in infancy, but skeletal deformities are not apparent until walking commences.

- Typical severe rickets, with short stature and bony deformity.
- Continues into adult life, with bone pain, deformity, and fracture in the absence of treatment.
- Proximal myopathy is absent.
- Adults suffer from excessive new bone growth, particularly affecting entheses and the longitudinal ligaments of the spinal canal. This can cause spinal cord compression which may need surgical decompression.

Oncogenic osteomalacia

Certain tumours appear to be able to produce FGF23 which is phosphaturic. This is rare and usually occurs with mesenchymal tumours (such as haemangiopericytomas, haemangiomata, or osteoid tumours) but has also been reported with a variety of adenocarcinomas (particularly prostatic cancer) and haematological malignancies (e.g. myeloma and chronic lymphocytic leukaemia). A similar picture can also be seen in some cases of neurofibromatosis. Clinically, such patients usually present with profound myopathy as well as bone pain and fracture. Biochemically, the major abnormality is hypophosphataemia, but this is usually accompanied by marked reduction in $1,25(OH)_2D$ concentrations. In some patients, other abnormalities of renal tubular function, such as glycosuria or aminoaciduria, are also present.

- FGF3 levels are elevated and fall with tumour removal.
- Tumour may be localized by CT, MRI or PET, or selective venous catheterization for FGF23.
- Medical treatment may include supplemental phosphate, 1,25OH vitamin D, or cinacalcet.

Complete removal of the tumour results in resolution of the biochemical and skeletal abnormalities. If this is not possible or if a causal tumour is not identified, treatment with vitamin D metabolites and phosphate supplements (as for X-linked hypophosphataemia) may help the skeletal symptoms.

Fanconi syndrome

The Fanconi syndrome is a combination of renal tubular defects which can result from several different pathologies. In particular, there is renal wasting of phosphate, bicarbonate, glucose, and amino acids. The combination of hypophosphataemia with renal tubular acidosis means that osteomalacia is a frequent accompaniment. This can be exacerbated by defective 1α-hydroxylation of vitamin D to its active form. The osteomalacia is treated by correction of the relevant abnormalities. This might involve the administration of phosphate, alkali, or $1,25(OH)_2D$ (calcitriol), depending on the precise circumstances.

Further reading

Carpenter TO (2003). Oncogenic osteomalacia—a complex dance of factors. *N Engl J Med* **348**, 1705–8.

Chong WH, et al. (2011). The importance of whole body imaging in tumor-induced osteomalacia. *J Clin Endocrinol Metab* **96**, 3599–600.

Holick MF, et al. (2011). Evaluation, treatment, and prevention of vitamin D deficiency: an Endocrine Society clinical practice guideline. *J Clin Endocrinol Metab* **96**, 1911–30.

Hypophosphataemia

Phosphate is important for normal mineralization of bone. In the absence of sufficient phosphate, osteomalacia results. Clinically, osteomalacia is often indistinguishable from other causes, although there may be features that will help distinguish the underlying cause of hypophosphataemia. In addition, phosphate is important in its own right for neuromuscular function, and profound hypophosphataemia can be accompanied by encephalopathy, muscle weakness, and cardiomyopathy. It must be remembered that, as phosphate is primarily an intracellular anion, a low plasma phosphate does not necessarily represent actual phosphate depletion. Several different causes of hypophosphataemia are recognized (see Box 6.13).

Treatment

- Mainstay is phosphate replacement, usually Phosphate-Sandoz®, each tablet of which provides 500mg of phosphate.
- Ideally, patients should receive 2–3g of phosphate daily between meals, but this is not easy to achieve. All phosphate preparations are unpalatable and act as osmotic purgatives, causing diarrhoea.
- Long-term administration of phosphate supplements stimulates parathyroid activity. This can lead to hypercalcaemia, a further fall in phosphate, with worsening of the bone disease due to the development of hyperparathyroid bone disease which may necessitate parathyroidectomy.
- To minimize parathyroid stimulation, it is usual to give one of the active metabolites of vitamin D in conjunction with phosphate. Typically, alfacalcidol or calcitriol in a dose of 1–2 micrograms daily is used.
- Patients receiving such supraphysiological doses of vitamin D metabolites are at continued risk of hypercalcaemia and require regular monitoring of plasma calcium, preferably at least every 3 months. The adequacy of calcitriol replacement can be assessed by maintaining 24h urinary calcium excretion >4–6mmol/day.
- In adults, the role of treatment for X-linked hypophosphataemia is probably confined to symptomatic bone disease.
  - There is little evidence that it will improve the long-term outcome.
  - There has even been some evidence that treatment might accelerate new bone formation.
- In children, treatment is usually given in the hope of improving final height and minimizing skeletal abnormality—the evidence that it is possible to achieve these goals is conflicting.

Box 6.13 Causes of hypophosphataemia

↓ *intestinal absorption*
- Phosphate binding antacids.
- Malabsorption.
- Starvation/malnutrition.

↑ *renal losses*
- Hyperparathyroidism:
  - 1°.
  - 2°, e.g. in vitamin D deficiency.
- Renal tubular defects:
  - Fanconi syndrome.
- X-linked hypophosphataemia.
- Oncogenic osteomalacia.
- Alcohol abuse.
- Poorly controlled diabetes.
- Acidosis.
- Drugs:
  - Diuretics.
  - Corticosteroids.
  - Calcitonin.

Shift into cells
- Septicaemia.
- Insulin treatment.
- Glucose administration.
- Salicylate poisoning.
- Catecholamine.
- Hyperventilation.

Further reading

Bergwitz C, Collins MT, Kamath RS *et al.* (2011) A 56-year old with hypophosphataemea *NEJM* **365**, 1625–35.
Liamis G, Milionis HJ, Elisaf M *et al.* (2010) Medication-induced hypophosphatemia. *QJM* **103**, 449–59.

Hypomagnesaemia

Introduction

- Low plasma magnesium levels are common in acutely ill patients. Clinical manifestations of this are less common. The most common clinical feature of magnesium deficiency is neuromuscular excitability, muscular weakness which is virtually indistinguishable from that associated with hypocalcaemia, which frequently coexists. Arrhythmias can also occur, as can coma.
- Positive Chvostek's and Trousseau's signs are seen.
- Is associated with hypocalcaemia and hypokalaemia.
- In the presence of magnesium deficiency, PTH secretion is inhibited and the peripheral action of PTH is also attenuated. Resultant hypomagnesaemia-induced hypocalcaemia will not respond to calcium treatment, unless the magnesium deficiency is corrected first. Hypokalaemia is also frequently seen in association with hypomagnesaemia. Treatment with potassium supplementation is often unsuccessful, unless magnesium is replaced at the same time.
- See Box 6.14 for causes.

Treatment

Symptomatic magnesium deficiency, especially if associated with hypocalcaemia or hypokalaemia, requires parenteral treatment.

- Magnesium sulfate 50% solution contains ~2mmol magnesium/mL. This should be administered IV, although IM is feasible but painful. An initial 4–8mmol should be given over 15min, followed by a slow infusion of 1mmol/h. The rate of the infusion can be adjusted in light of the response in plasma magnesium.
- In the presence of renal impairment, plasma magnesium can rise quickly, and so particular care must be undertaken if magnesium infusion is contemplated in the presence of renal failure.
- After repletion has been achieved intravenously, or in less severe cases, treatment can be continued orally.
- Various salts of magnesium have been used, including chloride, oxide, and glycerophosphate. Dosing is frequently limited by the purgative properties of magnesium salts.

Box 6.14 Causes of hypomagnesaemia
- GI losses:
  - Vomiting.
  - Diarrhoea.
  - Losses from fistulae.
  - Malabsorption.
- Renal losses:
  - Chronic parenteral therapy.
  - Osmotic diuresis.
  - Gitelman's syndrome.
- Diabetes.
- Drugs:
  - Alcohol.
  - Loop diuretics.
  - Proton pump inhibitors.
  - Aminoglycosides.
  - Cisplatin.
  - Ciclosporin.
  - Amphotericin.
- Metabolic acidosis.
- Hypercalcaemia.
- Other causes:
  - Phosphate depletion.
  - Hungry bone syndrome.

Further reading

Ayuk J, Gittoes NJ (2011). How should hypomagnesaemia be investigated and treated? *Clin Endocrinol (Oxf)* **75**, 743–6.

Osteoporosis

Introduction

Although the term osteoporosis refers to the reduction in the amount of bony tissue within the skeleton, this is generally associated with a loss of structural integrity of the internal architecture of the bone. The combination of both these changes means that osteoporotic bone is at high risk of fracture, even after trivial injury. The most common osteoporotic fractures are those of the hip, wrist (Colles'), and compression fractures of vertebral bodies. Patients who fracture ribs, the upper humerus, leg, and pelvis also have a higher incidence of osteoporosis.

Over recent years, there has been a change in focus in the treatment of osteoporosis. Historically, there has been a primary reliance on bone mineral density as a threshold for treatment, whereas currently there is far greater emphasis on assessing individual patients' risk of fracture that incorporates multiple clinical risk factors as well as bone mineral density.

See Box 6.15 for causes.

Box 6.15 Underlying causes of osteoporosis

- Gonadal failure:
  - Premature menopause (age <45).
  - Hypogonadism in men.
  - Turner's syndrome.
- Conditions leading to amenorrhoea, with low oestrogen (persisting >6 months):
  - Hyperprolactinaemia.
  - Anorexia nervosa.
  - Hypothalamic amenorrhoea.
- Endocrine disorders:
  - Cushing's syndrome.
  - GH deficiency.
  - Hyperparathyroidism.
  - Acromegaly with hypogonadism.
  - Hyperthyroidism (within 3 years).
  - Diabetes mellitus.
- GI disorders:
  - Malabsorption.
  - Post-gastrectomy.
  - Coeliac disease.
  - Crohn's disease.
- Liver disease:
  - Cholestasis.
  - Cirrhosis.

Box 6.15 (Continued)

- Neoplastic disorders:
    - Multiple myeloma.
    - Systemic mastocytosis.
- Inflammatory conditions:
    - Rheumatoid arthritis.
    - Cystic fibrosis.
- Nutritional disorders:
    - Parenteral nutrition.
    - Lactose intolerance.
- Drugs:
    - Systemic glucocorticoids.
    - Heparin (when given long-term, particularly in pregnancy).
    - Chemotherapy (primarily through gonadal damage).
    - Gonadotrophin-releasing hormone agonists.
    - Ciclosporin.
    - Anticonvulsants (long-term).
    - Aromatase inhibitors for breast cancer.
    - Androgen deprivation therapy (prostate cancer).
    - Proton pump inhibitors.
    - Selective serotonin reuptake inhibitors.
- Metabolic abnormalities:
    - Homocystinuria.
- Hereditary disorders.
    - Osteogenesis imperfecta.
    - Marfan's syndrome.
    - Hajdu–Cheney syndrome (autosomal dominant), with marked bone loss (acroosteolysis with osteoporosis and changes in skull and mandible).

Pathology of osteoporosis

Osteoporosis may arise from a failure of the body to lay down sufficient bone during growth and maturation; an earlier than usual onset of bone loss following maturity; or an ↑ rate of that loss.

See Table 6.7 for definitions and Box 6.16 for causes.

Peak bone mass
- Mainly genetically determined:
  - Racial effects (bone mass higher in Afro-Caribbean and lower in Caucasians).
  - Family influence on the risk of osteoporosis—may account for 70% of variation.
  - So far, >9 separate genetic associations described.
- Also influenced by environmental factors:
  - Exercise—particularly weight-bearing.
  - Nutrition—especially calcium.
- Exposure to oestrogen is also important:
  - Early menopause or late puberty (in ♂ or ♀) is associated with ↑ risk of osteoporosis.

Early onset of loss
- Early menopause.
- Conditions leading to bone loss, e.g. glucocorticoid therapy.

Increased net loss
- Ageing:
  - Vitamin D insufficiency.
  - Declining bone formation.
  - Declining renal function.
- Underlying disease states (see Box 6.15).

Lifestyle factors affecting bone mass
Increase
- Weight-bearing exercise.

Decrease
- Smoking.
- Excessive alcohol.
- Nulliparity.
- Poor calcium nutrition.

Table 6.7 WHO definitions for osteoporosis and low bone mass

T score	Fragility fracture	Diagnosis
–1		Normal
<–1 but ≥–2.5		Low bone mass (osteopenia)
<–2.5	No	Osteoporosis
<–2.5	Yes	Established (severe) osteoporosis

Box 6.16 Causes of increased bone mineral density

Artefacts
- Excess skeletal calcium.
- Extraskeletal calcium.
- Vertebral fracture.
- Radiodense material.

Focal increase in bone
- Paget's.
- Tumours.

Generalized increase
- Acquired osteosclerosis, e.g. renal osteodystrophy, fluorosis, mastocytosis, myelofibrosis, acromegaly.

Genetic
- Sclerosing bone dysplasias.
- Decreased absorption, e.g. osteoporosis, increased formation sclerosteosis, *LRP5* mutation.

Epidemiology of osteoporosis

- The risk of osteoporotic fracture increases with age. Fracture rates in ♂ are approximately half of those seen in ♀ of the same age. A ♀ aged 50 has approximately a 1:2 chance of sustaining an osteoporotic fracture in the rest of her life. The corresponding figure for a ♂ is 1:5.
- In the UK each year, in ♀, there are in excess of 25,000 vertebral fractures that come to clinical attention, together with over 40,000 wrist fractures and 50,000 hip fractures. The latter are a particular health challenge, as they invariably result in hospital admission. One-fifth of hip fracture victims will die within 6 months of the injury, and only 50% will return to their previous level of independence. It has been estimated that the overall cost of osteoporotic fractures in the UK is £2.1 billion annually.
- See Box 6.17 for investigations.

Box 6.17 **Investigations to consider an underlying cause of osteoporosis**

Useful in most patients
- FBC.
- ESR.
- Biochemical profile.
- Renal function.
- Liver function.
- Calcium.
- Thyroid function.
- Testosterone and LH (only in ♂).
- Vitamin D.

Useful in specific instances
- Oestradiol and FSH (in ♀ where menopausal status not clear).
- Serum and urine electrophoresis (if raised ESR or plasma globulin elevated).
- Anti-tissue transglutaminase antibodies (if any suggestion of coeliac disease).
- 24h urinary calcium excretion (to detect idiopathic hypercalciuria).
- Other investigations for specific diseases.

Low-trauma fractures associated with osteoporosis
Any fracture, other than those affecting fingers, toes, or face, which is caused by a fall from standing height or less is called a fragility (low-trauma) fracture, and underlying osteoporosis should be considered. Patients suffering such a fracture should be considered for investigation and/or treatment for osteoporosis.

Presentation of osteoporosis

- Usually clinically silent until an acute fracture.
- Two-thirds of vertebral fractures do not come to clinical attention.
- Typical vertebral fracture:
  - Sudden episode of well-localized pain.
  - May, or may not, have been related to injury or exertion.
  - May be radiation of the pain in a girdle distribution.
  - Pain may initially require bed rest but gradually subsides over 4–8 weeks; even after this time, there may be residual pain at the fracture site.
  - Osteoporotic vertebral fractures only rarely lead to neurological impairment.
- Any evidence of spinal cord compression should prompt a search for malignancy or other underlying cause.
- Following vertebral fracture, a patient may be left with persistent back pain, kyphosis, or height loss.
- Although height loss and kyphosis are often thought of as being indicative of osteoporosis, they are more frequently the result of degenerative disease, including disc disease. These changes cannot be attributed to osteoporosis in the absence of vertebral fractures.
- Peripheral fractures are also more common in osteoporosis.
- If a bone breaks from a fall from less than standing height, that represents a low-trauma fracture which might indicate underlying osteoporosis.
- Osteoporosis does not cause generalized skeletal pain.

Investigation of osteoporosis

Establish the diagnosis

- Plain radiographs are useful for determining the presence of fracture. Apart from this, they are of little utility in the diagnosis of osteoporosis. Bone density cannot be assessed reliably from a plain radiograph.
- *Bone densitometry.* In order to identify the presence of T score-defined osteoporosis, it is important to measure BMD appropriately. This is usually carried out at the hip and lumbar spine, using dual-energy X-ray absorptiometry (DXA). The presence of degenerative disease or arterial calcification can elevate the apparent bone density of the spine without adding to skeletal strength. ↑ reliance is, therefore, being placed on measurements derived from the hip. The diagnostic criteria for osteoporosis have been derived through the WHO (see Table 6.7).
- Biochemical markers of bone turnover may be helpful in the calculation of fracture risk and in judging the response to drug therapies, but they have no role in the diagnosis of osteoporosis.
- Use of fracture risk algorithms is now available to determine individuals' fracture risk (e.g. ℘ http://www.shef.ac.uk/FRAX). Such an approach can help tune therapies to those patients at heightened risk of fracture.

Exclude underlying causes

An underlying cause for osteoporosis is present in approximately 10–30% of women and up to 50% of men with osteoporosis. Many of the underlying causes (see Box 6.15) should be apparent from a careful history and physical examination. A few basic investigations are useful to exclude the more common underlying causes. Other investigations may be needed to exclude other specific conditions.

It is helpful to target investigations at those people who have a significantly lower than expected bone mass for their age (Z score <−2).

Monitoring therapy

- Repeat bone densitometry is not obligatory for monitoring, as there is no direct correlation between changes in bone density and the anti-fracture effects of drugs. This is an area of controversy.
- Minimum time interval should be 2 years between scans.
- Effective treatment leads to modest rise (~5% at spine) in bone density.
- Biochemical markers of bone turnover may be helpful in specific settings (e.g. P1NP and NTX).
- See Table 6.8 for efficacy for types of treatments

Table 6.8 Grade of evidence of anti-fracture efficacy of approved treatments for post-menopausal women with osteoporosis (when given with calcium + vitamin D)

Treatment	Vertebral fracture	Non-vertebral fracture	Hip fracture
Alendronic acid	A	A	A
Etidronate	A	B	NAE
Ibandronic acid	A	A#	NAE
Risedronate	A	A	A
Zoledronic acid	A	A	A
Denosumab	A	A	A
Calcitonin	A	B	B
Calcitriol	A	B	NAE
Raloxifene	A	NAE	NAE
Strontium ranelate	A	A	A#
Teriparatide	A	A	NAE
Recombinant human PTH (1-84)	A	NAE	NAE
HRT	A	A	A

NAE, not adequately evaluated; PTH, parathyroid hormone; HRT, hormone replacement therapy; #, in subsets of patients only.

Treatment of osteoporosis

Treatments should be considered according to their effect on fracture risk reduction and side effect profile.

In addition to pharmacological treatments aimed at reducing fracture risk, it must be remembered that non-pharmacological measures are also important. Thus, it is prudent to minimize the risk of falling by adjusting the home environment and reviewing the need for medications, such as hypnotics and antihypertensives, for instance.

Lifestyle measures

- Stop smoking.
- Avoid alcohol excess.
- Encourage weight-bearing exercise:
  - Lower-impact exercise, e.g. walking outdoors for 20min 3× weekly, may reduce fracture risk.
- Encourage well-balanced diet.
- Ensure adequate calcium and vitamin D intake.
- If necessary, give supplements to achieve calcium intake of ~1g daily.

Choice of therapy and who to treat

The National Institute for Health and Care Excellence (NICE) has produced guidance on the 2° prevention of osteoporotic fractures in post-menopausal women with a low-trauma fracture (⅏ http://guidance. nice.org.uk/TA161; ⅏ http://guidance.nice.org.uk/TA204). The guidelines focus on age, bone density, clinical risk factors, and cost effectiveness to derive recommendations.

The National Osteoporosis Guideline Group (NOGG) has also derived alternative clinical guidelines that are based on a fracture risk assessment tool (FRAX) that links into a web-based guideline tool to derive recommendations regarding prescribing (⅏ http://www.shef.ac.uk/FRAX; ⅏ http://www.shef.ac.uk/NOGG).

Therapy is given for 5 years in the first instance. Reassessment should occur at this time. If the T score at the femoral neck is below −2.5, then therapy should be continued. Consideration should also be given to continue therapy if there has been a previous vertebral fracture. Patients with a T score above −2.0 at the femoral neck are unlikely to benefit from continued treatment.

See Box 6.18 for vertebroplasty.

Glucocorticoid-induced osteoporosis

Glucocorticoid treatment is one of the major 2° causes of osteoporosis. Not all patients receiving steroid treatment do lose bone, and it is not clear what determines this. Patients who sustain fractures while taking glucocorticoids do so at higher bone density levels than in post-menopausal women, leading to the assertion that such patients should be treated at a higher bone density (T <−1.5) than would be the case for post-menopausal osteoporosis.

The Royal College of Physicians (UK) has produced guidelines for the management of glucocorticoid-induced osteoporosis (see Fig. 6.4).

Box 6.18 Vertebroplasty
- Percutaneous injection of bone cement into the fractured vertebral body.
- Effective at resolving pain in the short and longer term.
- Best for patients with acute fractures and persistent pain (>6 weeks).

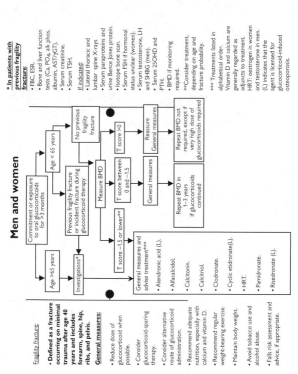

Fig. 6.4 Guidelines for the management of glucocorticoid-induced osteoporosis.

Men and women

Age >65 years

Age < 65 years

Commitment or exposure to oral glucocorticoids for >3 months

Previous fragility fracture or incident fracture during glucocorticoid therapy

No previous fragility fracture

Investigations*

Measure BMD

T score −1.5 or lower**

T score between 0 and −1.5

T score >0

General measures and advise treatment***

General measures

Reassure General measures

Repeat BMD in 1–3 years if glucocorticoids continued

Repeat BMD not required, except if very high dose of glucocorticoids required

• Alendronic acid (L).
• Alfacalcidol.
• Calcitonin.
• Calcitriol.
• Clodronate.
• Cyclic etidronate(L).
• HRT.
• Pamidronate.
• Risedronate (L).

Fragility fracture:

• **Defined as a fracture occurring on minimal trauma after age 40 years and includes forearm, spine, hip, ribs, and pelvis.**

General measures:

• Reduce dose of glucocorticoid when possible.

• Consider glucocorticoid-sparing therapy.

• Consider alternative route of glucocorticoid administration.

• Recommend adequate nutrition, especially with calcium and vitamin D.

• Recommend regular weight-bearing exercise.

• Maintain body weight.

• Avoid tobacco use and alcohol abuse.

• Falls risk assessment and advice, if appropriate.

* In patients with previous fragility fracture

• FBC, ESR.
• Bone and liver function tests (Ca, PO_4, alk phos, albumin, AST/γGT).
• Serum creatinine.
• Serum TSH.

If indicated:

• Lateral thoracic and lumbar spine X-rays.
• Serum paraproteins and urine Bence Jones protein.
• Isotope bone scan.
• Serum FSH if hormonal status unclear (women).
• Serum testosterone, LH and SHBG (men).
• Serum 25OHD and PTH.
• BMD if monitoring required.

**Consider treatment, depending on age and fracture probability.

*** Treatments listed in alphabetical order.

Vitamin D and calcium are generally regarded as adjuncts to treatment.

HRT: oestrogen in women and testosterone in men. (L) indicates that the agent is licensed for glucocorticoid-induced osteoporosis.

Complications of therapy for osteoporosis

(See Boxes 6.19 and 6.20 for special considerations.)

HRT

- Because of adverse effects (breast cancer, venous thromboembolism, coronary disease, and stroke), HRT is no longer regarded as a 1° treatment for osteoporosis in post-menopausal ♀.
- When a woman is receiving HRT for climacteric symptoms, however, there will be a beneficial effect on fracture risk reduction.
- Skeletal protection is rapidly lost on cessation of HRT.
- In ♀ with a premature menopause, HRT remains the most appropriate means of preventing bone loss in the absence of other contraindications.

Bisphosphonates

- Weekly (PO), daily (PO), monthly (PO), 3-monthly (IV), and annual (IV) preparations are available.
- Oral preparations require patients to follow strict dosing instructions. Oral bisphosphonates should be taken on an empty stomach, and 30–60min (dependent on drug) should pass prior to additional oral intake.
- GI disturbance, including nausea and oesophagitis, are common.
- Osteonecrosis of the jaw is a very rare side effect of bisphosphonates in doses given to treat osteoporosis (<0.5%). It may be treated with teriparatide.
- Flu-like symptoms occur in 20–30%, following IV administration of zoledronate (acute phase response commoner in younger patients).
- There is a possible association between atypical subtrochanteric femoral fractures in patients who have taken several years of bisphosphonates.
- If treated for 5 years, consider therapeutic holiday, unless T worse than 2.5 at the hips or, with existing history of vertebral fractures, T is worse than −2.0.

Calcium and vitamin D

- Constipation.
- Recent reports have raised queries of a link between exogenous calcium supplementation and increased risk of cardiovascular disease.

Calcitonin

- Very rarely used nowadays.
- Parenteral administration.
- Flushing.
- Nausea and diarrhoea.

Raloxifene

- Similar increase in risk of venous thrombosis as HRT.
- May induce/worsen climacteric symptoms.
- Reduces risk of breast cancer.

Strontium ranelate
- Diarrhoea.
- Venous thromboembolism.

Denosumab
- Effective for at least 6 years.
- Skin infections/eczema.
- Hypocalcaemia (ensure Ca and vitamin D levels normal prior).

Teriparatide
- Contraindications: hypercalcaemia, renal impairment, unexplained elevation of alkaline phosphatase—Paget's disease, prior irradiation.
- Risk of hypercalcaemia is not great. and no specific monitoring of treatment is recommended.
- Vomiting.
- Leg cramps.
- ↑ risk of osteosarcoma seen in rats given teriparatide for most of their life. It should be avoided in patients with ↑ risk of bone tumours (Paget's disease, raised alkaline phosphatase, previous skeletal radiotherapy).

Causes of increased bone mineral density

Artefacts
- Excess skeletal calcium (lumbar spondylosis, ankylosing spondylitis).
- Extraskeletal calcium (vascular, gallstones).
- Vertebral fracture.
- Radiodense material (surgical implants, strontium).

Focal increase in bone
- Paget's disease.
- Tumours (e.g. haemangioma, Hodgkin's, plasmacytoma).

Generalized increase in bone
Acquired osteosclerosis (general osteodystrophy, fluorosis, mastocytosis, hepatitis C, myelofibrosis, acromegaly).

Genetic sclerosing bone dysplasias
- ↓ absorption (e.g. osteopetrosis).
- ↑ formation (e.g. sclerosteosis).
- Disturbed balance of formation and resorption.

Box 6.19 Special considerations in men

(For algorithm, 📖 see Fig. 6.4, p. 500.)

- 2° causes of osteoporosis are more common in ♂ and need to be excluded in all ♂ with osteoporotic fracture.
- Bisphosphonates benefit bone mass in ♂ in a similar way to post-menopausal ♀.
- Hypogonadal ♂ show an improvement in bone mass on testosterone replacement. However, hypogonadal ♂ respond to bisphosphonates as do those with normal testosterone levels. Replacement testosterone along with bisphosphonate therapy is appropriate.

Box 6.20 Special considerations in premenopausal women

- 'Osteoporosis' in premenopausal ♀ is rare but well recognized.
- Younger women have a lower risk of fracture.
- It is important to exclude underlying causes of accelerated rates of bone loss.
- Osteoporosis can very rarely occur in conjunction with pregnancy or lactation. This is frequently self-limiting and usually requires little treatment other than calcium supplementation.
- In the absence of a pre-existing fracture, fracture risk is low. Advice regarding positive lifestyle factors is always prudent. Further assessment should be made around the age of natural menopause.
- In other situations, particularly where low-trauma fractures have occurred, other therapies may be carefully considered, recognizing there are no data to support the use of anti-fracture drugs in premenopausal women.
- Some caution needs to be exercised over the use of bisphosphonates in younger people:
  - Teratogenic in animals.
  - Long skeletal retention time.
  - In such patients, it may be worth considering alternative agents, such as calcitriol.

In general, the management of premenopausal women with osteoporosis and high fracture risk should be assessed by a clinician with a specialist interest in metabolic bone diseases.

Further reading

Black DM, Delmas PD, Eastell R, *et al.* (2007). Once-yearly zoledronic acid for treatment of post-menopausal osteoporosis. *N Engl J Med* **356**, 1809–22.

Boonen S, *et al.* (2012). Fracture risk and zoledronic acid therapy in men with osteoporosis. *N Engl J Med* **367**, 1714–23.

Ebeling PR (2008). Osteoporosis in men. *N Engl J Med* **358**, 1474–82.

Khosla S, *et al.* (2008). Osteoporosis in men. *Endocr Rev* **29**, 441–64.

Klazen CA, *et al.* (2010). Vertebroplasty versus conservative treatment in acute osteoporotic vertebral compression fractures (Vertos II): an open-label randomised trial. *Lancet* **376**, 108–92.

Meunier PJ, Roux C, Seeman E, *et al.* (2004). The effects of strontium ranelate on the risk of vertebral fracture in women with postmenopausal osteoporosis. *N Engl J Med* **350**, 459–68.

Ranney A, Tugwell P, Wells G, *et al.* (2002). Meta-analyses of therapies for postmenopausal osteoporosis. I. Systematic reviews of randomized trials in osteoporosis: induction and methodology. *Endocr Rev* **23**, 496–507.

Russell RGG (2011). Bisphosphonates: the first 40 years. *Bone* **49**, 2–19.

Sambrook P, Cooper C (2006). Osteoporosis. *Lancet* **367**, 2010–28.

Schilcher J, *et al.* (2011). Bisphosphonate use and atypical fractures of the femoral shaft. *N Engl J Med* **364**, 1728–37.

Watts NB, *at al.* (2012). Osteoporosis in men: an Endocrine Society clinical practice guideline. *J Clin Endocrinol Metab* **97**, 1802–22.

Weinstein RS (2011). Clinical practice. Glucocorticoid-induced bone disease. *N Engl J Med* **365**, 62–70.

Paget's disease

Paget's disease is the result of greatly ↑ local bone turnover, which occurs particularly in the elderly but can affect younger people.

Pathology

- The 1° abnormality in Paget's disease is gross overactivity of the osteoclasts, resulting in greatly ↑ bone resorption. This secondarily results in ↑ osteoblastic activity. The new bone is laid down in a highly disorganized manner and leads to the characteristic pagetic abnormality, with irregular packets of woven bone being apparent on biopsy and disorganized internal architecture of the bone on plain radiographs.
- Paget's disease can affect any bone in the skeleton but is most frequently found in the pelvis, vertebral column, femur, skull, and tibia. In most patients, it affects several sites, but, in about 20% of cases, a single bone is affected (monostotic disease). Typically, the disease will start in one end of a long bone and spread along the bone at a rate of about 1cm per year. Although it can spread within an affected bone, it appears that the pattern of disease is fixed by the time of clinical presentation, and it is exceedingly rare for new bones to become involved during the course of the disease.
- Paget's disease alters the mechanical properties of the bone. Thus, pagetic bones are more likely to bend under normal physiological loads and are thus liable to fracture. This can take the form of complete fractures, which tend to be transverse, rather than the more common spiral fractures of long bones. More frequently, fissure or incremental fractures are seen on the convex surface of bowed pagetic bones. These may be painful in their own right but are also liable to proceed to complete fracture. Pagetic bones are also larger than their normal counterparts. This can lead to ↑ arthritis at adjacent joints and to pressure on nerves, leading to neurological compression syndromes and, when it occurs in the skull base, sensorineural deafness.

Aetiology of Paget's disease

Unclear. There are two major theories:

- Familial:
  - Some genetic associations, especially with a sequestasome-1 mutation.
  - These are not invariable.
- Viral:
  - Inclusion bodies, similar to those seen in viral infections, have been identified in osteoclasts from patients with Paget's.
  - Some workers have found paramyxoviral (measles or canine distemper) protein or nucleic acid in pagetic bone; others have not been able to replicate this.

Epidemiology

Paget's disease is present in about 2% of the UK population over the age of 55. Its prevalence increases with age, and it is more common in ♂ than ♀. Only about 10% of affected patients will have symptomatic disease. It is most common in the UK or in migrants of British descent in North America and Australasia but rare in Africa. Studies in the UK and New Zealand have suggested that the prevalence may be declining with time.

Clinical features
- 90% asymptomatic.
- Most notable feature is pain. This is frequently multifactorial:
  - ↑ metabolic activity of the bone.
  - Changes in bone shape.
  - Fissure fractures.
  - Nerve compression.
  - Arthritis.
- Pagetic bones tend to increase in size or become bowed (16% cases): bowing can be so severe as to interfere with function.
- Fractures (either complete or fissure) present in 10%.
- Risk of osteosarcoma is increased in active Paget's disease but is a very rare finding.

Investigation
The diagnosis of Paget's disease is primarily radiological.

Radiological features of Paget's disease
- Early disease—primarily lytic:
  - V-shaped 'cutting cone' in long bones.
  - Osteoporosis circumscripta in skull.
- Combined phase (mixed lytic and sclerotic):
  - Cortical thickening.
  - Loss of corticomedullary distinction.
  - Accentuated trabecular markings.
- Late phase—primarily sclerotic:
  - Thickening of long bones.
  - Increase in bone size.
  - Sclerosis.

An isotope bone scan is frequently helpful in assessing the extent of skeletal involvement with Paget's disease. It is particularly important to identify Paget's disease in a weight-bearing bone because of the risk of fracture. The uptake of tracer depends on the disease activity, and isotope bone scans can also be used to assess the response to therapy.

In active disease, plasma alkaline phosphatase activity is usually (85%) elevated. An exception to this is in monostotic disease when there may be insufficient bone involved to raise the enzyme levels above normal. Alkaline phosphatase activity responds to successful treatment. There is little advantage in using the more modern markers of bone turnover over the total alkaline phosphatase activity for the monitoring of pagetic activity. A possible exception to this is in patients with liver disease where changes in bone alkaline phosphatase might be masked by the liver isoenzyme.

Complications

- Deafness is present in up to half of cases of skull base Paget's.
- Other neurological complications are rare. These can include:
  - Compression of other cranial nerves with skull base disease.
  - *Spinal cord compression.* Most common with involvement of the thoracic spine and is thought to result as much from a vascular steal syndrome as from physical compression. It frequently responds to medical therapy without need for surgical decompression.
  - Platybasia which can lead to an obstructive hydrocephalus that may require surgical drainage.
- Osteogenic sarcoma:
  - Very rare complication of Paget's disease.
  - Rarely amenable to treatment.
  - Presents with ↑ pain/radiological evidence of tumour, a mass, and very elevated alkaline phosphatase.
- Any increase of pain in a patient with Paget's disease should arouse suspicion of sarcomatous degeneration. A more common cause, however, is resumption of activity of disease.

Pagetic sarcomas are most frequently found in the humerus or femur but can affect any bone involved with Paget's disease.

Treatment

Treatment with agents that decrease bone turnover reduces disease activity, as indicated by bone turnover markers and isotope bone scans. There is evidence to suggest that such treatment leads to the deposition of histologically normal bone. Although such treatment has been shown to help pain, there is little evidence that it benefits the other consequences of Paget's disease. In particular, the deafness of Paget's disease does not regress after treatment, although its progression may be halted. Nonetheless, it has become generally accepted to treat patients in the hope that future complications of the disease will be avoided. Typical indications for treatment of Paget's disease are listed in Box 6.21.

Bisphosphonates have become the mainstay of treatment. IV zoledronate is the drug of choice and results in long-term normalization of alkaline phosphatase in the majority of patients. Calcitonin and plicamycin are no longer used.

Goals of treatment

- Minimize symptoms.
- Prevent long-term complications.
- Normalize bone turnover.
- Alkaline phosphatase in normal range.
- No actual evidence that treatment achieves this.

Box 6.21 Typical indications for treating Paget's disease

Evidence in this area is minimal.
- Pain likely due to Paget's.
- Neurological complications (e.g. deafness, spinal cord compression).
- Disease in weight-bearing bones.
- Disease in periarticular location.
- Prevention of long-term complications (e.g. bone deformation, osteoarthritis).
- Young patients.
- In preparation for surgery.
- Hypercalcaemia.
- Following fracture.

Monitoring therapy
- Plasma alkaline phosphatase every 6–12 months.
- Clinical assessment.

Re-treat if symptoms recur with objective evidence of disease recurrence (alkaline phosphatase or +ve isotope scan). There is no evidence that treating a raised alkaline phosphatase in the absence of symptoms affects outcome in Paget's.

Further reading

Albagha OM, et al. (2011). Genome-wide association identifies three new susceptibility loci for Paget's disease of bone. Nat Genet **43**, 685–9.

Ralston SH (2013). Clinical practice. Paget's disease of bone. N Engl J Med **368**, 644–50.

Ralston SH, et al (2008). Pathogenesis and management of Paget's disease of bone. Lancet **372**, 155–163.

Selby PL, Davie MW, Ralston SH, et al. (2002). National Association for the Relief of Paget's Disease: guidelines on the management of Paget's disease of the bone. Bone **31**, 366–73.

Inherited disorders of bone

Osteogenesis imperfecta

Osteogenesis imperfecta is an inherited form of osteoporosis where, in the vast majority of cases, there is a genetic defect in one of the two genes (*COLIA1* and *COLIA2*) encoding the α-chain of collagen type I collagen production. Several different mutations are recognized, and these produce different clinical pictures; these are generally separated into at least four types (see Table 6.9).

In addition to the osteoporosis and easy fracture, there may also be abnormalities of the teeth (dentinogenesis imperfecta), blue sclerae and hearing loss, hypermobility, and cardiac valvular lesions.

Radiological features include:
- Generalized osteopenia.
- Multiple fractures with deformity.
- Abnormal shape of long bones.
- Wormian bones in skull (Accessory skull bones completely surrounded by a suture line).

Diagnosis
- Features described in previous section and family history.
- Analysis of collagen type I genes (detect 90%).
- Three criteria:
  - Three fragility fractures aged <20 years.
  - At least one of: blue sclerae, scoliosis, hearing loss, joint laxity, dentinogenesis imperfecta, and family member.
  - Osteoporosis.

Recent studies have demonstrated that infusions of pamidronate lead to ↑ bone mass and reduced fracture incidence in affected children. Patients with milder disease might only be recognized in adulthood. There is no established role for bisphosphonates in young adults with osteogenesis imperfecta, although each case should be assessed on balance of risk factors for fracture. It is also noteworthy that fracture risk increases steeply with ageing in patients with osteogenesis imperfecta, and thus consideration should be given to interventions, including use of anti-fracture drugs.

Prenatal diagnosis of severe types is possible, and genetic counselling should be offered to all at-risk families.

Table 6.9 Classification of osteogenesis imperfecta

Type	Inheritance	Stature	Teeth	Sclerae	Hearing	Genetic defect
I	AD Mild	Normal	Normal	Blue	Variable loss	Substitution for glycine in COL1A1
II	AD/AR	Lethal deformity				Rearrangement of COL1A1 and COL1A2
III	AD/AR (Progressive deforming)	(Very short, severe scoliosis)	Abnormal	Variable	Loss common	Glycine substitution in COL1A1 and COL1A2
IV	AD	Mild	Abnormal	Normal	Occasional loss	Point mutations in a2(I) or a1(I)

Further reading

Bitton A, et al. (2009). Clinical problem-solving. A fragile balance. *N Engl J Med* **361**, 74–9.
Rauch F, Glorieux FH (2004). Osteogenesis imperfecta. *Lancet* **363**, 1377–85.

Paediatric endocrinology

Growth

Regulation of growth

Normal human growth can be divided into three overlapping stages (the Karlberg model), each under the control of different factors:

- *Infancy.* Growth is largely under nutritional regulation, and wide inter-individual variation in rates of growth is seen. Many infants show significant 'catch-up' or 'catch-down' in weight and length, and by 2 years, length is much more predictive of final adult height than at birth.
- *Childhood.* Growth is regulated by growth hormone (GH) and thyroxine. It is characterized by alternating periods of mini-growth spurts with intervening stasis, each phase lasting several weeks. However, over years, a child will tend to maintain their centile position on height charts, with a height velocity between the 25th and 75th centiles.
- *Puberty.* The combination of GH and sex hormones promotes bone maturation and a rapid growth acceleration or 'growth spurt'. In both sexes, oestrogen eventually causes epiphyseal fusion, resulting in the attainment of final height.

Sex differences

Adult heights differ between ♂ and ♀ by, on average, 13cm. However, during childhood, onset of the pubertal growth spurt is earlier in ♀, who are therefore, on average, taller than ♂ between the ages of 10–13 years.

Tempo

Within each sex, there may also be marked inter-individual differences in *tempo* of growth (or rate of attainment of final height) and the timing of puberty. Delay or advance of bone maturation is linked with timing of puberty. Constitutional delay in growth and puberty often runs in families, reflecting probable genetic factors. Comparison of *bone age* (estimated from a hand radiograph) with chronological age is, therefore, an important part of growth assessment.

Final height

Final height is estimated as the height reached when growth velocity slows to <2cm/year and can be confirmed by finding epiphyseal fusion on hand radiograph ± knee radiograph. Final height is largely genetically determined, and a target height can be estimated in each individual from their parent's heights.

Assessment of growth

Measurement

- From birth to 2 years old, supine length is measured ideally using a measuring board (e.g. Harpenden neonatometer). Two adults are needed to ensure that the child is lying straight and legs extended.
- From 2 years old, standing height is measured against a wall-mounted or free-standing stadiometer, with the measurer applying moderate upwards neck traction and the child looking forward in the horizontal plane.

- To minimize error in the calculation of height velocity (cm/year), height measurements should be taken at least 6 months apart, using the same equipment and ideally by the same person.
- Measurement of *sitting height* and comparison with *leg length* (*standing height – sitting height*) allows an estimate of body proportion.

Growth charts (see Figs. 7.1 and 7.2)

Height and weight velocity should be compared to age and sex appropriate reference data by plotting values on standard growth charts (e.g. the UK 1990 Growth Reference, Child Growth Foundation, London, UK). Charts based on the World Health Organization (WHO) child growth standards are becoming available and define the optimal growth for children who have been breastfed as a baby. The data are based on the UK90 and WHO data (http://www.rcpch.ac.uk/child-health/research-projects/uk-who-growth-charts/).

Mid-parental height (MPH)

MPH is an estimate of the child's genetic height potential and is calculated as:

[(Mother's height + father's height)/2] + 7cm (for boys)

or – 7cm (for girls).

It can be used to estimate a child's expected final height, but there is a wide target range (MPH ± 10cm for boys and ± 8.5cm for girls), and it is more commonly used to assess whether the child's current height centile is consistent with genetic expectation.

Bone age

Skeletal maturation proceeds in an orderly manner from the first appearance of each epiphyseal centre to the fusion of the long bones. From chronological age 3–4 years, bone age may be quantified from radiographs of the left hand and wrist by comparison with standard photographs (e.g. Greulich and Pyle method) or by an individual bone scoring system (e.g. Tanner–Whitehouse method). The difference between bone age and chronological age is an estimation of tempo of growth. The initiation of puberty usually coincides with a bone age around 10.5–11 years in girls and 11–11.5 years in boys, although the correlation between bone age and pubertal timing is approximate. Girls reach skeletal maturity at a bone age of 15 years and boys when bone age is 17 years. Thus, bone age allows an estimation of remaining growth potential and can be used to aid in the prediction of final adult height.

Final height prediction

Predictions of final height can be derived from information on current height, age, pubertal status, and bone age, using calculations described by Tanner and Whitehouse or Bayley and Pinneau, among others.[1]

Secular trends

Children's heights ↑ by >1cm in England and by >2cm in Scotland during the period from 1972–94, and similar trends are seen in many other countries. Population growth references used should be appropriate to the population studied and may occasionally need to be updated. However, secular trends in height over the last decade have reduced significantly in some countries.

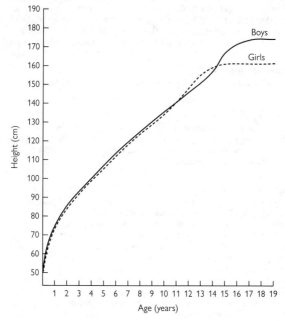

Fig. 7.1 Typical individual height-attained curves for boys and girls (supine length to the age of 2; integrated curves of Fig. 7.2).

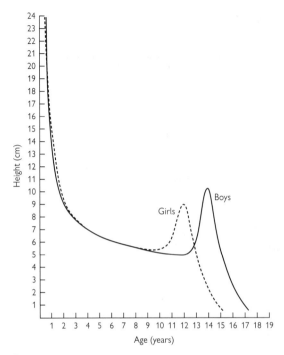

Fig. 7.2 Typical individual velocity curves for supine length or height in boys and girls. These curves represent the velocity of the typical boy and girl at any given instant.

Reference

1. De Waal WJ, Greyn-Fokker MH, Stijnen T, *et al.* (1996). Accuracy of final height prediction and effect of growth-reductive therapy in 362 constitutionally tall children. *J Clin Endocrinol Metab* **81**, 1206–16.

Short stature

Definition
Short stature is defined as height <2nd centile for age and sex on the UK 1990 growth chart. However, abnormalities of growth may be present long before attained height falls below this level and may be detected much earlier by assessing growth velocity and observing height measurements.

Assessment

History
- Who is concerned, child or parents?
- What are the parental heights?
- Has the child always been small or does the history suggest recent growth failure? Try to obtain previous measurements (e.g. from parents, GP, health visitor, school).
- Ask about maternal illness in pregnancy, drug intake and possible substance abuse in pregnancy, gestation at delivery, size at birth (weight/length/head circumference), childhood illnesses, medication, and developmental milestones.
- Systematic enquiry for headaches, visual disturbance, asthma/ respiratory symptoms, abdominal symptoms, and diet.
- Is there a family history of short stature or pubertal delay?
- What are the psychosocial circumstances of the child and the family?

Examination
- Assess height and height velocity over at least 6 months.
- Measure sitting height, and derive subischial leg length (standing height – sitting height (cm)) if skeletal disproportion suspected.
- Assess for the presence and severity of chronic disease. Low weight for height suggests a nutritional diagnosis, GI cause, or other significant systemic disease.
- Pubertal stage using Tanner's criteria (see 🕮 p. 537).
- Observe for dysmorphic features and signs of endocrinolopathy, presence and severity of chronic disease.
- Measure parents' heights, and calculate MPH.

Investigations
- Laboratory tests should include FBC, ESR, electrolytes, thyroid function, calcium, phosphate, antigliadin and antiendomysial antibodies, IGF-I level, karyotype (of particular importance in girls), and urinalysis.
- These tests may also be clinically indicated: GH provocation testing (e.g. arginine, glucagon, or ITT) (see Table 7.1) with other anterior pituitary function tests, MRI scan with specific reference to the hypothalamus and pituitary, skeletal survey (for bone dysplasia), and, very rarely, an IGF-1 generation test (for GH resistance, 🕮 see Growth hormone deficiency, p. 521).

Causes
- Genetic short stature.

Table 7.1 Comparison of GH provocation tests

	Insulin (IV)	Arginine (IV)	Glucagon (IM)
Age	>2 years	Any	<5 years and in neonates
Advantages	Gold standard	Safe, consistent response	Safe
	Also tests ACTH–cortisol axis		Also tests ACTH–cortisol axis
Disadvantages	Risk of severe hypoglycaemia but good safety record in experienced centres	Occasional nausea and vomiting	Nausea may last 3–4h
		Can cause skin irritation	Great care because of late hypoglycaemia

Other agents (e.g. L-dopa or clonidene) are less commonly used. Measurement of GH levels after exercise has poor sensitivity and specificity for detecting GH deficiency.

- Constitutional delay in growth and puberty—these first two together account for ~40% of cases.
- Chronic illness (including untreated coeliac disease, congenital heart disease, chronic renal failure, inflammatory bowel disease).
- Psychosocial deprivation (which may be associated with reversible GH deficiency, see 📖 p. 371).
- Small for gestational age (SGA), including intrauterine growth restriction (7.5%).
- Dysmorphic syndromes (e.g. Turner's syndrome, Noonan's syndrome (short stature, congenital heart defects, webbed neck), Down's syndrome).
- Malnutrition (1°, rare in the UK).
- GH deficiency (8%):
  - Undefined aetiology ('idiopathic', including those with abnormal pituitary morphology on MRI).
  - Congenital malformation in the hypothalamus/pituitary (HP) (e.g. septo-optic dysplasia) or acquired HP disorders (e.g. craniopharyngioma, trauma), the *GH*-1 gene or the GH-releasing hormone receptor gene, or rarely mutations in transcription factors controlling pituitary development (see 📖 p. 126).
  - GH resistance (rare genetic mutations in the GH receptor or GH-signalling molecules).
  - Endocrine disorders (hypothyroidism, hypoparathyroidism, Cushing's syndrome).
- Skeletal dysplasia (e.g. achondroplasia, hypochondroplasia).
- Metabolic bone disease (e.g. nutritional or hypophosphataemic rickets).
- Inhaled glucocorticoids.

Genetic short stature
Although stature does not follow strict Mendelian laws of inheritance, it does relate to parental height and is probably a polygenic trait. It should be remembered that short parents may themselves have an unidentified dominantly inherited condition (e.g. hypochondroplasia).

Constitutional delay of growth and puberty

Clinical features

- This condition often presents in adolescence but may also be recognized in earlier childhood, although it is more prevalent in ♂.
- Characteristic features include short stature and delay in pubertal development by >2 standard deviations (SD), and/or bone age delay in an otherwise healthy child. In the adolescent years, short sitting height percentile, compared to leg length, is typical.
- There is often a family history of delayed puberty.
- Bone age delay may also develop in a number of other conditions, but, in constitutional delay, bone age delay usually remains consistent over time and height velocity is normal for the bone age. Final height may not reach target height.
- GH secretion is usually normal, although provocation tests should be primed by prior administration of exogenous sex hormones if bone age is >10 years (see Box 7.1).

Management

Often only reassurance is necessary. Treatment is sometimes indicated in adolescent boys who have difficulty coping with their short stature or delayed sexual maturation.

- For the younger child with concerns about growth: low-dose *oxandrolone* (1.25mg/day for up to 12 months, oral). A synthetic derivative of testosterone which has significant growth-promoting, but minimal virilizing, actions and does not affect final height.
- For the older boy (>14 years) with concerns about puberty: *testosterone* (50–100mg IM, monthly for 3–6 months).
- For the older girl (>13 years) with concerns about puberty: ethinylestradiol (2 micrograms/day for 3–6 months).

See Box 7.1 for GH assessment.

Box 7.1 **GH assessment**

GH is normally secreted overnight in regular pulses (pulse frequency 180min). Frequently sampled overnight GH profiles are costly and laborious, and therefore standardized stimulation tests are more commonly useful. Peak GH <10 micrograms/L indicates GH deficiency (values >5 and <10 micrograms/L indicate partial GH deficiency). However, there can be large variation between different assay methods, and exact cut-offs must be locally validated. In late prepuberty, there is a physiological blunting of GH secretion, and when bone age is >10 years, sex steroid priming (testosterone 100mg IM in boys or oral ethinylestradiol 20 micrograms daily for 3 days in either sex) is necessary before GH testing.

A number of different agents may be used to stimulate GH secretion (arginine, insulin, or glucagon; see Table 7.1). All tests should be performed in the morning following an overnight fast, and serial blood samples are collected over 90–180min.

An IGF-1 level should also be measured in the baseline sample, as an additional marker of GH status.

IGF-I generation test
In those with high basal and stimulated GH levels, measurement of IGF-I levels before and following administration of GH (30 micrograms/kg/day) SC for 4 days allows an assessment of GH sensitivity/resistance. This test is rarely necessary.

Primary GH deficiency

1° GH deficiency is usually sporadic, but rarely it may be inherited as autosomal dominant, recessive, or X-linked recessive and may be associated with other pituitary hormone deficiencies. It may represent a defect in homeobox genes (e.g. *Pit1* (leading to GH, TSH, and PRL deficiency), *Prop1* (leading to GH, TSH, PRL, gonadotrophin, and later ACTH deficiencies), or *Hesx1*) which control HP development. Mutation in *Hesx1* has been associated with midline defects, such as optic nerve hypoplasia and corpus callosum defects (i.e. 'septo-optic dysplasia'). GH deficiency usually arises because of failure of release of GHRH from the hypothalamus.

Clinical features

- *Infancy*. GH deficiency may present with hypoglycaemia. Coexisting ACTH, TSH, and gonadotrophin deficiencies may cause prolonged hyperbilirubinaemia and micropenis. Size may be normal, as fetal and infancy growth is more dependent on nutrition and other growth factors than on GH.
- *Childhood*. Typical features include slow growth velocity, short stature, ↓ muscle mass, and ↑ SC fat. Underdevelopment of the mid-facial bones, relative protrusion of the frontal bones because of mid-facial hypoplasia, delayed dental eruption, and delayed closure of the anterior fontanelle may be seen. These children have delayed bone age and delayed puberty.

Secondary GH deficiency

Brain tumours and cranial irradiation

Pituitary or hypothalamic tumours may impair GH secretion, and deficiencies of other pituitary hormones may coexist. Cranial irradiation, used to treat intracranial tumours, facial tumours, and acute leukaemia, may also cause GH deficiency. Risk of HP damage is related to total dose administered, fractionation (single dose more toxic than divided), location of the irradiated tissue, and age (younger children are more sensitive to radiation damage).

GH secretion is most sensitive to radiation damage, followed by gonadotrophins, TSH, and ACTH. Central precocious puberty may also occur and may mask GH deficiency by promoting growth but will compromise final height if untreated. At-risk children should, therefore, be screened regularly by careful examination and multiple pituitary hormone testing.

These survivors of childhood cancer may also have other endocrine problems, including gonadal damage related to concomitant chemotherapy or radiation scatter, hypothyroidism related to spinal radiation, or glucose intolerance related to total body irradiation. It is recommended that all such patients should undergo endocrine surveillance.

Psychosocial deprivation

Severe psychosocial deprivation may cause reversible disturbance of GH secretion and growth failure. GH secretion improves within 3 weeks of hospitalization or removal from the adverse environment, and catch-up growth is often dramatic (see Fig. 7.3), although these children may continue to exhibit other features of emotional disturbance.

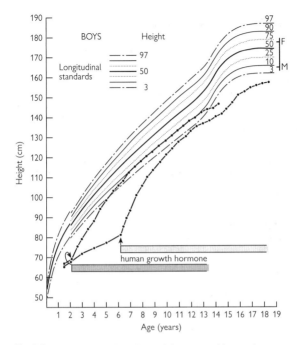

Fig. 7.3 Height of child with psychosocial short stature. Note catch-up on removal, marked by arrow, from parental home. Reproduced from Brook C (2001). Brook's Clinical Pediatric Endocrinology, Blackwell Publishing. With permission from Wiley Blackwell.

Treatment of GH deficiency

(See Fig. 7.4.)

Recombinant human GH has been available since 1985 and is administered by daily SC injection.

Dose

The replacement dose for childhood GH deficiency is 25–50 micrograms/kg/day (~0.7–1.4 micrograms/m^2 per day). Catch-up growth is optimized if GH is commenced early. A higher dose can be used in puberty, reflecting the normal elevation in GH levels at Tanner stage 3–4.

Side effects

Local lipoatrophy and benign intracranial hypertension occur rarely. Slipped upper femoral epiphyses are associated with GH deficiency, but the incidence is similar before or after GH treatment. Other pituitary hormone deficiencies may be unmasked by GH therapy, and thyroid function should be checked within 4–6 weeks of commencing therapy.

Retesting in adulthood

Once final height is achieved, GH secretion should be retested, as a significant percentage of subjects (25–80%) with GH deficiency in childhood subsequently have normal GH secretion in adulthood. In those with confirmed GH deficiency, continuation of GH treatment (at a dose of 0.2–0.5mg/day) through the late adolescent years into early adulthood (the transition phase) is recommended in order to complete somatic development (increasing lean body mass and muscular strength, reducing fat mass, improving bone density, and maintaining a healthy lipid profile). GH treatment may need to be continued beyond this phase as adult GH replacement.

The transition from paediatric to adult care is an important time, not only to re-evaluate GH status but also to reassess other pituitary function and management of any underlying disorder.

It is also recommended that assessment of bone mineral density, body composition, fasting lipid profile, and QoL by questionnaire should be undertaken at this time and repeated at 3–5-yearly intervals for those restarting GH treatment.

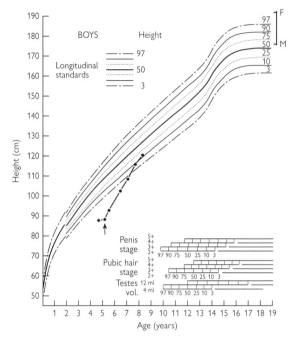

Fig. 7.4 Height of one brother with isolated growth hormone deficiency treated with human GH from age 6 years. Catch-up is partly by high velocity and partly by prolonged growth and is incomplete. F and M, parents' height centiles; vertical thick line, range of expected heights for family. Reproduced from Brook C (2001). Brook's Clinical Pediatric Endocrinology, Blackwell Publishing. With permission from Wiley Blackwell.

GH resistance

GH resistance may arise because of 1° GH receptor defects or post-receptor defects 2° to malnutrition, liver disease, type 1 diabetes, or, very rarely, circulating GH antibodies. *Laron syndrome* is a rare autosomal recessive condition caused by a genetic defect of the GH receptor. Affected individuals have extreme short stature, high levels of GH, low levels of IGF-I, and impaired GH-induced IGF-I generation (see Box 7.1, p. 521). Treatment with recombinant IGF-I is available.

Hypothyroidism

(See Fig. 7.5.)
- Congenital 1° hypothyroidism is detected by neonatal screening.
- Hypothyroidism presenting in childhood is usually autoimmune in origin.
- Incidence is higher in girls and those with personal or family history of other autoimmune disease.
- In childhood, hypothyroidism may present with growth failure alone, and bone age is often disproportionately delayed. Very rarely, early puberty may occur.
- Investigations show low T_4 and T_3, high TSH, +ve antithyroglobulin and antithyroid peroxidase (microsomal) antibodies.
- Replacement therapy with oral levothyroxine (100 micrograms/m^2 per day, titrated with thyroid function) results in catch-up growth, unless diagnosis is late.

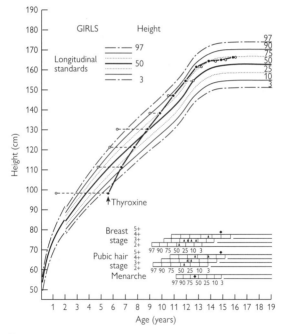

Fig. 7.5 Response of hypothyroid child treated with thyroxine. Solid circles, height for age; open circles, height for bone age. Reproduced from Brook C (2001). Brook's Clinical Pediatric Endocrinology, Blackwell Publishing. With permission from Wiley Blackwell.

Coeliac disease

More common in children with other autoimmune disorders. Although the classical childhood presentation is an irritable toddler with poor weight gain, diarrhoea, abdominal pain, and distension, in later childhood, poor growth with bone age delay may be the presenting feature. Measurement of tissue transglutaminase and antiendomysial and antigliadin antibodies are valuable screening tests, but diagnosis needs to be confirmed by small bowel biopsy. Catch-up growth usually follows commencement of a gluten-free diet.

Skeletal dysplasias

- This heterogeneous group of mostly dominantly inherited disorders includes *achondroplasia* and *hypochondroplasia*.
- These children usually have severe disproportionate short stature and a +ve or suspicious family history.
- Radiological assessment by skeletal survey often allows a specific diagnosis to be made.
- High-dose GH therapy has been used in these disorders, with variable success. Surgical leg lengthening procedures before and/or after puberty are also an additional option.

Small for gestational age (SGA) and intrauterine growth restriction (IUGR)

- SGA is defined as birthweight and/or length at least 2 SDs below the mean for gestational age. IUGR is defined as growth failure on serial antenatal US scans and would usually lead to a baby being born SGA. However, IUGR in late gestation may result in a baby who is within 2 SDs of the mean for birthweight or length.
- 90% of infants with SGA show catch-up growth by age 3 years. 8% of subjects born SGA will remain small at 18 years of age. Catch-up growth is more common in infants, with relative sparing of birth length and head circumference (>10th centile).
- In severe IUGR, length and head circumference are also reduced. Severe IUGR may be due to maternal factors, such as hypertension in pregnancy, placental dysfunction, or a wide range of chromosomal or genetic conditions in the fetus.
- Silver–Russell syndrome is characterized by severe IUGR, lateral asymmetry, triangular facies, clinodactyly (curvation of fifth finger), and extremely poor infancy feeding and post-natal weight gain.
- Children with severe IUGR who do not undergo catch-up growth may have early-onset puberty, despite bone age delay, and therefore achieve a very poor final height.
- Numerous epidemiological studies have shown a relationship between low birthweight and an ↑ risk of a number of disorders in later life, including hypertension, ischaemic heart disease, cerebrovascular disease, metabolic syndrome, and type 2 diabetes. The risk is ↑ with rapid post-natal weight gain. These associations relate to relatively low birthweight and not exclusively to those born SGA. It is recommended that those born SGA do not require any additional health surveillance above that indicated by clinical circumstances.

Management

GH therapy is used in the SGA/IUGR child who has failed to show catch-up growth by age 4 years. GH (at doses of 35–67 micrograms/kg/day) can increase growth velocity and final height. The effect of GH on later risk of insulin resistance as type 2 diabetes is not known.

Turner's syndrome

(□ also see Box 4.7, p. 337.)

Turner's syndrome should always be considered in a girl who is short for her parental target, and the classical dysmorphic features may be difficult to identify at younger ages. Karyotype usually confirms the diagnosis, although sufficient cells (>30) should be examined to exclude the possibility of mosaicism.

Clinical features

There may be a history of lymphoedema in the newborn period. Typically, growth velocity starts to decline from 3–5 years old (see Fig. 7.6), and gonadal failure, combined with a degree of skeletal dysplasia, results in loss of the pubertal growth spurt. Mean final height is consistently 20cm below the normal average within each population (143–146cm in the UK). GH secretion is normal, although IGF-I levels may be low. 10% progress through puberty spontaneously, but only 1% develop ovulatory cycles.

Management

- High-dose *GH therapy* (45 micrograms/kg/day) increases final height, although individual responses are variable. The height gained is related to time on GH treatment, and thus GH therapy should be commenced early; if the diagnosis has been made in early life, treatment is usually started from 3–5 years of age.
- The anabolic steroid oxandrolone can be used, in addition to GH, to promote growth from the age of 9 years. It has a positive effect on final height at a dose of 0.05mg/kg/day, max 2.5mg/day.
- Oral *oestrogen* is commenced between 12–14 years to promote 2° sexual development and pubertal growth. It should be started in low dose (ethinylestradiol 2 micrograms/day) and gradually ↑ with age. *Progesterone* should be added if breakthrough bleeding occurs or when oestrogen dose reaches 10 micrograms/day.

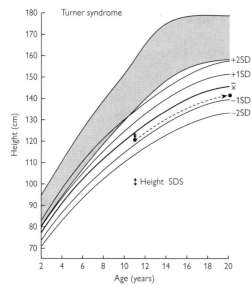

Fig. 7.6 Height SDS for chronological age extrapolated to final height. Reproduced from Brook C, (2001). Brook's Clinical Pediatric Endocrinology, Blackwell publishing. With permission from Wiley Blackwell.

Tall stature and rapid growth

Definition

Although statistically as many children have heights >2 SDs above the mean as have heights >2 SDs below the mean, referral for evaluation of tall stature is much less common than for short stature. Socially, for boys, heights up to 200cm are acceptable, whereas, for many girls, heights >182cm may be unacceptable. However, tall stature, and particularly accelerated growth rates in early childhood, can indicate an underlying hormonal disorder, such as precocious puberty. For causes, see Box 7.2.

Assessment

History

- Is tall stature long-standing or does the history suggest recent growth acceleration? Try to obtain previous measurements.
- Enquire about size at birth, infancy weight gain, intellectual development, and neurological development.
- Enquire about headaches, visual disturbance, and evidence of puberty.
- Is there a family history of tall stature or early puberty?

Examination

- Assess height and height velocity over at least 4–6 months.
- Measure sitting height and arm span.
- Pubertal stage?
- Dysmorphic features?
- Measure parents' heights, and calculate MPH (📖 see Assessment of growth, p. 514).

Investigations

The following investigations may be clinically indicated:

- Wrist radiograph for bone age.
- Sex hormone levels (testosterone, oestrogen, androstenedione, DHEAS), baseline and LHRH-stimulated LH and FSH levels.
- Karyotype.
- Serum IGF-I and IGFBP-3 levels.
- Oral glucose tolerance test—GH levels normally suppress to low or undetectable levels (<0.5 microgram/L).
- Specific molecular tests for overgrowth syndromes.

Management of tall stature

After excluding abnormal pathology, often only reassurance and information on predicted final height is necessary. In younger children, early induction of puberty, using low-dose sex steroids, advances the pubertal growth spurt and promotes earlier epiphyseal fusion. In older children already in puberty, high-dose oestrogen therapy in girls, or testosterone in boys, has been used to induce rapid skeletal maturation. However, theoretical side effects of high-dose oestrogen therapy include thromboembolic disease and oncogenic risk.

Box 7.2 Causes of tall stature in childhood

Normal variants
- Familial tall stature.
- Early maturation (largely familial but also promoted by early childhood nutrition and obesity. Height is not excessive for bone age which is advanced).

Hormonal
- 📖 see Precocious puberty, p. 538.
- GH or GHRH excess ('pituitary gigantism'), resulting from pituitary adenoma or ectopic adenomas, is a very rare cause of tall stature (📖 see p. 181).
- Other hormonal excess, e.g. hyperthyroidism, congenital adrenal hyperplasia (associated with signs of virilization), familial glucocorticoid deficiency.
- Rarely, oestrogen receptor or aromatase deficiencies delay puberty and epiphyseal fusion, resulting in tall adult height.

Chromosomal abnormalities
- XXY (Klinefelter's syndrome) (see 📖 p. 370).
- XYY, XYYY (each 'extra Y' confers, on average, 13cm additional height).

Other rare syndromes
Overgrowth and dysmorphic features are seen in Marfan's syndrome, homocystinuria, Sotos syndrome (early excessive growth ± autism), Beckwith–Wiedemann syndrome (overgrowth disorder and increased risk of childhood cancer), and Weaver's syndrome.

Further reading

Allen DB, Cuttler L, (2013). Clinical practice. Short stature in childhood - challenges and choices. *N Engl J Med* **368**, 1220–8.

Carel JC, Léger J (2008). Precocious puberty. *N Engl J Med* **358**, 2366–77.

Clayton PE, Cianfarani S, Czernichow P, *et al.* (2007). Management of the child born small for gestational age child (SGA) through to adulthood: a consensus statement of the International Societies of Paediatric Endocrinology and the Growth Hormone Research Society. *J Clin Endocrinology Metab* Epub 2 January.

Clayton PE, Cuneo RC, Juul A, *et al.* (2005). Consensus statement on the management of the GH-treated adolescent in the transition to adult care. *Eur J Endocrinol* **152**, 165–70.

Conway GS (2009). Adult care of pediatric conditions: lessons from Turner's syndrome. *J Clin Endocrinol Metab* **94**, 3185–7.

Dattani M, Preece M (2004). Growth hormone deficiency and related disorders: insights into causation, diagnosis, and treatment. *Lancet* **363**, 1977–87.

De Waal WJ, Greyn-Fokker MH, Stijnen T, *et al.* (1996). Accuracy of final height prediction and effect of growth-reductive therapy in 362 constitutionally tall children. *J Clin Endocrinol Metab* **81**, 1206–16.

Growth Hormone Research Society (2000). Consensus guidelines for the diagnosis and treatment of growth hormone (GH) deficiency in childhood and adolescence: summary statement of the GH Research Society. GH Research Society. *J Clin Endocrinol Metab* **85**, 3990–3.

Kelly WH, *et al.* (2012). Effect of inhaled glucocorticoids in childhood on adult height. *N Engl J Med* **367**, 904–12.

Saenger P, Wikland KA, Conway GS, *et al.* (2000). Recommendations for the diagnosis and management of Turner's syndrome. *J Clin Endocrinol Metab* **86**, 3061–9.

Normal puberty

Puberty is the sequence of physical and physiological changes occurring at adolescence, culminating in full sexual maturity.

Age at onset

Average age at onset of puberty is earlier in girls (~11 years) than in boys (~12 years) but varies widely (~±2 years from the mean age of onset) and is influenced by a number of factors:

- *Historical.* Age of menarche has ↓ this century from 17 years in 1900 to 12.8 years today, presumably as a result of improved childhood nutrition and growth.
- *Genetic.* Age at onset of puberty is partly familial.
- *Ethnicity.* Afro-Caribbean girls tend to have earlier puberty than Caucasians.
- *Weight gain.* Earlier puberty is seen in girls who are overweight, whereas girls who engage in strenuous activity and are thin often have delayed puberty.

Hormonal changes prior to and during puberty

- Adrenal androgens (DHEAS and androstenedione) rise 2 years before puberty starts ('adrenarche'). This usually causes no physical changes but occasionally results in early pubic hair and acne ('premature adrenarche').
- Pulsatile secretion of LHRH from the hypothalamus at night is the first step in the initiation of puberty and occurs well before physical signs of puberty. This results in pulsatile secretion of LH and FSH from the pituitary, and the gonadotrophin response to LHRH administration reverses from the prepubertal FSH predominance to a higher response in LH levels.

Physical changes

The first indication of puberty is breast development in girls and increase in testicular size in boys. In each sex, puberty then progresses in an orderly or 'consonant' manner through distinct stages (see Table 7.2). Puberty rating by an experienced observer involves identification of pubertal stage—particularly, breast development in girls and testicular volume (by comparison with an orchidometer) in boys.

Pubertal growth spurt

↑ oestrogen levels in both boys and girls leads to ↑ GH secretion. Peak height velocity occurs at puberty stages 2–3 in girls and is later in boys at stages 3–4 (testicular volume 10–12mL).

Table 7.2 The normal stages of puberty ('Tanner stages')

Boys

Stage	Genitalia	Pubic hair	Other events
I	Prepubertal	Vellus not thicker than on abdomen	TV[a] <4mL
II	Enlargement of testes and scrotum	Sparse, long pigmented strands at base of penis	TV 4–8mL Voice starts to change
III	Lengthening of penis	Darker, curlier, and spreads over pubes	TV 8–10mL Axillary hair
IV	Increase in penis length and breadth	Adult-type hair but covering a smaller area	TV 10–15mL Upper lip hair Peak height velocity
V	Adult shape and size	Spread to medial thighs (stage 6: spread up linea alba)	TV 15–25mL Facial hair spreads to cheeks Adult voice

Girls

Stage	Breast	Pubic hair	Other events
I	Elevation of papilla only	Vellus not thicker than on abdomen	
II	Breast bud stage: elevation of breast and papilla	Sparse, long pigmented strands along labia	Peak height velocity
III	Further elevation of breast and areola together	Darker, curlier, and spreads over pubes	
IV	Areola forms a second mound on top of breast	Adult type hair but covering a smaller area	Menarche
V	Mature stage: areola recedes and only papilla projects	Spread to medial thighs (stage 6: spread up linea alba)	

[a] TV, testicular volume: measured by size comparison with a Prader orchidometer. Adapted with permission from Tanner JM (1962) *Growth at adolescence*, 2nd edn. Blackwell Scientific Publications, Oxford.

Precocious puberty

Definition

- Early onset of puberty is defined as <8 years in girls and <9 years in boys.
- Gonadotrophin-dependent ('central' or 'true') precocious puberty is characterized by early breast development in girls or testicular enlargement in boys.
- Gonadotrophin-independent puberty occurs due to abnormal peripheral sex hormone secretion, resulting in isolated development of certain 2° sexual characteristics. This may involve autonomous testosterone production in a boy or autonomous oestrogen production in a girl. In addition, testosterone production from the adrenal or an ovarian tumour can induce virilization in a girl.

Assessment of precocious puberty

History

- Age when 2° sexual development first noted.
- What features are present and in what order did they appear? For example, virilization (pubic, axillary, or facial hair; acne; body odour), genital or breast enlargement, galactorrhoea (very rare), menarche, or cyclical mood changes?
- Is there evidence of recent growth acceleration?
- Family history of early puberty?
- Past history of adoption or early weight gain or prior CNS abnormality or insult (e.g. radiation)?

Examination

- Breast or genital and testicular size; degree of virilization (clitoromegaly in girls indicates abnormal androgen levels).
- Neurological examination, particularly visual field assessment and fundoscopy.
- Abdominal or testicular masses.
- Skin (? *café-au-lait* patches—McCune–Albright (📖 see Chapter 9, McCune–Albright syndrome, pp. 576–7) or NF-1578).
- Assess height and height velocity over 4–6 months.

Investigations

The following investigations may be clinically indicated:

- Wrist radiograph for bone age.
- Thyroid function.
- Sex hormone levels (testosterone, oestrogen, androstenedione, DHEAS).
- LH and FSH levels (baseline and 30 and 60min post-IV LHRH).
- 17αOH progesterone levels (baseline and 30 and 60min post-IV Synacthen®) if congenital adrenal hyperplasia suspected.
- Tumour markers (αFP, β-hCG).
- 24h urine steroid profile (see 📖 p. 230).
- Abdominal US scan (adrenal glands, ovaries).
- MRI scan (cranial, adrenal glands).
- For those with hypogonadotrophic hypogonadism, mutation screening for a monogenic cause (e.g. KA11, FGFRI, GnRHR, KISS1R) may be indicated (see 📖 p. 366).

Central precocious puberty

This is due to premature activation of pulsatile LHRH secretion from the hypothalamus, and the normal progression in physical changes is maintained ('consonance'). As precocious puberty is defined as occurring younger than 2 SDs before the average age, in a normal distribution, 2.5% of children will have early-onset puberty. In practice, in girls, central precocious puberty is more likely to be idiopathic or familial, whereas boys have a greater risk of intracranial or other pathology.

Causes

- Idiopathic or familial.
- Intracranial tumours, hydrocephalus, or other lesions.
- Post-cranial irradiation or trauma.
- Intracranial tumours (in particular, optic nerve glioma and hypothalamic germinoma), hamartoma, hydrocephalus, and non-specific brain injury (e.g. cerebral palsy).
- May also be triggered by long-standing elevation in sex hormones resulting from any peripheral source or adrenal enzyme defect (e.g. late-presenting simple virilizing CAH or inadequately treated CAH).
- Hypothyroidism (elevated TRH stimulates FSH release)—rare.
- Gonadotrophin-secreting tumours (e.g. pituitary adenoma or hepatoblastoma) are rare.

Treatment

Aims of treatment are:

- To avoid psychosocial problems for the child or family.
- To prevent reduced final height due to premature bone maturation and early epiphyseal fusion. A *final height prediction* is often necessary when considering the need for inhibition of puberty. Significant sparing of adult height is only likely to be achieved if presentation occurs and treatment is started ≤6 years of age.

Pituitary LH and FSH secretion can be inhibited by the use of LHRH analogues, e.g. *goserelin* 3.6mg SC monthly or 10.8mg SC 3-monthly, or *triptorelin* 3.75mg SC or deep IM (lower doses if weight <30kg) every 2 weeks for the first three injections, then 3–4-weekly thereafter. Treatment efficacy should be monitored regularly by clinical observation and ensuring that LH and FSH levels post-IV LHRH remain at low prepubertal levels. The dosing intervals may need to be reduced if there is evidence of inadequate suppression of pubertal development.

Gonadotrophin-independent precocious puberty

At least two genetic syndromes have been identified, both resulting in abnormal activation of gonadotrophin receptors, independent of normal ligand binding. Thus, in these conditions, the gonads autonomously secrete sex hormones, and levels of LH and FSH are suppressed by feedback inhibition.

McCune–Albright syndrome

(📖 also see McCune–Albright syndrome, pp. 576–7). This is a sporadic condition due to a somatic activating mutation of the GSα protein subunit which affects bones (polyostotic fibrous dysplasia), skin (café-au-lait spots), and potentially multiple endocrinopathies.

A number of different hormone receptors share the same G protein-coupled cyclic AMP second messenger system, and hyperthyroidism or hyperparathyroidism may also be present.

All cells descended from the mutated embryonic cell line are affected while cells descended from non-mutated cells develop into normal tissues. Thus, the phenotype is highly variable in physical distribution and severity.

Testoxicosis

This is a rare familial condition, resulting in precocious puberty only in boys due to an activating LH receptor mutation. Testes show only little increase in size, and, on biopsy, Leydig cell hyperplasia is characteristic. Treatment is by use of androgen receptor-blocking agents (cyproterone acetate) and aromatase inhibitors.

Peripheral sex hormone secretion

- Excessive peripheral androgen secretion may occur due to CAH, or androgen-secreting adrenal or gonadal tumours. These children usually have rapid growth, advanced bone age, and moderate-to-severe virilization in the absence of testicular or breast development.
(NB A testicular tumour may cause asymmetrical enlargement.)
- Peripheral oestrogen production from ovarian tumours is a rare cause of precocious breast development in girls.

Premature thelarche

Premature breast development, in the absence of other signs of puberty, may present at any age from infancy. Breast size may fluctuate and is often asymmetrical. The cause is unknown, although typically FSH levels (but not LH) are elevated, and ovarian US may reveal a single large cyst. Bone maturation, growth rate, and final height are unaffected.

'Thelarche variant'

This is an intermediate condition between premature thelarche and central precocious puberty. The aetiology is unknown. These girls demonstrate ↑ height velocity and rate of bone maturation, and ovarian US reveals a more multicystic appearance, as seen in true puberty. There is probably a whole spectrum of presentations between premature thelarche and true precocious puberty. Decision to treat should take into account height velocity and final height prediction as well as the rate of physical maturation and the severity of accompanying pubertal features (e.g. mood swings and difficult behaviour).

'Premature adrenarche' and 'pubarche'

The normal onset of adrenal androgen secretion ('adrenarche') occurs 1–2 years before the onset of puberty. 'Premature' or 'exaggerated' adrenarche is thought to be due to ↑ androgen production or sensitivity and presents with mild features of virilization, such as onset of pubic hair ('pubarche') or acne, in the absence of other features of puberty. NB Clitoromegaly in girls suggests a more severe pathology with excessive androgen production (e.g. CAH or androgen-secreting tumour).

The diagnosis is made in the presence of pubic hair and/or axillary hair; the absence of breast/testicular development in children aged <8 years. It is more common in girls.

Management

The management of premature adrenarche usually only requires reassurance after exclusion of other causes, as there is no significant impact on final height and onset/progression of puberty. Some of these girls may subsequently develop features of polycystic ovary disease. In these cases, treatment should be directed at the presenting feature (e.g. hirsutism, menstrual irregularities).

Delayed/absent puberty

Definition

Delayed puberty is defined as failure to progress into puberty by >2 SDs later than the average, i.e. >13 years in girls and >14 years in boys. Clinically, boys are more likely to present with delayed puberty than girls. In addition, some children present with delay in progression from one pubertal stage to the next for >2 years.

Psychological distress may be exacerbated by declining growth velocity relative to their peers. In the long term, severe delay may be a risk factor for ↓ bone mineral density and osteoporosis.

Causes

General

- Constitutional delay of growth and puberty (this is the most common cause; 📖 see Constitutional delay of growth and puberty, p. 520).
- Chronic childhood disease, malabsorption (e.g. coeliac disease, inflammatory bowel disease), or undernutrition.

Hypergonadotrophic hypogonadism

Gonadal failure may be:
- Congenital (e.g. Turner's syndrome in girls (📖 p. 336), Klinefelter's syndrome in boys (📖 p. 370)).
- Acquired (e.g. following chemotherapy, local radiotherapy, infection, torsion).

In these conditions, basal and stimulated gonadotrophin levels are raised.

Gonadotrophin deficiency

- Kallman's syndrome (📖 p. 362) (including anosmia).
- HP lesions (tumours, post-radiotherapy, dysplasia).
- Rare inactivating mutations of genes encoding LH, FSH (or their receptors).

These conditions may also present in the newborn period with micropenis and undescended testes in boys.

Investigation

The following investigations may be clinically indicated:
- LH and FSH levels (basal and post-IV LHRH stimulation).
- Plasma oestrogen or testosterone levels.
- Measurement of androgen levels before and after hCG therapy may be used to indicate presence of functional testicular tissue in boys.
- Karyotype.
- Pelvic US in girls to determine ovarian morphology.
- US or MRI imaging in boys to detect intra-abdominal testes.
- For those with hypogonadotropic hypogonadism, mutation screening for a monogenic cause (e.g. KALI, FGFRI, GnRHR, KISSIR) may be indicated.

It may be difficult to distinguish between constitutional delay and gonadotrophin deficiency, as gonadotrophin levels are low in both conditions. In these cases, induction of puberty may be indicated, with regular assessment of testicular growth in boys (which is independent of testosterone therapy), followed by withdrawal of treatment and reassessment when final height is reached.

Management

Depending on the age and concern of the child and parents, short-course exogenous sex steroids can be used to induce pubertal changes. If gonadotrophin deficiency is permanent or the gonads are dysfunctional or absent, then exogenous sex steroids are required to induce and maintain pubertal development (📖 see Constitutional delay of growth and puberty, p. 520).

Long-term treatment
(See Table 7.3.)

Table 7.3 Suggested schema for pubertal induction and maintenance in boys and girls

Testosterone dose	Testosterone interval	Duration	Ethinylestradiol dose (daily)	Duration
50mg	4 weeks	6 months	2 micrograms	6 months
100mg	4 weeks	6 months	5 micrograms	6 months
125mg	4 weeks	6 months	10 micrograms (+ a progesterone when bleed)	6 months
250mg	3–4 weeks	Onwards	20 micrograms 'pill'	Onwards

Treatment could be started at age 12–13 years in boys and 11–12 years in girls. Duration for each stage of treatment is determined by individual responses.

Boys
Testosterone (by IM injection) 50mg 4–6-weekly, gradually ↑ to 250mg 4-weekly.
• Monitor penis enlargement, pubic hair, height velocity, and adult body habitus.
• Side effects include severe acne and, rarely, priapism.

Girls
Oestrogen (oral). Start at low dose (*ethinylestradiol* 2 micrograms daily), and gradually increase.
• Promotes breast development and adult body habitus.
• *Progesterone* (oral) should be added if breakthrough bleeding occurs or when oestrogen dose reaches 10 micrograms/day.

Further reading

Hindmarsh PC (2009). How do you initiate oestrogen therapy in a girl who has not undergone puberty? *Clin Endocrinol (Oxf)* **71**, 7–10.
Miller JF (2012). Approach to the child with Prader-Willi syndrome. *J Clin Endocrinol Metab* **97**, 3837–44.
Palmert MR, Dunkel L (2012). Clinical practice. Delayed puberty. *N Engl J Med* **366**, 443–53.

Normal sexual differentiation

Gonadal development

- In the ♂ or ♀ embryo, the bipotential gonad develops as a thickening of mesenchymal cells and coelomic epithelium around the primitive kidney. This *genital ridge* is then colonized by primordial germ cells which migrate from the yolk sac to form the *gonadal ridge*. In the absence of a Y chromosome, the gonad will develop into an ovary.
- In the presence of a normal Y chromosome, immature Sertoli cells, germs cells, and seminiferous tubules can be recognized by 7 weeks, and testis differentiation is complete by 9 weeks. The *SRY* gene is an essential 'sex-determining region' on the Y chromosome which signals for testis differentiation.

Internal genitalia

- Embryonic *Müllerian* structures form the uterus, Fallopian tubes, and upper third of the vagina.
- In ♂, *anti-Müllerian hormone* is secreted by immature Sertoli cells in the testis by 6 weeks, and this causes regression of the Müllerian structures. Leydig cells appear in the testis at around day 60 and produce *testosterone* under placental hCG stimulation. Testosterone promotes growth and differentiation of the *Wolffian ducts* to form the epididymis, vas deferens, and seminal vesicles.

External genitalia

- In the absence of any androgen secretion, labia majora, labia minora, and clitoris develop from the embryonic genital swelling, genital fold, and genital tubercle, respectively.
- Development of normal ♂ external genitalia requires testosterone production from the testis and its conversion to *dihydrotestosterone* by the enzyme *5α-reductase*. In the presence of dihydrotestosterone, the genital tubercle elongates to form the corpora cavernosa and glans penis; the urethral fold forms the penile shaft, and the labioscrotal swelling forms the scrotum. This process commences around 9 weeks and is completed by 13 weeks. Testicular descent in ♂ occurs in the later two-thirds of gestation under control of fetal LH and testosterone.

Assessment of ambiguous genitalia

Most cases of ambiguous genitalia present at birth. Involvement of an experienced paediatric endocrinologist and surgeon should be sought as early as possible.

History

- Any maternal medication during pregnancy?
- Are parents consanguineous or is there a family history of ambiguous genitalia?
- Is there a neonatal history of hypoglycaemia or prolonged jaundice?

Examination

- Assess clitoris/phallus size; degree of labial fusion; position of urethra/urogenital sinus (anterior or posterior).
- Are gonads palpable? Check along line of descent.
- Are there any signs indicating panhypopituitarism? For example, midline defects/hypoglycaemia/hypocortisolaemia/prolonged jaundice.
- Dysmorphic features of Turner's syndrome may be seen in XO/XY mosaicism.

Investigations

- Bloods for karyotype, electrolytes, blood glucose, 17αOH progesterone.
- US of pelvis and labial folds (for Müllerian structures and gonads).
- Arrange for clinical photographs.
- After 48h old, when the neonatal hormonal surge has decreased, repeat bloods for 17αOH progesterone, cortisol, LH, FSH, and androgen levels. Collect a 2h urine sample to measure the steroid profile.
- Examination under anaesthesia (EUA) and cystogram may be required.

Specific tests

- Short Synacthen® test in a virilized XX (when CAH is suspected) may be required.
- 3-day hCG test in an undervirilized '♂' (testes present or 46,XY) assesses stimulated gonadal production of androgens and may be diagnostic of androgen biosynthesis defects or androgen insensitivity.
- LHRH test examines pituitary gonadotrophin secretion (this test is only informative in the neonatal period).
- Glucagon test examines cortisol and GH secretion.
- Androgen receptor function can be tested on cultured fibroblasts from a genital skin biopsy.
- DNA analysis for androgen receptor mutation, CAH mutations, and androgen biosynthesis mutations.

Disorders of sex development (DSD)

♂ and ♀ internal and external genitalia develop from common embryonic structures. In the absence of ♂ differentiating signals, normal ♀ genitalia develop. Genital ambiguity may, therefore, occur as a result of chromosomal abnormality, gonadal dysgenesis, biochemical defects of androgen synthesis, inappropriate exposure to external androgens, or androgen receptor insensitivity. See Box 7.3 for definitions.

46XX DSD

Disorders of ovarian development

Normal ♂ differentiation can occur if the *SRY* gene has been translocated onto an autosome.

Biochemical defects leading to androgen oversecretion

Congenital adrenal hyperplasia (CAH, 21-hydroxylase deficiency most commonly) is the most common cause of ambiguous genitalia in 46,XX.

Maternal hyperandrogenism

- The ♀ fetus may be virilized if maternal androgen levels exceed the capacity of placental aromatase to convert these to oestrogen.
- This may occur due to maternal disease (e.g. CAH, adrenal and ovarian tumours) or use of androgenic medication in pregnancy or, rarely, placental aromatase deficiency.

46XY DSD

Disorders of testis development

- XY gonadal dysgenesis can be caused by mutations in a number of genes controlling ♂ sexual differentiation, including *SRY, SF-1, WT-1* and *SOX*, and can present with normal external genitalia.
- Early testicular failure resulting from torsion or infarction.

Biochemical defects of androgen synthesis

Rare deficiencies of the enzymes 5α-reductase, 17β-hydroxysteroid dehydrogenase, or 3β-hydroxysteroid dehydrogenase, which is also associated with glucocorticoid and mineralocorticoid deficiencies, are autosomal recessively inherited and may result in variable degrees of undervirilization.

Androgen receptor insensitivity syndrome

(□ also see Androgen insensitivity syndrome, p. 416).

Defects of the androgen receptor gene on the X chromosome or autosomal post-receptor signalling genes may result in complete or partial androgen insensitivity.

- *Complete androgen insensitivity*. Results in normal ♀ external genitalia and usually only presents with testicular prolapse in childhood or primary amenorrhoea in adolescence.
- *Partial androgen insensitivity*. Presentation may vary from mild virilization to micropenis, hypospadias, undescended testes, or only ↓ spermatogenesis.

Box 7.3 Definitions

Disorders of chromosomes
Including:
- 45X Turner's and variants.
- 47XXY and variants.
- 45X/46XY mixed gonadal dysgenesis.
- 46XX/46XY gonadal chimera.

46XX DSD
Including:
- Disorders of gonadal (ovarian) development.
- Androgen excess.
- Structural disorders, e.g. cloacal exstrophy, vaginal atresia.

46XY DSD
Including:
- Disorders of gonadal (testicular) development.
- Disorders in androgen synthesis and action.
- Structural disorders, e.g. severe hypospadias, cloacal exstrophy.

Gonadotrophin defects
- Gonadotrophin deficiency may occur in *hypopituitarism* or may be associated with anosmia (*Kallmann's syndrome*). It usually presents with delayed puberty but is an occasional cause of micropenis and undescended testes.
- LH receptor gene defects are rare and result in complete absence of virilization, as the testes are unable to respond to placental hCG.

Anti-Müllerian hormone deficiency or insensitivity
Testes are usually undescended, and uterus and Fallopian tubes present.

Management of ambiguous genitalia
In the newborn period, the infant should be monitored in hospital for:
- Hypoglycaemia (until hypopituitarism is excluded).
- Salt wasting (until CAH is excluded).

Explain to the parents that the infant appears to be healthy but has a defect that interferes with determining sex. It is helpful to show the parents the physical findings as you explain this. Advise them to postpone the registration of the birth until after further investigations, and discuss what they will say to relatives and friends. The sex of the baby should be assigned as soon after birth as is practicable, given the need for accurate diagnosis.

Sex assignment

Decision on the sex of rearing should be based on the optimal expected outcome in terms of psychosexual and reproductive function. Parents should, therefore, be encouraged discussion with an endocrinologist, a surgeon specializing in urogenital reconstruction, a psychologist, and a social worker. Following the necessary investigations and discussions, early gender assignment optimizes the psychosexual outcome.

Further management

- If ♀ sex is assigned, any testicular tissue should be removed.
- Reconstructive surgery may include clitoral reduction, gonadectomy, and vaginoplasty in girls, and phallus enlargement, hypospadias repair, and orchidopexy in boys. In both sexes, multiple-stage procedures may be required.
- Topical or systemic *dihydrotestosterone* may enhance phallus size in ♂ infants, and a trial of therapy is sometimes useful before sex assignment.
- Hormone replacement therapy may also be required from puberty into adulthood.
- Continuing psychological support for the parents and children is very important.

Congenital adrenal hyperplasia

(📖 also see Chapter 4, Congenital adrenal hyperplasia (CAH) in adults, p. 320.)

A number of autosomally inherited enzyme deficiencies result in cortisol deficiency, excess pituitary ACTH secretion, and adrenal gland hyperplasia.

21-hydroxylase deficiency (>90%)

The most common cause of CAH results in cortisol and mineralocorticoid deficiency while the build-up of precursor steroids is channelled towards excess adrenal androgen synthesis. Different gene defects in the 21-hydroxylase gene (e.g. deletion, splice site or point mutation) result in different degrees of enzyme dysfunction and thus wide variation in phenotypes.

Clinical features

- Virilization of ♀ fetuses may result in clitoromegaly and labial fusion at birth. 75% have sufficient mineralocorticoid deficiency to cause renal salt wasting. Because ♂ have normal genitalia at birth, they may present acutely ill in the neonatal period with vomiting, dehydration, collapse, hyponatraemia, and hyperkalaemia. Non-salt-wasting boys present with early genital enlargement, pubarche, and rapid growth.
- If untreated or poorly treated, both sexes may develop pubic hair, acne, rapid height velocity, advanced bone maturation, and precocious puberty which may result in very short final height.
- 'Non-classical CAH' is due to milder 21-hydroxylase deficiency, and affected girls present in later childhood or adulthood with hirsutism, acne, premature/exaggerated adrenarche, menstrual irregularities, and infertility.

11β-hydroxylase deficiency (~5%)

This enzyme, which converts 11-deoxycortisol to cortisol, is the final step in cortisol synthesis. In addition to excess adrenal androgens, the overproduced precursor corticosterone has mineralocorticoid activity. Thus, in contrast to salt wasting in 21-hydroxylase deficiency, these subjects may have hypernatraemia and hypokalaemia. Hypertension is rarely seen in infancy but may develop during childhood and affects 50–60% of adults.

Specific investigations for CAH

(📖 see also Assessment of ambiguous genitalia, p. 545.)

- *Plasma 17αOH progesterone.* An elevated level indicates 21-hydroxylase deficiency. It may be difficult to distinguish this from the physiological hormonal surge which occurs in the first 2 days of life. This test should, therefore, be repeated (together with 11-deoxycortisol) after 48h of age.
- A 24h urine steroid profile (also collected after 48h of age) should confirm the diagnosis and allows detection of the rarer enzyme defects.
- A Synacthen® stimulation test may be required to discriminate between the different enzyme deficiencies.

- Plasma and urine electrolytes may need to be monitored over the first 2 weeks.
- Plasma renin level is also useful to confirm salt wasting in those with normal serum sodium and relatively mild 21-hydroxylase deficiency.

Other rare enzyme deficiencies

- *17α-hydroxylase deficiency*. Impairs cortisol, androgen, and oestrogen synthesis, but overproduction of mineralocorticoids leads to hypokalaemia and hypertension.
- *3β-hydroxysteroid dehydrogenase deficiency*. Impairs cortisol, mineralocorticoid, and androgen biosynthesis. ♂ have hypospadias and undescended testes; however, excess DHEA, a weak androgen, may cause mild virilization in ♀.

Steroid acute regulatory protein

- STAR mutation: 46XY sex reversal and severe adrenal failure. Heterozygous defect. Extremely rare.
- CYPIIAI (P450: side chain cleavage cytochrome enzyme): 46XY sex reversal and severe adrenal failure. Heterozygous defect. Extremely rare.
- P450 oxidoreductase deficiency: biochemical picture of combined 21-hydroxylase/17α-hydroxylase/17,20 lyase deficiencies. Spectrum of presentation from children with ambiguous genitalia, adrenal failure, and the Antley–Bixler skeletal dysplasia syndrome through to mildly affected individuals with polycystic ovary syndrome.

Management

- *Hydrocortisone* (15mg/m^2 per day orally in three divided doses). In addition to treating cortisol deficiency, this therapy suppresses ACTH and thereby limits excessive production of adrenal androgens. Occasionally, higher doses are required to achieve adequate androgen suppression; however, overtreatment may suppress growth.
- In salt losers, initial *IV fluid resuscitation* (10–20mL/kg normal saline) may be required to treat circulatory collapse. Long-term mineralocorticoid replacement (*fludrocortisone* 0.05–0.3mg/day) may have incomplete efficacy, particularly in infancy, and *sodium chloride* supplements are also needed. Up to 10mmol/kg per day may be needed in infancy.
- *Reconstructive surgery* (clitoral reduction, vaginoplasty). Often performed in infancy, and further procedures may be required during puberty. Needs experienced surgeon.
- Patients and families need to be aware of the need for extra hydrocortisone during intercurrent illness or significant stress. Instructions on what to do for mild, moderate, and severe illnesses ('Sick Day Rules') and for operative procedures should be made available (see 📖 Addison disease treatment, p. 266). Patients and families should have parenteral hydrocortisone available to give in emergency situations.

Monitoring of hormonal therapy

- *Height velocity and bone age*. If hydrocortisone therapy is insufficient, growth rate will be above normal and bone age will be advanced. Conversely, if hydrocortisone therapy is excessive, growth is suppressed.
- *17αOHP*. Blood levels should be assessed several times each year. Levels should be measured before and after each hydrocortisone dose; these may be collected at home by the parents, using 'spot' capillary blood samples. In girls and prepubertal boys, androgen levels (testosterone and androstenedione) can be measured if there is concern about poor control and/or virilization.
- *Mineralocorticoid and sodium replacement*. Should be monitored by measuring plasma electrolytes and renin levels, and by regular blood pressure assessments.

Genetic advice

- The inheritance of CAH is autosomal recessive, and parents should be informed of a 25% risk of recurrence in future offspring.
- If the mutation is identifiable on DNA analysis in the child and parents, chorionic villus sampling may allow prenatal diagnosis.
- Maternal *dexamethasone* therapy from around 5–6 weeks of pregnancy is used to prevent virilization of the ♀ fetus without significant maternal complications (see 🕮 p. 446).

Further reading

Brook CGD (ed.) (1995). *Clinical Paediatric Endocrinology*, 3rd edn. Blackwell Science, Oxford.

Consensus Statement on 21 hydroxylase deficiency. Joint LWPES/ESPE Working Group (2002). *J Clin Endocrinol Metab* **87**, 4048–53.

Fluck CE, Miller WL (2006). P450 oxidoreductase deficiency: a new form of congenital adrenal hyperplasia. *Curr Opin Paediatric* **18**, 435–41.

Hochberg Z (ed.) (1998). *Practical Algorithms in Pediatric Endocrinology*. Karger, Basel.

Hughes IA (1989). *Handbook of Endocrine Investigations in Children*. John Wright & Sons, Bristol.

Hughes IA, Houk C, Ahmed SF, *et al.* (2006). Consensus statement on management of intersex disorders. *Arch Dis Child* **91**, 554–63.

Wilkins L (1994). In Kappy MS, Blizzard RM, Migeon CJ (eds.) *The diagnosis and treatment of endocrine disorders in childhood and adolescence*, 4th edn. Charles C Thomas, Springfield, Illinois.

Neuroendocrine disorders

The neuroendocrine system

Introduction

- Neuroendocrine cells are found in many sites throughout the body. They are particularly prominent in the GI tract and pancreas and share a common embryological origin. These cells have the ability to synthesize, store, and release peptide hormones.
- Due to the prevalence of neuroendocrine cells, the majority of neuroendocrine tumours occur within the gastroenteropancreatic axis. Of these tumours, >50% are traditionally termed carcinoid tumours and have been usually subclassified into foregut, midgut, and hindgut lesions, with the remainder largely comprising pancreatic islet cell tumours.
- Carcinoid and islet cell tumours are generally slow-growing.

Further reading

Barakat MT, Meeran K, Bloom SR (2004). Neuroendocrine tumours. *Endocr Relat Cancer* **11**, 1–18.

Classification of neuroendocrine neoplasias (NENs)

- There is a move towards standardizing the terminology of these tumours; the European Neuroendocrine Society (ENETS) recommends the use of the umbrella term neuroendocrine neoplasia (NEN). The term NEN includes low- and intermediate-grade neoplasia (previously referred to as carcinoid or atypical carcinoid) which are now referred to as neuroendocrine tumours (NETs) and high-grade neoplasia (neuroendocrine carcinoma, NEC). There is a confusing array of classifications of NENs, based on anatomical origin, histology, and secretory activity.
- Many of these classifications are well established and widely used.
- The WHO classifications of lung and thymic NETs and gastroenteropancreatic (GEP) NETs are shown in Table 8.1.
- The name carcinoid continues to be used in the WHO classification of lung and thymic NETs. See Table 8.1.
- It is important to understand the differences between 'differentiation', which is the extent to which the neoplastic cells resemble their non-tumourous counterparts, and 'grade', which is the inherent aggressiveness of the tumour.
- The grades (low, intermediate, or high grade) in lung and thymic NETs are based on mitoses and necrosis. In GEP NETs, in addition to mitoses, the Ki67 index (a marker of proliferation) determines the grade.
- Neuroendocrine carcinomas are the most aggressive NENs and can either be small or large cell type.

Clinical features of NENs

NENs are diagnosed based on histological features of biopsy specimens. The presenting features of the tumours vary like any other tumour, based on their anatomical location, such as abdominal pain, intestinal obstruction. Many are incidentally discovered during endoscopy or imaging for unrelated conditions. In a database study, 49% of NENs were localized, 24% had regional metastases, and 27% had distant metastases. The NENs most associated with metastases are pancreatic, followed by caecal, colonic, and small intestine in reducing frequency. These tumours rarely manifest themselves due to their secretory effects.

Table 8.1 WHO classification of neuroendocrine tumours

Grade	WHO lung and thymic NETs	WHO GEP NETs
Low grade	Carcinoid	NET G1
Intermediate grade	Atypical carcinoid	NET G2
High grade (neuroendocrine carcinoma)	Small/large cell carcinoma	NET G3

Diagnostic investigations of NENs

Pathology

- Macroscopically, the exact anatomical site, distance from margins, and the size of the tumour need to be described.
- Histological characterization comprises of structure and presence of necrosis.
- Immunohistochemistry needs to be performed, including neuroendocrine markers chromogranin A and synaptophysin.
- Mitotic counts and the Ki67 index are used to grade tumours. The standards for these depend on the anatomical location of the primary tumour.

Biochemical investigations

- Only a third of patients with neuroendocrine tumours develop symptoms due to hormone secretion.
- Relatively common neuroendocrine syndromes are hyperinsulinaemic hypoglycaemia associated with insulinomas, Zollinger–Ellison syndrome associated with gastrinomas, and the carcinoid syndrome which is characterized by flushing, diarrhoea, hypo- or hypertension, arrhythmias, and wheezing.
- 5HIAA (a serotonin metabolite) has been the traditional mainstay in screening for, and in the follow-up of, HIAA-secreting NENs.
- 5HIAA levels are only elevated in GEP NETs after metastasis to the liver, with the exceptions of ovarian and lung NENs or retroperitoneal metastases.
- Elevated 5HIAA levels have 75% sensitivity and near 100% specificity, as long as false +ves due to dietary sources of serotonin, such as bananas, avocados, pineapples, and chocolate, are excluded.
- 5HIAA levels correlate well with the carcinoid syndrome and are a useful guide to monitoring treatment.
- Serum chromogranin A is a useful diagnostic indicator and also a marker of disease progression and response to treatment.
- False +ves—renal failure, liver failure, PPI, atrophic gastritis, inflammatory bowel disease.
- False –ves—levodopa, phenothiazines.

Imaging

- The current approach to visualizing primary tumours and secondaries involves the use of high resolution CT and MRI.
- The *RECIST* criteria are used to assess tumour burden, disease progression, and response to treatment.
- The involvement of the GI wall is best visualized by endoscopic ultrasonography and endomicroscopy.
- Somatostatin receptor scintigraphy involves the use of the radiotracers ^{111}In, ^{68}Ga, and ^{99}Tc and can help identify somatostatin-avid lesions.
- PET CT or PET MRI may replace somatostatin receptor scintigraphy in the future.
- The availability of these techniques varies considerably across different centres.

Treatment of NENs

A multidisciplinary approach to the treatment of NENs is essential.

Surgical treatment

- Surgery is the treatment of choice for NENs grades 1 and 2, except in the presence of widespread distant metastases and extensive local invasion.
- Preoperative octreotide may prevent carcinoid crisis.
- In patients with widespread local disease or distant metastases, surgery could still be beneficial by reducing tumour bulk. When debulking liver metastases, intraoperative ablation may be used as adjunctive treatment. This is helpful in symptom control.
- Surgery may be required to alleviate intestinal obstruction.
- There are surgical standards (ENETS) for the treatment of GEP NENs.
- There are limited data to set standards for the surgical management of bronchial and extra-gastrointestinal tumours.

Ablative therapies

- For NENs with liver metastases, radiofrequency ablation or transarterial chemoembolization are used.

Medical management

- The endpoints of clinical trials are either progression-free survival or time to progression due to their slow growth. This is a fundamental difference compared with adenocarcinomas.
- For neuroendocrine carcinomas, chemotherapeutic options are similar to those for small cell lung cancer.
- Medical management for symptom control and disease progression is applicable when potentially curative surgery and ablative procedures are not possible.

See Box 8.1 for non-functioning pancreatic NENs.

Medical therapies that are available are:

Somatostatin analogues

- Somatostatin analogues (SSA) have relatively minor side effects and provide long-term symptom control.
- Octreotide and lanreotide and their longer-acting analogues reduce the level of biochemical tumour markers in the majority of patients and control symptoms in around 70% of cases.
- SSAs may be beneficial in functioning and non-functioning metastatic small intestinal G1 NET for tumour stabilization. They are not recommended for use in metastatic G3 NEC.
- Radiolabelled somatostatin analogues with yttrium-90 alleviate symptoms of metastatic tumours and may improve quality of life.
- Pasireotide, a newer somatostatin analogue which has a high binding affinity to four out of the five human somatostatin receptor subtypes, has a longer half-life. This drug is being investigated for use in NENs in conjunction with newer molecular targeted therapies.

Box 8.1 Non-functioning pancreatic NENs

These are defined by the absence of a hormone secretion syndrome. They may present as incidental small tumours or large neoplasia, with symptoms related to tumour burden. At presentation, 30–70% have liver metastases, and this is associated with poorer prognosis. Treatment includes curative surgery for localized tumours ≥2cm or those that show evidence of growth on follow-up under this size. Palliative surgery may be offered to patients with inoperable primaries. In advanced disease, the treatment options include chemotherapy, PRRT (see 📖 p. 560), molecular targeted therapy.

Interferon α

- There is reasonable biochemical response (about 45%), with improvement in symptoms.
- A combination of interferon with octreotide has been shown to produce biochemical and symptomatic improvement in patients who have previously had no significant benefit from either drug alone.

Chemotherapy

Cytotoxic chemotherapy may be considered in patients with progressive, advanced, or uncontrolled symptomatic disease. It is recommended in metastatic pancreatic NET, foregut metastatic G2 NET, and NEC G3 of any primary. It is not recommended in well-differentiated midgut NET.

- Streptozotocin-based combinations, such as with fluorouracil, have been historically in use. Three-drug regimens, including cisplatin or doxorubicin, show superior response rates compared to the two-drug regimen.
- Capecitabine (prodrug of 5FU) is administered orally and may offer more antitumour effect.
- Like streptozotocin, dacarbazine is an alkylating agent and has shown to be of benefit in the treatment of pancreatic NETs.
- Temozolomide, another alkylating agent and an orally administered analogue of dacarbazine, is associated with less toxicity. However, data are limited.

Molecular therapies

These therapies target signalling pathways, such as tyrosine kinase (TK) and mammalian target of rapamycin (sirolimus) (mTOR), which have a regulatory role in neuroendocrine cell growth.

- The small molecule TK inhibitor sunitinib has been shown to significantly increase progression-free survival in patients with malignant pancreatic NETs when compared with placebo.
- The mTOR inhibitor everolimus has been shown to reduce the risk of progression by 65% vs placebo in a recent study. It may also be used with octreotide.

Peptide receptor radioligand therapy (PRRT)

- In a large study using ^{90}Y-DOTA tyr3-octeotide in patients with metastatic neuroendocrine tumours with uptake on pretreatment somatostatin receptor scintigraphy, 34% had a measurable decrease in tumour size, 15% had a biochemical response, and 30% improved symptomatically.
- In another trial using ^{177}Lu-DOTA, there was a tumour response rate of 30%.
- These are relatively newer modalities of treatment, with few long-term data.

Radiolabelled MIBG

- MIBG is structurally related to noradrenaline, and, after IV injection, a proportion of NETs concentrate significant amounts of the compound.
- In retrospective studies, reduction in 5HIAA excretion was seen in 37% of patients with GEP NETs and objective tumour responses seen in 15–30% of patients. Symptomatic benefit was achieved in 25–50% of patients treated with radiolabelled MIBG.

▶▶ Carcinoid crisis

Despite the changes in nomenclature of NENs and the tumours that were traditionally described as carcinoids being included under the classification of NENs, the 'carcinoid crisis' is still an important descriptive term. It is a potentially life-threatening condition that should be prevented, where possible, and treated as an emergency.

- Clinical features include hypotension, tachycardia, arrhythmias, flushing, diarrhoea, bronchospasm, and altered sensorium.
- The carcinoid crisis can be triggered by manipulation of the tumours, such as during biopsy, surgery, or palpation.
- These result in the release of biologically active compounds from the tumours.
- Preoperatively, the risk of a crisis can be reduced by the administration of SC octreotide (300 micrograms).
- During a crisis, commence an IV infusion of octreotide at a rate of 50–150 micrograms/h, in addition to fluid resuscitation and supportive management.

Carcinoid heart disease

Carcinoid heart disease is characterized by thickening of valve leaflets, valvular cups, and chordae. These result in valvular stenosis or regurgitation and eventually heart failure.

This condition is seen in 40–50% of patients with carcinoid syndrome and 3–4% of patients with neuroendocrine tumours, typically with right-sided involvement (tricuspid regurgitation or pulmonary regurgitation). Left side is involved in <10%.

Patients with carcinoid syndrome and carcinoid heart disease should have an annual echocardiographic assessment. During the first evaluation, a patent foramen ovale should be sought, and, in the presence of this condition, there can be left-sided valve disease. The timing of valve replacement should be made by experienced cardiologists and cardiac surgeons.

Further reading

European Neuroendocrine Tumour Society. Available at: ✆ http://www.enets.org.

Pavel ME, et al. (2011). Everolimus plus octreotide long-acting repeatable for the treatment of advanced neuroendocrine tumours associated with carcinoid syndrome (RADIANT-2): a randomised, placebo-controlled, phase 3 study. *Lancet* **378**, 2005–12.

Raymond E, et al. (2011). Sunitinib malate for the treatment of pancreatic neuroendocrine tumors. *N Engl J Med* **364**, 501–13.

Yao JC, et al. (2011). Everolimus for advanced pancreatic neuroendocrine tumors. *N Engl J Med* **364**, 514–23.

Insulinomas

Definitions and background

- An insulinoma is a functioning neuroendocrine tumour of the pancreas that causes hypoglycaemia through inappropriate secretion of insulin.
- Unlike other neuroendocrine tumours of the pancreas, more than 90% of insulinomas are benign.
- >80% of insulinomas are solitary, but some are multiple, either simultaneously or consecutively, a situation likely to be associated with MEN-1 in approximately 10%.
- Insulinomas are found with equal frequency throughout the head, body, and tail of the pancreas.

Epidemiology

- The annual incidence of insulinomas is of the order of 1–2 per million population.
- There is a slight female preponderance in the fifth decade of life.
- 5–10% of insulinomas are associated with MEN-1.

Clinical presentation

- Patients may present with neuroglycopenic symptoms, including headaches, diplopia, blurred vision, altered behaviour, and sometimes seizures.
- Whipple's triad remains as useful as ever in diagnosing insulinoma: symptoms of hypoglycaemia, plasma glucose (laboratory glucose—and not fingerprick readings) of 2.2mmol/L or less, and resolution of symptoms with glucose.

Biochemical investigations

- The gold standard investigation for establishing the diagnosis of insulinomas is the 72h fast.
- Shorter durations of fast (15h), repeated on three separate occasions, may be used as a screening tool.

Diagnostic criteria

- Laboratory blood glucose of ≤2.2mmol/L.
- Concomitant inappropriate insulin elevation.
- Elevated C-peptide and proinsulin.
- β-hydroxybutyrate of <2.7mmol/L.
- Absence of sulfonylureas and metabolites in plasma or urine.

Tumour localization

(See Table 8.2.)

- Islet cell tumours are often small and may not be detected by any imaging technique. The available radiological modalities have a wide reported range of sensitivity which is frequently dependent on the equipment and the operator.
- MRI or spiral CT correctly detects >60% of tumours, but preoperative localization can be difficult in tumours <1cm in diameter.
- Arterial stimulation (with calcium or secretin), followed by venous sampling, can localize approximately 90% of insulinomas but carries the risks of a more invasive technique.
- Endoscopic US, which requires specialized equipment and expertise, may identify tumours as small as 5mm. The head of the pancreas is visualized with the probe in the duodenum, and the body and tail with it in the stomach.
- Intraoperative US, using a transducer applied directly to the pancreas, improves the sensitivity of US to ~90%.
- Experienced surgeons can frequently identify the lesions intraoperatively by palpation alone, and the risk of multiple tumours makes a thorough examination of the whole pancreas essential at operation.
- Somatostatin receptor scintigraphy has been shown to be useful in detecting insulinomas, but it is dependent on somatostatin receptor subtype expression by the tumour.
- Glucagon-like peptide-1 receptor imaging has also been shown to be useful.

Table 8.2 Radiological localization of pancreatic insulinomas

Localization technique	Reported sensitivity (%)
Transabdominal US	30–61
Endoscopic US	80
Intraoperative US	90
CT	42–78
MRI	20–100
Octreotide scanning	68–86
Pancreatic arteriography	29–90
Venous sampling	84

Treatment of insulinomas

- The treatment of choice in all, but poor, surgical candidates is operative removal.
- Surgical options include enucleation of tumours, partial pancreatectomy, Whipple procedure, or rarely total pancreatectomy.
- In experienced surgical hands, the mortality is less than 1%. The mortality is largely influenced by the incidence of acute post-operative pancreatitis and peritonitis.
- Post-operative hyperglycaemia may occur, even following partial pancreatectomy.
- Medical treatment to control symptoms may be achieved using diazoxide alone or in combination with octreotide pending surgery or in those patients who have high surgical risk.
- Radiolabelled somatostatin analogue therapy may induce a biochemical and symptomatic response in patients with malignant insulinomas.
- Everolimus, the M Tor inhibitor, may be useful in metastatic insulinoma but has significant side-effects.

Prognosis of insulinomas

- Following the removal of a solitary insulinoma, life expectancy is restored to normal.
- Malignant insulinomas, with metastases usually to the liver, have a natural history of years, rather than months, and may be controlled with medical therapy or specific antitumour therapy using streptozotocin and fluorouracil. The management goals are targeted at managing blood glucose and tumour load.
- Average 5-year survival estimated to be approximately 35% for malignant insulinomas.

Further reading

Carl Pallais J, et al. (2012). Case records of the Massachusetts General Hospital. Case 33-2012. A 34-year-old woman with episodic paresthesias and altered mental status after childbirth. *N Engl J Med* **367**, 1637–46.

de Herder WW, et al. (2011). New therapeutic options for metastatic malignant insulinomas. *Clin Endocrinol (Oxf)* **75**, 277–84.

Placzkowski KA, et al. (2009). Secular trends in the presentation and management of functioning insulinoma at the Mayo Clinic, 1987-2007. *J Clin Endocrinol Metab* **94**, 1069–73.

Gastrinomas

Definitions
- Gastrin, synthesized in the G cells, predominantly in the gastric antrum, is the principal gut hormone stimulating gastric acid secretion.
- The Zollinger–Ellison (ZE) syndrome is characterized by gastric acid oversecretion and manifests itself as severe peptic ulcer disease (PUD), gastro-oesophageal reflux, and diarrhoea.

Incidence
The incidence of gastrinomas is 0.5–2/million population/year.

Sites of origin
- Gastrinomas are the most common functional malignant pancreatic endocrine tumours.
- The most common extrapancreatic site of origin is the duodenum in 50–80% of sporadic ZE and 70–100% of patients with MEN-1.
- Less common sites are stomach, liver, bile duct, heart, and small cell lung cancer.
- Pancreatic tumours are more aggressive than duodenal tumours.

Clinical presentation
- The mean age of presentation of patients with sporadic gastrinomas is 48–55 years and is almost equally found in ♂ and ♀.
- Most patients with ZE syndrome present with a single duodenal ulcer or gastro-oesophageal reflux.
- Abdominal pain is a presenting feature (due to PUD) in 75–98% of patients.
- Diarrhoea is present at diagnosis in 30–70%.
- 20–30% of patients with gastrinomas have MEN-1.
- At diagnosis, 5–10% of duodenal gastrinomas and 20–25% of pancreatic gastrinomas have hepatic metastases.
- Suspect ZE syndrome when there is severe PUD without *Helicobacter pylori*, resistance to PPIs, or in the presence of hypercalcaemia.

Diagnosis of Zollinger–Ellison syndrome

- The diagnosis rests on demonstrating an inappropriate elevation of fasting gastrin levels in the presence of hyperchlorhydria (pH ≤2).
- Patients should have antisecretory treatment stopped prior to the test (3 days for H$_2$ blockers and 2 weeks for PPIs), as these drugs are associated with hypergastrinaemia. However, gastrin levels above 250pmol/L are rarely due to PPI therapy alone.
- A gut hormone profile may identify elevated plasma levels of pancreatic polypeptide or other gut hormones.
- The tumour localization techniques described for insulinomas are also relevant for gastrinomas (see Table 8.3).
- Very small tumours or duodenal tumours can be very hard to localize, and even small tumours are frequently associated with local lymph node disease.
- Selective arterial angiography may be combined with a provocative test for gastrin release, using a bolus of calcium gluconate or secretin for elusive small tumours. 3mL calcium gluconate is injected into the gastroduodenal, superior mesenteric, splenic, and hepatic artery, in turn, with a 5min gap in between. After 30s at each site, sampling is undertaken.
- For causes of hypergastrinaemia, see Box 8.2.

Box 8.2 Causes of hypergastrinaemia

Low or normal gastric acid production
- H$_2$ blockers.
- PPIs.
- Vagotomy.
- Hypochlorhydria.
- Short gut syndrome.
- Renal failure.
- Hypercalcaemia.

Elevated gastric acid production
- Gastrinoma.
- G cell hyperplasia.

Treatment of gastrinomas

(See Table 8.3.)
- The treatment of choice is complete surgical tumour removal, although this is usually only considered after the tumour has been identified preoperatively.
- Surgery is rarely justified in patients with known hepatic metastases, although some small studies have raised the possibility of benefit from tumour debulking.
- Where preoperative imaging has failed to identify a tumour, the patient is often best maintained on high-dose PPI therapy (e.g. 60mg of omeprazole), with regular imaging to reassess. Check B_{12} annually.
- Somatostatin analogues do not appear to be more effective at controlling gastric acid hypersecretion and relieving symptoms than PPIs or H2 blockers.
- The data are currently few, but, as for insulinomas, radiolabelled somatostatin analogues may be a future treatment option for gastrinomas.
- In patients with MEN-1, management is more controversial, but the usual policy is to operate when a well-defined tumour can be identified.

Table 8.3 Treatment options for gastrinomas

Medical treatment	Surgery	Palliation
PPIs	Tumour resection	Chemotherapy
H2 blockers	Tumour debulking	Hepatic artery embolization
Octreotide	Liver transplant	

Prognosis of gastrinomas

- 10-year survival without liver metastases is 95%.
- 10-year survival with single or limited metastases in both lobes is approximately 80%.
- Where there are diffuse metastases, the outlook is less favourable, with a 10-year survival of approximately 15%.

Further reading

Simmons LH, et al. (2013). Case records of the Massachusetts General Hospital. Case 6-2013. A 54-year-old man with recurrent diarrhea. N Engl J Med **368**, 757–65.

Glucagonomas

Definitions

- Glucagonomas are neuroendocrine tumours that usually arise from the α cells of the pancreas and produce the glucagonoma syndrome through the secretion of glucagon and other peptides derived from the preproglucagon gene.
- The large majority of glucagonomas are malignant, but they are also very indolent tumours, and the diagnosis may be overlooked for many years.
- Up to 90% of patients will have lymph node or liver metastases at the time of presentation.
- They are classically associated with the rash of necrolytic migratory erythema.

Epidemiology

- The annual incidence is estimated at 1 per 20 million population.
- Glucagonomas are uncommon in MEN-1.

Clinical presentation

(See Table 8.4.)

- The characteristic rash—necrolytic migratory erythema—occurs in >70% of cases and usually manifests initially as a well-demarcated area of erythema in the groin before migrating to the limbs, buttocks, and perineum.
- Mucous membrane involvement is common, with stomatitis, glossitis, vaginitis, and urethritis being frequent features.
- Glucagon antagonizes the effects of insulin, particularly on hepatic glucose metabolism, and glucose intolerance is a frequent association (>90%).
- Sustained gluconeogenesis also causes amino acid deficiencies and results in protein catabolism which can be associated with unrelenting weight loss in >60% of patients.
- Glucagon has a direct suppressive effect on the bone marrow, resulting in a normochromic normocytic anaemia in almost all patients.

Biochemical investigations

- The diagnosis is confirmed on finding raised plasma glucagon levels.
- A gut hormone profile may also show elevated neuroendocrine markers, such as pancreatic polypeptide, chromogranin A.
- Impaired glucose intolerance and hypoaminoacidaemia may be present.

Tumour localization

- At the time of diagnosis, 50–100% of glucagonomas will have metastasized to the liver, and most 1° tumours will be >3cm in diameter.
- These tumours rarely present problems of radiological localization, and transabdominal US and CT scanning are usually adequate.
- Small tumours may require more sophisticated imaging techniques, including endoscopic ultrasound (see Table 8.4). Octreotide scanning probably offers the best means of evaluating the extent of metastatic disease.

Table 8.4 Clinical features of the glucagonoma syndrome

Site	Clinical features
Skin	Necrolytic migratory erythema
Mucous membranes	Angular stomatitis
	Atrophic glossitis
	Vulvovaginitis
	Urethritis
Nails	Onycholysis
Scalp	Alopecia
Metabolism	Glucose intolerance
	Protein catabolism and weight loss
Haematological	Anaemia
	Venous thromboses
Psychiatric	Depression
	Psychosis

Treatment
- Surgery is the only curative therapeutic option, but the potential for a complete cure may be as low as 5%.
- Somatostatin (SST) analogues are the treatment of choice, with excellent response rates in treating the necrolytic migratory erythema. They are less effective at reversing the weight loss and have an inconsistent effect on glycaemic control such that diabetes mellitus may need to be managed with insulin therapy.
- If SST analogues fail, the rash may be improved using IV amino acids and fatty acids.
- Experience with chemotherapy is limited. However, palliative chemotherapy, using streptozotocin and fluorouracil, has been shown to produce a 50% reduction in glucagon levels in 75% of patients, but the benefit is frequently only temporary. Antitumour activity has also been shown with the alkylating agent temozolomide.
- Hepatic artery embolization may result in a dramatic relief of symptoms, with remissions of several months recorded.
- As for the other pancreatic islet cell tumours, there are data to suggest that radiolabelled somatostatin analogues may be therapeutic in the glucagonoma syndrome.
- Nutritional support is essential, as patients may experience a prolonged catabolic state.

VIPomas

Definitions
- In 1958, Verner and Morrison[1] first described a syndrome consisting of refractory watery diarrhoea and hypokalaemia, associated with a neuroendocrine tumour of the pancreas.
- The syndrome of watery diarrhoea, hypokalaemia, and acidosis (WDHA) is due to secretion of vasoactive intestinal polypeptide (VIP).
- Tumours that secrete VIP are known as VIPomas.
- VIPomas account for <10% of islet cell tumours and mainly occur as solitary tumours.
- >60% are malignant and metastasize to the lymph nodes, liver, kidneys, and bone.

Clinical presentation
- The most prominent symptom in most patients is profuse watery diarrhoea which is secretory in nature and, therefore, rich in electrolytes (see Box 8.3).
- Other causes of secretory diarrhoea should be considered in the differential diagnosis (see Box 8.4).
- VIPomas are rare in MEN-1 patients, occurring in <1% of cases.

Biochemical investigations
- Elevated levels of plasma VIP are found in all patients with the VIPoma syndrome, although false +ves may occur in dehydrated patients due to diarrhoea from other causes.
- A gut hormone profile may identify other raised tumour markers, such as pancreatic polypeptide, and aid detection of some other causes of watery diarrhoea, e.g. gastrinomas.
- A phaeochromocytoma screen should be performed, especially in children in whom it is common to find the tumours residing in the adrenal medulla.

Box 8.3 Clinical features of the VIPoma syndrome
- Watery diarrhoea.
- Hypokalaemia.
- Achlorhydria.
- Metabolic acidosis.
- Hypercalcaemia.
- Hyperglycaemia.
- Hypomagnesaemia.
- Facial flushing.

Box 8.4 Differential diagnosis of secretory diarrhoea

- Infection e.g. *Escherichia coli* or cholera toxins.
- Laxative abuse.
- Villous adenoma.
- Other gut neuroendocrine tumours, e.g. carcinoid tumours or gastrinomas.
- Carcinoma of the lung.
- Medullary carcinoma of the thyroid.
- Systemic mastocytosis.
- Immunoglobulin A deficiency.

Tumour localization

- The majority of tumours secreting VIP originate in the pancreas while others arise from the sympathetic chain.
- 1° VIPomas have very rarely been reported to arise from a variety of other sites, such as the lung, oesophagus, small bowel, colon, and kidney.
- Most patients present with large tumours which can be easily identified by transabdominal US or CT, although small tumours may require additional methods of tumour localization, as previously discussed (see Table 8.2).

Treatment

- Severe cases require IV fluid replacement and careful correction of electrolyte disturbances.
- Surgery to remove the tumour is the treatment of first choice, if technically possible, and may be curative in around 40% of patients. Surgical debulking may also be of palliative benefit.
- Somatostatin analogues produce effective symptomatic relief from the diarrhoea in most patients. Long-term use does not result in tumour regression.
- Glucocorticoids in high dosage have also been shown to provide good relief of symptoms.
- A trial of lithium may be warranted in resistant cases, and this therapy may be combined with octreotide.
- Chemotherapy using streptozotocin, in combination with fluorouracil, has resulted in response rates of >30%.
- Hepatic artery embolization can offer temporary respite from severe diarrhoea.

Reference

1. Verner JV, Morrison AB (1958) Islet cell tumor and a syndrome of refractory watery diarrhea and hypokalemia. *Am J Med* **25**, 374–380.

Somatostatinomas

Definitions
- Somatostatinomas are very rare neuroendocrine tumours, occurring both in the pancreas and in the duodenum.
- >60% are large tumours located in the head or body of the pancreas.
- The clinical syndrome may be diagnosed late in the course of the disease when metastatic spread to local lymph nodes and the liver has already occurred.

Clinical features
(See Box 8.5.)
- Glucose intolerance or frank diabetes mellitus may have been observed for many years prior to the diagnosis and retrospectively often represents the first clinical sign. It is probably due to the inhibitory effect of somatostatin on insulin secretion.
- A high incidence of gallstones has been described similar to that seen as a side effect with long-term somatostatin analogue therapy.
- Diarrhoea, steatorrhoea, and weight loss appear to be consistent clinical features and may be associated with inhibition of the exocrine pancreas by somatostatin.
- Small duodenal somatostatinomas may occur in association with NF-1, and, although these rarely cause the inhibitory clinical syndrome, they present with obstructive biliary disease through local spread of the tumour.
- Somatostatinomas are infrequently associated with MEN-1 (7%).

Biochemical investigations
- Plasma somatostatin levels will be raised and may also be associated with raised levels of other neuroendocrine tumour markers, including ACTH and calcitonin.
- Multisecretory activity is commoner with pancreatic (33%) than with duodenal (16%) somatostatinomas.

Tumour localization
- Transabdominal US and CT scanning may demonstrate the tumour since metastatic disease is often apparent at presentation.
- Additonal methods of tumour localization, as previously described, may also be required (see Table 8.2).

Treatment
- Surgery should be considered as first-line treatment as, although a cure is rare, even debulking surgery may result in significant palliation.
- Hepatic embolization can be considered, and chemotherapy with streptozotocin and fluorouracil may be used to control malignant disease.

Box 8.5 Clinical features of the somatostatin syndrome
- Glucose intolerance/diabetes mellitus (95%).
- Gallstones (68%).
- Diarrhoea and steatorrhoea.
- Weight loss (25%).
- Anaemia (14%).
- Hypochlorhydria.

Inherited endocrine syndromes and MEN

McCune–Albright syndrome

Definitions

The syndrome is characterized by:
- Polyostotic fibrous dysplasia.
- *Café-au-lait* pigmented skin lesions.
- Autonomous function of multiple endocrine glands.

A clinical diagnosis requires two of these pathologies.

Epidemiology

The condition affects 1:100,000 to 1:1,000,000 people.

Genetics

- A genetic, but not an inherited, condition due to a post-zygotic somatic mutation in the gene (*GNAS1*) that encodes the α-chain of the stimulating G protein of adenyl cyclase (GSα mutation). This results in activation of adenyl cyclase.
- The somatic mutation results in mosaicism, and consequently the proportion and distribution of affected cells in a tissue will be determined by the precise stage in development at which the mutation occurred.
- Mutational analysis of the *GNAS1* gene from affected tissues or blood is available in some centres in the UK.

Clinical features

Polyostotic fibrous dysplasia

- Solitary or multiple expansile bony lesions which can cause fracture deformities and nerve entrapment typically develop before the age of 10 years.
- The femora and the pelvic bones are most frequently affected, and radiographs of these bones are useful for screening.
- Osteosarcomas are a rare complication.
- For treatment, see Box 9.1.

Café-au-lait pigmentation

The lesions are characterized by an irregular border (in neurofibromatosis, the border is smooth), do not cross the midline, and tend to be ipsilateral to the bone lesions.

Endocrinopathies

See Table 9.1.

Involvement of other organs

- Hepatobiliary complications, such as neonatal jaundice, elevated transaminases, and cholestasis are relatively common.
- Cardiomegaly, tachyarrhythmias, and sudden cardiac death may occur.
- Gastrointestinal polyps, splenic hyperplasia, and pancreatitis are reported complications.
- Recognized CNS associations include microcephaly, failure to thrive, and developmental delay.

Table 9.1 Endocrinopathies in McCune–Albright syndrome

Condition	Presentation	Treatment
Precocious puberty	Frequent initial presentation Typically aged 1–9 years Low gonadotrophins Adults fertile Less frequent in boys	Cyproterone acetate
Thyroid nodules	Present in almost 100% of patients 50% become toxic due to autonomous nodule function	Antithyroid drugs, radioiodine, surgery
GH-secreting pituitary tumours and prolactinomas	Present with features of acromegaly or hyperprolactinaemia	Somatostatin analogues, dopamine agonists, surgery
Cushing's syndrome	Adrenal hyperplasia or adenoma	Adrenalectomy
Hypophosphataemic rickets	↓ phosphate ↓ 1,25 vit D ↑ ALP Normal calcium, 25OH vit D, and PTH	Calcitriol, phosphate supplements

Box 9.1 Treatment of polyostotic fibrous dysplasia
- Surgery may be complicated by bleeding, and radiotherapy has a limited effect.
- There is some recent evidence to support the use of bisphosphonates, particularly pamidronate, for both symptomatic pain relief and the radiological healing of bone.

Prognosis
- Most patients live well beyond reproductive age.
- Bone deformities may reduce life expectancy.
- Sudden cardiac death, although recognized, is uncommon.

Further reading

Lumbroso S, Paris F, Sultan C (2002). McCune–Albright syndrome: molecular genetics. *J Paediatr Endocrinol Metab* **15**, 875–82.

Spiegel AM, Weinstein LS (2004). Inherited diseases involving G proteins and G protein-coupled receptors. *Annu Rev Med* **55**, 27–39.

Neurofibromatosis

Definitions

- Neurofibromatosis type 1 (NF1) is also known as von Recklinghausen disease and refers to the occurrence of multiple neurofibromas, *café-au-lait* spots, and Lisch nodules (pigmented hamartomas nodules of aggregated dendritic melanocytes) affecting the iris.
- Endocrinopathies are sometimes associated with NF1.
- NF type 2 (NF2) is characterized by the presence of bilateral acoustic neuromas, typically resulting in deafness.
- Other features of NF2 include posterior subcapsular cataracts, retinal gliomas, pigmented retinopathy, and gaze palsies.
- NF2 has no common associated endocrinopathies.
- NF2 is rare, with an estimated frequency of 1 in 40,000 live births.

NF1

Genetics

- NF1 is a highly penetrant, autosomal dominant condition.
- The NF1 gene is located on chromosome 17 and encodes a GTPase-activating protein (neurofibromin).
- Neurofibromin promotes cleavage of GTP to GDP.

Epidemiology

- The incidence of NF1 is 1 per 3,000 of the population.
- NF1 is nearly 100% penetrant but shows variable clinical expression.
- Approximately 50% of cases are sporadic.

Clinical features

- Diagnosis is generally apparent by the age of 1 year.
- The *café-au-lait* spots become visible shortly after birth (95%); 70% have axillary or groin freckling.
- The multiple cutaneous and subcutaneous neurofibromas appear around puberty (95%).
- Lisch nodules, affecting the iris, start to appear typically after the age of 5 years (95%).
- The endocrine features are detailed in Box 9.2.
- Learning disabilities occur in 60% of patients with NF1.
- Gliomas may be found in around 15% of patients, most commonly affecting the optic pathways.
- Neurofibrosarcomas complicate around 6% of cases.
- Skeletal dysplasias (e.g. sphenoid wing dysplasia, scoliosis, tibial pseudoarthrosis, pectus excavatum, etc.) may be found in up to 5% of cases.
- Vascular dysplasia may occur, with the commonest region affected being the renal vasculature, resulting in renovascular hypertension in up to 3% of cases.
- Macrocephaly (16%), seizures (5%), and short stature (6%) are all reported features of NF1.
- Associated phaeochromocytomas are seen in <5% of NF1 patients.

Box 9.2 Endocrine features of NF1

- Puberty and pregnancy:
  - Both are associated with a change in size of neurofibromas.
- Hypothalamus and pituitary:
  - Optic gliomas impinge on adjacent tissues and may affect hypothalamic and/or pituitary function.
- Phaeochromocytoma 0.1–5.0%:
  - Serious complication of NF1.
  - Uncommon before age 20 years.
  - Most commonly adrenal (20% bilateral), but extra-adrenal lesions are reported.
- Gut neuroendocrine tumours:
  - Found in around 1% of NF1 patients.

Further reading

Arun D, Gutmann DH (2004). Recent advances in neurofibromatosis type 1. *Curr Opin Neurol* **17**, 101–5.

Rose VM (2004). Neurocutaneous syndromes. *Mo Med* **101**, 112–16.

von Hippel–Lindau disease

Definitions

Characterized by:
- CNS haemangioblastomas.
- Retinal angiomas.
- Renal cysts and carcinomas.
- Phaeochromocytomas.
- Pancreatic neuroendocrine tumours (less common) and pancreatic cysts.
- Occasional endolymphatic sac tumours.

See Box 9.3.

Clinical diagnosis established by:
- Two or more haemangioblastomas.
- A haemangioblastoma and a visual manifestation.
- A haemangioblastoma or visual manifestation and a family history of haemangioblastoma.

- The condition occurs in approximately 1 in 36,000 live births.
- The average age of presentation is 27 years, and the condition is nearly 100% penetrant by the age of 65 years.
- VHL may be subdivided into type 1 and type 2 disease.
- Type 1 VHL is the commonest form of the disease and is characterized by a tendency to develop tumours in the eyes, brain, spinal cord, kidney, and pancreas.
- Affected family members with VHL type 2 are also susceptible to developing phaeochromocytomas, and this may be further subdivided into VHL type 2A (develop phaeochromocytomas and renal cell carcinomas).

Genetics
- VHL is a highly penetrant autosomal dominant condition.
- The *VHL* gene is on chromosome 3 and is a tumour suppressor gene.
- Mutations which result in loss of the VHL protein lead to VEGF expression in normoxia as well as hypoxia, thus enhancing the growth of these tumours which are often very vascular.
- Mutational analysis of the VHL gene is available in the UK.
- Genetic testing in affected families is recommended from the age of 5 years.
- With appropriate counselling, prenatal diagnosis with amniocentesis and chorion villous sampling is an option.

See Table 9.2 for surveillance.

Box 9.3 Less common manifestations of von Hippel–Lindau disease

Pancreas	Cysts
	Adenomas
Epididymis	Cystadenoma
CNS	Syringomyelia
	Meningioma
Liver	Adenoma
	Haemangioblastoma
	Cysts
Lung	Angioma
	Cysts
Spleen	Angioma

Table 9.2 Surveillance in VHL

Condition	Screening test
Retinal angiomas	Annual ophthalmic examination from infancy/early childhood
CNS haemangioblastomas	MRI head ± spine every 12–36 months, starting from adolescence
Renal cell carcinoma	MRI abdomen 12-monthly from the age of 16 years
Phaeochromocytoma	Plasma/urine metanephrines from early childhood
	Imaging if biochemical abnormalities detected

Clinical features

- Retinal angiomas are the initial manifestation of VHL in 40% of patients. They are uncommon before the age of 10 years but continue to develop throughout life. They tend to be peripheral in the retina, appearing as red oval lesions. Bleeding and retinal detachment may occur, and treatment is with laser therapy.
- 75% of haemangioblastomas occur in the cerebellum, and they are the initial presenting feature in 40% of VHL patients. Treatment is with surgery or radiotherapy.
- Renal carcinoma is the commonest cause of death in VHL patients. By the age of 60 years, 70% of VHL patients will be affected, with a mean age of presentation of 44 years. The lesions tend to be multifocal. The management of choice is surgical resection.

- Phaeochromocytomas occur in up to 20% of VHL families and are bilateral in 40% of cases. The frequency of this condition varies widely between families, as certain mutations are particularly associated with a high risk of phaeochromocytoma. Regular biochemical screening is essential in these high-risk families.
- The majority of pancreatic tumours associated with VHL are non-functioning, but they may secrete VIP, insulin, glucagons, or calcitonin. They occur in 10–20% of VHL patients and should be treated expectantly, unless symptomatic, enlarging, or >2–3cm.

Prognosis

- Until recently, the median survival for a VHL patient was 40–50 years of age, with the majority of deaths attributable to renal cell carcinoma.
- Currently, the prognosis for individual patients depends upon the location and complications of the tumours but overall is improving as a result of the institution of screening programmes and consequent earlier therapeutic interventions.
- For surveillance in VHL, see Table 9.2.

Further reading

Kaelin WG Jr (2003). The von Hippel–Lindau gene, kidney cancer and oxygen sensing. *Am Soc Nephrol* **14**, 2703–11.

Lonser RR, *et al.* (2003). Von Hippel-Lindau disease. *Lancet* **361**, 2059–67.

Maher RM, Hartmut PH, Richard S (2011). Von Hippel–Lindau disease: a clinical and scientific review. *Eur J Hum Genet* **19**, 617–23.

Richard S, Graff J, Lindau J, *et al.* (2005). Von Hippel–Lindau disease. *Lancet* **363**, 1231–4.

Carney complex

Definitions
A clinical diagnosis is made by finding two of the clinical features listed in Clinical presentation below or one of these features plus either an affected first-degree relative or an inactivating mutation in the gene *PRKARI*α.

Genetics
- Autosomal dominant.
- An inactivating mutation of the *PRKARI*α gene on the long arm of chromosome 17q2 can be identified in approximately 50% of families.

Clinical presentation
- Spotty skin pigmentation.
- Cardiac, skin, or mucosal myxomas.
- Endocrine tumours (see Box 9.4).
- Psammomatous melanotic schwannoma.

> **Box 9.4 Endocrine tumours associated with Carney complex**
> - The commonest endocrine manifestation is 1° pigmented nodular adrenocortical disease (PPNAD), causing Cushing's syndrome.
> - Large cell calcifying Sertoli cell tumour (LCCSCT).
> - GH/PRL-secreting pituitary adenoma (also somatotroph/mammotroph hyperplasia).
> - Thyroid adenoma.
> - Ovarian cysts.

Further reading
Bertherat J, *et al.* (2009). Mutations in regulatory subunit type 1A of cyclic adenosine 5'-monophosphate-dependent protein kinase (PRKAR1A): phenotype analysis in 353 patients and 80 different genotypes. *J Clin Endocrinol Metab* **94**, 2085–91.

Sandrini F, Stratakis C (2003). Clinical and molecular genetics of Carney complex. *Mol Genet Metab* **78**, 83–92.

Stergiopolous SG, Abu-Asab MS, Tsokos M, *et al.* (2004). Pituitary pathology in Carney complex patients. *Pituitary* **7**, 73–82.

Stratakis CA, Kirschner LS, Carney JA (2001). Clinical and molecular features of the Carney complex. *J Clin Endocrinol Metab* **86**, 4041–6.

Cowden syndrome

Clinical presentation
(Also see Box 9.5.)
- The condition is characterized by multiple hamartomas, involving organ systems derived from all three germ cell layers.
- Patients are also at risk from breast, thyroid, and endometrial carcinomas.
- Thyroid pathology occurs in >75% of patients, and the lesions may be multifocal.
- Weight gain is common.

Epidemiology
Estimated to affect 1 in 200,000 individuals.

Genetics
- Autosomal dominant condition.
- Inactivating mutations in the *PTEN* tumour suppressor gene can be identified in approximately 80% of affected probands.

> **Box 9.5 Endocrine features of Cowden syndrome**
> - Non-medullary thyroid carcinomas, especially follicular thyroid carcinoma.
> - Multinodular goitre.
> - Thyroid adenomas.
> - Parathyroid adenomas are extremely rare.

Further reading
Pilarski R, Eng C (2004). Will the real Cowden syndrome please stand up (again)? Expanding mutational and clinical spectra of the PTEN hamartoma tumour syndrome. *J Med Genet* **41**, 323–6.

POEMS syndrome

Definitions
Progressive polyneuropathy, organomegaly, endocrinopathy, monoclonal gammopathy, and skin changes (POEMS) is a rare disorder of unclear pathogenesis which is probably mediated by ↑ production of lambda light chains from abnormal plasma cells.

Clinical presentation
- Progressive polyneuropathy.
- Organomegaly, especially hepatosplenomegaly and lymphadenopathy.
- Common endocrinopathies (84%) (multiple in 65%) include hypogonadotrophic hypogonadism (70%—2/3 central, 1/3 1°), hypothyroidism (60%), hypoadrenalism (60%), diabetes mellitus (50%), hyperprolactinaemia (20%).
- Monoclonal gammopathy.
- Skin changes.

Treatments
Include chemotherapy, irradiation, and surgery.

Further reading
Dispenzieri A, Gertz MA (2004). Treatment of POEMS syndrome. *Curr Treat Options Oncol* **5**, 249–57.

MEN type 1

Definitions

Characterized by:

- Parathyroid tumours/hyperplasia.
- Anterior pituitary adenomas.
- Pancreatic neuroendocrine tumours.

A clinical diagnosis of MEN-1 is made by the presence of two out of three of these tumours or one of these tumours in the context of a family history of MEN-1.

The prevalence of MEN-1 has been estimated at 1 in 10,000 of the population.

Genetics

- MEN-1 is an autosomal dominant condition, with an estimated penetrance of 99% by the age of 50 years.
- The *MEN-1* gene is located on the long arm of chromosome 11 (11q13) and is a tumour suppressor gene. The function of the encoded protein MENIN is under investigation.
- The mutations causing MEN-1 are inactivating in nature.
- More than 1,300 mutations in the *MEN-1* gene have been described in affected families, and there is no clear genotype–phenotype correlation.
- Mutational analysis is available in the UK, although it is important to note that up to 10% of patients will not have mutations identifiable within the coding region of the *MEN-1* gene.

Clinical features

- The disease has been reported to manifest itself from the ages of 5 to 80 years.
- MEN-1 is associated with a high mortality due to aggressive tumours or biochemical sequelae of the tumours.
- 1° hyperparathyroidism is the commonest presenting feature in MEN-1 and occurs in 85–95% of patients with MEN-1. The next commonest presenting features are insulinomas or prolactinomas.
- Pituitary adenomas are found in approximately 30% of MEN-1 patients (see Table 9.3).
- The incidence of pancreatic endocrine tumours varies between 30% and 80% in different series (see Table 9.4).
- Other lesions are also associated with MEN-1 (see Table 9.5).

Table 9.3 Pituitary tumours in MEN-1

Tumour	Frequency (%)
Prolactinoma	60
Acromegaly	25
Non-functioning tumour	1
Cushing's disease	<1

Table 9.4 Pancreatic tumours in MEN-1

Tumour	Frequency (%)
Gastrinoma	60
Non-functioning tumour	30–80
Insulinoma	30
Glucagonoma	2
PPoma	<1
VIPoma	<1

Table 9.5 Other lesions in MEN-1

Tumour	Frequency (%)
Adrenal cortical tumours (including carcinoma)	5
Carcinoid tumours	4
Lipomas	1
Phaeochromocytoma	0.5
Malignant melanoma	0.5
Testicular teratoma	0.5
Multiple (>3) angiofibromas	75 (specificity 95%)

Management of MEN type 1

Primary hyperparathyroidism

- The hypercalcaemia is frequently mild, with an early age of onset, and is the first manifestation of the disease in 85–95% of patients.
- Multiple gland disease (adenomas or hyperplasia) is common, in contrast with sporadic 1° hyperparathyroidism where usually a single adenoma is found.
- Surgical management is the gold standard. However, the timing of surgery remains controversial.
- In view of the potential for multigland disease, total parathyroidectomy with lifelong oral calcitriol replacement should always be considered.
- One surgical approach is a 3.5 gland parathyroidectomy. Other options include total parathyroidectomy, with autotransplantation of parathyroid tissue into the forearm.
- Cinacalcet may be used where surgery fails or in patients with high surgical risk.
- Due to the risk of malignant tumours, a near total transcervical thymectomy at the time of parathyroidectomy should be considered.

Pituitary tumours

These are managed with surgery, medical therapies, or radiotherapy, as per sporadic pituitary tumours (📖 see Chapter 2, Pituitary tumours, p. 136).

Gastrinomas

- These can be pancreatic or extrapancreatic.
- Most of these gastrinomas are malignant and frequently metastatic.
- The role of surgery in the management of gastrinomas in the setting of MEN-1 is controversial. For non-metastatic disease, surgery is the ideal treatment.
- Surgery for tumours >2cm has been recommended and has been shown to improve disease-related survival.
- An experienced surgeon is essential if these tumours are to be resected.
- Gastrinomas are a significant cause of morbidity and mortality in MEN-1 patients and respond to medical therapy with high-dose proton pump inhibitors (PPI) at a dose of omeprazole 40–60mg bd. The aim of PPI therapy is to reduce basal gastric acid output. The prognosis of patients with MEN-1 has improved considerably with the use of PPIs to manage the Zollinger–Ellison syndrome.

Non-functioning pancreatic neuroendocrine neoplasia

- Non-functioning pancreatic neuroendocrine neoplasia (NEN) can occur in patients <15 years.
- Due to advances in imaging, these tumours are being more frequently diagnosed than before.
- Malignant pancreatic NENs are now the commonest cause of death in patients with MEN-1.

- Endoscopic ultrasound is the most sensitive technique for detecting these tumours, and somatostatin receptor scintigraphy the most sensitive for diagnosing metastases.
- The timing of surgery for these tumours is controversial. Some centres recommend removing tumours >2cm or growing tumours and surveillance for tumours under this size. However, malignancy can be missed in smaller tumours with this approach.

Mutational analysis

The criteria for performing mutational analysis are controversial and vary from centre to centre in the UK. One approach is to recommend assessing the following categories of patient:

- Patients with two MEN-1 tumours.
- First- and second-degree relatives of patients with MEN-1.
- Consider screening in patients with 1° hyperparathyroidism <40 years of age, particularly in the presence of multigland disease.
- Consider screening in patients with isolated pancreatic neuroendocrine tumours, especially gastrinomas.
- Mutational analysis should be considered in patients with parathyroid adenomas under the age of 30 years.
- Within a family known to have MEN-1, mutational analysis should still be offered to people with hyperparathyroidism or hyperprolactinaemia, as 'phenocopies' (those with disease manifestation without mutations) have been reported to occur in 5–10% of MEN-1 kindreds. Biochemical diagnosis alone should not be relied upon. These phenocopies do not have MEN-1 and can be reassured.

Screening for MEN type 1

(See Box 9.6 and Table 9.6.)

- Screening is relevant for affected patients, asymptomatic mutation carriers, and first- and second-degree relatives in families with a clinical diagnosis of MEN-1, but where a mutation has not been identified.
- Manifestations of MEN-1 are very rare before the teenage years but have been described as young as 5 years. Careful parental counselling can encourage some childhood monitoring which ideally should include a careful history for symptoms (e.g. hypoglycaemia) and height and weight assessment, in addition to calcium and prolactin measurements.
- Screening involves both careful clinical history and examination as well as biochemical assessment and imaging modalities (see Table 9.6).
- Age-related penetrance: age 10–7%, 20–52%, 30–87%, 40–99%, 60–100%.
- Current evidence supports commencing screening for pituitary lesions and insulinomas from the age of 5 years, hyperparathyroidism from the age of 8, gastrinomas and other NETs from the age of 20.

Table 9.6 Screening adults in MEN-1

Test	Frequency
Calcium, phosphate, and PTH	Annual
Basal anterior pituitary function (particularly prolactin and IGF-1)	Annual
Fasting gut hormones	Annual
Fasting glucose	Annual
24h urinary 5HIAA and chromogranin A	Annual
MRI abdomen ± endoscopic ultrasound	Annual to 3-yearly
MRI pituitary	Baseline, 3-yearly

Box 9.6 Prognosis

MEN-1 is associated with a mortality of nearly 50% by the age of 50 years. The commonest cause of death is metastatic pancreatic NENs. With modern management of gastrinomas, improved surveillance, and timely intervention, patients with MEN-1 are living longer.

Further reading

Brandi ML, Gagel AF, Angeli A, et al. (2001). Guidelines for diagnosis and therapy of MEN type 1 and 2. *J Clin Endocrinol Metab* **86**, 5658–71.

Thakker RV, Newey PJ, Walls GV, et al. (2012). Clinical practice guidelines for multiple endocrine neoplasia type 1 (MEN1). *J Clin Endocrinol Metab* **97**, 2990–3011.

MEN type 2

Definitions
MEN-2 may be divided into three forms:
- MEN-2A comprises of familial medullary thyroid carcinoma (FMTC) in combination with phaeochromocytoma and parathyroid tumours. MEN-2A accounts for nearly 90–95% of all MEN-2 cases.
- MEN-2B is defined as the occurrence of FMTC in association with phaeochromocytoma, mucosal neuromas, and a marfanoid habitus.
- FMTC may also occur in isolation.
- See Table 9.7 for classification.

Genetics
- MEN-2 is an autosomal dominant condition.
- The *C-RET* proto-oncogene, activating mutations of which cause MEN-2, is located on the long arm of chromosome 10 (10q11.2).
- This gene encodes RET which is a transmembrane receptor with an extracellular cysteine-rich domain and an intracellular tyrosine kinase domain. The protein plays a role in the development of the neural crest and the enteric nervous system.
- The *C-RET* proto-oncogene is also involved, via inactivating mutations, in the aetiology of Hirschsprung's disease.
- Different germline mutations cause different clinical syndromes. In contrast to MEN-1, MEN-2 shows a strong genotype–phenotype correlation.
- Approximately 50% of MEN-2A is caused by a codon 634 mutation, and nearly all MEN-2B is caused by the Met918Thr mutation.
- Mutational analysis is available in the UK.

Clinical features—MEN-2A
MTC
- MTC is often the initial manifestation and is generally multifocal.
- Phaeochromocytoma and parathyroid disease typically develop later.
- Diagnosis of MTC requires histological analysis which reveals C cell hyperplasia and stromal amyloid.
- Circulating calcitonin levels are generally elevated, but hypocalcaemia is not seen.
- CEA is also elevated and is a useful tumour marker.
- With metastatic disease, diarrhoea is common (30%).
- Rarely, these tumours secrete ACTH, resulting in Cushing's syndrome due to ectopic ACTH secretion.

Phaeochromocytoma
- Usually presents later than MTC.
- Most commonly associated with codon 634 mutations.
- 50% will be bilateral, but malignancy is rare (<10%).
- These lesions must be excluded prior to surgery for any other indication.

Table 9.7 Classification and presentation of MEN-2

Pathology	MEN-2A	MEN-2B	FMTC
MTC	95%	~100%	~100%
Phaeochromocytoma	50%	50%	Not present
Parathyroid neoplasia	20–30%	Not present	Not present
Marfanoid habitus	Not present	75%	Not present
Mucosal neuromas	Not present	10–20%	Not present
Intestinal ganglioneuromatosis	Not present	~40%	Not present

Primary hyperparathyroidism
- Generally results from hyperplasia of the glands.
- Mainly associated with codon 634 mutations, less commonly with other *RET* mutations.
- Can present as early as 5 years with codon 634 mutations, and commencement of early screening is recommended.

Clinical features—MEN-2B
- Mucosal neuromas can be found on the distal tongue, conjunctiva, and throughout the gastrointestinal tract (may cause malabsorption).
- A marfanoid habitus is typically evident.
- MTC tends to present earlier than in MEN-2A and frequently follows a more aggressive course.

Management of MEN type 2

(See Box 9.7 for prognosis.)

MTC

- The definitive treatment is adequate surgery by total thyroidectomy and careful lymph node dissection by an experienced surgeon. (Check calcitonin 3 months post-operatively.)
- Post-operative levothyroxine is administered to all patients. These tumours are not TSH-driven, therefore TSH suppression is not recommended.
- Tumour spread is usually local, but distant metastases do occur.
- Regular post-operative calcitonin assessment (first 3 months, then 6–12-monthly) is used to monitor for disease recurrence.
- MRI, octreotide scanning, and venous catheterization may all be helpful in staging disease recurrence.
- Treatment of recurrent disease responds poorly to radiotherapy or chemotherapy and, consequently, is generally surgical, if appropriate.
- Somatostatin analogues may help symptom control, e.g. diarrhoea, but do not appear to have an antitumour effect.
- Few data are available to date, but therapy with radiolabelled MIBG or somatostatin analogues appears to offer significant symptomatic improvement, although tumour stabilization and/or regression was observed only rarely.
- Molecular therapies that inhibit RET and other tyrosine kinases may be of benefit in metastatic MTC, e.g. vandetanib.
- Children with MEN-2 should be considered for early prophylactic surgery. This should generally be performed before the age of 5 years and before the age of 1 year in patients with the highest risk of mutations.
- Different mutations are associated with specific phenotypes. Risk stratifications of mutations should guide planning of management in terms of screening, timing, and extent of surgery, in conjunction with clinical, imaging, and biochemical data.

Phaeochromocytoma

- These tumours are best treated medically with α- and β-blockade, followed by surgical removal.
- The risk of multifocal and/or recurrent disease must be considered, although malignant phaeochromocytomas are rare.
- Screening has resulted in the earlier detection of these lesions.

Primary hyperparathyroidism

The criteria for diagnosis and the indications for surgery are broadly similar to those for sporadic 1° hyperparathyroidism.

Mutational analysis

- First- and second-degree relatives of patients with MEN-2 and genetic analysis should be performed as early as possible in at-risk children so that appropriate treatment can be planned early.
- Consider screening in patients with sporadic MTC or sporadic phaeochromocytoma or in patients with mucosal neuromas or other phenotypic features compatible with MEN-2B.
- Somatic *RET* oncogene mutations confer a worse prognosis in sporadic medullary carcinoma.

Screening for MEN type 2

Biochemical and radiological screening is relevant for affected patients, asymptomatic mutation carriers, and first- and second-degree relatives in families with a clinical diagnosis of MEN-2, but where a mutation has not been identified (see Table 9.8).

Table 9.8 Screening in MEN-2

Test	Frequency
Calcitonin, CEA	Annual
Phaeochromocytoma screen	Annual
Calcium ± PTH	Annual
MRI adrenals	Annual to 3-yearly

Box 9.7 Prognosis

- Variable.
- Overall, 10-year survival rate for MEN-2B is 65% and for MEN-2A 80%. The outcomes depend on the presence of metastases from MTC.
- The prognosis for these patients is improving with earlier screening and intervention.
- Children who have had timely and appropriate thyroidectomy are leading healthy lives.

Further reading

Brandi ML, Gagel AF, Angeli A, et al. (2001). Guidelines for diagnosis and therapy of MEN type 1 and 2. *J Clin Endocrinol Metab* **86**, 5658–71.

Carling T (2005). Multiple endocrine neoplasia syndrome: genetic basis for clinical management. *J Curr Opin Oncol* **17**, 7–12.

Constante G, Meringolo D, Durante C, et al. (2007). Predictive value of serum calcitonin levels for preoperative diagnosis of medullary thyroid carcinoma in a cohort of 5817 consecutive patients with thyroid nodules. *J Clin Endocrinol Metab* **92**, 450–5.

Marx SJ (2005). Molecular genetics of multiple endocrine neoplasia types 1 and 2. *J Nat Rev Cancer* **5**, 367–75.

Waguespack SG, Rich TA, Perrier ND, et al. (2011). Management of medullary thyroid carcinoma and MEN2 syndromes in childhood. *Nat Rev Endocrinol* **7**, 596–607.

Wirth LJ, et al. (2013). Case records of the Massachusetts General Hospital. Case 5-2013. A 52-year-old woman with a mass in the thyroid. *N Engl J Med* **368**, 664–73.

Inherited primary hyperparathyroidism

Definitions
- Parathyroid tumours affect 1 per 1,000 population.
- 1° hyperparathyroidism is inherited in up to 10% of patients.

Causes
- MEN-1.
- MEN-2A.
- Hyperparathyroidism-jaw tumour syndrome (HPT-JT).
- Familial isolated hyperparathyroidism (FIHP).

HPT-JT
- Autosomal dominant condition.
- Characterized by pathology in three main tissues:
  - Parathyroid tumours which show a high penetrance in these patients and, in up to 15% of cases, will be parathyroid carcinomas.
  - Ossifying fibromas which affect the maxilla and/or mandible in around 30% of HPT-JT patients.
- Renal manifestations may also occur, the commonest are bilateral renal cysts (19% of patients) but also include hamartomas and Wilms' tumours.
- Benign and malignant uterine pathology is seen in up to 75% of women with HPT-JT and reduces reproductive fitness.
- In sporadic parathyroid cancer, *HRPT2* somatic mutations have been identified in 75% of tumours.
- Other tumours have also been reported in these patients, including pancreatic adenocarcinomas, testicular mixed germ cell tumours, Hürthle cell thyroid adenomas, and benign and malignant uterine tumours.
- The gene (*HRPT2*), inactivating mutations of which are responsible for HPT-JT, has been identified on the long arm of chromosome 1 (1q31.2), and mutational analysis is available in the UK.
- The function of the protein product (parafibromin) encoded by this tumour suppressor gene is unknown.

FIHP
- Affected individuals within a kindred suffer only from 1° hyperparathyroidism as an isolated endocrinopathy.
- In some kindreds, mutations in the *MEN-1* or *HRPT2* genes have been identified, but, in the majority, the cause is still unknown.

Further reading
Carpten JD, Robbins CM, Villablanca A, *et al.* (2002). HRPT2, encoding parafibromin, is mutated in hyperparathyroidism-jaw tumor syndrome. *Nat Genet* **32**, 676–80.

Marx SJ (2002). Hyperparathyroidism in hereditary syndromes: special expressions and special managements. *J Bone Miner Res* **17**, N37–43.

Inherited renal calculi

Definitions

- Renal calculi affect 12% of ♂ and 5% of ♀ by the 7th decade of life.
- Renal calculi arise due to a reduced urine volume or ↑ excretion of stone-forming components, such as calcium, oxalate, urate, cystine, xanthine, and phosphate.
- A variety of causes for renal stones are established (see Box 9.11 for general causes of nephrolithiasis), but the commonest aetiology is hypercalciuria.
- Calcium stones account for >80% of all renal calculi.
- Uric acid stones comprise 5–10% of all renal calculi.
- The commonest cause of hypercalciuria is hypercalcaemia, and this, in turn, is most frequently 2° to 1° hyperparathyroidism.
- Nephrolithiasis is frequently a recurrent condition, with a relapse rate of 75% in 20 years.
- Features associated with recurrence include early age of onset, +ve family history, and lithiasis related to infection or underlying medical conditions.

Genetics

- Renal calculi generally arise from complex multifactorial disease resulting from an interaction between genetic and environmental factors.
- The disorder may be familial in up to 45% of patients.
- The majority of causative genes are probably, as yet, unidentified and account for much of 'idiopathic' calcium nephrolithiasis.
- Many cases of hypercalciuria are likely to be polygenic, but two examples of monogenic causes are Dent's disease and autosomal dominant hypocalcaemic hypercalciuria (ADHH).

Dent's disease

- X-linked condition.
- Due to inactivating mutations in a chloride channel (*CLC5*) gene.
- Characterized by hypercalciuria, nephrocalcinosis, β2 microglobinuria, progressive glomerular disease, and mild rickets due to renal phosphate loss in affected ♀.

Familial hypocalciuric hypercalcaemia (FHH)

- Autosomal dominant condition.
- Due to activating mutations in the calcium-sensing receptor gene.
- May be asymptomatic or present early with neonatal or childhood seizures.

See Box 9.8 for causes and Box 9.9 for mutational analysis.

Box 9.8 Causes of renal calculi
- Hypercalciuria.
- Hyperoxaluria.
- Hyperuricosuria.
- Hypocitraturia.
- Urinary tract infection, e.g. *Proteus*, *Pseudomonas*, *Klebsiella*.
- 1° renal disease, e.g. polycystic kidney disease.
- Drugs, e.g. indinavir (protease inhibitor-antiretroviral), diuretics, salicylates, allopurinol, some chemotherapeutic agents.

Box 9.9 Mutational analysis
- Currently, largely a research tool.
- Mutations in a variety of genes have been reported to result in renal calculi due to hypercalciuria, hyperoxaluria, cystinuria, or hyperuricosuria.
- As these research tests move into the clinical domain, then family screening will become increasingly relevant.

Investigation of renal calculi (see also Table 9.9)
- 24h urine volume and urine osmolarity (low urine volume raises production of solutes).
- 24h urinary calcium excretion.
- Urine pH.
- Stone composition, if possible.
- Exclude causes of hypercalcaemia (hyperparathyroidism, immobilization, or renal tubular acidosis).
- Exclude hypercalciuria (excess chloride, excess sodium, malignancy, sarcoidosis, renal calcium leak, and drugs, e.g. levothyroxine or loop diuretics).
- Exclude causes of hyperoxaluria (1° hyperoxaluria, vitamin B6 deficiency, short bowel syndrome, and excess dietary oxalates).
- Exclude urinary tract infection.
- Exclude causes of hyperuricosuria (gout, dietary, uricosuric drugs, binge drinking, or myeloproliferative disorders).
- Exclude causes of hypocitraturia—citrate is the 1° agent for removal of excess calcium (renal tubular acidosis, potassium or magnesium deficiency, urinary tract infection, renal failure, and chronic diarrhoea).
- Exclude cysteine (usually genetic in origin) or xanthine (usually 2° to allopurinol treatment) stones.

Management
- Increase fluid intake.
- Appropriate dietary modifications.
- Treat underlying cause.

Table 9.9 Acid load test for diagnosis of renal tubular acidosis

Side effects	Nausea
Procedure	Normal breakfast
	Fluid intake 200–300ml/h
	08.00 empty bladder
	Hourly collection of urine for pH over 10h
	10.00 ammonium chloride capsules 0.1g/kg taken over 1h to avoid gastric irritation
Sampling	Urine hourly–pH
	Electrolytes 10:00 14:00 18:00
Interpretation	Urine pH should fall <5.2
	Plasma bicarbonate should fall (ammonium chloride absorbed)

Causes of hypercalciuria

With hypercalcaemia

- Primary hyperparathyroidism.
- Granulomatous disease.
- Vitamin D excess.
- Malignancy (rare as a cause of stone).
- Hyperthyroidism.

With normocalcaemia

- Distal renal tubular acidosis.
- Granulomatous disease.
- Cushing's disease.
- Idiopathic hypercalciuria.
- Dent's disease.
- Bartter syndrome.
- Hypocalcaemic hypercalciuria.
- Hereditary hypophosphataemic rickets.
- Acromegaly.

Further reading

Langman CB (2004). The molecular basis of kidney stones. *Curr Opin Paediatr* **16**, 188–93.

Sakhaee K, *et al.* (2012). Clinical review. Kidney stones 2012: pathogenesis, diagnosis, and management. *J Clin Endocrinol Metab* **97**,1847–60.

Thakker RV (2004). Diseases associated with the extracellular calcium-sensing receptor. *Cell Calcium* **35**, 275–82.

Worcester EM, Coe FL. (2010). Clinical practice. Calcium kidney stones. *N Engl J Med* **363**, 954–63.

Endocrine surgery

Transsphenoidal surgery/craniotomy

Preoperative assessment

Confirm the following:

- Anterior and posterior pituitary function normal or on adequate replacement:
  - Short Synacthen® test (note both the 0 and 30min values), and/or normal ACTH/9 a.m. cortisol. NB Patients with recent loss of ACTH will have a normal response to SST, as adrenal atrophy will not have evolved. If in any doubt, replace with glucocorticoids.
  - FT_4.
  - LH, FSH, oestradiol, or testosterone.
  - Prolactin.
  - Serum and urine osmolality, and electrolytes if polyuric.
- Recent (<3 months) MRI pituitary.
- Formal visual field perimetry and visual acuity assessment.
- Document extraocular muscle movements.
- Urea and electrolytes (<1 week presurgery).
- Group and save serum.
- MRSA screen should be done at least 2 weeks prior to admission for surgery if the patient has been in hospital within the last year.
- Record therapeutic options discussed with patient, including:
  - Risks of surgery (e.g. CSF leakage, meningitis, bleeding, partial or total hypopituitarism, including diabetes insipidus, and potential effects on fertility and visual deterioration).
  - Risk of recurrence requiring further surgery or radiotherapy.
  - Warn patients that a sample of fat may be taken from their thigh or abdomen for packing of the pituitary fossa.
  - Reiterate the need for lifelong follow-up.
- Ensure antibiotic prophylaxis is given prior to surgery (the precise regimen may vary, depending on the centre and patient, e.g. flucloxacillin 500mg qds and amoxicillin 500mg tds PO/IV; use erythromycin if penicillin-allergic). Some surgeons advocate a prolonged course of antibiotics if CSF leakage occurs whilst others recommend close surveillance and prompt treatment if concern regarding possible meningitis (NB lower threshold for patients with Cushing's disease).
- MRSA +ve patients require prophylaxis with IV vancomycin.
- If steroid-deficient, steroid reserve is unknown, or if a patient has Cushing's disease (inadequate stress response), give *hydrocortisone* 20mg orally with morning premedication.
- If on levothyroxine preoperatively (for 2° hypothyroidism), change to equivalent dose of T_3.

Post-operative

- Start hydrocortisone (20mg at 8 a.m./10mg at 12 noon/10mg at 6p.m.) after surgery. Reduce to hydrocortisone 10mg/5mg/5mg on day 3 post-operatively.
- Watch for: headache, fever/photophobia/other signs of meningitis, CSF leak, deterioration of vision, diplopia, bleeding, symptoms of hyponatraemia.
- Fluid balance—watch for diabetes insipidus:
  - Review the clinical status of the patient at regular intervals (? euvolaemic/hypovolaemic/hypervolaemic).
  - Record fluid input/output assiduously (NB fluid replacement in theatre may be excessive; therefore, always include perioperative fluids in fluid balance charts, and note sodium content).
  - Check U&Es, plasma and urine osmolalities on a regular basis (at least once daily and more frequently if clinical concerns).
  - Post-operatively, restrict to 2L total fluid input (IV and PO).
  - If patient becomes polyuric, i.e. >200mL/h for ≥3 consecutive hours (in the context of a 2L/24h fluid restriction), then urgently check plasma U&Es, plasma and urine osmolalities, and urinary sodium. While waiting for results, allow free fluids; aim to replace the fluid deficit.
  - If diabetes insipidus confirmed by the results, give a single dose of *desamino-D-arginine vasopressin* (desmopressin) (1 microgram SC).
  - When fluid deficit has been replaced (usually orally), restart 2–3L fluid restriction (again, include IV and PO routes).
  - If polyuria recurs, treat as before.
  - Regular U&Es, plasma and urine osmolalities required.
  - If polyuria continues to recur up to and after 96h post-operatively, consider regular DDAVP orally or intranasally, if possible (not if a transsphenoidal approach is used).
- Hyponatraemia occurring 1 week after a transsphenoidal adenectomy is most commonly due to SIADH; rarely, cerebral salt wasting may occur. Check urinary sodium, and assess fluid status (cerebral salt wasting causes very high urinary sodium and is associated with dehydration and a high urine volume).
- Check for CSF leakage: bedside-test nasal fluid with Glucostix® and send a sample for beta-transferrin/tau-protein (abundant in neurons) for confirmation (+ve if CSF).
- If patients sent home on day 3 post-operatively, they should be advised to watch for a fever, headache, excessive sensitivity to light, confusion, drowsiness, vomiting, nasal discharge, deterioration of vision, excessive urination (>200mL/h for ≥3 consecutive hours).
- In patients with Cushing's disease, check 9 a.m. cortisol concentrations on day 7, having omitted hydrocortisone dose on the evening before and on the morning of the test. 9 a.m. cortisol <50nmol/L suggests cure; occasionally, cortisol takes a few days to fall to undetectable levels.
- For all patients on day 7, recheck visual acuity and formal visual field perimetry and eye movements, along with FBC, ESR, LFTs, U&Es,

plasma and urine osmolalities, glucose, TFTs (for those patients not on T_3).
- Comment on results:
  - If FT_4 and FT_3 low, offer T_3 and recheck TFTs in 6 weeks.
  - If serum cortisol >450nmol/L, stop hydrocortisone.
  - If serum cortisol 150–450nmol/L, stop hydrocortisone and cover with steroids in times of stress.
  - If serum cortisol <150nmol/L, continue on hydrocortisone.
- Recheck HPA axis 6 weeks post-operatively.
- Give information to patient, including advice on driving:
  - For an ordinary driving licence (group 1, car or motorcycle), a minimum horizontal field of 120 degrees is required as well as no significant defect within the central 20 degrees. For a licence to drive a group 2 vehicle (bus or lorry), then normal binocular field is required. Taxi driver licence regulations vary locally.
  - If an individual has normal visual fields and acuity and an uncomplicated transsphenoidal operation, they may restart to drive once recovered from the surgery (group 1 and group 2 licences).
  - Following a craniotomy, group 2 licence holders are suspended for 6 months; however, group 1 licence holders can restart driving once recovered, providing their vision is satisfactory and there is no history of seizures.
  - All patients should inform their insurance company about the pituitary tumour and pituitary surgery.
- Give information to patient on contact details for the Pituitary Foundation support group and DVLA:
  - The Pituitary Foundation, 17/18 The Courtyard, Woodlands, Bradley Stoke, Bristol BS12 4NQ. Tel: 01454 201612.
  - Medical Adviser, The Drivers' Medical Branch, 2 Sandringham Park, Swansea Vale, Llansamlet, Swansea SA6 8QD. Tel: 0870 0600 0301.

Thyroidectomy

Preoperative

- Ensure euthyroidism. Surgery in the presence of poorly controlled hyperthyroidism is associated with an increased post-operative mortality (often by precipitation of a thyroid storm).
- If surgery is required in the presence of hyperthyroidism, give *potassium iodide* (60mg 3× a day for 10 days); this reduces thyroid hormone release and probably decreases perioperative blood loss. The radiographic contrast agent iopanoic acid, which is rich in iodine, provides a useful alternative and has the additional benefit of potently inhibiting the 5-deiodinase, thus reducing T_4 to T_3 conversion. Oral *propranolol* (40–120mg 3× a day) reduces clinical manifestations of thyrotoxicosis. Steroids (e.g. hydrocortisone 100mg IV 4× a day) can be used to decrease T_4 to T_3 conversion.
- Check vocal cord function by indirect laryngoscopy.
- Warn of post-operative risks: recurrent laryngeal nerve damage <1%, keloid scarring, haemorrhage, permanent hypoparathyroidism <0.5%, and hypothyroidism (10% of partial thyroidectomy patients).

Post-operative

- Risk of haemorrhage in first 24h, particularly major haemorrhage deep to the strap muscles leading to airway compression. Watch for stridor, respiratory difficulties, and wound swelling. Drainage from wound drains is unhelpful. Treat by evacuating the haematoma; consider intubation or a tracheostomy. Clip removers and artery forceps should be kept to hand on the ward.
- Recurrent laryngeal nerve damage is permanent in <1% and transient in 2–4%. Patient's voice is often husky for about 3 weeks post-operatively and may be treated with lozenges and humidified air.
- Symptomatic unilateral damage can be treated by stabilization of the affected cord in adduction by submucosal Teflon® injection under direct laryngoscopy.
- Bilateral damage leads to unopposed adductor action of the cricothyroid muscle which causes glottis closure and airway obstruction. Treatment involves reintubation, paralysis, hydrocortisone (100mg 4× a day IM for oedema), and extubation at 24h—if that fails, a tracheostomy should be performed.
- If recurrent laryngeal nerve damage is persistent at 9 months, an attempt can be made to resuture the nerve.
- Monitor calcium. Transient hypoparathyroidism is usually evident within 7 days (for treatment, 📖 see Hypoparathyroidism, p. 478).
- Patients undergoing thyroidectomy are at high risk of post-operative nausea and vomiting.
- Following total thyroidectomy for malignancy, the patient should be converted to T_3, which should be stopped at least 10 days prior to the post-operative radioiodine uptake scan to allow the TSH to rise (📖 see Follow-up of papillary and FTC, p. 100). Alternatively, recombinant TSH can be used for the scan.

- If total thyroidectomy is performed for hyperthyroidism, levothyroxine (~1.6 micrograms/kg) should be commenced 4–5 days post-operatively, as, during the operation, handling of the thyroid results in release of stored thyroid hormones, and levothyroxine has a long half-life. Check TSH in 6–8 weeks.
- Following partial thyroidectomy, transient biochemical hypothyroidism may occur during the first 2 months and does not warrant treatment, unless the patient is symptomatic or it becomes persistent.

Parathyroidectomy

Parathyroidectomy of one or two glands undertaken for 1° hyperparathyroidism may result in transient and self-limiting hypocalcaemia. Total parathyroidectomy (e.g. for MEN-1 or as part of surgical management of advanced head and neck malignancy) may be complicated by severe and permanent hypocalcaemia which may be very difficult to manage.

Post-operative care for patients undergoing parathyroidectomy of 1–2 glands

- Check calcium, phosphate, magnesium, albumin on the evening of surgery and daily thereafter. Calcium begins to fall post-operatively after about 4–12h; the nadir is usually reached by 24h. Calcium may recover spontaneously; however, one-third of patients will require calcium support perioperatively. With the advent of minimally invasive parathyroidectomy and short hospital stays (<24h), many centres advocate prophylactic calcium and vitamin D replacement in all cases in the immediate aftermath of surgery, which is continued until the patient is reviewed 1–2 weeks later in the outpatient clinic.
- *Symptoms of hypocalcaemia* (mainly due to neuromuscular irritability): perioral paraesthesiae, Chvostek's sign, Trousseau's sign, tetany, laryngospasm, bronchospasm, seizures, prolonged QT interval on ECG, extrapyramidal movement disorders, and delirium. Calcium levels often <1.75mmol/L before symptoms manifest, although rapid changes in calcium result in more pronounced symptomatology.
- Magnesium deficiency is common due to previous hyperparathyroidism (causes renal wasting of magnesium). Chronic magnesium deficiency impairs release of PTH and causes functional hypoparathyroidism and hypocalcaemia.

Causes of hypocalcaemia post-1–2 gland removal

- *'Functional hypoparathyroidism'* common. Causes: delayed recovery of the other parathyroid glands due to long-term suppression; parathyroid gland ischaemia; parathyroid gland 'stunning' by intraoperative handling; hypomagnesaemia. PTH level will be detectable; phosphate should be normal. Usually spontaneously improves over days to weeks. Management of symptomatic hypocalcaemia (Ca usually <1.8mmol/L) with calcium (up to 2g/day in divided doses). Add in vitamin D/vitamin D metabolites if persistent hypocalcaemia. Replace magnesium, as necessary. Gradual withdrawal of therapy to assess recovery.
- *'Hungry bone syndrome'* due to extensive skeletal remineralization once skeleton released from PTH excess. Ongoing ↑ ALP, ↓ calcium, ↓ PO_4, ↓ Mg. PTH levels may be normal or high. Pre-existing vitamin D deficiency will exacerbate hypocalcaemia. May require large doses of calcium and vitamin D/vitamin D metabolites for weeks to months.
- *Permanent hypoparathyroidism.* Rare (<2% of cases). Check PTH level after day 3; level will be undetectable (<1pg/mL). Replace with oral calcium and vitamin D/vitamin D metabolites long-term.

- Other complications:
  - Recurrent laryngeal nerve palsy (<1%).
  - Failure to correct hypercalcaemia.
- Overall, both minimally invasive and conventional parathyroidectomy are very safe operations, with low morbidity and mortality.

Calcium management following total parathyroidectomy

- Hypocalcaemia is inevitable unless management instituted.
- Pre-emptive treatment is worth considering (e.g. 1α-calcidol 1–2 micrograms/day—this dose may be insufficient to completely prevent hypocalcaemia but may prevent life-threatening hypocalcaemia and is unlikely to cause serious toxicity in the short term).
- Acute management in patients with life-threatening hypocalcaemia (e.g. Trousseau's sign, laryngospasm, seizures):
  - 10mL of 10% calcium gluconate, diluted 1 in 10 in normal saline or glucose 5%, infused into large vein over 10min. Monitor cardiac rhythm.
  - Repeat, as necessary, to control acute emergency.
  - Patients will need ongoing calcium replacement: 100mL of 10% calcium gluconate in 1L of 5% glucose or 0.9% sodium chloride, infused over 24h (monitor calcium regularly (4–6-hourly), and adjust rate as necessary).
  - Start oral vitamin D analogues and oral calcium.

Vitamin D analogues (1α-calcidol; calcitriol)

- Potent and effective in acute hypocalcaemia due to rapid correction of calcium. Short half-lives allows for rapid and careful titration of dose in response to calcium levels. Narrow therapeutic window (but hypercalcaemia much shorter lived if it develops).
- Dose for dose, calcitriol twice as efficacious as 1α-calcidol (i.e. 1 microgram calcitriol equivalent to 2 micrograms 1α-calcidol). 1α-calcidol can be given down an NG tube.
- Starting doses usually high (e.g. 4–8 micrograms/day of 1α-calcidol in divided doses), rapidly weaned to maintenance doses (typically 1–2 micrograms/day 1α-calcidol).
- Reassess often (at least every 1–2 days) in early stages of management. Longer-term options include ergocalciferol or colecalciferol, but hypercalcaemia will be more prolonged if it develops.

Calcium

- 1–2g/daily in divided doses. A maximum daily absorbable dose of calcium is probably 3g day.
- Absorption may vary from different types of calcium salts and may be greater when calcium is given away from food.
- The long-term aim is to manage without calcium, just on vitamin D/vitamin D metabolites.

Long-term goal of management is to prevent symptoms of hypocalcaemia without toxicity. Aim for lower half of normal range (2.0–2.3mmol/L), with normal urinary calcium excretion (to minimize risk of nephrolithiasis and nephrocalcinosis).

Phaeochromocytoma

Preoperative

- Check for bilateral disease or metastases: MRI chest and abdomen, and an MIBG scan (10% multiple).
- Ensure adequate α- and β-blockade once the diagnosis is made.
- Start β-blockade only AFTER patient has been adequately α-blocked (unopposed β-blockade can lead to marked vasoconstriction, ischaemic damage, and hypertension).
  - α-*blockade*. Start *phenoxybenzamine* (10–20mg PO, 3–4× day)—an irreversible α-blocker. Adequacy of dose assessed by monitoring haematocrit and postural BP drop (reflex vasodilation). Side effects include dizziness, lethargy, and ankle swelling. Some centres use doxazosin; others are concerned that this does not offer both α1- and α2-blockade.
  - Start treatment at least 1 week before surgery, ideally >3 weeks.
  - β-*blockade*. Start *propranolol* (20–80mg PO, 3× day) when patient adequately α-blocked. Titrate to maximum tolerated or a total dose of 240mg/day in divided doses.
- Control BP: α- and β-blockers often sufficient; if not, add a calcium channel blocker or an ACE inhibitor; α-methyltyrosine 1–4g/day (a false catecholamine precursor which inhibits tyrosine hydroxylase, the rate-limiting step for catecholamine synthesis) is rarely used to control BP.
- Some centres advocate the use of additional IV phenoxybenzamine (0.5–1.0mg/kg in 250mL 5% dextrose, given over 2h) for 3 days prior to surgery (titrate the dose according to BP; often, 0.5mg/kg is sufficient).
- Monitor haemoglobin/haematocrit (because of haemodilution, preoperative blood transfusions may be necessary) and postural BP.
- Group and save serum, and cross-match 2 units of blood.
- Ensure that the patient is well hydrated (if necessary, use an IV infusion of saline) prior to going to theatre.

Post-operative

- Stop α- and β-blockers.
- Watch for ↓ BP: sudden withdrawal of catecholamines leads to marked arterial and venous dilatation. This is worsened by inadequate volume loading and should initially be treated with volume replacement rather than by pressor agents.
- If hypertension persists 2 weeks post-operatively, then residual tumour or metastases must be considered.
- Long-term monitoring required, as approximately 14% recur.
- If bilateral adrenalectomy performed, see next section.

Bilateral adrenalectomy

- Give hydrocortisone (100mg, 4× day IM) post-operatively; this will provide adequate mineralocorticoid as well as glucocorticoid cover. Continue this until eating and drinking (often <48h). Monitor U&Es.
- From day 3, give hydrocortisone PO (double usual replacement dose, e.g. 20mg/10mg/10mg), and add fludrocortisone PO (100 micrograms daily).
- Long-term replacement with hydrocortisone 10mg/5mg/5mg, and fludrocortisone 50–150 micrograms daily.

Phaeochromocytoma in pregnancy (see p. 447)

- Rare condition; may present as paradoxical supine hypertension, with pressure from the gravid uterus causing release of catecholamines, and normal blood pressure in the supine and erect positions.
- Start α-blockade, then β-blockade; phenoxybenzamine can cross the placenta but is generally safe for the fetus (may cause perinatal CNS depression and transient hypotension). Propranolol has been reported to be associated with intrauterine growth retardation, fetal bradycardia and hypoglycaemia, and premature labour.
- Surgery is more controversial, although some authors advocate surgery in the first and second trimesters up to 24 weeks' gestation.
- Caesarian section is advocated, with a combined tumour resection. Vaginal delivery carries a significant maternal risk.

Endocrinology and ageing

Endocrinology and ageing

Introduction

- Ageing causes changes in many hormonal axes. How much of this change is normal physiology associated with ageing and how much represents true endocrine dysfunction, and thus warrants treatment, is unclear.
- Concomitant disease and polypharmacy are common in the elderly population, with frequent 2° effects upon the endocrine system.

Fluid and electrolyte homeostasis in the elderly

- Elderly patients are particularly prone to fluid and electrolyte disturbances due to changes associated with ageing, concomitant disease, and drug usage.
- Elderly patients have ↓ renal function compared with younger patients:
  - ↓ glomerular filtration rate, with creatinine clearance ↓ by 8mL/min/1.73m^2 per decade after age 30.
  - ↑ renovascular disease.
  - ↓ renal sensitivity to circulating hormones:
    — Aldosterone.
    — Vasopressin.
    — Atrial natriuretic peptide (probable).
  - ↓ ability to dilute or concentrate urine.
- Elderly patients have ↓ renin levels, with 2° decreases of aldosterone levels (both basal and stimulated levels). Aldosterone levels may be <50% normal by 70 years of age. ↓ renal sensitivity to aldosterone may result in isolated mineralocorticoid deficiency (distal renal tubular acidosis (type 4) with hyponatraemia, hyperkalaemia, hyperchloraemia, and normal anion gap acidosis); this is more common with diabetes mellitus.

Vasopressin/ADH

- Unlike many other hormones, vasopressin (ADH) responses are potentiated in elderly patients, with ↑ release from the neurohypophysis in response to an osmotic stimulus and less effective suppression. Normal vasopressin release is a balance of inhibitory and stimulatory effects at baroreceptors and osmoreceptors. It may be that loss of inhibition with ageing due to degenerative changes results in relatively unopposed stimulation of ADH and a ↓ ability to suppress ADH release.
- In addition, altered renal sensitivity to vasopressin results in ↓ ability to excrete free water.

Hypernatraemia and dehydration

- Perception of thirst is altered in elderly persons (in younger people, thirst is perceived at plasma osmolalities >292mOsm/kg, whereas in older people, thirst is perceived at plasma osmolalities >296mOsm/kg). Elderly patients may also be unable to ingest fluids because of other disabilities and/or effects of medications.
- Thus, elderly persons are particularly susceptible to dehydration when there are increased fluid losses (e.g. during hot summers). This is exacerbated by impaired renal concentrating ability.

Hyponatraemia

- Common. Hyponatraemia affects 7% of healthy elderly people, 15–18% of elderly people in residential care facilities, and 53% of elderly people in nursing care facilities.
- Mortality rates in hospitalized elderly patients with hyponatraemia are high (in patients aged >65 years, 16% mortality in those with hyponatraemia, compared with 8% without hyponatraemia).
- Often associated with medication (e.g. diuretics).
- Commonest electrolyte disturbance in cancer (📖 see SIADH due to ectopic vasopressin production, p. 648).
- Symptoms include confusion, lethargy, coma, seizures.
- Overall approach to investigation and management is similar to that of hyponatraemia in younger patients (📖 see Hyponatraemia, p. 216).
- Mild idiopathic hyponatraemia is also recognized in elderly patients, without necessarily having sinister cause or consequence, and is thought to be 2° to altered threshold for ADH secretion.

Further reading

Ayus JC (1996). Abnormalities of water metabolism in the elderly. *Semin Nephrol* **16**, 277–88.
Beck LH (1998). Changes in renal function with ageing. *Clin Geriatr Med* **14**, 199–209.

Bone disease in the elderly

Osteoporosis

Osteoporosis is not an inevitable part of ageing, but it is a common disease in elderly people and is associated with high morbidity and mortality in both males and females (☐ see Osteoporosis, p. 490).

Vitamin D deficiency (☐ p. 484)

- Very common in the elderly.
- Vitamin D insufficiency (evidence of 2° hyperparathyroidism, ↑ bone turnover, BMD loss) occurs at levels of 25OH vitamin D <50nmol/L.
- Vitamin D deficiency usually defined as concentrations <25nmol/L.
- Vitamin D deficiency and/or insufficiency is common, particularly in elderly institutionalized patients, in extreme latitudes, and in fracture patients.
- Supplementation in free-living elderly patients (>65 years of age) ↓ fracture risk.

Primary hyperparathyroidism

- Prevalence of 1° hyperparathyroidism is 10/100,000 in ♀ <40 years old, rising to 190/100,000 in ♀ >65 years old. Half of all cases of 1° hyperparathyroidism occur in ♀ >60 years old.
- Elderly people are more prone to symptoms (weakness, fatigue, confusion) at relatively mild levels of hypercalcaemia (2.8–3.0mmol/L).
- Other causes of hypercalcaemia must be excluded.
- Coexisting vitamin D insufficiency and deficiency is common.
- Management is similar to that described in ☐ Chapter 6, Hypercalcaemia, p. 460.
- Surgery is not contraindicated by age alone.

Paget's disease

☐ see Chapter 6, Paget's disease, pp. 506–9.

Further reading

Mosekilde L (2005). Vitamin D and the elderly. *Clin End* **62**, 265–81.

GH and IGF-1 in the elderly

- Many of the features of normal ageing resemble those of growth hormone deficiency in younger patients.
- Changes in body composition with ageing include ↓ lean body mass (↓ body water, ↓ muscle mass, and ↓ bone mass) and ↑ total body fat and visceral fat mass, associated with abnormal lipid profile (↑ total and LDL cholesterol, ↑ TGs), insulin resistance, and ↓ exercise and cardiac capacity.
- Overall, integrated GH concentrations show a decrease with age, with ↓ GH pulse amplitude and duration, but pulse frequency unchanged. For ♂ over 25 years old, GH secretion ↓ by ~50% every 7 years.
- IGF-1 ↓ with ↑ age (reflected in age-adjusted normative ranges).
- IGFBP-3 ↓ with ↑ age (and is also GH-dependent).
- The ↓ in GH concentration with age is likely to be related to altered hypothalamic regulation, rather than a decreased secretory capacity.
- Other factors may also ↓ GH/IGF-1 concentrations with ageing, such as ↓ physical fitness, ↓ production of sex hormones, fragmented sleep (GH is secreted mainly during slow-wave sleep), and malnutrition (inhibiting IGF-1 synthesis).
- The use of replacement GH therapy in healthy elderly people has been debated.
- A systematic review of the use of GH in healthy elderly patients found fat mass ↓ by 2.1kg and lean body mass ↑ by 2.1kg. There were no clear benefits to serum lipid measurements or bone density. Side effects were frequently observed (oedema, arthralgias, carpal tunnel syndrome, glucose intolerance), and theoretical concerns of malignancy related to raised IGF-1 levels remain. Furthermore, no functional benefits have been demonstrated.
- Older patients with GH deficiency related to pituitary disease are usually easily differentiated from other subjects with age-related decline in IGF-1, using standard provocative testing (GH response to insulin-induced hypoglycaemia, arginine, or glucagon).
- A systematic review of the use of GH in elderly patients (aged 60–80 years) with GH deficiency found ↓ total cholesterol (4–8%), ↓ LDL-C (11–16%), ↓ waist circumference (~3cm), and increased quality of life (measured by AGHDA score). No effects have been clearly demonstrated on HDL-C or TG concentrations, BP, or bone density. Data on the effects of GH on body composition were conflicting in studies.
- Few data exist on the benefits of GH in patients with GH deficiency over the age of 80.
- GH is not licensed in the UK for healthy elderly people without clear evidence of clinical and biochemical GH deficiency.

Further reading

Kokshoorn N (2011). GH replacement therapy in elderly GH-deficient patients: a systematic review. *Eur J Endocrinol* **164**, 657–65.

Liu H (2007). Systematic review: the safety and efficacy of growth hormone in the healthy elderly. *Ann Int Med* **146** 104–15.

Gonadal function in the elderly

Women

- The mean age of menopause is 51 years (range 35–58 years) and is defined retrospectively after 12 months of amenorrhoea as the permanent cessation of menstruation due to loss of ovarian follicular activity.
  - FSH 10–15× higher than premenopausal levels.
  - LH 3–5× higher.
  - Oestrogen 10% of previous level (often lower than ♂ of similar age).
  - Inhibin often undetectable.
- The adrenal gland is the major source of sex steroids post-menopausally, with oestrogen production mainly from aromatization of adrenal androgens (androstenedione) in adipose tissue.
- Low FSH/LH may indicate hypopituitarism, although gonadotrophins may be depressed by serious illness.
- For further discussion, 📖 see Chapter 4, Menopause, p. 342.

Men

- ♂ may remain potent and fertile until their death. However, sexual activity, libido, and potency decline gradually and progressively from midlife.
- As with GH deficiency, there is an overlap between clinical features of hypogonadism and 'normal ageing' (↓ lean body mass and muscle function, ↑ fat mass, ↓ virility, ↓ libido, and ↓ overall well-being). Functional 2° hypogonadism is common in serious chronic illness, especially when associated with malnutrition and debilitation.
- Normal ranges for testosterone in ♂ of different ages have not been well established.
- Free testosterone levels ↓ slowly from age 20 to 80, but there is significant intra- and inter-individual variation. The underlying mechanism is that of ↓ testosterone production, rather than ↑ clearance of testosterone. Testosterone production ↓ with ageing, as testicular weight, Leydig cell function, and FSH/LH response to GnRH stimulation ↓.
- The extent to which lower testosterone *per se* and/or a lower free androgen index explain the age-related decline in sexual function is not clear. Although testosterone concentrations may be lower than in younger ♂, testosterone concentrations are still sufficient for normal libido and sexual function. Profoundly low testosterone concentrations (<8nmol/L in a 9 a.m. blood sample) in the appropriate clinical setting should prompt investigation for hypoandrogenism. Gonadotrophins should be raised in 1° testicular failure, and low levels associated with low testosterone should prompt a search for 2° causes, though gonadotrophins may be low because of other serious disease.

- Fat body mass increases more than lean body mass with age; thus, there is ↑ aromatization of androgens to oestrogens. The effects of this are unclear.
- Hypoandrogenism may also result from hyperprolactinaemia due to pituitary/hypothalamic disease, renal dysfunction, hypothyroidism, drugs (psychotropic and anti-dopaminergic agents); all more common in the elderly population.

Testosterone therapy (📖 p. 378)
- Few small studies in elderly ♂, either as replacement in patients with clear hypogonadism or in healthy ♂.
- Data point towards a +ve effect on well-being, muscle mass and strength, and ↓ fat mass in elderly patients, with greatest effect in patients with clear hypogonadism.
- Risk of 2° polycythaemia, liver dysfunction (particularly if testosterone taken orally), prostatism, exacerbation of prostate adenocarcinoma, and possibly dyslipidaemia.

Erectile dysfunction (📖 p. 388)
- Common in elderly ♂. 50% of ♂ >60 have erectile dysfunction; 90% of these ♂ have concurrent medical problems or are on medication potentially causing impotence.
- Aetiology often multifactorial:
  - Atherosclerosis—commonest cause with both macro- and microvascular disease.
  - Penile denervation—autonomic neuropathy (most commonly due to diabetes mellitus); pelvic surgery (including prostatectomy—30% of ♂ >75 develop erectile dysfunction after prostatectomy (compared with 7% of younger ♂ after prostatectomy)).
  - Drugs (β-blockers, calcium channel antagonists, other antihypertensive agents, psychotropic drugs).
  - Psychogenic.

Delayed/absent ejaculation
- ↑ common with age due to autonomic nerve dysfunction, drugs, previous surgery, and usually the harbinger of erectile dysfunction.
- Evaluation similar to that of younger patients (📖 see Evaluation of erectile dysfunction, p. 390).
- Management similar to younger patients, with caveat that phosphodiesterase inhibitors may interact with nitrates and antihypertensive agents.

Fertility
- Testicular morphology, semen production, and testicular steroidogenesis are maintained into old age.
- There is some evidence for a small increase in specific genetic disorders in the children of older men.

Adrenal function in the elderly

Cortisol
- Overall, cortisol secretion generally very similar in elderly persons to younger persons.
- Dynamic testing shows more prolonged release of ACTH and cortisol to stress (physiological, insulin-induced hypoglycaemia, and/or CRH administration) and slower inhibition of ACTH secretion by cortisol.

Dehydroepiandrosterone sulphate
- DHEA and DHEAS levels peak in humans aged 20–30 years and thereafter decline with age (20% of peak values in ♂ and 30% of peak values in ♀ by age 70 years). Responsiveness to ACTH-stimulated secretion also reduces with age.
- The physiological relevance of the fall of DHEA and DHEAS levels with age is not established.
- Although DHEA therapy is sometimes used in patients with adrenal insufficiency, its use in, otherwise healthy, elderly patients (who experience an age-related ↓ in DHEA) is not recommended; there have been no demonstrated clinical benefits (in terms of longevity, well-being, bone density, cognitive function, body mass composition, or cardiovascular status).

Aldosterone
📖 see Fluid and electrolyte homeostasis in the elderly, p. 614.

Thyroid disease in the elderly

Thyroid disease is twice as common in the elderly as in younger patients (see Table 11.1).

Abnormal thyroid function tests

- Concomitant disease and polypharmacy are common in the elderly and may alter the interpretation of results. For example, glucocorticoids (prescribed to 2.5% of the population aged 70–79 years) cause decreased TSH, ↓ thyroid hormone release, ↓ concentration of thyroid hormone-binding proteins, ↓ T_4 to T_3 conversion.
- Sick euthyroid syndrome is more common in the elderly due to frequent concurrent non-thyroidal illness (see 📖 p. 24), with reduced free triiodothyronine (FT_3), ↑ reverse free tri-iodothyronine, and (less commonly) reduced free thyroxine (FT_4), with inappropriately normal or suppressed TSH levels.
- See Table 1.4 for effects on thyroid function of drugs frequently prescribed for elderly patients.

Hypothyroidism (see 📖 p. 74)

- Commonest thyroid problem in elderly people.
- 7–17% of elderly people.
- ♂:♀ ratio increases with ageing.
- Commonest causes are autoimmune thyroiditis, previous surgery, or radioiodine therapy (post-ablative hypothyroidism occurs more frequently in people >55 years old than in younger patients).
- 25% present with classical symptoms of hypothyroidism. 50% complain of fatigue and weakness. Elderly patients with hypothyroidism report cold intolerance, weight gain, paraesthesiae, and muscle cramps less frequently than do younger patients with hypothyroidism.
- The elderly are more susceptible to hypothyroid (myxoedema) coma than younger people; it remains rare, however.
- Elderly patients with unrecognized hypothyroidism may be at greater risk of the development of perioperative and intraoperative complications (including intraoperative hypotension, heart failure, and post-operative gastrointestinal and neuropsychiatric complications).
- Hypothyroidism should be considered in elderly patients with ↑ CK or transaminases, ↓ Na, macrocytic anaemia, or dyslipidaemia.
- Thyroid replacement therapy should be done cautiously, as ischaemic heart disease may be unmasked or exacerbated, e.g. 12.5–25 micrograms/day of levothyroxine, ↑ by 12.5–25 micrograms increments every 3–8 weeks until TSH is normalized.
- Total replacement T_4 dose is lower in the elderly than in younger patients (in younger patients, approximately 1.6 micrograms/kg is required, but older patients require 20–30% less).
- Compliance may be problematic. Supervised therapy or administration using a Dosette® box may help. Alternatively, calculate the total weekly dose of levothyroxine, and give 70% of the total dose once a week or 50% of the total dose twice weekly.

Table 11.1 Changes in thyroid-related investigations with ageing

TSH	No significant change; secretion remains pulsatile, but loss of physiological nocturnal TSH rise is blunted
T_4	Unchanged overall (both secretion and clearance ↓)
T_3	10–50% decrease; occurs at an earlier age in ♀ than in ♂
rT_3	↑
Thyroid antibodies	Prevalence ↑ with age; significance uncertain (2% at age 25, 15–32% at age 75)
24h radioactive iodine uptake	Unchanged

Hyperthyroidism (see 📖 p. 26)

- 0.3–2% of elderly people.
- Presentation is often atypical, often with few signs or symptoms.
- Clinical symptoms of hyperthyroidism are different in the elderly; non-specific symptoms, such as weight loss, depression, or agitation, predominate. Consider the diagnosis with muscle weakness; heart failure, arrhythmias, atrial fibrillation; weight loss; and osteoporotic fracture.
- An isolated suppressed TSH concentration is associated with an ↑ cardiovascular mortality and a 3-fold higher risk of atrial fibrillation in the next 10 years. 2–24% of elderly patients with atrial fibrillation are hyperthyroid, and 9–35% of elderly patients with hyperthyroidism have atrial fibrillation.
- Underlying cause may be toxic multinodular goitre; Graves's disease.
- Treatment options are similar to those in younger patients (📖 see Treatment, p. 30).
- Radioactive iodine is favoured because it is definitive and it avoids risks of surgery. Hypothyroidism is common after radioiodine therapy in elderly people.

Goitre

- Diffuse goitre becomes less frequent with age in both ♂ and ♀ (found in 31% of ♀ aged <45 years, compared with 12% of ♀ aged >75 years on clinical examination).
- Multinodular goiter, as assessed by both clinical and US examination, increases with age (incidence of US-detected multinodular goitre 90% of ♀ >70 years, 60% of ♂ >80 years).
- Management similar to that of multinodular goitre in younger patients (📖 see Multinodular goitre and solitary adenomas, pp. 64–7).

Thyroid cancer (see 📖 p. 91)

- Total incidence rate for all thyroid cancers is unchanged, but the relative frequencies are altered.
- Papillary carcinoma is more common in young and middle-aged patients and accounts for only 50% of thyroid cancers in patients over 60 years old. Older patients have a higher mortality rate.
- Follicular carcinoma: peak incidence in 6th decade of life. Prognosis is poorer in older patients, possibly due to the increased frequency of extraglandular recurrences in older patients.
- Anaplastic thyroid carcinoma: peak incidence in 7th decade. Two-thirds of all cases occur in patients >65 years. It presents with a rapidly growing hard mass which is often locally invasive and may be associated with metastatic lesions. The prognosis is poor.
- Sarcomas and 1° thyroid lymphomas are more common in elderly patients.
- Medullary thyroid cancer: sporadic forms have a mean age at presentation of 47 years; hereditary forms more common in younger patients. Older age at diagnosis and more advanced stage are independent markers of a poorer prognosis.
- Overall evaluation and treatment is similar to that of younger patients, but accurate preoperative histology is very important, as tumours not treated surgically (e.g. anaplastic carcinoma and lymphoma) are relatively more common.

Further reading

Grimley Evans J, Williams TF, Michel J-P, *et al.* (eds.) (2000). *Oxford Textbook of Geriatric Medicine*. Oxford University Press, Oxford.
Vermeulen A (ed.) (1997). Endocrinology of ageing. *Ballière's Clin Endocrinol Metab* **11**, 223–50.

Endocrinology aspects of other clinical or physiological situations

Hypoglycaemia

Definition (Whipple's triad)
- Plasma glucose of <2.2mmol/L, *associated with*
- Symptoms of neuroglycopenia, *and*
- Reversal of symptoms with correction of glucose levels.

Epidemiology
Uncommon in adults, apart from patients with diabetes being treated with certain agents, either alone or in combination (e.g. insulin, sulfonylureas).

Pathophysiology
Physiology of glucose control
Plasma glucose concentrations are usually kept within narrow limits (~3.3–5.6mmol/L), providing an uninterrupted supply of glucose to the brain (which can consume up to 50% of hepatic glucose output).

The liver is the major regulator (80–85%) of circulating blood glucose concentrations in healthy individuals and responds to changes in circulating insulin, GH, cortisol, glucagon, and adrenaline.
- *Postprandial state:* hepatic glucose production is inhibited by ↑ plasma glucose and ↑ insulin concentrations.
- *Fasting state:* plasma glucose ↓ with consequent ↓ in insulin secretion, stimulating hepatic glucose efflux (due to ↑ cortisol, GH, and glucagon).

Mechanisms of hypoglycaemia
- *Excessive/inappropriate action of insulin (or IGF-1):* inhibiting hepatic glucose production, despite adequate glycogen stores, while peripheral glucose uptake is enhanced.
- *Impaired neuroendocrine response* with inadequate counter-regulatory response (e.g. cortisol) to insulin.
- *Impairment of hepatic glucose production* due to either structural damage or abnormal liver enzymes.

Classification of hypoglycaemia
Traditionally, hypoglycaemia has been classed as fasting or postprandial.
- *Fasting hypoglycaemia:* occuring several hours (typically >5h) after food (e.g. early morning, following prolonged fasting or exercise).
- *Postprandial (reactive) hypoglycaemia:* occuring 2–5h after food.

Causes of hypoglycaemia can fit into both categories, so another classification has been proposed, based on whether the patient is unwell (see Box 12.1.)

Box 12.1 Causes of hypoglycaemia in adults

Ill or medicated individual

- Drug-induced (commonest cause; both accidental and non-accidental):
  - Insulin or insulin secretagogue.
  - Alcohol (impairs hepatic gluconeogenesis and is often associated with poor glycogen stores).
  - Others (e.g. pentamidine, quinine, indometacin, glucagon (during endoscopy)).
- Organ failure or critical illness:
  - Liver failure (over 80% of liver needs to be destroyed/removed).
  - Chronic renal failure.
  - Sepsis, e.g. malaria, Gram -ve, or meningococcal; related to high metabolic requirements, reduced energy intake, and possibly cytokines from the inflammatory process.
- Hormone deficiency:
  - Cortisol deficiency, e.g. Addison's disease, hypopituitarism.
- Non-islet cell tumours:
  - Excessive IGF-II secretion from large mesenchymal tumours (non-islet cell tumour hypoglycaemia), e.g. fibrosarcoma, mesothelioma (~1/3 retroperitoneal, 1/3 intra-abdominal, and 1/3 intrathoracic).

Seemingly well individual

- Insulinoma:
  - Benign 85%, malignant 15%.
  - Occasionally, part of MEN-1 (~10%).
- Non-islet cell tumours:
  - Adrenal carcinoma, phaeochromocytoma.
  - Hepatocellular carcinoma
  - Lymphoma, myeloma, leukaemia.
  - Advanced metastatic malignancy.
- Functional β-cell disorders (nesidioblastosis):
  - Non-insulinoma pancreatogenous hypoglycaemia (typically after eating).
  - Post-gastric bypass hypoglycaemia (incidence and mechanisms unclear; may require treatment with α-glucosidase inhibitor, diazoxide, or octreotide).
- Autoimmune:
  - Antibodies to insulin (antibody-bound insulin dissociates, leading to elevated free insulin; typically associated with late postprandial hypoglycaemia; mainly reported amongst people of Japanese or Korean descent).
  - Insulin receptor-activating antibodies (rare; may require treatment with plasmapheresis or immunosuppression).
- Accidental or surreptitious hypoglycaemia (e.g. insulin or insulin secretagogue administration).

From Cryer PE (1997).

Symptoms of hypoglycaemia

- See Table 12.1 for classification of symptoms.
- Adrenergic symptoms have been identified at arterialized plasma glucose concentrations of 3.3mmol/L (equivalent to a venous plasma concentration of 3.1mmol/L).
- Neuroglycopaenic symptoms have been identified at arterialized plasma glucose concentrations of 2.8mmol/L (equivalent to a venous plasma concentration of 2.6mmol/L).
- EEG changes occur at 2.0mmol/L.
- The majority of symptoms of acute hypoglycaemia are adrenergic, but neuroglycopaenic symptoms occur with subacute and chronic hypoglycaemia.
- The rate of decrease in the plasma glucose concentration does not influence the occurrence of the symptoms.
- Patients with recurrent hypoglycaemia may not get symptoms until glucose concentrations are very low (so-called 'hypo unawareness'), whilst patients with poorly controlled diabetes mellitus may experience hypoglycaemic symptoms at 'normal' blood glucose levels.

Table 12.1 Classification of symptoms and signs of hypoglycaemia

Adrenergic	Neuroglycopaenic
Sweating	Visual disturbance (e.g. diplopia, blurred vision)
Hunger	Poor concentration
Tingling	Drowsiness
Trembling	Lethargy
Palpitations	Unusual behaviour
Anxiety	Personality change
	Confusion
	Focal neurological abnormality
	Seizures
	Coma

Investigations of hypoglycaemia

- Glucose (BM) strip: unreliable for low glucose concentrations.
- Liver and renal function tests.
- Blood ethanol concentration.
- Synacthen® test.
- Insulin, C-peptide, pro-insulin, and glucose during hypoglycaemia (see Table 12.2).
- Inappropriately elevated insulin in presence of hypoglycaemia suggests insulinoma, self-administration of insulin/sulfonylurea, post-gastric bypass hypoglycaemia, non-insulinoma pancreatogenous hypoglycaemia syndrome, or insulin autoimmune hypoglycaemia.
- Absence of C-peptide, but the presence of insulin, during hypoglycaemia suggests exogenous insulin administration or raised IGF-II.
- Insulinomas often associated with elevated pro-insulin:insulin ratio.
- Consider assay for presence of sulfonylureas.
- Fasting β-hydroxybutyrate (elevated in most causes of hypoglycaemia but suppressed if insulin present, e.g. insulinoma, self-administration of insulin, or sulfonylureas).
- Consider IGF-I and II and pro-IGF-II. IGF-II may be normal in non-islet cell hypoglycaemia, but this is in association with suppressed IGF-I and GH; usual IGF-II:IGF-I ratio 3:1, ratio >10 seen in non-islet cell hypoglycaemia. Tumours tend to secrete pro-IGF-II, leading to a raised pro-IGF-II:IGF-II ratio.
- Chest and abdominal radiographs/CT.
- Consider insulin and insulin receptor antibodies.

Further investigation of fasting hypoglycaemia

- *15h fast:*
  - Measure plasma glucose and insulin after fasting for 15h.
  - Glucose <2.2mmol/L and insulin >5mU/L is inappropriate.
  - Good screening test if repeated 3 times.
  - 75% of patients with an insulinoma will develop hypoglycaemia within 18h of beginning a fast.
- *72h fast:*
  - The most reliable test for hypoglycaemia (detects 98% patients with insulinoma, compared with >70% at 24h).
  - The patient should remain hydrated and active.
  - Measure plasma glucose, insulin, C-peptide, and pro-insulin 6-hourly (unless the patient is symptomatic or the glucose level is <3.5mmol/L when measurements are made every 1–2h); the test is terminated if the laboratory glucose <2.2mmol/L or after 72h.
  - β-hydroxybutyrate should be measured at the end of the fast (its presence makes insulinoma unlikely).
- *C-peptide suppression test:*
  - Rationale: insulin administration to induce hypoglycaemia should suppress endogenous insulin secretion. C-peptide serves as a measure of endogenous insulin secretion and is suppressed during hypoglycaemia to a lesser degree in people with an insulinoma than in normal persons.

Table 12.2 Biochemical features of insulinoma and factitious hypoglycaemia

Plasma marker	Insulinoma	Sulfonylurea	Insulin injection
Glucose	↓	↓	↓
Insulin	↑	↑	↑
C-peptide	↑	↑	↓

- Useful when 72h fast test is inconclusive.
- Method: IV insulin administered over 2h and measurements of plasma C-peptide and glucose made.
- Results should be interpreted using age- and BMI-matched normative data.

Further investigation of postprandial hypoglycaemia

- *Prolonged oral glucose tolerance test:*
  - Not physiological.
  - 10% of the normal (asymptomatic) population have a +ve response, with blood glucose levels <2.6mmol/L.
- *Mixed meal test over 5h:*
  - More physiological.
  - Uses foods with a medium-to-low glycaemic index ('hyperglucidic').
  - 47% of patients with suspected postprandial hypoglycaemia have a +ve test vs 1% of asymptomatic subjects.
  - However, diagnostic criteria not formally agreed for this test.
- *Ambulatory glucose sampling:*
  - Gaining favour, as it may correlate symptoms with low sugar readings and improvement of symptoms with recovery from hypoglycaemia.

Other investigations may be indicated if there is clinical and biochemical evidence of an insulinoma (e.g. 📖 see Tumour localization, p. 563).

Management of hypoglycaemia

Acute hypoglycaemia

- *If conscious:*
  - 15–20g oral carbohydrate (ideally food and a sugary drink) should be administered as soon as possible.
  - Dextrogel®/Glucogel® (formerly known as Hypostop Gel®), a glucose-containing gel which is absorbed by the buccal mucosa, may be used in drowsy, but conscious, individuals.
- *If unconscious:*
  - 75–80mL of 20% glucose intravenously into a large vein (over 10–15min), followed by a saline flush as the high concentration of glucose is an irritant and may even lead to venous thrombosis. A maintenance infusion of 5% or 10% dextrose is often required thereafter, especially if there is an ongoing risk of recurrent hypoglycaemia (e.g. overdose of a long-acting insulin/analogue).
  - 1mg glucagon IM may be administered if there is no IV access. This increases hepatic glucose efflux, but the effect only lasts for 30min, allowing other means of blood glucose elevation (e.g. oral) before the blood glucose falls again. It is ineffective with hepatic dysfunction and if there is glycogen depletion, e.g. ethanol-related hypoglycaemia, and is relatively contraindicated in patients with known insulinoma, as it may induce further insulin secretion. Glucagon is ineffective if given within 3 days of a previous dose of glucagon.
- 2° *cerebral oedema* may complicate hypoglycaemia and should be considered in cases of prolonged coma despite normalization of plasma glucose. Mannitol and/or dexamethasone may be helpful.

Recurrent chronic hypoglycaemia

If definitive treatment of the underlying condition is unsuccessful or impossible, symptoms may be alleviated by frequent (e.g. 4-hourly) small meals, including overnight. Diazoxide, administered by mouth, is useful in the management of patients with chronic hypoglycaemia from excess endogenous insulin secretion due to an insulinoma or islet cell hyperplasia.

Postprandial reactive hypoglycaemia (PRH)

Definition

Hypoglycaemia following a meal, due to an imbalance between glucose influx into (exogenous from food and endogenous glucose production) and glucose efflux out of the circulation.

Pathophysiology and causes

- *Exaggerated insulin response.* Related to rapid glucose absorption, e.g. post-gastrectomy dumping syndrome. This results in a delayed insulin peak with respect to the peak blood glucose, probably related to an exaggerated GLP-1 (glucagon-like peptide-1) response.
- *Incipient diabetes mellitus.* Occasionally presents with postprandial hypoglycaemia, possibly related to disordered insulin secretion.
- *Insulin resistance-related hyperinsulinaemia*, e.g. obese subjects with or without impaired glucose tolerance.
- *Impaired glucagon sensitivity and secretion.* In response to hypoglycaemia; involved in the pathogenesis of PRH.
- *Renal glycosuria.* Accounts for up to 15% of patients with PRH.
- *Body composition:*
  - 20% of very lean people are prone to PRH.
  - Massive weight reduction increases the risk of PRH.
  - Lower body obesity (especially in ♀) is associated with high normal insulin sensitivity and PRH.
- *Diet:*
  - High-carbohydrate, low-fat diet, by ↑ insulin sensitivity.
  - Prolonged very low calorie diets (>2 weeks) by reducing counter-regulatory hormones, especially GH.
- *Alcohol:*
  - Inhibits hepatic glucose output.
  - Increases insulin secretion in response to glucose and sucrose.
- Idiopathic.

Investigation

- *Prolonged oral glucose tolerance test.* Not physiological; 10% of the normal (asymptomatic) population have a +ve response with blood glucose levels <2.6mmol/L.
- *Hyperglucidic mixed meal test.* More physiological; 47% of patients with suspected PRH have a +ve test vs 1% of asymptomatic subjects.
- *Ambulatory glucose sampling.* Gaining favour, as it may correlate symptoms with low sugar readings and improvement of symptoms with recovery from hypoglycaemia.

Management

Diet

- Frequent, small, low-carbohydrate, high-protein meals.
- Avoid rapidly absorbed carbohydrates.
- Avoid sugary drinks, especially in combination with alcohol.
- Addition of soluble dietary fibres, e.g. 5–10g guar gum or pectin or hemicellulose per meal, delays absorption and lowers the glycaemic and insulinaemic indices (especially effective in rapid gut transit time).

Drugs

- Acarbose, an intestinal α-glucosidase inhibitor, delays sugar and starch absorption, thus reducing the insulin response to a meal.
- Metformin can be useful, 500mg with meals.
- Supplemental chromium is reported to downregulate β-cell activity and increase glucagon secretion.
- In exceptional cases, with debilitating PRH, diazoxide (side effects— water retention, hypertrichosis, digestive disorders) or somatostatin analogues may be required.
- Propranolol and calcium antagonists have been used; however, controlled studies are lacking.

Further reading

Brun JF, Fedou C, Mercier J (2000). Postprandial reactive hypoglycaemia. *Diabet Metab* **26**, 337–51.

Cryer PE (1997). Hypoglycemia: pathophysiology, diagnosis, and treatment. Oxford University Press, New York.

Cryer PE, Axelrod L, Grossman AB, Heller SR, Montori V, Seaquist ER, Service FJ (2009). Evaluation and management of adult hypoglycaemic disorders: an Endocrine Society clinical practice guideline. *J Clin Endocrinol Metab* **94**, 709–28.

de Groot, *et al.* (2009). Non-islet cell tumour-induced hypoglycaemia: a review of the literature including two new cases. *Endocr Relat Cancer* **14**, 979–93.

Gama R, Teale JD, Marks V (2003). Clinical and laboratory investigation of adult spontaneous hypoglycaemia. *J Clin Path* **56**, 641–6.

Service FJ (1995). Hypoglycaemic disorders. *N Engl J Med* **350**, 2272–9.

Mastocytosis

Background and definitions

Mastocytosis is a heterogenous group of disorders characterized by the pathological accumulation of mast cells in tissues. The main types of mastocytoses are cutaneous and systemic. Systemic mastocytosis is frequently diagnosed but seldom established as a differential diagnosis in the work-up of flushing (sensation of warmth, usually on the face and neck, due to vasodilation and increased cutaneous circulation). Flushing due to neurogenic stimuli are likely to be associated with sweating (wet flushing), and flushing due to vasodilator substances associated with 'dry' flushing. Systemic mastocytosis usually features in the latter category.

See Box 12.2 for causes of raised tryptase.

Classification

Mastocytosis is broadly classified into cutaneous and systemic mastocytosis (see Box 12.3).

Clinical features

- Urticaria pigmentosa and dermographism are the usual cutaneous manifestations (exacerbated when rubbed—Darier's sign).
- Systemic manifestations include flushing, anaphylaxis, abdominal pain, and diarrhoea.
- Anaemia, hepatosplenomegaly, peptic ulceration, and steatorrhoea can occur due to mast cell infiltration.

Epidemiology

- It is a rare disorder.
- Affects both sexes equally.
- Children usually have cutaneous mastocytosis, and adults the systemic variety.

Investigations

- Serum tryptase, which is predominantly produced in mast cells, is usually elevated.
- Skin biopsy stained with Giemsa and immunohistochemical staining for tryptase and c-kit (mast cell growth factor receptor).
- Bone marrow biopsy is warranted for adults with evidence of mastocytosis to diagnose systemic mastocytosis.

Box 12.2 Causes of raised tryptase level
- Acute myeloid leukaemia.
- Myelodysplastic disorders.
- Hypereosinophilic syndrome.
- Asthma (mild elevation).

Box 12.3 WHO classification of systemic mastocytosis
- Indolent systemic mastocytosis.
- Systemic mastocytosis with clonal haematological non-mast cell lineage disease.
- Mast cell leukaemia.
- Mast cell sarcoma.
- Extracutaneous mastocytosis.

Treatment
- Avoidance of triggers (e.g. alcohol, aspirin).
- Treat anaphylaxis as a medical emergency.
- Preparation of patients appropriately before surgery and other medical procedures with antihistamines, glucocorticoids, H2 blockade, and montelukast.
- Antihistamines, such as cetirizine, fexofenadine, can be used to reduce flushing and itching.
- H2 blockers and proton pump inhibitors, such as ranitidine and omeprazole, can help with abdominal symptoms, such as pain and heartburn.
- In patients who are not intolerant of NSAIDs, aspirin may help reduce flushing.
- Additional antileukotriene agents, such as montelukast, may help some with ongoing symptoms.
- Other treatment options, including tyrosine kinase inhibitors, have been assessed, but their effectiveness is not convincing.

Further reading
Liu AY, et al. (2010). Clinical problem-solving. A rash hypothesis. N Engl J Med **363**, 72–8.
Murali MR, et al. (2011). Case records of the Massachusetts General Hospital. Case 9-2011. A 37-year-old man with flushing and hypotension. N Engl J Med **364**, 1155–65.

Cancer

Chemotherapy and radiotherapy may have endocrine effects.

Anticancer chemotherapy

There are three types of anticancer chemotherapeutic agents:

- *Cytotoxics*. These have no direct hormonal sequelae. Alkylating agents are more likely to induce permanent ♂ sterility (without affecting potency), and, in ♀, they may induce premature menopause which may increase the likelihood of osteoporosis.
- *Immunomodulators*. Prednisolone in excess causes Cushing's syndrome, and acute withdrawal may precipitate adrenal insufficiency. *Cyclophosphamide*, in particular, may cause early menopause. Thyroid dysfunction has been reported rarely with *tacrolimus* and *interferon* therapy.
- *Hormones*:
  - *Progestagens* are used in breast cancer; of these, *megestrol acetate* has potent glucocorticoid activity and thus may cause Cushing's syndrome in excess or adrenal insufficiency if abruptly withdrawn.
  - *Aromatase inhibitors*, such as *aminoglutethimide*, may cause adrenal insufficiency, and corticosteroid replacement is necessary.
  - *Trilostane*, which inhibits 3β-hydroxysteroid dehydrogenase, may also cause adrenal insufficiency.
  - *Gonadorelin analogues*, used for prostatic cancer and breast cancer, cause an initial increase in LH levels and then suppression and cause side effects similar to orchidectomy in ♂ and the menopause in ♀.
  - *Antiandrogens*, used in prostatic cancer, have predictable side effects, such as gynaecomastia, hot flushes, impotence, and impaired libido.

Radiotherapy

- Cranial radiotherapy, whose field encompasses the hypothalamo–pituitary area, may result in hypopituitarism (📖 see Chapter 2, Hypopituitarism, p. 202). The most radiosensitive axis is the GH axis, followed by the FSH/LH axis, then the ACTH and TSH axes. Even low radiation doses of <40Gy can affect the GH axis. Panhypopituitarism is generally seen with doses of >60Gy, doses often used in the presence of nasopharyngeal or skull base tumours.
- Head and neck irradiation may result in hypothyroidism and hypoparathyroidism.
- After 5 or more years of follow-up, 50% of patients treated with radiotherapy only for laryngeal and pharyngeal carcinoma will develop hypothyroidism; combined surgery and radiotherapy results in roughly 90% of patients developing hypothyroidism. The rates for hypoparathyroidism were 88% and 90%, respectively.
- Radiotherapy affects the testes dose-dependently. Fertility is affected much more than androgen-synthesizing capacity so that most ♂ have normal testosterone levels unless given testicular doses >20–30Gy.
- The effects of radiotherapy to both ovaries are amplified with age. Premature menopause may be elicited by doses >10Gy.

Endocrine sequelae of survivors of childhood cancer

Background

It is estimated that approximately 1:900 adults in the developed world has survived a childhood cancer. The treatment of childhood malignancies in the form of surgery, chemotherapy, and, perhaps most important of all, supportive care is now more advanced than ever and has resulted in very significant improvements in survival. For example, the 5-year survival of the commonest childhood and adolescent malignancies acute lymphoblastic leukaemia (ALL) and Hodgkin's lymphoma is >80% and 90%, respectively.

Basic concepts and definitions

Alkylating agents (e.g. cyclophosphamide, busulfan, procarbazine) work by damaging DNA in rapidly dividing cancer calls. Non-neoplastic cells can also be subjected to damage by these agents.

Gray (Gy) is the unit of absorbed dose of ionizing radiation corresponding to 1 joule/kg. Like alkylating agents, ionizing radiation causes damage to the DNA of proliferating cancer cells (and other normal tissues in the way).

The dose of radiation measured in Gy depends on the type of cancer and its stage. For example, for solid tumours of epithelial origin, the dose can vary between 60 and 80Gy, and the dose for lymphomas could be 20–40Gy. To put this in perspective, the dose of radiation to the stomach from an AP chest X-ray is approximately 0.25mGy, and from a CT scan of the abdomen, it is at least 12.5mGy.

Children who survive cancers are at risk of a number of hormone deficiencies and sometimes overactivity of some endocrine organs, such as hyperthyroidism. The common endocrine complications include growth hormone deficiency, hypothyroidism, and disrupted puberty. Awareness of these hormonal imbalances has increased, and they need to be actively sought and treated in order to improve quality of life.

The endocrine sequelae of craniopharyngiomas specifically has been covered in Chapter 2 (📖 see p. 188).

Growth hormone deficiency

Adult short stature is common in survivors of childhood cancers (📖 pp. 130 and 524). The disease and its treatment, precocious puberty, growth hormone deficiency (GHD), primary hyperthyroidism, depression, or a combination of all of these could result in short stature.

GHD could be due to direct tumour invasion or as a consequence of surgery, as in the case of craniopharyngiomas (📖 see p. 188). GHD is a common, and sometimes the only, anterior pituitary deficit after cranial irradiation. The risk of developing GHD is 90% within 5 years of external beam radiotherapy of doses ≥30Gy. With doses between 18 and 24Gy, it may take 10 years to develop GHD. The likelihood of developing GHD with chemotherapy is low.

Clinical assessment

- Growth velocity.
- Weight and BMI.
- Sitting height (radiotherapy can cause vertebral dysplasia).
- Arm span.
- Pubertal assessment for evidence of precocious puberty (precocious puberty can result in a falsely reassuring growth spurt).

Investigations

The diagnosis can be difficult to make. GHD is suspected when a decreased growth velocity is found over a 6-month period. The diagnosis is made using a combination of clinical features and investigations.

- Bone age to assess skeletal maturation.
- Insulin tolerance test (📖 see p. 114).
- GHRH with arginine may lack sensitivity in patients who have received radiotherapy.
- IGF-1 and IGFBP-3 are not reliable markers of GH secretion following radiotherapy or those with CNS lesions.

Treatment

- There is no clear evidence of either increased risk of recurrence of the original tumour or death associated with GH therapy, despite the anti-apoptotic and pro-proliferative effects of GH and IGF-1.
- There is evidence to suggest an increased risk of a secondary tumour in survivors of acute leukaemia. Meningiomas are the commonest second neoplasms.
- GH therapy in survivors of childhood cancers for adult GHD has been shown to improve quality of life and modest improvements in metabolic parameters.
- See section on growth hormone replacement (📖 see p. 134).

Thyroid abnormalities

Thyroid abnormalities are common endocrine sequelae in survivors of childhood cancers.

Primary hypothyroidism

Primary hypothyroidism can develop up to 25 years after radiotherapy. It is usually seen after mantle irradiation for Hodgkin's lymphoma and craniospinal irradiation for HS tumours. It is more likely to occur in girls. Long-term surveillance with thyroid function tests, early detection, and treatment are important.

Central hypothyroidism

Rare and usually associated with irradiation to the hypothalamic/pituitary area of doses >30Gy. There is a small association between chemotherapy and central hypothyroidism.

Hyperthyroidism

Much rarer than hypothyroidism and associated with doses of ≥35Gy to the thyroid.

Thyroid neoplasia

There is an increased likelihood of developing papillary and follicular cancers of the thyroid after radiotherapy. Children treated before the age of 10 and with doses between 20 and 30Gy are at highest risk. There can be a very long latent period before the development of thyroid cancers; therefore, ongoing long-term follow-up is essential.

Thyroid cancers secondary to radiotherapy do not behave more aggressively than those occurring in people without radiotherapy.

Disruption of puberty

Puberty can be affected in survivors of childhood cancers in terms of precocious puberty, accelerated rate of progression through puberty, delayed progression through puberty, or hypogonadotrophic hypogonadism.

Precocious puberty (see 📖 *p. 538)*

Precocious puberty (<8 years for girls and <9 years for boys) is caused by premature activation of the hypothalamo–pituitary–gonadal axis and is associated with irradiation. It is more likely in girls and those who are overweight and is associated with radiotherapy at an early age.

Clinical assessment

- Height and weight on growth charts, assessing growth velocity.
- An early sign of precocious puberty is an increase in growth velocity. However, this can be masked either by concomitant GHD or hypothyroidism.
- Tanner staging—in girls, evidence of breast development <8 years is a sign of precocious puberty; in boys, however, testicular volume is an unreliable marker, as there may be concomitant seminiferous dysfunction.
- A bone age on X-ray of >2 SDs for the chronological age is a consistent finding.

Management

Delaying the progression of puberty with GnRH agonists results in better outcomes for height, especially in conjunction with GH where appropriate for GHD (📖 see section on Precocious puberty, p. 538).

Hypogonadotrophic hypogonadism

Gonadotrophin deficiency is less common than GH deficiency and is dependent on the dose of radiotherapy received to the hypothalamic–sellar area. Whether chemotherapy alone results in gonadatrophin deficiency is uncertain.

Assessment and management

📖 see section on delayed puberty, p. 542.

Male gonadal dysfunction

- Leydig cells are vulnerable to radiation damage but relatively tolerant of chemotherapy due to their slow turnover. Children who receive >24Gy for testicular relapse of ALL have a high risk of developing testosterone deficiency.
- Germ cells, on the other hand, are at risk of damage from both chemo- and radiotherapy.
- Fertility is impaired in 40–60% of ♂ survivors of childhood cancer.
- Alkylating agents are associated with highest risk in terms of chemotherapeutic agents.
- Relatively low doses, such as 0.15Gy, are associated with ♂ subfertility.

Female gonadal dysfunction

- Ovarian failure can occur either acutely or as a delayed effect, following the treatment of cancer.
- In young girls, if ovarian dysfunction occurs before the onset of puberty, there can be delayed puberty and primary amenorrhoea.
- During puberty, ovarian failure can result in arrested pubertal development, secondary amenorrhoea, and menopausal symptoms.
- Alkylating agents are associated with a high risk of developing ovarian failure.
- Abdominopelvic irradiation increases the risk of ovarian failure. This risk is higher when used in conjunction with alkylating agents.
- Women with ovarian failure are at higher risk of osteoporosis and cardiovascular disease.

Osteoporosis

- Survivors of childhood cancers are at risk of osteopenia, osteoporosis, and consequently fractures as a result of the primary disease, glucocorticoids, chemotherapy, hypogonadism, and GHD.
- DEXA scans should be interpreted with caution, taking into consideration age, pubertal stage, and height.

Obesity

Obesity is strongly associated with craniopharyngiomas and other CNS tumours and their treatment. Hypothalamic damage can result in morbid obesity. For other cancers, a combination of GHD, steroids, and other undetermined factors are also believed to cause obesity. Insulin resistance is also common, and the risk of type 2 diabetes is increased.

Syndromes of ectopic hormone production

Definition

The secretion into the systemic circulation of a hormone or other biologically active molecule by a neoplasm (benign or malignant) that has arisen from a tissue that does not normally produce that hormone or molecule, resulting in a clinically significant syndrome. See Table 12.3 for common syndromes associated with ectopic hormone production.

Table 12.3 Common syndromes associated with ectopic hormone production

Syndrome	Ectopic hormone	Typical tumour types
Hypercalcaemia of malignancy	PTHrP	Squamous cell lung carcinoma
		Other squamous cell carcinoma (skin, oesophagus, head and neck)
		Renal cell carcinoma
		Breast adenocarcinoma
		Adult T-cell lymphoma associated with HTLV-1
	1,25(OH)$_2$ colecalciferol	Lymphomas
SIADH	Vasopressin/ADH	Small cell lung carcinoma
		Squamous cell lung carcinoma
		Bronchial carcinoid
		Mesothelioma
		Pancreatic or gut carcinoid
		Adenocarcinoma of the duodenum, pancreas, prostate
		Phaeochromocytoma
		Medullary thyroid carcinoma
		Haematopoietic malignancies (lymphoma, leukaemia)

Table 12.3 (Continued)

Syndrome	Ectopic hormone	Typical tumour types
Cushing's syndrome	ACTH (most commonly)	Small cell lung carcinoma
		Thymic carcinoid tumour
		Bronchial carcinoid tumour
		Pancreatic endocrine tumours (including carcinoid tumours)
		Carcinoid tumours of the gut
		Phaeochromocytoma
		Medullary thyroid carcinoma
		Other lung cancers (adenocarcinoma, squamous cell carcinoma)
	CRH (rarely)	Carcinoid tumour
	Ectopic expression of receptors for GIP; LH	Macronodular adrenal hyperplasia
Non-islet cell hypoglycaemia	IGF-2	Mesenchymal tumours
		Mesothelioma
		Fibrosarcomas
Oncogenic osteomalacia	FGF23	Sarcomas
		Haemangiomas
		Fibromas
		Prostate adenocarcinoma
		Osteoblastomas
Male feminization	hCG	Testicular neoplasms (seminomas, teratomas)
		Germinomas
		Choriocarcinomas
Acromegaly	GHRH	Pancreatic islet cell tumours
		Carcinoid tumours
	GH	Lung, pancreatic islet cell tumours

SIADH due to ectopic vasopressin production

Diagnosis

- Hyponatraemia (plasma Na <130mmol/L).
- Dilute plasma (serum osmolality <270mOsm/kg).
- Inappropriately concentrated urine (in the face of hyponatraemia and plasma hypo-osmolality, any urine osmolality > plasma osmolality is inappropriate).
- Persistent renal Na excretion (urinary Na >20mmol/L).
- Euvolaemia (or very mild hypervolaemia).
- Normal renal, adrenal, and thyroid function.
- Plasma urea and uric acid levels can be helpful markers of plasma dilution.
- The commonest tumours causing SIADH are tumours with neuroendocrine features, most commonly small cell lung carcinoma and carcinoid tumours. Small cell lung carcinomas have usually metastasized by the time SIADH is present.
- Lung diseases and neurological disorders (including malignancies) may cause SIADH due to aberrant hypothalamic vasopressin release, rather than vasopressin release from the tumour *per se*. In SIADH due to ectopic hormone secretion, release of vasopressin from the neurohypophysis may be suppressed.
- Other causes of SIADH must be excluded (⬚ see Syndrome of inappropriate ADH (SIADH), p. 220).

Management

Hyponatraemia

- The initial management is fluid restriction, with daily monitoring of the plasma sodium and osmolality. Hyponatraemia has usually developed gradually, and its correction should be similarly gradual. Fluid restriction to 500mL total fluid intake per day may be needed for several days. Urate levels can be useful as a marker of water intoxication and its resolution. As hyponatraemia is corrected, fluid restriction can be relaxed, depending on the plasma sodium. 1500–2000mL/day is usual.
- For patients in whom fluid restriction is insufficient or not possible, demeclocycline (150–300mg tds–qds) can be used to produce a nephrogenic diabetes insipidus to achieve a normal plasma sodium. Demeclocyline can result in photosensitivity, and patients should be warned to avoid prolonged exposure to sunlight.
- Life-threatening hyponatraemia (e.g. convulsions) may rarely require hypertonic saline and furosemide; however, rapid correction of hyponatraemia may result in central pontine myelinolysis, and, in the vast majority of cases, water restriction is safe, effective, and sufficient.
- Tolvaptan (see ⬚ p. 221): a competitive vasopressin V2-receptor antagonist may also be useful.

Management of the underlying tumour

Curative surgery will also cure the SIADH, as will curative chemotherapy and/or radiotherapy. Chemotherapy and radiotherapy may have an important palliative role, as the tumour is usually incurable by the time hyponatraemia is detected.

Humeral hypercalcaemia of malignancy

Hypercalcaemia is a common complication of malignancy; may be due to ectopic hormone secretion (PTHrP; rarely $1,25(OH)_2$ colecalciferol); cytokine and inflammatory mediators that activate osteoclastic bone resorption (such as IL-6 and RANK-L production by myeloma cells); or due to bone destruction by metastases.

Parathyroid hormone-related peptide (PTHrP)

- PTHrP binds to and activates PTH/PTHrP receptor type 1, resulting in osteoclast-mediated bone resorption and reduced renal excretion of calcium.
- The biochemical picture of hypercalcaemia and hypophosphataemia may be indistinguishable from 1° hyperparathyroidism. However, PTH levels are suppressed in PTHrP-mediated hypercalcaemia (NB 1° hyperparathyroidism can coexist with malignancy).
- PTHrP secretion by metastatic cells within bone also causes hypercalcaemia by causing local osteolysis.
- PTHrP can be measured directly and is elevated in 80% of cancer patients with hypercalcaemia.
- Tumours that metastasize to bone are more prone to produce PTHrP than tumours that do not metastasize to bone (50% of 1° breast cancer express PTHrP, compared with 92% of metastases of breast cancer to bone). This may be due to induction of PTHrP secretion by the bone microenvironment; alternatively, PTHrP production by tumour cells may enhance their ability to metastasize to bone.
- For tumours associated with humeral hypercalcaemia, 🕮 see Table 12.3, p. 646.

Management

- As per normal management of hypercalcaemia (🕮 see Other causes of hypercalcaemia, p. 469).
- Glucocorticoids may be particularly effective in treatment of hypercalcaemia associated with malignancy. This may be due to direct effects of glucocorticoids on the tumour cells (e.g. haemopoietic malignancies) and/or because of downregulation of production of $1,25(OH)_2$ colecalciferol.
- Bisphosphonates may also have antitumour effects in myeloma as well as control osteoclastic destruction of bone.

Cushing's syndrome due to ectopic ACTH production

- Ectopic ACTH production is responsible for 10–20% of all endogenous Cushing's syndrome.
- Commonest tumour types are those with neuroendocrine features. 50% of ectopic ACTH secretion is due to small cell lung carcinoma. Carcinoid tumours are also very common (thymic carcinoid 15%; pancreatic endocrine tumours, including pancreatic carcinoids, 10%; bronchial carcinoid 10%). Ectopic CRH production has been described but is extremely rare.

Diagnosis

- Despite often extremely high cortisol levels, patients often do not manifest central weight gain due to the underlying malignant process with its rapid progress and associated cachexia.
- Hypertension, hypokalaemia, metabolic alkalosis are common features (overwhelming of the 11β-hydroxysteroid dehydrogenase enzyme, resulting in exposure of the mineralocorticoid receptor to high circulating glucocorticoids).
- Glucose intolerance, susceptibility to infection, thin skin, poor wound healing, and steroid-associated mood disturbance are all common features.
- Patients may be pigmented due to MSH arising from high POMC levels.
- ACTH levels may be extremely high (usually >100pg/mL).
- In 90% of ectopic ACTH-secreting tumours, high-dose dexamethasone testing (2mg qds) shows a failure of cortisol levels to drop to 50% of baseline values due to a lack of any normal physiological feedback upon ACTH production. However, some carcinoid tumours may behave indistinguishably from pituitary-dependent ACTH production. CRH testing and/or inferior petrosal sinus sampling may be necessary to distinguish these conditions (see 📖 p. 162).
- Ectopic ACTH-producing tumours can be extremely difficult to localize and may require multiple modalities of imaging.

Management

Excision of the underlying tumour may be possible. Other options include medical management using metyrapone and/or ketoconazole, although very high doses may be needed (📖 see Table 2.10, p. 171). Bilateral adrenalectomy with glucocorticoid and mineralocorticoid replacement is also an option.

Macronodular adrenal hyperplasia

- A rare cause of ectopic Cushing's syndrome.
- Most are sporadic; a few are familial.
- Most commonly due to synthesis of ectopic GIP receptors in adrenal tissues.
- GIP secretion associated with meals results in activation of adrenal glands and food-related hypercortisolaemia.
- Other ectopic receptors reported include β-adrenergic receptors and LH receptors.

Carcinoid tumours and ectopic hormone production

📖 See p. 556 and Table 12.3, p. 646.

Endocrine dysfunction and HIV/AIDS

Adrenal

Subclinical changes can be detected, including elevated basal cortisol concentrations and lower DHEA concentrations.

Adrenal insufficiency

Uncommon (<4% of patients with AIDS). In patients with clinical signs suggestive of hypoadrenalism (hyponatraemia and hypovolaemia), 30% incidence of inadequate response to Synacthen®.

Causes

- *Infection*. Histologically common. Adrenal function usually maintained (10% of residual adrenal tissue is adequate for normal function).
  - CMV (adrenalitis found post-mortem in 40–90% of patients with advanced disease).
  - *Mycobacterium avium intracellulare* (MAI) complex, tuberculosis.
  - *Cryptococcus*.
- *Neoplasm*. Lymphoma, Kaposi's sarcoma.
- *Haemorrhage*.
- *Drug-induced*:
  - Rifampicin induces ↑ hepatic metabolism of corticosteroids. In subjects with already compromised adrenal reserve, this may precipitate an Addisonian crisis.
  - Ketoconazole inhibits cortisol synthesis.
  - Megestrol acetate possesses glucocorticoid activity and may cause 2° adrenal insufficiency. Abrupt cessation after long-term treatment may precipitate an adrenal crisis.
- *2° adrenal insufficiency*:
  - Drugs (megestrol acetate).
  - Hypopituitarism 2° to toxoplasmosis, *Cryptococcus*, CMV.
  - Idiopathic anterior pituitary necrosis.

Hypercortisolism

Mild hypercortisolaemia common in all stages of HIV infection, without clinical manifestation of Cushing's syndrome.

Possible causes

- Chronic stress.
- Proinflammatory cytokines.
- Binding protein dysfunction.
- Glucocorticoid resistance.
- Concomitant use of ritonavir and inhaled fluticasone.

Gonads

Males

- SHBG concentrations are often elevated; this can lead to normal total testosterone concentrations but low free testosterone concentrations.
- Testosterone deficiency common in ♂ patients with AIDS (6% of patients with asymptomatic HIV infection, compared with 50% of patients with AIDS).
- Hypogonadism is associated with wasting, ↓ muscle mass, fatigue, loss of libido, and impotence. Hypogonadism may be 1° or 2°; up to 75% of patients with hypogonadism have low or inappropriately normal gonadotrophins.

Causes

- 1° *hypogonadism:*
  - *Testicular destruction/infiltration.* Due to infection (CMV most commonly, MAI, toxoplasmosis, TB) or neoplasm (lymphoma, Kaposi's sarcoma, germ cell tumours).
  - *Drug-induced.* Ketoconazole (inhibits steroidogenesis, causing lowered testosterone levels), megestrol acetate, other glucocorticoids.
- 2° *hypogonadism.* Due to malnutrition, severe acute illness, destructive disorders of pituitary/hypothalamus (CMV, toxoplasmosis, lymphoma); medications, such as megestrol acetate (glucocorticoid-like action causes hypogonadotrophic hypogonadism).

Females

- Hypogonadism in ♀, as evidenced by oligo-/amenorrhoea, less common than in ♂ unless advanced disease. Fertility rates not affected until advanced disease.
- Hypoandrogenism (testosterone, DHEA) common in ♀ with wasting syndrome.

Electrolyte disturbance due to endocrine perturbation in HIV/AIDS

Hyponatraemia

Very common in advanced disease. Due to SIADH in 50%; adrenal insufficiency also a common cause.

Calcium disorders

- *Hypocalcaemia.* Common (18% of patients with AIDS). Main cause is vitamin D deficiency. Other causes: severe illness; hypomagnesaemia; altered PTH secretion/metabolism; malabsorption of calcium and vitamin D due to GIT opportunistic infection; medications (foscarnet (complexes with calcium), pentamidine (induces renal magnesium wasting and 2° PTH deficiency)).
- *Hypercalcaemia.* Rare. May relate to lymphoma or granulomatous disease.

Thyroid

- Overt thyroid dysfunction is uncommon. Most common thyroid dysfunction is sick euthyroid syndrome (non-thyroidal illness). ↑ thyroid-binding globulin often observed (significance unknown).
- Subclinical hypothyroidism may occur during HAART (highly acitve antiretroviral therapy).
- *Infections.* Rare; usually post-mortem diagnoses. Thyroid function usually euthyroid or sick euthyroid.
  - *Pneumocystis carinii (*may also cause a thyroiditis).
  - Mycobacteria.
  - *Cryptococcus neoformans.*
  - *Aspergillosis.*
- *Neoplasm.* Rare. Usually eu- or sick euthyroid; may be hypothyroid due to infiltrative destruction.
  - Kaposi's sarcoma.
  - Lymphoma.

Pituitary

- *Anterior hypopituitarism.* Very rare.
- *Posterior pituitary dysfunction,* causing diabetes insipidus (DI). Common.
- *Infection.* Toxoplasmosis, TB.
- *Neoplasm.* Cerebral lymphoma.

Wasting syndrome

Definition

The involuntary loss of >10% of baseline body weight, in combination with diarrhoea, weakness, or fever. Wasting is an AIDS-defining condition.

Cause

Unknown but, in part, reflects ↓ calorie intake due to anorexia associated with 2° infection. Underlying ↑ resting energy expenditure associated with HIV infection *per se.* Hypogonadism common in ♂ with wasting syndrome.

Treatment

- *Highly active antiretroviral therapy* (HAART). Associated with overall weight gain, though lean body mass may remain unchanged.
- *Nutritionally-based strategies.* Adequate caloric intake to meet metabolic demands. Efficacy limited, as refeeding generally increases fat body mass, with little/less effect on lean body mass.
- *Appetite stimulants.* Megestrol acetate increases caloric intake and weight compared to placebo, though most of weight gain due to ↑ fat mass. Dronabinol stimulates appetite, but weight gain is minimal.
- *Exercise.* Although exercise can increase total and lean body mass in patients with AIDS, its role in patients with wasting syndrome is not known.
- *Androgen therapy.* In hypogonadal ♂ patients with wasting syndrome, testosterone increases overall weight and, in particular, lean body mass. Both IM and transdermal testosterone effective. Testosterone therapy not indicated in eugonadal ♂ with wasting.

- *Growth hormone therapy.* Patients with the wasting syndrome generally have GH resistance, as suggested by high serum GH and low IGF-I levels. The most likely cause for this is undernutrition. High-dose GH has shown improvements in lean body mass and protein balance in patients with acquired GH deficiency or severe catabolic states. Side effects (peripheral oedema, arthralgias, myalgias) common due to high doses required. GH may improve fat redistribution that occurs with refeeding.
- *Cytokine modulators.* Although many inflammatory cytokines are ↑ during acute illness and sepsis, their specific role in wasting syndrome is not known. Thalidomide, a potent inhibitor of TNF, can increase body weight and reduce protein catabolism but has a very high rate of serious side effects and is contraindicated in ♀ of childbearing age due to phocomelia (limit malformation).

Lipodystrophy

- Loss of SC fat, particularly in the face, peripheries, and buttocks; in some cases, with concomitant subcutaneous fat deposition, particularly in the abdominal area, neck, dorsocervical area ('buffalo hump'). Visceral fat deposition also occurs.
- Associated dyslipidaemia with hypertriglyceridaemia, low HDL cholesterol, insulin resistance, glucose intolerance, and (less commonly) frank diabetes mellitus. ↑ cardiovascular mortality from myocardial infarction.
- Associated with HIV-1 protease inhibitors (PIs), used as part of HAART. 40% of patients treated with PIs will develop lipodystrophy by 1 year. HIV protease inhibitor-naive patients have similar body composition and fat distribution to that of non-HIV-infected men. Indinavir may be less potent in inducing lipodystrophy than ritonavir and saquinavir.
- Abnormal body composition and hypertriglyceridaemia may be part of refeeding phenomenon consequent upon improved well-being and loss of anorexia *per se*.
- Nucleoside reverse transcriptase inhibitors may be associated with fat loss and accumulation also, but this may be a separate phenomenon to that seen with PIs.

Management
- Observation in mild cases.
- Very low-fat diets and exercise (particularly resistance exercise).
- Withdrawal or switching of PIs in some circumstances may be warranted.
- Anabolic agents (testosterone, GH) not effective.
- Liposuction from areas of fat accumulation; fat pad insertions for areas of lipoatrophy also used.
- Standard lipid-lowering agents for hypertriglyceridaemia (e.g. gemfibrozil).
- HMG CoA reductase inhibitors metabolized by P4503A4 (which is inhibited by PIs), so risk of myopathy may be ↑.
- Role for thiazolidinediones unclear.

Liver disease and endocrinology

Sex hormones—males
(See Table 12.4.)
- Hypogonadism occurs in 70–80% of ♂ with chronic liver disease. There is a combination of 1° testicular failure and failure of hypothalamo–pituitary regulation.
- Alcohol acts independently to produce hypogonadism. There is a combination of 1° testicular failure and failure of hypothalamo–pituitary regulation.
- The effects of elevated oestrogens result in ↑ loss of the ♂ escutcheon, loss of body hair, redistribution of body fat, palmar erythema, spider naevi, and gynaecomastia.
- The ↑ conversion of testosterone and androstenedione to oestrone is attributed, at least in part, to portosystemic shunting. In addition, the large increase in SHBG concentration will increase the oestrogen/testosterone ratio, as testosterone has a higher affinity for SHBG.
- Spironolactone may result in iatrogenic feminization by inhibiting testosterone action.
- There is no evidence that exogenous administration of androgens reverses hypogonadism in chronic liver disease.

Sex hormones—females
(See Table 12.4.)
- Alcoholism increases the frequency of menstrual disturbances and spontaneous abortion but does not affect fertility.
- Liver dysfunction of whatever aetiology is associated with an early menopause.
- Alcohol, rather than liver disease, is the prime cause of hypogonadism. Non-alcoholic liver disease is only associated with hypogonadism in advanced liver failure when it is accompanied by encephalopathy and impaired GnRH secretion.
- Plasma testosterone and oestrone concentrations are usually normal; androstenedione concentration is ↑, and dehydroepiandrostenedione and dehydroepiandrostenedione sulphate levels are reduced.

Thyroid
- The liver synthesizes albumin, T_4-binding prealbumin (TBPA), and T_4-binding globulin (TBG), all of which bind thyroid hormones covalently and reversibly.
- Thyroid function tests must be interpreted with caution in patients with liver disease. In acute liver disease, e.g. acute viral hepatitis, TBG levels are ↑ which increases the measured total circulating T_4 and T_3 levels. In biliary cirrhosis and chronic active hepatitis, TBG may be ↑. In other chronic liver disease and in hepatomas, TBG is also ↑. In severe cases of acute liver disease, TBG may be low due to reduced synthesis. The liver deiodinates T_4 to T_3, and this is impaired in liver disease. T_4 is preferentially converted to rT_3, and there is an increase in the rT_3/T_3 ratio.

Table 12.4 Sex hormone changes in liver disease

Hormone	Level
Testosterone	↓↓
SHBG	↑
Oestrone	↑
Oestradiol	↑/normal
LH	Inappropriately low/normal
FSH	Inappropriately low/normal
Prolactin	↑/normal
IGF-1	↓
IGFBP-3	↓

Table 12.5 Thyroid function changes in liver disease

Hormone	Acute hepatitis	CAH/PBC	Cirrhosis
T_4	↑ ↓	↑	↓
fT_4	↑ →	→	↑
T_3	↓	↑	↓
fT_3	↓	↓	↓
rT_3	↑	→	↑ →
TSH	↑	↑	↑ →
TBG	↑	↑	↓

CAH, chronic active hepatitis; PBC, primary biliary cirrhosis.

- In liver cirrhosis, TBG, T_4, and T_3 are low.
- Table 12.5 summarizes the changes in TFTs with liver disease. Free T_4 and T_3 assays are essential for the accurate interpretation of thyroid status in liver disease.

Adrenal hormones

- Patients who abuse alcohol may develop a clinical phenotype of Cushing's syndrome, with moon facies, centripetal obesity, striae, and muscle wasting, and may have increased plasma cortisol concentrations. This is termed *pseudo-Cushing's syndrome*.
- Reversible (on abstention) adrenocorticoid hyperresponsiveness occurs in alcoholics. In liver disease, cortisol metabolism may be impaired, leading to elevated plasma cortisol levels, loss of diurnal cortisol variation, and failure to suppress with dexamethasone.

Further reading

Malik R, Hodgson H (2002). The relationship between the thyroid gland and the liver. *QJM* **95**, 559–69.

Renal disease and endocrinology

Calcitriol
There is impaired renal conversion of 25-hydroxyvitamin D_3 to $1,25(OH)_2D_3$ in end-stage renal failure (ESRF), leading to metabolic bone disease (📖 see Table 6.6, p. 482).

Parathyroid hormone and renal osteodystrophy
- Serum parathyroid hormone (PTH) secretion is stimulated by low serum calcium in ESRF. This is due to:
  - ↓ renal phosphate clearance (resulting in ↑ calcium/phosphate mineral ion product, precipitation of vascular calcification with consequent hypocalcaemia triggering PTH release). Vascular calcification is a major contributor to vascular death in ESRF. High phosphate *per se* may increase PTH secretion directly, but evidence of the mechanism for this is lacking.
  - Impaired renal calcitriol secretion.
- As renal function declines, an elevated PTH and a ↓ calcitriol can be detected, with creatinine clearance of 50mL/min. This rise in PTH is initially sufficient to maintain the serum calcium in the normal range.
- In ESRF, patients are markedly hyperphosphataemic and hypocalcaemic. The degree of hyperparathyroidism progresses inversely with the fall in renal function. Tertiary hyperparathyroidism occurs when PTH secretion becomes autonomous, and hypercalcaemia will persist even after renal transplantation.
- Hyperparathyroid bone disease and osteomalacia are the main mechanisms behind the development of high turnover bone disease in renal osteodystrophy. Hypogonadism is also common in both ♂ and ♀ with ESRF. Adynamic bone disease also contributes, probably due to direct toxic effects from urea and other nitrogenous compounds upon bone cells. Renal osteodystrophy causes bone pain and fractures.

Treatment of renal osteodystrophy
- Maintenance of normal phosphate levels with phosphate binders (such as calcium carbonate) and the treatment of osteomalacia. The ↑ use of calcium carbonate has been suggested as the cause of the ↑ incidence of adynamic renal osteodystrophy, but intensive vitamin D therapy and peritoneal dialysis are probably also contributory.
- Alfacalcidol or calcitriol (which do not require renal 1α-hydroxylation) are effective in treating osteomalacia.
- Calcitriol at a dose of 1–2 micrograms/day is used for established renal osteodystrophy. Lower doses of calcitriol (0.25–0.5 micrograms/day) are used in early ESRF to prevent the development of renal osteodystrophy.
- Parathyroidectomy is advocated in bone disease uncontrolled by vitamin D therapy or the development of tertiary hyperparathyroidism.
- Cinacalcet acts directly at the calcium-sensing receptor to lower PTH secretion. This markedly improves 2° hyperparathyroidism, calcium and phosphate levels, and renal osteodystrophy. Improvement in mortality due to ↓ vascular calcification has not yet been demonstrated.

Prolactin

Hyperprolactinaemia is common in ESRF but is usually mild, i.e. <1,000mU/L. The cause is both ↑ secretion and ↓ renal clearance.

Gonadal function

- Hypogonadism—clinical and biochemical—is common in ESRF.
- In ♂, there is impaired pulsatile release of LH, although basal LH levels are usually elevated due to impaired renal clearance. Serum FSH is usually normal or mildly elevated.
- In ♀, levels of oestradiol, progesterone, and FSH are reported to be within the normal range in the early follicular phase but fail to show the usual cyclical changes. Menstrual disturbance is common. Amenorrhoea, polymenorrhoea, and menorrhagia can also occur on dialysis. Infertility is the rule, and conception on dialysis is the exception.
- Sexual dysfunction is common in both sexes but has been better studied in ♂. 60% of ♂ have some degree of impotence, and examination yields 80% to have testicular atrophy and 14% to have gynaecomastia.
- Treatment of hypogonadism in ESRF is suboptimal. Testosterone therapy is not associated with any clinical benefit in ♂.

Growth hormone and growth retardation

- Basal GH levels are normal, but there is impaired secretion following an adequate hypoglycaemic stimulus in 40–70% of patients with ESRF.
- There is impaired growth in children, particularly during periods of greatest growth velocity, and puberty is delayed. This combination leads to short stature. The improved growth velocity after renal transplantation is often too little too late in order to attain a normal stature.
- Recombinant human GH (rhGH) has been shown to be an effective treatment for growth retardation in children with stable chronic renal failure (CRF) and ESRF as well as after renal transplantation.

Thyroid

The 'sick euthyroid' finding is common in CRF (□ see Sick euthyroid syndrome, p. 24).

Adrenal

- The adrenal axis is not impaired clinically by CRF.
- There is evidence of blunted cortisol response to hypoglycaemia, but this is not relevant clinically.
- Patients with amyloidosis are at risk of hypoadrenalism due to adrenal amyloid infiltration.

Endocrinology in the critically ill

(See Table 12.6.)

ACTH and cortisol

- CRH, ACTH, and cortisol increase rapidly during all forms of acute illness.
- Low albumin and CBG cause free cortisol to be substantially higher.
- This physiological adaptation results in:
  - Provision of substrates for major organ energy expenditure (via catabolism).
  - Haemodynamic advantages (enhanced sensitivity to angiotensin II, ↑ vasopressor and inotropic response to catecholamines).
  - Prevention of an excessive immune response.
- Inflammatory cytokines result in ↑ cortisol metabolism and reduced receptors, i.e. peripheral cortisol resistance.
- After moderate-to-severe injuries, plasma cortisol starts to fall after a day or two but only reach normal levels after a week.
- Cortisol is elevated for at least 2 weeks in patients with severe burns.
- Prolonged critical illness results in low CRH and ACTH, with a 'normal' or slightly raised cortisol, perhaps driven by an alternative pathway involving endothelin.
- Cortisol deficiency should be suspected in an acutely ill patient with a plasma cortisol of <690nmol/L or an increment of <250nmol/L on a 250 micrograms short Synacthen® test.
- Drugs used in intensive care may contribute to adrenal insufficiency by:
  - Reducing cortisol metabolism, e.g. etomidate (frequently used in induction of anaesthesia) and ketoconazole.
  - Promoting cortisol metabolism, e.g. phenytoin, carbamazepine, and rifampicin.

Metabolism

- Hyperglycaemia is common in critical illness (even in non-diabetic subjects) due to ↑ cortisol, catecholamines, GH, and glucagon.
- These hormones and inflammatory cytokines also contribute to insulin resistance.
- IV insulin, titrated to maintain normoglycaemia (glucose <6.1mmol/L), reduces mortality by >40%.

TSH and thyroid hormones

- TSH levels usually remain stable in acute injury. Total T_4 and T_3 tend to fall but may remain within the normal range.
- Enhanced thyroid hormone metabolism by ↑ activity of liver deiodinase type 3 (peripheral hormone deactivator).
- With prolonged illness, total T_4 tends to fall below the normal range. FT_4 remains in the normal range.
- Total and free T_3 levels fall after injury and may remain suppressed for 2–3 weeks after a severe injury. The rT_3 level rises.
- In prolonged critical illness, the thyroid function conforms to the 'sick euthyroid syndrome' (☐ see Sick euthyroid syndrome, p. 24).

Gonadotrophins and gonadal steroids

In prolonged illness, hypogonadotrophic hypogonadism occurs.

Table 12.6 Endocrine and other changes seen in the ill

Acute illness	
ACTH/CRH	↑↑↑
Albumin/CBG	↓
Free cortisol	↑↑
Catabolism	↑↑
Immune response	↓
Inflammatory response	↑↑
Cortisol resistance	↑
Glucose	↑
Insulin resistance	↑↑
TSH	→
FT_4 and FT_3	→ ↓
IGF-1, IGFBPs, GHBPs	↓
Prolonged critical illness	
ACTH/CRH	↓ ↓
Free cortisol	→ or ↑
TSH, total T_4	↓
rT_3	↑
LH/FSH/T/oestradiol	↓
GH	↓
Response to GHRH	↓

Growth hormone

- In critical illness, the GH axis is profoundly affected, with initially raised GH secretion but low IGF-1, IGFBPs, and GHBP related to peripheral GH resistance.
- Prolonged critical illness >5–7 days results in low GH and a blunted response to GHRH.
- Recombinant GH was proposed as a beneficial agent for critical illness; however, the evidence is lacking, and there are reports of a detrimental effect.

Hormone replacement and critical illness

There is no evidence that, other than insulin, hormonal supplementation in the critically ill improves outcome.

Further reading

Elleger B, Debaveye Y, Van den Berghe G (2005). Endocrine interventions in the ICU. *Eur J Intern Med* **16**, 71–82.

Isidori AM, Kaltsas GA, Pozza C, et al. (2006). The ectopic adrenocorticotropin syndrome: clinical features, diagnosis, management, and long-term follow-up. *J Clin Endocrinol Metab* **91**, 371–7.

Syndromes of hormone resistance

Definition

Reduced responsiveness of target organs to a particular hormone, usually secondary to a disorder of the receptor or distal signalling pathways. This leads to alterations in feedback loops and elevated circulating hormone levels.

Thyroid hormone resistance

📖 see Resistance to thyroid hormones, pp. 10, 50.

Androgen resistance

📖 see Androgen insensitivity syndrome, pp. 416, 546.

Glucocorticoid resistance

- Autosomal dominant and recessive forms have been described.
- The resistance can be generalized or tissue-specific, partial or complete, and transient or permanent.
- Several mutations of the human glucocorticoid receptor gene have been described.
- Diminished sensitivity to glucocorticoid leads to reduced glucocorticoid feedback on CRH and ACTH, leading to ↑ CRH, ACTH, and cortisol concentrations.
- The clinical features are not due to excess glucocorticoid, as there is reduced peripheral tissue sensitivity. However, elevated ACTH leads to ↑ secretion of mineralocorticoid (e.g. deoxycorticosterone) and androgens (DHEA and DHEAS). This may lead to hypertension and hypokalaemic alkalosis, hirsutism, acne, oligomenorrhoea in ♀, and sexual precocity in ♂.
- Glucocorticoid resistance may be differentiated from Cushing's syndrome as, despite evidence of ↑ urinary cortisol, abnormal suppression with dexamethasone, and ↑ responsiveness to CRH, the diurnal rhythm of cortisol secretion persists, there are no clinical features of Cushing's syndrome, BMD is normal or ↑, and there is a normal response to insulin-induced hypoglycaemia.
- Low-dose dexamethasone treatment (1–3mg/day) may efficiently suppress ACTH and androgen production.

ACTH resistance

- Rare autosomal recessive disorders where the adrenal cortex fails to respond to ACTH in the presence of an otherwise normal gland (mineralocorticoid secretion is preserved under angiotensin II control). Very rarely can be due to autoantibodies blocking the ACTH receptor.
- The presenting clinical features include hypoglycaemia, which is often neonatal, neonatal jaundice, ↑ skin pigmentation, and frequent infections.
- Occasionally, ACTH resistance is a component of the *triple A syndrome* of alacrima (absence of tears), achalasia of the cardia, and ACTH resistance plus neurological disorders.

- *Biochemical features.* Undetectable or low 9 a.m. cortisol, with grossly elevated ACTH (often >1,000ng/mL), and normal renin, aldosterone, and electrolytes, and impaired response to short Synacthen® test.
- *Treatment.* Steroid replacement.

Mineralocorticoid resistance (see 📖 p. 262)

Also known as type 1 pseudohypoaldosteronism, this is a rare inherited disorder which usually presents in children with vomiting and anorexia, soon after birth, failure to thrive, salt loss, and dehydration. Both autosomal dominant and recessive forms have been described.

- *Biochemical features:*
  - ↓ serum sodium.
  - ↑ serum potassium (hyperkalaemic acidosis).
  - ↑ urinary sodium (despite hyponatraemia).
  - ↑ plasma and urinary aldosterone.
  - ↑ plasma renin activity.
- Diagnosis requires proof of unresponsiveness to mineralocorticoids (no effect of fludrocortisone on urinary sodium).
- Treatment is with sodium supplementation, and carbenoxolone has been used successfully. With time, treatment can often be weaned, and salt wasting is unusual following childhood.

Further reading

Charmandari E, Kino T, Ichijo T, *et al.* (2008). Generalized glucocorticoid resistance: clinical aspects, molecular mechanisms, and implications of a rare genetic disorder. *JCEM* **93**, 1563–72.

Differential diagnosis of possible manifestations of endocrine disorders

Sweating
- Menopause/gonadal failure.*
- Thyrotoxicosis.*
- Intoxication.*
- Drug/alcohol withdrawal.*
- Phaeochromocytoma.
- Acromegaly.
- Carcinoid syndrome.
- Hypoglycaemia.
- Diabetes mellitus.
- Parkinsonism.
- Autonomic neuropathy (gustatory sweating).
- Renal cell carcinoma.
- Chronic/subacute infection (e.g. TB, endocarditis).
- Haematological malignancy (e.g. lymphoma).
- Anxiety.
- Idiopathic.
- Drugs, e.g. fluoxetine, tricyclics, aspirin, NSAIDs, tamoxifen, omeprazole.
- Fabry's disease (most commonly causes anhidrosis).

Investigation of sweating
- History.
- Clinical examination.
- Thyroid function tests, serum gonadotrophin levels, blood glucose level.
- Specific investigations, according to clinical suspicion.

Management of sweating
- Treat the underlying cause where possible.
- Antiperspirants.
- Topical aluminium chloride ± ethanol.
- Anticholinergics—glycopyrronium bromide (oral or topical).
- Clonidine—taken at night to avoid sedation.
- Iontophoresis.
- Botulinum toxin A injections into affected areas (inhibits the release of acetylcholine at the synaptic junction of local nerves).
- Local excision of axillary sweat glands.
- Sympathetic denervation:
  - Video-assisted endoscopic thoracic sympathectomy: excision or radioablation.
  - Sympathotomy (chain disconnection between T2 ganglion and stellate ganglion).

* Commonest causes.

Palpitations (often associated with sweating)

- Thyrotoxicosis.
- Hypoglycaemia (insulinoma).
- Phaeochromocytoma.
- Anxiety states.
- Cardiac arrhythmia.
- Caffeine excess.
- Alcohol/drug withdrawal.

General malaise, tiredness

- Addison's disease.
- Hypo- or hyperthyroidism.
- Hypogonadism.
- Hypopituitarism/GH deficiency.
- Osteomalacia.
- Diabetes mellitus.
- Cushing's syndrome.
- Anaemia.
- Drugs (prescription and recreational drugs):
  - Antihistamines, antidepressants, antihypertensives (β-blockers, methyldopa, clonidine), neuroleptics, corticosteroids.
- Malignancy.
- Chronic fatigue syndrome (may be associated with reduced cortisol output, both basally and in response to a variety of challenges).
- Chronic illness (cardiac, respiratory, hepatic).
- Chronic pain.
- Fibromyalgia.
- Depression.
- Sleep disorders (obstructive sleep apnoea).
- Infection.
- Musculoskeletal/neurological disease (myasthenia gravis).
- Toxins.
- Idiopathic.

Investigation of fatigue

- Careful history-taking:
  - Duration, onset, recovery, and type of fatigue.
  - Person's usual activity level.
- Clinical examination.
- Serum electrolytes.
- Haemoglobin ± serum ferritin level.
- Inflammatory markers (ESR, CRP).
- Liver function tests.
- Serum calcium and phosphate levels.
- Thyroid function tests.
- Short Synacthen® test.

Flushing
- Gonadal failure (with flushing and sweats).
- Drugs.
  - Chlorpropamide.
  - Nicotinic acid.
  - Antioestrogens.
  - LHRH agonists.
- Carcinoid (dry flushing—no sweats).
- Mastocytosis.
- Medullary thyroid cancer.
- Anaphylaxis.
- Pancreatic cell carcinoma.
- Phaeochromocytoma (more often pallor).
- Fever.
- Alcohol.
- Autonomic dysfunction.
- Some foods:
  - Fish.
  - Tyramine-containing food (cheese).
  - Nitrites (cured meat).
  - Monosodium glutamate.
  - Spicy food.
- Gustatory flushing.
- Benign cutaneous flushing.
- Idiopathic.

Initial evaluation of patients with flushing
- Careful history.
- Physical examination (ideally during a flush although not often possible):
  - Examine skin carefully.
  - Pulse rate.
  - BP.
  - Thyroid examination.
  - Respiratory examination (wheeze).
  - Careful abdominal examination.
  - Urine dipstix.
- Biochemistry:
  - Gonadotrophin levels.
  - 2× 24h urinary 5HIAA measurements.
  - Serum chromogranin A.
  - 2× 24h urinary catecholamine measurements.
  - Plasma metanephrines (if high level of suspicion).
  - Serum tryptase level (if suspecting mastocytosis).
  - Calcitonin level (if suspecting medullary thyroid cancer).
  - Plasma VIP (if suspecting pancreatic carcinoma).
  - Immunoglobulin levels (raised IgE may suggest allergies).
- Specific investigations, according to suspected diagnosis.

Management of flushing

- Treat the underlying cause.
- Nadolol (non-selective β-blocker) effective in some cases of benign cutaneous flushing.
- Somatostatin analogues can be used to treat flushing associated with carcinoid syndrome.
- Antihistamines may be effective in some histamine-secreting carcinoid tumours.

Further reading

Cleare A (2003). The neuroendocrinology of chronic fatigue syndrome. *Endocr Rev* **24**, 236–52.

Cornuz J, Guessous I, Favrat B (2006). Fatigue: a practical approach to diagnosis in primary care. *CMAJ* **174**, 765–7.

Eisenach J, Atkinson J, Fealey R (2005). Hyperhidrosis: evolving therapies for a well established phenomenon. *Mayo Clin Proc* **80**, 657–66.

Izikson L, English J, Zirwas M (2006). The flushing patient: differential diagnosis, workup and treatment. *J Am Acad Derm* **55**, 193–208.

Paisley AN, Buckler HM (2010). Investigating secondary hyperhidrosis. *BMJ* **341**, c4475.

Stress and the endocrine system

Definition
Stress may be considered as a state of threatened, or perceived as threatened, homeostasis. The principal effectors of the stress response are corticotrophin-releasing hormone (CRH), glucocorticoids (GCs), catecholamines, arginine vasopressin (AVP), and POMC-derived peptides (especially α-melanocyte-stimulating hormone) and β-endorphins.

Endocrine effects of stress
The endocrine response to stress is mediated by CNS and peripheral components. The CNS components mediating the endocrine response to stress are located in the hypothalamus and brainstem and consist of the neurons releasing CRH, AVP, and the noradrenergic cell groups in the medulla/pons. Peripheral components of the endocrine stress response include the sympathetic–adrenal medulla system, the parasympathetic system, and the hypothalamo–pituitary–adrenal axis.

Hypothalamo–pituitary axis
- ↑ amplitude of synchronized pulsatile release of CRH and AVP (potent synergistic factor of CRH) into the hypophyseal portal system.
- ↑ stimulated ACTH production.
- ↑ adrenal glucocorticoid and androgen secretion.
- GCs also play a role in termination of the normal stress response by −ve feedback at the pituitary, hypothalamus, and extrahypothalamic regions.

Growth hormone axis
- GCs suppress GH production and inhibit the effects of IGF-1 (thus, children with anxiety disorders may have short stature).
- CRH increases somatostatin production, inhibiting GH production.
- GH response to IV glucagon is blunted.

Thyroid axis
- GCs reduce the production of TSH and limit the conversion of T_4 to the more active T_3 by reducing deiodinase activity.
- Somatostatin suppresses both TRH and TSH release.
- 📖 see Sick euthyroid syndrome, p. 24.

Reproductive axis
- CRH reduces GnRH secretion.
- GCs suppress GnRH neurons and pituitary gonadotrophs and render the gonads resistant to gonadotrophins.
- GCs also render peripheral tissues resistant to oestradiol.
- Chronic stress leads to amenorrhoea in ♀ and low LH and testosterone in ♂.
- Oestrogens increase CRH expression via an oestrogen response element in the promoter region of the CRH gene. This may account for the sex-related differences in the stress response and HPA axis activity.
- CRH is produced by the ovary, endometrium, and placenta during the latter half of pregnancy, leading to physiological hypercortisolism.

Metabolism
- GCs, via their direct effect and via reduced GH and sex hormone activity, result in muscle and bone catabolism and fat anabolism.
- Chronic activation of the stress system is associated with ↑ visceral adiposity, ↓ lean body mass, and suppressed osteoblastic activity (which may ultimately lead to osteoporosis).
- GCs induce insulin resistance and other features of the metabolic syndrome.

Other effects
- Immune: activation of the HPA axis inhibits the immune/inflammatory response; most components of the immune response are inhibited by glucocorticoids (>20% of genes expressed in human leukocytes are regulated by glucocorticoids), increasing the susceptibility to infections.

Further reading

Charmandari E, Tsigos C, Chrousos G (2005). Endocrinology of the stress response. *Annu Rev Physiol* **67**, 259–84.

Endocrinology of exercise

Exercise and the hypothalamo–pituitary axis

Exercise presents a significant challenge to physiological homeostasis. The endocrine system is integral to the body's ability to adapt to exercise, allowing the mobilization of metabolic fuels and also assisting in key cardiorespiratory responses.

- A 'stress' response is a significant part of this, with both CRH and ADH stimulating the release of ACTH and hence cortisol. This response promotes gluconeogenesis and helps to limit exercise-induced inflammation. Chronically trained athletes demonstrate a background hypercortisolaemia, although an attenuated cortisol rise in response to exercise is also seen.
- GH is released in response to acute exercise and remains ↑ until around 2h afterwards, although the mechanisms underlying this are not clear. The response is proportional to both the intensity and duration of the exercise. In longer term, both 24h GH secretion and IGF-1 levels correlate well with physical activity and VO_{2max}.
- In order that fluid homeostasis can be maintained, ADH is released in response to exercise by osmotic stimuli. However, non-osmotic stimuli can also affect ADH release, and this may contribute to the development of exercise-associated hyponatraemia.
- Prolactin is secreted in response to an exercise bout, although regular exercise does not seem to affect prolactin levels long-term. The role of prolactin in exercise is not clear, but it may impact on immune function.
- Both prolactin and cortisol suppress GnRH secretion, and hence LH/FSH secretion, which may explain why exercise can suppress gonadal function. Potential effects of this are discussed in The female athlete triad on 📖 p.673.
- TSH is rapidly stimulated in response to acute exercise, but longer-term effects are not clear. Exercise training can inhibit peripheral thyroid hormone metabolism, leading to increased levels of reverse T_3 and increased levels of T_3.

Exercise and bone health

- Physical activity has been shown to ↑ bone mass, especially at load-bearing sites. Approximately 26% of total adult bone mass is gained in 2 years around the time of peak bone gain (12.5 years in girls and 14.1 years in boys), meaning that physical activity may be particularly important around this time.
- Bone strength may be a more important measure than bone mass. Small, but significant, exercise-related ↑ in bone strength have also been seen in the lower extremities in children.
- In older adults, bone mass is improved with weight-bearing exercise, compared with controls, in general due to the attenuation of normal bone loss rather than an ↑ in bone mass in the intervention group.
- Rates of stress fracture in athletes have been ↓ with calcium and vitamin D supplementation, although the evidence is not yet strong enough for supplementation to be recommended routinely. Dosing is also not clear.

The female athlete triad

This has been recognized since the 1990s and is defined as the interplay between:

- Energy deficit (with or without an eating disorder).
- Amenorrhoea.
- Osteoporosis.

Hypothalamic amenorrhoea can develop in the context of stress, weight loss, and exercise. An energy deficit (between intake and expenditure) appears to be essential for weight loss and exercise-related forms, with leptin also playing a key role. Problems with bone health may result from a combination of poor intake of calcium and vitamin D and disruption of gonadal function.

▶ It is vital to ask about energy intake, weight, and menstrual function in young female athletes. A detailed history is key to diagnosis of amenorrhoea, and investigation should rule out alternative causes,

Successful management often takes a multidisciplinary approach, including both dietetic and psychological input. Strategies include:

- Exercise reduction and dietary modification to eliminate the energy deficit and ensure adequate nutrient intake are important. Weight gain may be required.
- For bone health, ensuring an adequate intake of calcium and vitamin D is important. Whether supplemental doses are required (and if so, what they should be) is not clear. There is no clear evidence for OCP use in this context, although it is widespread.
- Bone densitometry is likely to be helpful both to assess bone health and to evaluate the effectiveness of interventions.

Doping

Unfortunately, a small, but significant, number of athletes use banned performance-enhancing substances in order to gain a competitive advantage. Many of these are endocrine in origin. While their effects can be advantageous, side effects are also a significant issue. Some of the most popular are:

- Androgenic anabolic steroids. These improve performance by increasing muscle mass and strength. The main side effects are endocrine dysfunction, including virilization, hepatotoxicity, adverse cardiac effects, and psychiatric problems.
- EPO. This improves performance by improving oxygen delivery to muscle. The main side effect is an increased risk of thrombosis.
- GH. This results in improved muscle mass and reduced fat mass, although there is limited evidence of a performance benefit. Adverse effects are similar to those seen in acromegaly.
- Insulin. This can have beneficial anabolic effects, although side effects, such as hypoglycaemia and weight gain, may make it less attractive.

Further reading

Gordon CM (2010). Clinical practice. Functional hypothalamic amenorrhea. *N Engl J Med* **363**, 365–71.

Mastorakos G, Pavlatou M, Diamanti-Kandarakis E, Chrousos GP (2005). Exercise and the stress system. *Hormones (Athens)* **4**, 73–89.

McGrath JC, Cowan D (2008). Drugs in sport. *Br J Pharmacol* **154**, 493–5.

Complementary and alternative therapy and endocrinology

Introduction

- Many patients use natural products alongside, or instead of, conventional therapy. Products and information are available from many sources, but in particular the Internet.
- Patients need to be asked specifically about usage.
- Hospital pharmacists can be extremely helpful in sourcing information about natural products, including interactions with conventional medicines.
- Quality control of natural products is usually poor, with content ranging anywhere from 0% of stated level to several fold higher.
- Safety data are often absent or inadequate. Some preparations may also contain pharmacologically active compounds which can interact with other treatments or worsen comorbidities (e.g. alternative and complementary therapies for menopausal symptoms have been shown to contain oestrogenic properties which would be a concern for women with hormone-dependent diseases, such as breast cancer).
- Discussion of any natural products listed here is not intended *in any way* to imply efficacy or safety of these products or to recommend their usage, but rather to illustrate the compounds being promoted for these conditions by alternative information sources.

Alternative therapy used in patients with diabetes mellitus

A major concern with natural products used by patients with diabetes mellitus is that of interaction with conventional medicines, placing the patient at risk of hypoglycaemia.

Hypoglycaemic agents

These work by ↑ insulin secretion from the pancreas or due to direct insulin-like action at the insulin receptor.

- Banaba (*Lagerstroemia speciosa*)—crepe myrtle. Banaba extracts contain corosolic acid and ellagitannins, which may have direct insulin-like effects at insulin receptors.
- Bitter melon (*Momordica charantia*). Contains a polypeptide with insulin-like effects. Used as juice, powder, extracts, and fried food. Often part of Asian and Indian foods.
- Fenugreek (*Trigonella foenum-gracum*). Used as powder, seeds, or as part of dietary supplement. May enhance insulin release and may also decrease carbohydrate absorption due to laxative effect. May also inhibit platelets and thus increase bleeding diathesis.
- Gymnema (*Gymnema sylvestre*), 'gurmar' in Hindi ('sugar-destroying'). Extract 'GS4' also used. May increase endogenous insulin secretion (↑ C-peptide levels noted in users). In some preliminary studies, gymnema improved HbA1c and ↓ insulin or OHA requirements.
- Berberine (from *Coptis chinensis*). AMP kinase activator and promotes GLUT4 translocation to the cell membrane. Some studies suggest an HbA1c-lowering effect.

Insulin sensitizers

- Cassia cinnamon (*Cinnamomum aromaticum*)—also known as Chinese cinnamon (*Cinnamomum verum* is the usual cinnamon used in the UK, although cassia cinnamon may be contained in ground cinnamon mixes). May increase insulin sensitivity and lower fasting blood glucose levels. Appears safe and well tolerated.
- Chromium. Chromium deficiency is associated with impaired glucose tolerance, hyperglycaemia, and ↓ insulin sensitivity. Chromium forms part of a 'glucose tolerance factor' complex, and therefore supplements are sometimes labelled 'chromium GTF'. In patients with diabetes and chromium deficiency, addition of chromium improves glycaemic control. However, the role of chromium in patients without deficiency is not clear. The American Diabetes Association only recommends chromium usage in patients with documented chromium deficiency. Excessive chromium may cause renal impairment.
- Vanadium. Thought to stimulate hepatic glycogenolysis; inhibit gluconeogenesis, lipolysis, and intestinal glucose transport; increase skeletal muscle glucose uptake, utilization, and glycogenolysis. High-dose vanadium (taken as vanadyl sulphate) may improve insulin sensitivity and glycaemic control in patients with type 2 diabetes, with large doses of elemental vanadium required for these effects—however, doses >1.8mg/day vanadium may cause renal impairment.

- Ginseng (both *Panax ginseng* and American ginseng (*Panax quinquefolius*)). Contain ginsenoisides which may improve insulin sensitivity. Efficacy and safety not established.
- Prickly pear cactus (*Opuntia ficus-indica*), also called opuntia or 'nopals' (referring to the cooked leaves of the cactus). Prominent in Mexican folk medicine as a treatment for diabetes. *Opuntia streptacantha* stems may improve glycaemic control, either acting as an insulin sensitizer or by slowing carbohydrate absorption; however, this is not observed with other prickly pear cactus species.
- Reservatrol. Extracted from grapes and red wine. Activates sirtuin 1 (with an indirect effect on substrates, including PPARγ) and AMP kinase.
- Cannabinoids activate AMPK and PPARγ. Only anecdotal data on glucose lowering available; formal trials ongoing.

Carbohydrate absorption inhibitors

- *Soluble fibre*. Increases viscosity of intestinal contents, thus slowing gastric emptying time and carbohydrate absorption, resulting in lower postprandial blood glucose levels.
- The following products have some evidence of reducing postprandial blood glucose levels and may also improve total and LDL cholesterol levels in patients. They may also interfere with absorption of drugs and, therefore, should not be taken at the same time as conventional medicines:
  - Blond psyllium seed (*Plantago ovata*).
  - Guar gum (*Cyamopsis tetragonoloba*).
  - Oat bran (*Avena sativa*).
  - Soy (*Glycine max*)—contains both soluble and insoluble fibre and may improve insulin resistance, fasting BM, lipid profile, and HbA1c in type 2 diabetes.
- *Insoluble fibre*. Glucomannan (*Amorphophallus konjac*)—can delay glucose absorption.

Other products used by patients with diabetes mellitus

- Alpha-lipoic acid. Antioxidant. May improve insulin resistance. May help symptoms of diabetic neuropathy (? mechanism).
- Stevia (*Stevia rebaudiana*). May enhance insulin secretion. May be toxic.
- Huangqi (*Radix astragali*). Used to treat hypoglycaemia unawareness. May increase neural activation in central glucose-sensing regions in response to hypoglycaemia.

Alternative therapy used in menopause

Phytoestrogens

- Main types are isoflavones (most potent and most widespread), lignans, and coumestans.
- Sources:
  - Isoflavones: legumes (soy, chickpea, garbanzo beans, red clover, lentils, beans). Main active isoflavones are genistein and daidzein.
  - Lignans: flaxseed, lentils, whole grains, beans, many fruits and vegetables.
  - Coumestans: red clover, sunflower seeds, sprouts.
- Other phytoestrogens: chasteberry (*Vitex agnus-castus*).
- Not structurally similar to oestrogen or to selective oestrogen receptor modulators (SERMs) but contain a phenolic ring that allows binding to oestrogen receptors-α and -β. Effects of binding depend upon ambient oestrogen levels, relative ratio and concentration of ER-α and ER-β; tissue type and location. Relatively much less potent than endogenous oestrogen (by 100–10,000-fold).
- Phytoestrogens *in vitro* stimulate proliferation of normal human breast tissue and of oestrogen-sensitive breast tumour cells. Theoretically, phytoestrogens may stimulate ER +ve breast cancer and other oestrogen-sensitive tumours. Phytoestrogens may also antagonize the effects of tamoxifen or other SERMs. Phytoestrogens have not been shown to stimulate endometrial growth; however, they are not usually taken with progestagenic compounds. It is not known whether the other serious side effects of conventional oestrogens (e.g. DVT, pulmonary emboli, IHD, stroke) occur with phytoestrogen use. Many sources of phytoestrogens (e.g. coumestans) interfere with warfarin.
- Soy protein (20–60mg/day, containing 34–76mg isoflavones) modestly decreases frequency and severity of vasomotor symptoms in a proportion of menopausal women.
- Synthetic isoflavones (ipriflavone) do not have antivasomotor activity.
- Phytoestrogens from red clover have not shown consistent improvement in vasomotor symptoms. Other sources of phytoestrogens have not shown improvement in menopausal symptoms.
- Compounds with oestrogenic activity should not be used in women who should not take oestrogen (e.g. in women with breast cancer).
- For use in osteoporosis, 🕮 see Alternative therapy used by patients with osteoporosis, pp. 680–1.

Other compounds with oestrogenic activity

- Kudzu (*Pueraria lobata*).
- Alfalfa (*Medicago sativa*).
- Hops (*Humulus lupulus*).
- Liquorice (*Glycyrrhiza glabra*).
- *Panax ginseng* (ginseng)—*in vitro* evidence of stimulation of breast cancer cells.

Other substances used

- Black cohosh (*Actaea racemosa*, formerly *Cimicifuga racemosa*)—not to be confused with blue cohosh and white cohosh which are entirely separate plants. Widely used in menopause. Although often advertised as such, black cohosh does not bind to oestrogen receptors or have oestrogen effects and little evidence for efficacy for hot flushes.
- Dong quai (*Angelica sinensis*)—not clear if oestrogenic. *In vitro* evidence of promotion of breast cancer cells.

Alternative therapy used by patients with osteoporosis

Calcium

- Hundreds of preparations available.
- Several types of calcium salts available (including citrate, carbonate, lactate, gluconate, phosphate), with little evidence of superiority of absorption, etc. between different compounds, other than calcium citrate useful in patients with low gastric acidity (e.g. on concomitant proton pump inhibitors or H2 antagonists).

Magnesium

- Necessary for release of PTH.
- In itself, not effective in treating osteoporosis, unless patients are deficient in magnesium.

Fluoride

Increases bone density but not strength—bones less elastic, more brittle—with resultant ↑ fracture rate.

Trace elements

- For example, manganese, zinc, boron, copper.
- Whilst many trace elements are important for multiple enzyme systems, including those in bone, most patients are not deficient, and thus supplements have negligible +ve effect upon osteoporosis. Moreover, many minerals in high doses cause serious side effects (e.g. manganese doses >11mg/day can cause extrapyramidal side effects).

Vitamin D

Multiple preparations available, mainly as ergocalciferol or colecalciferol (vitamin D metabolites require prescription). Tablets containing >200IU vitamin D require a prescription in the UK.

Isoflavones

- For more detail about the mechanism of action of phytoestrogens, 🕮 see Alternative therapy used in menopause, p. 678.
- Soy protein in doses >80mg/day may improve bone mineral density, but no studies of soy have shown improvement in fracture rate. Possible adverse effects upon oestrogen-sensitive tissues, such as ER +ve breast cancer.
- Ipriflavone—semisynthetic isoflavone, produced from daidzein. No oestrogenic effects. No evidence of improved fracture outcome. Some studies of ipriflavone with calcium have reported improved BMD, although other studies have not shown an improvement. Ipriflavone can cause serious lymphopenia ($<1 \times 10^9$mL) which may take up to a year to recover.

Tea

- Tea consists of green tea (unfermented), oolong tea (partially fermented), and black tea (completely fermented).
- All teas contain fluoride and have high isoflavonoid content, in addition to caffeine.
- Coffee (with a high caffeine content) has been associated with ↑ hip fracture risk. However, tea-drinking of all types has been associated with higher BMD, although no fracture outcome has been reported.

DHEA

see Miscellaneous alternative therapy p. 682.

Wild yam

Wild yam contains diosgenin which is used commercially as a source for DHEA synthesis; however, this does not occur in humans.

Other compounds used by patients for osteoporosis

- Flaxseed (alpha-linolenic acid and lignans).
- Gelatin.
- Dong quai.
- *Panax ginseng*.
- Alfalfa.
- Liquorice.

There is no evidence of a +ve effect upon bone of these compounds.

Miscellaneous alternative therapy

Iodine and the thyroid

- Sources: kelp, shellfish-derived products.
- Effects: iodine-induced goitre or hypothyroidism, particularly in patients with underlying thyroid disease (may have a Wolff–Chaikoff effect in patients with Graves's disease, causing inhibition of iodide organification and thus thyroid hormone production).
- Iodine-induced hyperthyroidism in areas of endemic goitre and iodine deficiency.

DHEA—'elixir of youth'

- Reported to slow or improve changes associated with ageing, including general well-being, cognitive function, sexual function, energy levels, body composition, muscle strength, and to aid weight loss and treat the metabolic syndrome.
- Mechanism of action: DHEA is secreted by the adrenal glands and interconverted to DHEAS. Both DHEAS and DHEA are converted to androgens and oestrogens that then act directly at their receptors.
- DHEA and DHEAS may play a role in replacement of adrenal androgens in patients with adrenal insufficiency, resulting in improved well-being, particularly with respect to sexual function.
- Not proven in controlled trials to improve health in other patients without adrenal insufficiency.
- Risks of androgenic effects in women when taken at high doses (100–200mg/DHEA daily). Theoretical risk of promoting hormone-sensitive cancers, such as prostate and breast cancers. DHEA may also interfere with antioestrogen effects of anastrazole and other aromatase inhibitors.

Further information

Natural Medicines Comprehensive Database. Available at: ᴍ http://www.naturaldatabase.com (requires subscription).

Chapter 13

Diabetes

Classification and diagnosis of diabetes

Background
Diabetes mellitus (DM) is a metabolic disorder characterized by chronic hyperglycaemia due to defects in insulin secretion and/or insulin action. Currently, 4–6% of the UK population have diabetes. Worldwide, 285 million people were diagnosed with diabetes in 2010, and this number is predicted to exceed 400 million by 2030.

Diagnosis
DM is a biochemical diagnosis based on fasting and postprandial (2h) glucose levels during a 75g OGTT. In 1997, the American Diabetes Association (ADA) proposed lowering the normal fasting plasma glucose level to <6.1mmol/L and the threshold for diabetes to ≥7.0mmol/L. They also recommended that fasting plasma glucose was the preferred diagnostic test (outside of pregnancy) in order to reduce the number of OGTTs needed. Table 13.1 describes the plasma glucose thresholds associated with different stages of dysglycaemia; these range from normal glucose tolerance through impaired glucose tolerance (IGT), impaired fasting hyperglycaemia (IFG), and on to frank DM. In 2010, the ADA and WHO introduced HbA1c ≥48mmol/mol or 6.5% as a diagnostic criterion for DM. A diagnosis of diabetes is confirmed in any person with typical hyperglycaemic symptoms (e.g. polyuria, polydipsia, weight loss), with a random or postprandial blood glucose ≥11.1mmol/L or fasting plasma glucose ≥7mmol/L. In asymptomatic patients or those with intercurrent illness, a second abnormal result is necessary to establish a definitive diagnosis of diabetes.

Table 13.1 WHO glucose thresholds for diagnosis of diabetes mellitus and other stages of dysglycaemia

		Venous plasma glucose (mmol/L)
Normal	Fasting	<6.1
	and 2h glucose during an OGTT	<7.8
Diabetes	Fasting	≥7.0
	or 2h glucose during an OGTT	≥11.1
IGT	Fasting	<7.0
	and 2h glucose during an OGTT	≥7.8 and <11.1
IFG	Fasting	≥6.1 and <7.0

Classification

During the 1980s, the WHO published the first widely accepted classification of diabetes. Diabetes was classified as insulin-dependent DM (IDDM) or type 1 diabetes, and non-insulin-dependent DM (NIDDM) or type 2 diabetes. In 1997, the updated classification of diabetes retained the terms type 1 and type 2 diabetes, discarding the terms IDDM and NIDDM. The updated classification system focused on the specific underlying aetiology of diabetes. These aetiological groups are listed in Box 13.1.

Box 13.1 Aetiological classification of diabetes mellitus[1]

1. **Type 1 diabetes** (5–10% of cases): β-cell destruction.
   - Includes autoimmune and idiopathic forms.
2. **Type 2 diabetes** (90% of cases): defective insulin secretion, usually with defective insulin action.
3. **Other specific types:**
   - Genetic defects of β-cell function:
     - Maturity onset diabetes of the young (MODY).
     - Mitochondrial DNA mutations.
     - Neonatal diabetes.
   - Genetic defects of insulin action:
     - Lipodystrophies.
     - Insulin receptor mutations (includes type A insulin resistance, leprechaunism, Rabson–Mendenhall syndrome).
     - Rare downstream insulin-signalling defects.
     - Monogenic obesity/hyperphagia (e.g. leptin deficiency).
   - Diseases of the exocrine pancreas:
     - Pancreatitis, trauma, pancreatectomy, neoplasia, pancreatic destruction (including cystic fibrosis and haemochromatosis), others.
   - Endocrinopathies:
     - Cushing's syndrome, acromegaly, phaeochromocytoma, glucagonoma, hyperthyroidism, autoimmune polyglandular syndrome 1 and 2, others.
   - Drug- or chemical-induced:
     - Glucocorticoids, thyroid hormone, diazoxide, β-adrenergic agonists, thiazides, γ-interferon, antiretroviral treatment (HIV).
   - Infections:
     - Congenital rubella, cytomegalovirus (CMV), others.
   - Uncommon forms of immune-mediated diabetes:
     - 'Stiff man' syndrome (type 1 diabetes, rigidity of muscles, painful spasms), anti-insulin receptor antibodies, others.
   - Other genetic syndromes associated with diabetes:
     - Down's syndrome, Klinefelter's syndrome, Turner's syndrome, Wolfram syndrome (or DIDMOAD—diabetes insipidus, DM, optic atrophy, and sensorineural deafness), Friedreich's ataxia, Huntington's chorea, Lawrence–Moon–Biedl syndrome, myotonic dystrophy, Prader–Willi syndrome, others.
4. **Gestational diabetes mellitus.**

[1] Adapted from ADA classification.

The vast majority of patients with diabetes have either type 1 diabetes (secondary to autoimmune-mediated β-cell destruction and absolute insulin deficiency) or type 2 diabetes (due to insulin resistance and defects of insulin secretion). Table 13.2 outlines the key differences. Although the remaining aetiological subtypes account for <10% of all diabetes cases, it is important to consider these rarer causes of diabetes, which comprise the entire differential diagnosis, in order to facilitate personalized management of these patients. Rarer forms, such as maturity onset diabetes of the young (MODY), largely arise in young adults. These individuals are often assumed to have type 1 or type 2 diabetes and frequently experience long delays before the correct diagnosis is reached. Fig. 13.1 illustrates a suggested diagnostic algorithm for young adults.

Table 13.2 Differences between type 1 and type 2 diabetes

	Type 1 diabetes	Type 2 diabetes
Peak age of onset (years)	12	60
UK prevalence	0.25%	5–7% (10% of those >65 years of age)
Initial presentation	Polyuria, polydipsia, weight loss, ketoacidosis	Hyperglycaemic symptoms, often with complications of diabetes
Aetiology	Autoimmune β-cell destruction	Combination of insulin resistance, β-cell destruction, and β-cell dysfunction
Presence of β-cell antibodies	>90%	No
Insulin-dependent	Yes	No
Diabetic ketoacidosis	Common	Rare
Obesity	Uncommon	Common
Insulin resistance	Uncommon	Common
Treatment	Insulin from outset	Diet ± oral hypoglycaemic agents ± insulin

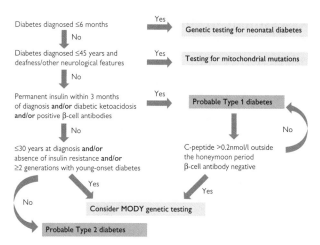

Fig. 13.1 Aetiological diagnosis in diabetes diagnosed <45 years.

Assessment of the newly diagnosed patient

There are two issues to address in a patient with a new diagnosis of diabetes: firstly, what the immediate management (inpatient vs outpatient, optimal treatment) is and, secondly, what the underlying aetiology is. Assigning aetiology is usually most challenging in those diagnosed in the second to fourth decades of life where there is overlap of clinical features between the common and rarer forms of diabetes. Reassessment over the first year or so after diagnosis can be helpful. If in any doubt over whether this is type 1 diabetes, be safe and commence insulin.

Fig. 13.1 suggests an algorithm for the investigation of young adults.

- *History:* acute or insidious onset, family history of diabetes, presence of other autoimmune diseases, ethnic origin.
- *Examination:* BMI, acanthosis nigricans, vitiligo. Evaluation of precipitating cause or infection.
- *Investigations:* HbA1c; renal, liver, and thyroid function; lipid profile. Ketones (urine or blood) and venous bicarbonate to assess for DKA. Test for β-cell antibodies in younger patients (<45 years at diagnosis).

Causes of diagnostic confusion

- *Latent autoimmune diabetes of adulthood (LADA).* This presents like type 2 diabetes but is a form of type 1 diabetes with insidious onset, defined by the presence of any β-cell antibody. Treat like type 2 diabetes, but progression to insulin is usually more rapid.
- *Ketosis-prone diabetes (KPD).* This presents with DKA or ketosis, but insulin requirements decline over weeks → months, and insulin can often be stopped. Most commonly seen in patients of African origin who are antibody −ve. Patients should be advised that they may develop ketosis again during illness and be given ketone-monitoring equipment.
- *Monogenic diabetes.* see p. 691.

Genetics

Type 1 diabetes

The overall lifetime risk of developing type 1 diabetes in a Caucasian population is currently 0.4%. This risk increases to:

- 1–2% if your mother has type 1 diabetes.
- 3–6% if your father has type 1 diabetes.
- 5–6% if a sibling has type 1 diabetes.
- Monozygotic twins have ~50% concordance rate by age 40 years.

Early linkage studies identified the importance of the human leukocyte antigen (HLA) genes of the major histocompatibility complex (MHC) in type 1 diabetes susceptibility. These variants account for half of the heritability of type 1 diabetes. The HLA class II DR and DQ loci (respectively encoded by genes *DRB* and *DQB*) account for almost all type 1 diabetes susceptibility from this region. >90% of patients with type 1 diabetes carry at least one copy of the *DRB**301-*DQB**201 or *DRB**401-*DQA**301-*DQB**302 (allele numbers after asterisk).

Other susceptibility loci include variants in the gene encoding insulin (*INS*) which confers a 2-fold increased risk. More recent genome-wide association studies (GWAS) have increased the total number of loci associated with type 1 diabetes to >40; however, these loci have much lower effect size than the *HLA* or *INS* genes.

These genetic studies have confirmed that the pathogenesis of type 1 diabetes involves disordered immune regulation. Indeed, ↑ levels of islet cell antibodies (ICA), anti-glutamic acid decarboxylase (GAD) antibodies, and anti-tyrosine phosphatase antibodies (anti-IA-2 antibodies) are usually detected at diagnosis. The presence of all three antibodies give a non-diabetic individual an 88% chance of developing type 1 diabetes over the next 10 years.

Type 2 diabetes

The importance of genetic background in the aetiology of type 2 diabetes is well established from family and twin studies (concordance between monozygotic twins is 60–100%). Heritability of type 2 diabetes is estimated at ~25%.

- So far, >70 genetic susceptibility variants for type 2 diabetes have been detected, largely through GWAS.
- *TCF7L2* (encoding transcription factor 7-like 2 protein) in chromosome 10q is the susceptibility locus, with the largest effect on type 2 diabetes risk, described to date, with a per-allele odds ratio of ~1.4.
- Together, the genetic loci found so far only explain a small proportion (~10%) of the overall heritable risk for type 2 diabetes.
- Ongoing research is focused on identifying rare genetic variants which might account for the missing heritability in type 2 diabetes.
- Potential areas of clinical translation include risk prediction, prevention, pharmacogenetics, and development of novel therapeutics.

Maturity onset diabetes of the young (MODY)

MODY, the commonest cause of monogenic β-cell dysfunction, is estimated to be the underlying cause in 0.5–1% of all patients with diabetes. A typical 'MODY patient' has young age of onset (<45 years, frequently <25 years), autosomal dominant family history of diabetes, absence of autoimmune markers, absence of insulin resistance and remains C-peptide +ve, even if insulin-treated. Mutations in ten different genes have been associated with the MODY phenotype; however, in clinical practice, the vast majority of MODY cases are due to heterozygous mutations in genes encoding the enzyme glucokinase (GCK) and the nuclear transcription factors hepatocyte nuclear factor 1α (HNF1A), hepatocyte nuclear factor 4α (HNF4A), and hepatocyte nuclear factor 1β (HNF1B).

HNF1A-MODY (previous name MODY3)

- Accounts for 30–70% of MODY cases.
- Associated with a progressive defect of insulin secretion which can be complicated by severe hyperglycaemia (1/3 patients eventually require insulin therapy) and frequent microvascular complications.
- Low renal threshold for glucose.
- Importantly, these patients are exquisitely sensitive to sulfonylureas. Low doses (e.g. gliclazide 40mg od) are recommended as first-line pharmacological therapy, often maintaining excellent glycaemic control for years. Insulin can be stopped in those who were assumed to have type 1 diabetes at onset of diabetes.
- Low C-reactive protein (<0.5mg/L).

HNF4A-MODY (previous name MODY1)

- Accounts for 5–10% of MODY cases.
- Clinical presentation similar to HNF1A-MODY (except normal renal glucose threshold).
- Also sensitive to sulfonylureas (📖 see HNF1A-MODY above).
- Neonatal hyperinsulinaemia and hypoglycaemia associated with macrosomia in affected neonates.

GCK-MODY (previous name MODY2)

- Accounts for 30–70% of MODY cases.
- Results in a raised threshold for glucose-stimulated insulin secretion, but importantly insulin secretion remains regulated.
- Lifelong, mild, stable fasting hyperglycaemia (fasting plasma glucose 5.5–8mmol/L and HbA1c <8%). Low increment of glucose rise following a carbohydrate challenge.
- GCK-MODY can be diagnosed at any age. Patients are often asymptomatic, with hyperglycaemia found during screening.
- Diabetes-related microvascular complications are not observed.
- Patients should be managed on diet alone (insulin is usually only required during pregnancy if the fetus is macrosomic).
- Secondary care follow-up is not usually required.

HNF1B-MODY (previous name MODY5)

- Also known as renal cysts and diabetes (RCAD) syndrome.
- Accounts for 5–10% of cases of MODY.

- Clinical features include malformations of the genitourinary system (commonly renal cysts and other renal developmental abnormalities), pancreatic atrophy, and exocrine insufficiency.
- Patients or family members may present to renal physicians first.
- Not sensitive to sulfonylureas.

Management of MODY in pregnancy

Although MODY is an uncommon cause of GDM, women with MODY often present with dysglycaemia in pregnancy. Most will be managed according to routine guidelines, but for those known to have MODY prior to pregnancy, specific advice on management can be sought from the MODY UK diagnostic centre (℡ http://www.diabetesgenes.org).

For those with HNF1A/HNF4A-MODY already well controlled on low-dose SU agents prior to pregnancy, there is a good argument for using glibenclamide pre-conception (safe in type 2 diabetes) and continuing as long as good control is maintained.

In HNF4A-MODY, an affected fetus can develop hyperinsulinaemia, macrosomia, and neonatal hypoglycaemia. Seek specialist advice on fetal monitoring.

In GCK-MODY, treatment (with insulin) is only recommended if macrosomia is developing. Seek specialist advice.

Neonatal diabetes

- Affects ~1 in 100,000–150,000 live births.
- Diabetes diagnosed before 6 months is likely to be one of the monogenic subtypes of neonatal diabetes, rather than type 1 diabetes. *Refer those diagnosed before 6 months for genetic investigation, even if many years later and attending adult clinics.* Diagnosis could change management.
- Transient neonatal diabetes (TNDM): diabetes usually remits within 3 months—chromosome 6q24 imprinting abnormalities (70% cases), mutations in the K_{ATP} channel genes (20% cases).
- Permanent neonatal diabetes (PNDM): mutations in *KCNJ11* and *ABCC8* genes, respectively encoding the Kir6.2 and SUR1 subunits of the K_{ATP} channel (50% cases); insulin gene mutations (10–15% cases).
- Patients with *KCNJ11* and *ABCC8* mutations can be effectively treated with high-dose sulfonylureas and insulin stopped.
- ~20% cases with K_{ATP} channel gene mutations have additional neurological features (DEND syndrome—developmental delay, epilepsy, and neonatal diabetes).
- *INS* mutations should be treated with insulin sensitizers or insulin.
- Seek specialist advice for management (℡ http://www.diabetesgenes.org).

Mitochondrial diabetes

- Due to mutations in mitochondrial DNA (most common is an A-to-G point mutation at position 3243 in the tRNA leucine gene).
- Maternal inheritance.
- Commonly associated with sensorineural deafness (MIDD: maternally inherited diabetes and deafness).

- Clinical features include CNS disease, ophthalmic disease (e.g. macular retinal dystrophy), myopathy, cardiac disease (e.g. LVH), and renal disease—patients should have echos, and consider neurology referral.
- Clinical phenotype can be variable, even within the same family, due to heteroplasmy.
- Patients should be referred to clinical genetics team for advice.

Genetic causes of severe insulin resistance

- Characterized by young onset of severe insulin resistance, e.g. acanthosis nigricans, dyslipidaemia, hypertension, hepatic steatosis, PCOS. This constellation of features, particularly in non-obese patients, should raise suspicion of a genetic cause. Treatment can be challenging. Exercise and insulin sensitizers are first line, then high-dose insulin (concentrated U-500 insulin may be helpful).
- *Lipodystrophies.* Insulin resistance plus abnormal fat distribution, e.g. loss of fat from limbs and increased central and ectopic fat. The classic Dunnigan familial partial lipodystrophy is caused by mutations in *LMNA*. Mutations in *PPARG* present with a similar phenotype. The lipodystrophies are more readily diagnosed in female patients.
- *Insulin receptor mutations.* Present with a range of severities but, in addition to severe insulin resistance, can present initially with fasting hypoglycaemia and growth defects and hyperandrogenism in women.

Diagnostic genetic testing

Diagnostic testing is available for the MODY subtypes, neonatal diabetes, mitochondrial mutations (particularly, the common A3243G variant), and the lipodystrophies (LMNA/PPARG). Although testing can be expensive, a clinical diagnosis is not a substitute for a definitive genetic test, especially where treatment decisions, such as stopping insulin, might depend on the outcome. Involve clinical genetics services to help with family screening. In the UK, the Genetic Diabetes Nurses network can provide help and expertise, and there is also an online MODY probability calculator; access both through ℘ http://www.diabetesgenes.org/.

Further reading

American Diabetes Association (2012). Diagnosis and classification of diabetes mellitus. *Diabetes Care* 35(S1), S64–71.

Greeley SAW, Naylor RN, Philipson LH, Bell GI (2011). Neonatal diabetes: An expanding list of genes allows for improved diagnosis and treatment. *Curr Diab Rep* **11**, 519–32.

Murphy R, Turnbull DM, Walker M, Hattersley AT (2007). Clinical features, diagnosis and management of maternally inherited diabetes and deafness (MIDD) associated with the 3243A>G mitochondrial point mutation. *Diabet Med* **25**, 383–99.

Semple RK, Savage DB, Cochran EK, Gorden P, O'Rahilly S (2011). Genetic syndromes of severe insulin resistance. *Endocr Rev* **32**, 498–514.

Thanabalasingham G, Owen KR (2011). Diagnosis and management of maturity onset diabetes of the young (MODY). *BMJ* **343**, 837–42.

Visscher PM, Brown MA, McCarthy MI, Yang J (2012). Five years of GWAS discovery. *Am J Hum Genet* **90**, 7–24.

Expert management of type 1 diabetes

Background

This condition is characterized by absolute insulin deficiency secondary to T-cell-mediated autoimmune destruction of the insulin-producing islets. This is characterized by the presence of T1-associated autoantibodies to glutamic acid decarboxylase (GAD), islet autoantigen (IA-2), and insulin which can often be detected for a few years prior to diagnosis and frequently declines from the time of diagnosis. They are often absent in long-standing disease and are not thought to be pathogenic themselves. 80–95% of patients will have demonstrable autoantibodies at diagnosis. Type 1 diabetes typically presents in children but can present much later in life. Age at presentation is bimodal, with a peak around puberty and another peak between 20–30 years of age. Incidence rates in those under 5 years have been rising sharply.

Some patients of Afro-Caribbean descent may present with diabetes and ketones but are antibody –ve and have ketosis-prone type diabetes (KPD, 🕮 see p. 688). Patients who develop type 1 diabetes later in life frequently have a more insidious presentation, often termed latent auto-immune diabetes in adults (LADA, 🕮 see p. 688).

Soon after diagnosis with type 1 diabetes, patients commonly go through the 'honeymoon period' when insulin requirements reduce dramatically and patients can even come off insulin for a short duration. This phase can last from a few weeks to a few years (longer with increasing age), but it is important to monitor blood glucose carefully and reinstate insulin treatment as soon as blood glucose starts to rise. At the time of diagnosis, patients usually have between 10–20% of β-cell function left, which can sustain the patient through this phase.

Management

In type 1 diabetes, insulin therapy is mandatory, along with dietary advice and standard diabetes education. The aim of treatment is to mimic physiological insulin production as far as possible, given limitations of current insulin delivery. Physiological studies suggest normal insulin requirements are around 0.5–0.6 units/kg/day, split equally between background (basal) and mealtime (bolus) requirements.

An initial education package will include:

- An explanation as to what diabetes is and what it means to the patient.
- Aims of treatment, e.g. rationale of reducing complications and suggested values to aim for (see Box 13.2).
- Self-monitoring, e.g. both the method(s) of doing this, the reasons for doing it, and what to do with the results.
- Injection technique.
- Advice about hypoglycaemia detection and treatment.
- Dietary advice with information on carbohydrate counting.
- Information about annual screening (review) for complications of diabetes, including referral to their local eye screening service.

Box 13.2 Suggested aims of treatment

Pre-meal blood glucose	4.5–7.5mmol/L
Post-meal blood glucose (at 2h)	8–10mmol/L
HbA1c	42–58mmol/mol (6.0–7.5%) WITHOUT Recurrent or debilitating hypoglycaemia
Blood pressure	<130/80mmHg
Body mass index	20–25 ideally
Home monitoring	Ideally required before each meal (to help judge the dose of insulin required) and pre-bed

- Advice regarding DVLA, insurance companies, and Diabetes UK.
- Advice regarding pregnancy (for women of childbearing age).

All patients with type 1 diabetes should be offered structured education in flexible insulin therapy within their first year with diabetes. There are a number of programmes available across the UK, the most widely available is called DAFNE (Dose Adjustment For Normal Eating), but a variety of local programmes offer training along similar principles.

Types of insulin

- Physiological insulin replacement depends on dividing the insulin into basal (background) and bolus (mealtime/quick-acting) insulin.
- Background insulin is affected by weight, stress, exercise, alcohol.
- Quick-acting insulin is adjusted, according to carbohydrate intake and exercise, and is used to correct high readings.
- Inhaled insulin. This was available briefly but was withdrawn in 2010. Some newer preparations are under evaluation but are not currently commercially available.
- Currently available insulins are listed in Box 13.3.

Insulin regimens

Basal bolus regimen

This is the most widely used regimen and the basis of most structured education programmes for type 1 diabetes. Once or twice daily isophane or analogue insulin is used to cover basal requirements, which can be adjusted in response to exercise, alcohol, or illness. Ideally, the basal insulin is titrated so that, if the patient did not eat, blood glucose would remain stable. This is often done using carbohydrate-free days. Soluble or rapid-acting analogue insulin is used to cover meals and also to correct high blood glucose readings. This regimen, combined with patient education that trains patients to adjust the doses in response to food, exercise, and illness, provides patients with flexibility to be able to lead a more normal life.

Box 13.3 Summary of types of insulin available

Type of insulin	Examples	Peak activity (h)	Duration of action (h)
Bolus (quick-acting) insulin			
Rapid-acting analogues	Humalog® (insulin lispro)	0–2	3–4
	NovoRapid® (insulin aspart)	1–3	3–4
	Apidra® (insulin glulisine)	1–3	3–4
Soluble	Actrapid®	1–3	6–8
	Humulin S®	1–3	6–8
	Insuman Rapid®	1–4	7–9
Basal (background) insulin			
Isophane (NPH)	Insulatard®	2–8	10–16
	Humulin I®	2–8	10–16
	Insuman Basal®	3–4	11–20
Long-acting analogues	Levemir® (insulin detemir)	Peakless	12–16
	Lantus® (insulin glargine)	Peakless	18–24
	*Tresiba® (insulin degludec)	Peakless	42
Mixed insulin			
Isophane with soluble insulin	Humulin M3®		
	Insuman Comb 15®		
	Insuman Comb 25®		
	Insuman Comb 50®		
Biphasic analogue insulin	Humalog Mix 25®		
	Novomix 30®		
Animal insulin	Display similar characteristics to the human insulin above		
	Hypurin® Bovine Neutral		
	Hypurin® Porcine Neutral		
	Hypurin® Bovine Isophane		
	Hypurin® Porcine Isophane		
	Hypurin® Porcine 30/70 mix		

* Available in standard U100 and U200 strength

Twice daily fixed mixture

These are pre-prepared mixtures of soluble and isophane insulin, most commonly in the ratio of 30% soluble/70% isophane (e.g. Humulin M3®). Insuman mixes are available in other ratios. Newer mixes with biphasic analogue insulin are also available (e.g. Novomix 30®, Humalog Mix 25®). These have the advantage of only two injections a day but offer less flexibility in terms of ability to respond to changes in food, exercise, or illness. These may be used in patients who are unable to inject more often or live a very fixed lifestyle and are more commonly used in those with type 2 diabetes.

Twice daily free mixing

Historically, before insulin pens were available, this was a standard regimen, with patients drawing up insulin from vials in syringes. Usually, they would use 2/3 isophane, 1/3 soluble, with 2/3 of the total daily dose given pre-breakfast and 1/3 given pre-evening meal. This regime allows very little flexibility in timing or quantity of meals and little ability to adjust for changes in insulin requirements due to exercise or illness.

Insulin pump: continuous subcutaneous insulin infusion (CSII)

This involves continuous infusion of quick-acting insulin (usually rapid-acting analogue insulin), using a small pager-sized pump through a small subcutaneous cannula. The cannula is replaced by the patient every 2–3 days. The pump is programmed to deliver basal insulin, as required, through the day and can be increased in response to illness or decreased/suspended in response to exercise or alcohol. Most modern pumps have in-built bolus calculators that use pre-programmed values for insulin: carbohydrate ratios, insulin sensitivity, and blood glucose targets to calculate insulin doses. They can also store information on blood glucose readings entered into the pump and insulin delivered for download and review. This is discussed in more detail in the next section.

Structured education in flexible insulin therapy

The Diabetes Control and Complications Trial (DCCT) demonstrated that intensive control of blood glucose reduced the risks of microvascular complications. However, in this study, this was associated with a 3-fold increase in severe hypoglycaemia (episodes requiring third-party assistance). Subsequent studies in which patients were trained to adjust their own insulin doses on the basis of their current blood glucose levels, expected carbohydrate intake, and activity allowed them to achieve similar blood glucose control, with a reduction in hypoglycaemia. There are a number of similar programmes available (DAFNE, BERTIE, EXPERT, etc.) which are based around the following key principles:

- Separation of meal (quick-acting) and background (basal) insulin.
- Adjustment of mealtime insulin, based on carbohydrate intake.
- Correction doses, based on a correction factor.

Basal insulin

Basal insulin is usually long-acting insulin, either regular (Insulatard® or Humulin I®) or analogue (glargine or detemir). This replaces background requirements and should produce stable glucose levels if the patient does not eat carbohydrate. This should be adjusted in response to alcohol or exercise. Commonly split into morning and evening doses if blood sugars are seen to rise towards end of a 24h dose period.

Quick-acting insulin

This may be regular (Humulin S®, Insuman Rapid®) or analogue (NovoRapid®, Humalog®, or Apidra®). This is adjusted, based on carbohydrate intake and current blood glucose levels.

Insulin-to-carbohydrate ratio

This is the amount of insulin required for a fixed amount of carbohydrate (usually 10g). This is sometimes also expressed as number of grams of carbohydrate required to neutralize 1 unit of insulin. A common starting point for a normal weight adult would be 1 unit/10g.

Rule of 500. A simple rule to calculate insulin-to-carbohydrate ratio is to divide 500 by the total daily dose (TDD).

For example, for a TDD of 50 units, insulin-to-carbohydrate ratio will be 500/50 = 10g/unit. For a total daily dose of 80 units, insulin to carbohydrate ratio will be 500/80 = 6.25.

This can be tested by checking blood glucose levels 2h post-meal. If these are above target (usually set for <10mmol/L), then this can be increased.

Insulin sensitivity (correction factor)

This is the degree to which 1 unit of insulin will drop the blood glucose. A common starting point for an adult is 1 unit to drop the glucose by 3mmol/L.

Rule of 100. 100/TDD = correction factor in mmol/L.

For example, for a TDD of 50 units, correction factor = 100/50 = 2. (This is the '1800 rule' when measuring glucose in mg/dL.)

Principles of dose adjustments

Patients are advised to test blood glucose before meals and before bed. Reflect on blood glucose readings at regular intervals to look for patterns over the previous 5–7 days. The only exception to waiting for a pattern is when overnight or fasting hypoglycaemia occurs, when patients should reduce their night-time background insulin by 10–20% the following night.

Some simple rules of adjustment are:
- Make one change at a time.
- Use carbohydrate-free days to adjust the daytime basal.
- Adjust the bedtime basal insulin, based on the fasting glucose.
- If a correction dose is required at the same time every day, consider changing the insulin-to-carbohydrate ratio or basal insulin active at that time.
- Reduce evening basal insulin after alcohol or exercise by 25–50%.
- Do not correct post-hypo highs.
- If high post-meal readings, increase insulin-to-carbohydrate ratio.
- Reduce bedtime basal insulin in response to recurrent unexplained nocturnal hypoglycaemia.

Dawn phenomenon

Most people have a surge in insulin requirements 3–4h before waking up. This is mainly due to increased amplitude and frequency of GH pulses but also coincides with a natural rise in cortisol levels. In about 30% of people, this causes >30% increase in insulin requirements. In patients on NPH insulin, this coincides with a reduction in activity of the insulin, leading to fasting hyperglycaemia. Increases in bedtime NPH lead to overnight hypoglycaemia. This effect is less pronounced with analogue basal insulins, which do not wane in function in the early hours. However, a large proportion of patients with type 1 diabetes experience rising glucose between 4 and 8 a.m., leading to consistent fasting hyperglycaemia. These issues can only be properly controlled by an insulin pump which can be programmed to increase basal rates at the required time overnight.

Sick day rules

When unwell, patients become more insulin-resistant and can sometimes develop ketosis. If severe enough, this can progress to ketoacidosis. A third of admissions for DKA are precipitated by illness, and some may be avoided by appropriate use of 'sick day rules'.

- Never stop basal insulin.
- Continue mealtime insulin with addition of extra insulin, as described in the box on Minor illness and Severe illness below.
- Drink sugar-free fluids to remain hydrated—100mL/h.

Minor illness

KETONES urine –/+ OR blood <1.5mmol/L.

- If blood glucose >8mmol/L, increase all insulin doses by 10–20%.
- Check blood glucose and ketones every 4–6h.
- Take correction insulin (quick-acting insulin at usual correction doses) every 4–6h, even if not eating.

Severe illness

KETONES urine ++/+++ OR blood >1.5mmol/L.

- Increase background insulin by 30–40%.
- KETONES 1.5–3mmol/L: take 10% of total daily insulin dose every 2h as quick-acting insulin until ketones go away.
- KETONES >3mmol/L: take 20% of total daily insulin dose every 2h as quick-acting insulin until ketones go away.
- If ketones do not fall after 2–4h, seek medical advice.

When ketones –ve/trace or <1.5mmol/L, carry on as for 'minor illness'. Try to eat 10–20g carbohydrate 4-hourly. Test frequently.

Calculation example

A patient has a standard regimen of basal insulin 12 units bd and 1 unit/10g CHO, giving an average TDD of 50 units.

- If unwell and hyperglycaemic but ketones <1.5mmol/L, increase basal insulin to 13–14 units bd, and take regular correction doses.
- If blood ketones are 1.5–3mmol/L, take 10% of TDD = 5 units 2-hourly till ketone –ve.
- If blood ketones are >3mmol/L, take 10 units 2-hourly till ketone –ve.

▶▶ *If ketones do not fall with these approaches and patients become more ill or cannot take fluids due to nausea and vomiting, they should seek urgent medical advice and will usually require admission.*

Hypoglycaemia

Management of hypoglycaemia (□ see p. 746)

Hypoglycaemia (low blood glucose) is defined as blood glucose below 3.9 mmol/L, resulting from an imbalance between glucose supply, glucose utilization, and current insulin levels. This is characterized by typical symptoms (see Table 13.3).

Autonomic symptoms are associated with a release of catecholamines, cortisol, glucagon, and growth hormone. They typically occur at a blood glucose level of around 3.8mmol/L while neuroglycopenic symptoms occur when glucose levels drop below 3mmol/L. In the elderly or those with long diabetes duration, autonomic symptoms are less pronounced and occur at lower blood glucose levels, often resulting in delay in detecting hypoglycaemia. This can also result in neuroglycopenia and confusion, causing failure of recognition of hypoglycaemia.

Risk factors and causes of hypoglycaemia are listed in Box 13.4.

Severe hypoglycaemia

- This is defined as an episode that requires assistance from another person, or that requires hospitalization or parenteral glucose administration or treatment with glucagon.
- This occurs when blood glucose drops to a level inadequate to support consciousness, usually below 1.5mmol/L.
- It is thought that, in some cases, this is associated with seizures or cardiac arrhythmias and can be associated with death. The term 'dead in bed' describes the scenario seen in about 6% of deaths in young people with type 1 diabetes where the patient is found dead in an undisturbed bed. There is often a history of recent susceptibility to nocturnal hypoglycaemia.

Impaired awareness of hypoglycaemia

Recurrent hypoglycaemia can reduce the hormonal and symptomatic responses to subsequent hypoglycaemia, and, over time, after exposure to multiple episodes, patients can lose the ability to recognize hypoglycaemia. This is termed hypoglycaemia unawareness. Those with impaired awareness of hypoglycaemia have a 3–5-fold greater risk of severe hypoglycaemia, compared to those with normal awareness. Often, other people will recognize hypoglycaemia before the patient does.

A simple score to assess awareness of hypoglycaemia is called the GOLD score (see Fig. 13.2).

Table 13.3 Typical symptoms of hypoglycaemia

Autonomic	Neuroglycopenic	General
Sweating	Confusion	Headache
Palpitations	Drowsiness	Nausea
Shaking	Odd behaviour	
Hunger	Speech difficulty	
	Incoordination	

Box 13.4 Hypoglycaemia: risk factors and causes

Risk factors	Causes
• Impaired awareness of hypoglycaemia.	• Insulin doses are excessive, ill timed, or of the wrong type of insulin.
• Previous exposure to severe hypoglycaemia.	• Inadequate exogenous carbohydrate.
• Increasing age.	• Endogenous glucose production is decreased (e.g. alcohol ingestion).
• Increasing duration of diabetes.	• Glucose utilization is increased.
• Strict glycaemic control.	• Insulin clearance is decreased (e.g. renal failure).
• Sleep.	
• C-peptide negativity.	

Ask patient: "How often are you aware of episodes of hypoglycaemia (capillary blood glucose <3.5mmol/L)?"

Always   Never

1   2   3   4   5   6   7

A score of 1 or 2 implies good awareness. A score of 3 denotes borderline awareness, and a score of 4 or above denotes impaired awareness.

Fig. 13.2 GOLD score.

Insulin pump therapy

As per NICE guidance in the UK, insulin pump therapy is recommended as a treatment option for adults and children 12 years and older with type 1 diabetes provided:

- Attempts to achieve target HbA1c with MDI result in disabling hypoglycaemia, OR
- HbA1c remains above 69mmol/mol or 8.5%, despite a high level of care.

CSII is also recommended for children younger than 12 years with type 1 diabetes provided:

- MDI therapy is considered impractical or inappropriate.

Following initiation of CSII, it should only be continued if it results in sustained improvement in terms of improved HbA1c or reduced hypoglycaemia. CSII therapy in the UK is used by about 3.5% of patients with type 1 diabetes, compared to 20–35% in France, Germany, and the USA. NICE guidance recommends that up to 15% of those in the UK would be eligible under current guidance.

It is recommended that insulin pump therapy should only be started by a trained team, comprising a physician, nurse, and dietitian with special interest in pump therapy.

Key advantages of pump therapy are based around the ability to adjust or alter basal insulin delivery through the day and to take recurrent boluses, as required, to cover food intake. The pump uses rapid-acting insulin (usually an analogue) which is infused continuously through an infusion set. The pump usually contains a disposable reservoir which is replaced every 2–3 days. The patient can deliver boluses to cover meals, using buttons on the pump or on a remote handheld which communicates with the pump.

Pump start

This is often done in groups, and often patients are started on saline to ensure that they can change sets and use the pumps safely before converting to insulin. Patients often require daily contact with the healthcare team over the first few days as their basal rates are adjusted.

Starting doses can be calculated by a number of methods, but usually total daily dose is reduced by 30%. Usually, patients will be started on one or two basal rates through the day which will then be adjusted, according to blood glucose levels.

Adjusting basal rates

Changes in basal rates take between 2 and 4h to produce a change in plasma insulin levels. In clinical practice, it is common to adjust a basal rate 2h before the effect is desired, i.e. if a patient is often hypoglycaemic at around 4 p.m., the basal rate would be lowered at 2 p.m.

To test if a basal rate is appropriate, it is common to perform carbohydrate-free days where the patient takes no carbohydrate (they may take other food) and tests blood glucose every 2–3h. Based on a rise or fall in glucose, basal rates can be adjusted appropriately.

Using downloads

All available insulin pumps allow all their data to be downloaded to a computer. This allows the user and the healthcare professional to analyse the information and look for patterns that may be associated with either hyper- or hypoglycaemia.

Bolus calculators

All currently available pumps have in-built bolus calculators. These can be programmed with insulin-to-carbohydrate ratio, insulin sensitivity, and target blood glucose values. The calculator then takes into account the effect of any previous boluses that were administered that may still be having a glucose-lowering effect and provides a recommendation for a bolus. This prevents 'stacking' of insulin and reduces the risk of hypoglycaemia.

Advanced pumping

Temporary basal rates

These allow the patient to increase or decrease the basal rate for a limited duration of time. For example, to avoid the risk of hypoglycaemia during exercise, the patient can reduce the basal rate to 50% of usual during exercise. Similarly, if stressed or unwell and blood glucose is running high, the patient can increase the basal rate by 70% to bring them under control.

Altered wave boluses (see Box 13.5)

Pumps offer the ability to deliver the bolus over different time periods to cover different types of food.

Square wave bolus: this delivers the bolus over a given period of time and is useful if someone plans to eat gradually over a given time period, e.g. grazing on popcorn during a movie.

Box 13.5 Types of bolus dose deliverable by pump

Type of bolus	Diagrammatic representation	Suggested use
Normal wave		Standard meals
Square (extended) wave		Extended meals—benefits not proven and the lack of early insulin action may be problematic
Dual wave		Variable amounts as normal bolus, followed by the remainder as an extended bolus—suggested, but not proven, to improve postprandial glucose excursions after high carbohydrate, low glycaemic index, or high-fat meals

Dealing with pump failure

Non-delivery of insulin from a pump is a major risk, and there have been a few deaths with ketoacidosis due to this. Occasionally, if infusion sets are not changed every 3 days, blood glucose levels rise due to non-delivery of basal insulin. Patients should keep a supply of SC insulin for use in the event of pump failure.

Pump manufacturers technical support helpline

- Medtronic: 01923 205 167.
- Roche: 0800 701 000.
- Animas: 0800 055 6606.

Continuous glucose monitoring

Continuous glucose monitoring (CGM) systems consist of small sensors inserted subcutaneously, usually on the abdominal wall, that measure glucose in the interstitial fluid and display the value along with trend information, and various alarms on the pump or a monitor. Interstitial fluid glucose lags 6–15min behind blood glucose, and CGM need to be calibrated, using capillary glucose values 1–4 times/day.

Retrospective CGM systems are downloaded and analysed after wearing and can be used to provide detailed information about glucose excursions over a 6-day period. Combined with detailed information about carbohydrate, insulin, and activity, they can be used to adjust therapy to help improve glucose control or reduce hypoglycaemia.

CGM systems are increasingly used to provide a constant readout of (interstitial) glucose and trends (e.g. rising or falling). In the UK, funding for CGM is on an individual patient basis and varies between centres.

The JDRF-CGM study and STAR-3 have shown that CGM can help reduce HbA1c by up to 0.5% in motivated patients without any increase in hypoglycaemia. Results have been less robust in adolescents and children, possibly reflecting the ease of use and ability to assimilate and utilize the extra information.

Alarms

Low alarm

This is usually set somewhere between 3 and 5mmol/L. Given the delay between blood glucose and sensor glucose, by the time sensor glucose reads 3mmol/L, blood glucose is often below 2mmol/L. However, setting the alarm too high leads to a high false +ve alarm rate, which can be intrusive. Many patients sleep through alarms, mainly at night.

High alarm

This alerts the patient when blood glucose is high and should trigger a correction bolus delivered through the bolus calculator.

Predictive alarm

Predictive alarms alert the patient to impending hypoglycaemia. Often, patients will have to respond to a predictive alarm when their sensor glucose is >6mmol/L in order to prevent blood glucose dropping below 4mmol/L.

Low glucose suspend

One of the pump systems (Medtronic Paradigm Veo®) automatically suspends insulin delivery for up to a maximum of 2h if the patient fails to respond to a 'low alarm'. Basal insulin can be manually restarted at any point within the 2h. This should usually be set to kick in at a glucose of 3.5–4.5mmol/L and has been shown to significantly reduce the duration of hypoglycaemia.

Use of downloads

Most modern home blood glucose meters and all currently available insulin pumps have the capability to download data to a computer. These data can then be used to obtain statistics, such as mean glucose, standard deviation, and number of hypo- or hyperglycaemic excursions. They can also be used to look for trends or patterns that can be used to inform changes to therapy.

Pump downloads can be used to evaluate total daily dose, frequency of set changes, and number of boluses/day and, when combined with data from a meter, can provide very useful data on patterns.

Patients can download their pumps and/or meters and send the information electronically to their diabetes team, allowing remote consultations and making it easier for the diabetes team to provide dose adjustment advice.

Suggested use of downloads

- Look for mean tests/day.
- Look for mean boluses/day.
- Look for mean total daily dose and basal/bolus split.
- Pattern management:
  - Look at different time periods (overnight/post-breakfast/post-lunch and post-evening meal), and try to identify patterns.
  - Look for low blood glucose readings, and use the download to identify possible causes (high insulin-to-carbohydrate ratio, correction bolus, basal rate too high).
  - Look for very high blood glucose, and look for possible causes (missed bolus, inadequate insulin-to-carbohydrate ratio, overtreatment of hypo).

Emerging therapies

Closed-loop systems

The latest generation of sensor-augmented pumps can suspend insulin delivery for up to 2h if the patient fails to respond to a hypoglycaemia alarm. This is particularly useful in preventing prolonged nocturnal hypoglycaemia and has been shown to reduce the duration of nocturnal hypoglycaemia in those most at risk. Currently, multiple groups are developing further generations of closed-loop systems, testing algorithms that adjust insulin delivery through the pump, based on glucose data obtained from CGM.

Immune modulation

Risk of type 1 diabetes can be predicted in siblings of patients with type 1 diabetes. Currently, immune modulation with anti-CD3 agents is in clinical trials to try and stop the progression of the condition. To date, these studies have produced small, but significant, protection of endogenous insulin production and reduction in insulin doses, but the data do not currently justify clinical use outside of clinical trials. For more information on trials on immune modulation in type 1 diabetes ℅ http://www.bris.ac.uk/trialnet-uk/index.html

Islet cell transplantation

Following the first reports of insulin independence following islet cell transplant in 2000, this has become an established procedure for patients with type 1 diabetes fulfilling any one of the following criteria:

• Recurrent disabling hypoglycaemia despite optimal medical therapy.
• Already on immunosuppression for a renal transplant.
• Progressive microvascular complications.
• Hypoglycaemia unawareness.

Patients must have type 1 diabetes, be aged 18–65 years, and must have insulin requirements <0.6 units/kg, with body weight <85kg and BMI <28kg/m². Creatinine clearance must be >60mL/min.

Islets are separated from the donor pancreas and infused intraportally into the liver. The patient requires immunosuppression. Outcomes include improved glucose control, protection against hypoglycaemia, and slowing down in deterioration of nephropathy. Latest data show 70% patients are insulin-independent at 1 year, dropping to 50% at 4 years. For details on islet transplantation in the UK ℘ http://www.youngdiabetologists.org.uk/etools/guidelines/islet

Pancreas transplantation

Pancreas transplantation is most commonly performed simultaneously with renal transplant in patients with type 1 diabetes and renal failure. Occasionally, it may be performed alone for similar indications as islet cell transplant in whom islet cell transplantation is considered inappropriate. This procedure has a 4% operative mortality, with 10–15% risk of re-laparotomy. At 1 year, 95% are insulin-independent, with between 65 and 70% insulin-independent at 5 years. The outcomes are better for simultaneous pancreas kidney transplant (SPK) than pancreas transplant alone (PTA) or pancreas after kidney (PAK). These procedures should be carried out at centres with expertise in transplantation and diabetes management following multidisciplinary assessment.

Further reading

American Diabetes Association (2005). Defining and reporting hypoglycemia in diabetes: a report from the American Diabetes Association Workgroup on Hypoglycemia. *Diabetes Care* **28**, 1245–9.

DAFNE Study Group (2003). Training in flexible, intensive insulin management to enable dietary freedom in people with type 1 diabetes: dose adjustment for normal eating (DAFNE) randomized controlled trial. *Diabet Med* **20** Suppl 3, 4–5.

Hovorka R, *et al.* (2010). Manual closed-loop insulin delivery in children and adolescents with type 1 diabetes: a phase 2 randomised crossover trial. *Lancet* **375**, 743–51.

JDRF CGM Study Group (2008). Continuous glucose monitoring and intensive treatment of type 1 diabetes. *N Engl J Med* **359**, 1464–76.

National Institute for Health and Clinical Excellence (2004). NICE Guidelines, type 1 diabetes in adults. Available at: ℘ http://guidance.nice.org.uk/CG15/Guidance//Adults.

National Insitute for Health and Clinical Excellence (2008). NICE Guidelines, diabetes insulin pump therapy. Available at: ℘ http://publications.nice.org.uk/continuous-subcutaneous-insulin-infusion-for-the-treatment-of-diabetes-mellitus-ta151/guidance.

Effect of intensive therapy on the development and progression of diabetic nephropathy in the Diabetes Control and Complications Trial. The Diabetes Control and Complications (DCCT) Research Group (1995). *Kidney Int* **47**, 1703–20.

Hypoglycemia in the Diabetes Control and Complications Trial. The Diabetes Control and Complications Trial Research Group (1997). *Diabetes* **46**, 271–86.

Pickup J, Mattock M, Kerry S (2002). Glycaemic control with continuous subcutaneous insulin infusion compared with intensive insulin injections in patients with type 1 diabetes: meta-analysis of randomised controlled trials. *BMJ* **324**, 705.

Shapiro AM, *et al.* (2006). International trial of the Edmonton protocol for islet transplantation. *N Engl J Med* **355**, 1318–30.

Expert management of type 2 diabetes

Background

Type 2 diabetes is associated with multiple vascular risk factors and a wide range of complications such that its management draws on many areas of primary and secondary healthcare. Treatment is, therefore, complex and time-consuming. Patient education and self-care are crucial parts of management. The NICE clinical guideline, focusing on the management of type 2 diabetes, and its regular updates provide clear advice for healthcare professionals on all aspects of care across the disease continuum, including when to use specific diabetes therapies.

Key priorities of care

Offer a structured diabetes education programme (that meets the Department of Health and Diabetes UK Patient Education Working Group criteria) to every person and/or their carer at or around the time of diagnosis, with annual review and reinforcement.

Provide individualized and ongoing culturally sensitive nutritional advice. Set individualized target glycated haemoglobin (HbA1c) with the patient, and provide a level of care to achieve and maintain that target.

Offer self-monitoring of blood glucose as an integral part of self-management, and agree when it should be performed and how it should be interpreted and acted upon. When starting insulin therapy, employ a structured training programme with active dose titration.

Dietary/lifestyle advice

Encourage high-fibre, low glycaemic index sources of carbohydrate, such as fruit, vegetables, wholegrains, and pulses; include low-fat dairy products and oily fish; control the intake of foods containing saturated and trans fatty acids. This should be integrated with other aspects of lifestyle modification, including physical activity and losing weight. For the overweight, an initial weight loss target of 5–10% is advised whilst remembering any weight loss is beneficial. Remember that alcohol is a significant source of calories, and advise accordingly.

Glucose targets

Early intensive management of blood glucose has long-term benefits in terms of reductions in all diabetes-related complications, including cardiovascular disease. Whilst many patients will perform and should act on self-monitored plasma glucose values (<7.0mmol/L pre-meal and <8.5mmol/L post-meal), the HbA1c is generally used as the measure of overall control and usually serves as the trigger for treatment change. Although 48mmol/mol or 6.5% is recommended for people on single oral therapy and/or diet and lifestyle, and 58mmol/mol or 7.5% for people on more complex regimens, individualized targets should be agreed upon with the patient, and pursuing highly intensive levels of less than 48mmol/mol should be avoided. HbA1c may be increased in iron deficiency anaemia and decreased in haemolytic anaemia, secondary anaemia due to cirrhosis. Haemoglobinopathy may also affect it up or down.

Oral glucose control therapies

(See Table 13.4 for summary.)

Biguanides

Metformin is first-line therapy for the majority of patients, particularly the obese or overweight. It is also used in some insulin-treated, insulin-resistant, overweight subjects to reduce insulin requirements. The UKPDS showed significantly better results from metformin for complications and mortality, compared to other therapies in the overweight patient with type 2 diabetes. With long-term use, a 0.8–2.0% (or 9–22mmol/mol) reduction in HbA1c can be expected.

Mode of action

Works by reducing hepatic gluconeogenesis and increasing muscle glucose uptake/metabolism.

Side effects/contraindications

Contraindicated in patients with renal (creatinine >130nmol/L), hepatic, or cardiac impairment, or who consume significant amounts of alcohol. GI side effects occur in up to half of patients in the first 1–2 weeks of treatment but are usually transient. If the starting dose is low (e.g. 500mg once daily), most people develop tolerance and are able to take higher doses; <5% are totally intolerant. Consider a trial of extended absorption metformin where GI tolerability prevents continued use. Rarely, skin rashes and lactic acidosis occur.

Special precaution

Using radiological contrast media with metformin is associated with an increased risk of lactic acidosis, and therapy should be stopped at the time of, or prior to, such investigations and restarted 2 days after the test, unless renal function has been affected by the procedure, in which case delay until this has resolved.

Insulin secretagogues

Sulfonylureas include gliclazide, glipizide, glimepiride, glibenclamide, tolbutamide, and chlorpropamide. Consider as first-line in non-obese patients, those unable to tolerate metformin, or if a rapid response to therapy is required because of hyperglycaemic symptoms. Can be used as second-line agents when blood glucose control is inadequate with metformin.

Mode of action

Stimulate β-cell potassium ATP channel, closing the potassium channel which leads to membrane depolarization, calcium influx, and subsequent insulin release. A doubling of glucose-stimulated insulin secretion can be expected. Results in a 1–2% (or 11–22mmol/mol) reduction in HbA1c long term.

Table 13.4 Oral hypoglycaemic agents: summary

Class	Mechanism of action	Expected HbA1c reduction	Weight effect
Biguanide	Increase muscle glucose uptake and metabolism, decrease hepatic gluconeogenesis	0.8–2.0% 9–22mmol/mol	Neutral
Sulfonylurea	Stimulate insulin secretion	1.0–2.0% 11–22mmol/mol	Increase
Prandial glucose regulator	Stimulate insulin secretion	0.6–2.0% 7–22mmol/mol	Increase
Alpha-glucosidase inhibitor	Inhibits digestive enzyme	0.4–0.7% 5–8mmol/mol	Decrease
Thiazolidinedione	Activate PPAR-γ receptor	0.6–1.5% 7–17mmol/mol	Increase
DPP-4 inhibitor	Inhibits enzymic degradation of incretin hormones (GIP, GLP-1)	0.4–1.0% 5–11mmol/mol	Neutral ? decrease

Side effects
Predominantly hypoglycaemia and weight gain. In the UKPDS, the mean weight gain seen after 10 years of therapy was 2.3kg. Hypoglycaemia is grossly under-reported with sulfonylurea therapies, with recent data suggesting that up to 50% of patients experience at least one episode of low blood sugar each year. The elderly are at particular risk. The longer-acting agents, such as glibenclamide, should, if possible, be avoided.

Special precaution
Avoid in patients with porphyria.

Rapid-acting insulin secretagogues
These agents, whilst more commonly used in East Asian countries, are not frequently prescribed in the UK. They include repaglinide, a carbamoylmethyl benzoic acid derivative, and nateglinide, a D-phenylalanine derivative, both of which stimulate insulin secretion with a short duration of action. They are given 3 times a day and often referred to as prandial glucose regulators. The short duration of action is associated with low rates of hypoglycaemia, and they have been shown to reduce HbA1c by 0.6–2% (7–22mmol/mol). They should not be used in people with renal and hepatic impairment.

Thiazolidinediones (glitazones)

Pioglitazone is generally only used as an alternative to insulin in people suboptimally controlled on metformin and/or sulfonylurea because of its side effects. Its indication does, however, vary around the world, and, in the UK, it is also considered in combination with insulin. The recent introduction of incretin-based therapies (see Oral and injectable incretin-based therapies, Table 13.5) appears to have limited its use even further. A reduction of 0.6–1.5% (7–17mmol/mol) in HbA1c can be expected, with low rates of hypoglycaemia.

Mode of action

Insulin-sensitizing agents by activating the peroxisome proliferator activated receptor (PPAR-γ) which stimulates gene transcription for glucose transporter molecules, such as Glut 1 and Glut 4.

Side effects

Patients should be warned about the possibility of significant oedema and weight gain. Pioglitazone should not be used in people with evidence of heart failure and those at a higher risk of bone fracture and osteoporosis. In contrast to troglitazone, improvements in liver function, especially with non-alcoholic steatohepatitis (NASH), have been reported.

Special precaution

Troglitazone was withdrawn soon after its UK launch because of reports of hepatotoxicity. The second of these agents, rosiglitazone, whilst not associated with hepatotoxicity, was associated with other significant side effects, including ischaemic heart disease and increased cardiovascular morbidity, and was withdrawn in 2011.

Alpha-glucosidase inhibitors

Acarbose is generally only considered in patients unable to tolerate other oral glucose-lowering agents. When taken with food, it reduces postprandial glucose peaks by inhibiting the digestive enzyme α-glucosidase which normally breaks carbohydrates into their monosaccharide components, thus retarding glucose uptake. The passage of undigested carbohydrates into the large intestine results in bacterial breakdown and the development of common unpleasant GI side effects.

Oral and injectable incretin-based therapies

(See Table 13.5 for comparison.)

GLP-1 receptor analogues

Exenatide and liraglutide are licensed for the use in people with type 2 diabetes, in combination with other oral therapies and basal insulin, and are available as subcutaneous injections. They are associated with an HbA1c reduction of 1–2% or 11–22mmol/mol and are particularly attractive as glucose-lowering agents because of low rates of hypoglycaemia and a weight loss over 6 months of ~3–4kg.

Table 13.5 Comparison between the incretin-based therapies (GLP-1 receptor agonists and DPP-4 inhibitors)

	Sitagliptin 100mg od	Vildagliptin 50mg bd	Exenatide 10 micrograms bd	Liraglutide 1.2 or 1.8mg od
Administration	Oral	Oral	SC injection	SC injection
Reduction in HbA1c	0.3–1.0%	0.4–0.7%	0.8–0.9%	1.0–1.5%
	3–11mmol/mol	5–8mmol/mol	9–10mmol/mol	11–17mmol/mol
Reduction in fasting plasma glucose (mmol/L)	0.9–1.1	0.3–1.0	0.6–1.6	1.6
Change in weight (kg)	−1.1 to +0.8	−0.23 to +1.3	~3–4	~3–4
Hypoglycaemia	Low	Low	Low	Low

Mode of action
The incretin hormones glucagon-like polypeptide-1 (GLP-1) and gastric intestinal polypeptide (GIP), released from the GI tract in response to nutrient ingestion, stimulate insulin and suppress glucagon secretion in a glucose-dependent manner. Their extrapancreatic effects include a slowing of gastric emptying and central effects on the brain, leading to satiety and reduced appetite.

Side effects
Mainly gastrointestinal, with generally mild and transient nausea, vomiting, and diarrhoea. Headaches and dizziness are also reported. Increased risk of hypoglycaemia when used with sulfonylureas.

Special precautions
Should not be used in people with a history of pancreatitis.

Dipeptidyl peptidase-4 (DPP-4) inhibitors
Oral therapies that are being used increasingly after metformin in many patients. Sitagliptin has the broadest indication for use and can be used with insulin. Lead to a 0.4–1.0% or 5–11mmol/mol reduction in HbA1c over a 12-month period, with very low rates of hypoglycaemia, and are weight-neutral (maybe even helping to reduce weight).

Mode of action
Inhibition of enzymic degradation of incretin hormones GLP-1 and GIP.

Side effects
Few major side effects reported. Skin rashes and nasopharyngitis.

Special precautions
Should not be used in people with history of pancreatitis. Liver function test monitoring with vildagliptin.

Insulin therapy

The majority of patients with type 2 diabetes will require insulin injections at some point in their lives. Most guidelines recommend the addition of a basal insulin when other therapies are unable to achieve or maintain adequate glycaemic control. When using a basal insulin, existing oral therapies should be continued. The use of a sulfonylurea should be reviewed if hypoglycaemia occurs. Many patients initiated on a basal insulin will require further intensification within 12 months to either a basal bolus regimen or twice daily pre-mix.

Insulin can also be initiated as twice daily pre-mix insulin, and sulfonylureas are usually discontinued. Insulin can be used with sitagliptin and pioglitazone, although the latter should be discontinued if clinically significant fluid retention develops.

The newer analogue insulins offer certain advantages over the older human and animal insulins. They are, however, more expensive, and many national and international guidelines suggest that their use in type 2 diabetes should be restricted to people with difficulties on human and animal insulin, in particular, hypoglycaemia.

For different insulin preparations in the management of type 1 diabetes, see Box 13.3, p. 696.

Bariatric surgery

Gastric bypass appears to have significant, and usually persistent, effects on the metabolic abnormalities of type 2 diabetes, including glucose tolerance, dyslipidaemia, and hypertension. Further randomized controlled trials with predefined metabolic entry criteria and detailed follow-up are required. (For a full discussion of bariatric surgery, see Chapter 15, Obesity p. 862.)

The delivery of diabetes care

The increasing global prevalence of diabetes is placing substantial pressures on healthcare systems and economies, leading to reviews of how diabetes care can be delivered in a most cost-effective manner. Although care has traditionally been delivered from a diabetes centre and this model may still be preferred in many developing countries with large rural communities, there is an increasing move towards community-based service for routine care (primary care), with only the more complex care being delivered in hospitals by specialists (secondary care).

Chronic disease care models

In most European countries and the USA, diabetes care provision is planned and based upon a system of insurance, with differing splits between national and private schemes. Drugs are approved onto national formularies and reimbursed.

Many countries are basing care on 'chronic care models' whose key components are:
- Self-management.
- Decision support systems.
- Delivery system design.
- Clinical information systems.
- Healthcare organization and community resources.

Comprehensive, well-organized intensive diabetes management, incorporating planned diabetes visits, telephone contacts, and group education, has been shown to reduce:
- Hospital admissions.
- Unplanned outpatient attendances.
- Healthcare costs.

A number of countries with limited diabetes care infrastructure have worked with the World Diabetes Foundation to establish new strategic national diabetes management projects.

In the UK, the template defining the important components of care is the National Service Framework (NSF). To provide guidance on its implementation, healthcare professionals and service users, as part of the National Diabetes Support Team (NDST), have developed 'The Levels of Care' approach to help with the service design process.

Levels of diabetes care

- Level 1: includes generic, essential components—'the must haves'.
- Level 2: outlines core principles of level 1 components and important quality standards, including, for example, those in NICE guidance.
- Level 3: covers how to design and organize local services.
- Level 4: focuses on care pathways.

Whilst levels 1 and 2 are considered national or generic, levels 3 and 4 describe activity at a local level and should be designed to make sure that the patient is always seen by the most appropriate healthcare professional with the most appropriate level of training and skills at the most appropriate time and healthcare setting, including, when necessary, access to secondary and tertiary care specialists.

Commissioning

To ensure a high-quality service for all patients which is best value for money, the concept of commissioning is now being developed in many countries, such as the UK. For the process to be effective, it should involve collaboration between all interested parties, including healthcare professionals, patients, and local government.

Minimum requirements of the commissioning process should involve:

- Assessment of local needs.
- Design of specification to meet the needs.
- Procurement of local services.
- Proactive monitoring and audit of services.

The vast majority of routine diabetes care in the future will be delivered in the community. Increasingly, both oral and injectable glucose-lowering therapies are being initiated and intensified in the community, with the involvement of specialist support, when needed and called upon by primary healthcare professionals. The management of other cardiovascular risk factors, including weight, blood pressure, and lipids, and also the different components of the annual clinical and biochemical review can also largely take place in the community.

Further reading

Drucker DJ, Sherman SI, Bergenstal RM, Buse JB (2011). The safety of incretin-based therapies--review of the scientific evidence. *J Clin Endocrinol Metab* **96**, 2027–31.

Farmer AJ (2012). Use of HbA1c in the diagnosis of diabetes. *BMJ* **345**, 10.

Gerstein HC, Miller ME, Genuth S, *et al.* (2011). Long-term effects of intensive glucose lowering on cardiovascular outcomes. ACCORD Study Group. *N Engl J Med* **364**, 818–28.

Gough SC (2011). Organising a diabetes service. In: Stewart PM, Wass J (eds.) *Oxford textbook of endocrinology and diabetes*, 2nd edn, pp. 2005–11. Oxford University Press, Oxford.

Holman RR, Paul SK, Bethel MA, Matthews DR, Neil HA (2008). 10-year follow-up of intensive glucose control in type 2 diabetes. *N Engl J Med* **359**, 1577–89.

Lebovitz HE (2011). Type 2 diabetes mellitus-current therapies and the emergence of surgical options. *Nat Rev Endocrinol* **7**, 408–19.

Nathan DM, Buse JB, Davidson MB, Ferrannini E, Holman RR, Sherwin R, Zinman B; American Diabetes Association; European Association for Study of Diabetes (2009). Medical management of hyperglycemia in type 2 diabetes: a consensus algorithm for the initiation and adjustment of therapy: a consensus statement of the American Diabetes Association and the European Association for the Study of Diabetes. *Diabetes Care* **32**, 193–203.

National Institute for Health and Clinical Excellence (2008). NICE Guidelines Type 2 diabetes. Available at: ℘ http://www.nice.org.uk/nicemedia/live/11983/40803/40803.pdf.

Shyangdan DS, Royle P, Clar C, Sharma P, Waugh N, Snaith A (2011). Glucagon-like peptide analogues for type 2 diabetes mellitus. *Cochrane Database Syst Rev* **10**, CD006423.

Tahrani AA, Bailey CJ, Del Prato S, Barnett AH (2011). Management of type 2 diabetes: new and future developments in treatment. *Lancet* **378**, 182–97.

Zinman B (2011). Initial combination therapy for type 2 diabetes mellitus: is it ready for prime time? *Am J Med* **124** (1 Suppl), S19–34.

Diabetes and life

Driving

Diabetes is said to influence the ability to drive safely because of hypoglycaemia or complications, such as a reduction in visual acuity or fields. It has been found to carry a similar risk of accidents to epilepsy, and restrictions are placed on some drivers with diabetes. This can be a difficult subject for people with diabetes, but the DVLA (Driver and Vehicle Licensing Agency) in the UK sets legal requirements which must be met. If the DVLA is not informed appropriately, a driving licence and insurance may be invalid. Different standards apply for Northern Ireland and are administered by the DVA (Driver and Vehicle Agency, ℠ http://www.dvani.gov.uk).

Box 13.6 summarizes good practice for driving with diabetes.

Medical standards of fitness to drive

The guidance outlined here was produced by the DVLA Drivers Medical Unit and came into effect from October 2011. Full details are available on the DVLA website (℠ http://www.nidirect.gov.uk/index/information-and-services/motoring/driver-licensing/telling-dva-about-a-condition.htm). It is important to check for the latest information, as the standards are reviewed every 6 months. Different standards apply for licensing to drive group 1 vehicles (cars and motorcycles) and group 2 vehicles (large lorries and buses).

▶ Hypoglycaemia

Group 1

Hypoglycaemia is a significant risk factor for accidents while driving. For group 1 licences, the following should be notified to the DVLA immediately if licensed. If any of these arise, revocation or refusal of a licence is likely until the situation has been satisfactorily resolved:

- There has been >1 episode of hypoglycaemia requiring the assistance of a third party in the previous 12 months.
- Awareness of hypoglycaemia becomes impaired.
- A driver suffers a disabling episode of hypoglycaemia while driving.

Group 2

The situation is similar, except there must not have been a single episode of hypoglycaemia requiring third-party assistance in the previous 12 months.

Holding a group 1 licence (cars and motorcycles)

Those not treated with insulin

As long as there are no problems with hypoglycaemia and there are no other contraindications to driving (e.g. from neuropathy/visual problems), the DVLA does not need to be informed. Drivers on any treatment, other than diet alone, need to be under regular medical review.

Those treated with insulin

Must inform the DVLA of their diabetes. As long as there are no problems with hypoglycaemia, short-term (1–3 years) licences are issued under the following conditions:

- Must perform appropriate blood glucose monitoring.

Box 13.6 Good practice for driving with diabetes

- Test blood glucose before driving, even short distances, and every 2h during longer journeys if there is any possibility of hypoglycaemia.
- If blood glucose <4.0mmol, carbohydrate (CHO) should be taken and driving delayed for at least 45min to allow any cognitive deficit to recover.
- If glucose is <5mmol/L before driving, extra carbohydrate should be strongly considered.
- Keep a source of rapid-acting CHO (e.g. glucose tablets) easily available in the vehicle to treat symptoms of hypoglycaemia arising while driving.
- Do not continue to drive once symptoms of hypoglycaemia develop.
- Move out of the driver's seat to treat hypoglycaemia.

- Must not be regarded as a likely source of danger to the public whilst driving.
- Must meet standards for visual acuity and visual field.

Temporary insulin treatment

The DVLA does not need to be informed initially as long as under medical supervision and not advised to be at risk of disabling hypoglycaemia. The DVLA must be informed if:

- Disabling hypoglycaemia develops.
- Treatment continues for longer than 3 months (3 months post-partum in the case of gestational diabetes).

Holding a group 2 licence (large lorries and buses)

Those managed using agents carrying a risk of hypoglycaemia (including insulin)

A recent change in the law means that this group will now be able to apply for a group 2 licence as long as they meet the qualifying conditions. For those on insulin, they must also undergo an independent medical examination and sign a commitment to follow medical advice. The procedure for application is detailed on the DVLA website.

Qualifying conditions are:

- Has full awareness of hypoglycaemia.
- No episode of hypoglycaemia requiring the assistance of a third party in the last 12 months.
- Demonstrates an understanding of the risk of hypoglycaemia.
- Tests appropriately (and, if on insulin, can produce results from the last 3 months, using a meter with a memory function).
- There are no other debarring complications of diabetes.

Those using other treatment with no other contraindications

If on diet alone, the DVLA does not need to be informed. For other treatment, drivers must be under regular medical review and test glucose regularly. The DVLA must be informed but will usually issue a licence.

Sport and exercise and diabetes

The suggested amount of exercise is the same for those with diabetes as for the general population (see Box 13.7). The health benefits, such as ↓ in blood pressure and lipids, may be particularly helpful in diabetes. However, metabolic changes during exercise can make the management of diabetes difficult. When encouraging people with diabetes to exercise, it is important to take account of any complications. For example, weight-bearing exercise is unlikely to be appropriate for an individual with significant peripheral neuropathy. Cardiovascular risk should also be assessed and formal assessment arranged, if appropriate.

For advice on sport and diabetes, see ✍ http://www.runsweet.com/.

Type 1 diabetes

Lower intensity (aerobic) exercise

In those without diabetes, insulin levels ↓ during exercise of lower intensity and longer duration. The difficulty of achieving this with exogenous insulin therapy means that the most common problem in diabetes is hypoglycaemia. Fear of hypoglycaemia is recognized as the most important factor limiting people with type 1 diabetes for adopting a more active lifestyle. Post-exercise hypoglycaemia is a real concern, particularly in young men sleeping alone.

Higher intensity (anaerobic) and resistance exercise

In contrast, high intensity exercise and resistance exercise (particularly involving the upper body) can cause significant ↑ glucose through ↑ catecholamines. This is often unexpected and can cause confusion and frustration.

General advice

- Avoid hypoglycaemia before exercise.
- Test blood glucose before, during, and after exercise where possible.
- Aim to keep blood glucose between 7 and 10mmol/L before and during exercise.
- Ensure a supply of fast-acting CHO is freely available.
- Ensure safety—make sure those around are aware and can treat hypoglycaemia. If alone, ensure somebody knows where you are supposed to be and expected time of return.

Strategies for dealing with hypoglycaemia

- Avoid bolus insulin injection near exercising muscle (e.g. legs if running/cycling).
- Adequate dietary energy consumption is important. This will vary with factors, such as body weight and duration and intensity of exercise.
- If exercise is within 2h of a meal, bolus insulin dose with that meal should be ↓ by 25–75%.
- Extra rapid-acting CHO can be taken during exercise. Up to 1g/kg body weight/h may be needed, although absorption of >60g/h can be problematic. Ideally taken from around 15–20min into exercise and gradually in small amounts thereafter.

Box 13.7 **Physical activity recommendations for health**
- At least 150min each week of moderate intensity physical activity in blocks of at least 10min (e.g. 30min on at least 5 days each week), 75min of vigorous activity each week, or a combination of the two.
- At least two sessions of muscle strengthening activity each week. These should not be on consecutive days.

- A post-exercise snack may be needed, with a reduced insulin bolus. Insulin requirements with an evening meal post-exercise may also be reduced.
- A ↓ in basal insulin injection of 10–20% may be required on the night after exercise to avoid nocturnal hypoglycaemia.
- CSII therapy can be very useful for exercise. Basal rate should be ↓ to 20–50% of normal around 30min before exercise and then ideally returned to normal around 30min before the end. Insulin pumps can be removed for exercise, although there is a significant risk of hyperglycaemia ± ketosis.
- Post-exercise CSII basal rate should be ↓ by 20% from bedtime to around 4 a.m.

Strategies for dealing with hyperglycaemia
- A small insulin bolus (often only 0.5–1 unit) may be needed immediately before or after exercise. If given before, a snack may be required afterwards.

Type 2 diabetes
Both aerobic and resistance exercise are beneficial in type 2 diabetes. There is also a benefit in reducing the risk of 'pre-diabetic' states (IFG and IGT) developing into diabetes.

The main benefits are:
- Improvement in glycaemic control.
- Insulin sensitivity ↑ acutely with a single bout of exercise and chronically with sustained exercise, leading to ↓ insulin requirements.
- Cardiovascular risk factors improve.
- Help with weight control, both through better energy balance and a reduction in insulin requirements.
- Improvements in general well-being and functional capacity.

Alcohol and diabetes

People with diabetes can continue to drink alcohol without problems as long as they do so sensibly. Excess alcohol should be avoided (see Box 13.8). It is best to avoid or limit sweet alcoholic drinks, such as sweet wines and alcopops, and mixers should be of the 'sugar-free' or 'diet' varieties.

▶ Alcohol increases the risk of hypoglycaemia, with larger amounts increasing the risk. The risk can persist for up to 16h.

- Avoid drinking alcohol on an empty stomach—starchy snacks may be helpful if drinking throughout an evening.
- Alcoholic drinks contain carbohydrate but should not be used to replace meals or snacks.
- After consuming larger amounts of alcohol, ensure that some CHO is eaten before going to bed (especially if treated with insulin). Healthy snacks are better, but chips or pizza, for example, are an alternative. Breakfast should be eaten the following morning.
- Alcohol intoxication may reduce hypoglycaemic symptoms. Remember a hypo could be confused with drunkenness if alcohol is on the breath.

Box 13.8 Diabetes UK recommended alcohol limits
- ♀—no more than 2 units/day.
- ♂—no more than 3 units/day.

Recreational drug use and diabetes

In questionnaire surveys:
- 5–25% of those aged 12–20 and 29% of those aged 16–30 admitted to recreational drug use during their lifetime.
- >50% of young people with DKA admitted into a tertiary centre over a 10-month period admitted to drug use, although only 20% volunteered this on initial questioning.

The index of suspicion for drug use needs to be high, as drug use is significantly associated with risk of death from acute diabetes-related events (OR 5.7). In those where there is significant suspicion, urinary drug screening should be considered. Box 13.9 lists some of the adverse effects reported with recreational drugs in diabetes.

Mechanisms by which recreational drugs affect diabetes are variable:
- Effects on judgement and decision-making. For example:
  - Missed insulin doses, resulting in hyperglycaemia/DKA.
  - Alterations in food intake, resulting in hyper- or hypoglycaemia.
  - Reduced ability to recognize hyper- or hypoglycaemia and treat appropriately due to impaired perception.
- Catecholamine toxicity.
- Increased lipolysis.
- Altered renal handling of ketones and bicarbonate.

Advice about being as safe as possible when using recreational drugs should be made available to people with diabetes. This may include:
- Being as well informed as possible about potential effects.
- Choosing as safe an environment as possible.
- Never experimenting the first time alone.
- Carrying something identifying you as having diabetes.
- Ensuring at least one person present knows you have diabetes and ideally knows how to handle any emergency and remains capable of providing assistance.

Box 13.9 Observed consequences of common recreational drugs
- MDMA (ecstasy): diabetic ketoacidosis (DKA) and hyponatraemia.
- Ketamine: DKA (acidosis out of proportion to ketosis), rhabdomyolysis.
- Heroin: hyperglycaemic hyperosmolar state (HHS), following heroin OD; lethal levels of methadone in a patient who died of DKA.
- Cocaine: HHS and DKA (one study has shown cocaine use to be a strong independent risk factor for recurrent DKA).
- Cannabis: direct effects minimal, although may lower blood glucose in large amounts.

Travel and diabetes

People with diabetes need to plan ahead prior to travelling on holiday or for business (see Box 13.10). If possible, take more medication (especially insulin) than should be required in case there is a problem. When obtaining insulin abroad, it is important to remember that not every country uses U100 (i.e. 100 units/mL) insulin which is the standard in the UK. Some countries use U40 or U80.

Crossing time zones can be complex. The day is longer travelling east to west, and extra insulin doses may be required. Travelling west to east, the day is shorter, so doses of basal insulin may overlap and require reduction. Insulin requirements may alter when on holiday due to increased temperature (↓), unaccustomed exercise (↓), and a change in diet (↑ or ↓).

Box 13.10 Travelling by plane with diabetes
- Contact the airport and airline well in advance.
- Have a letter from the healthcare team, explaining the need to carry medication, delivery devices (including needles), and monitoring equipment in hand luggage.
- Carry CHO-containing food for the journey.
- Ensure insulin does not travel in the hold—temperatures may cause degradation, and there will be problems if luggage is lost.
- Inform airlines in advance of use of CSII/CGM technology.
  - Wireless functionality may interfere with aircraft systems.
  - Might need alternative insulin delivery for the journey.
- Should not go through X-ray machines or full body scanners.

Ramadan and diabetes

Fasting during Ramadan, the holy month of Islam, is a duty for all healthy adult Muslims. Evidence from Islamic countries shows that ~43% with T1DM and 79% with T2DM fast, leading to an estimate of 50 million worldwide. Many Muslims also fast for 1–2 days each week throughout the year. Fasting includes omission of all oral intake, including liquids and medications, during daylight hours. Fasting is not meant to create excessive hardship, and advice should be sought from healthcare professionals as to the risks. Healthcare providers must advise honestly, but be sensitive to an individual's spiritual views, with advice sought from religious leaders where appropriate.

The main risks during Ramadan are:
- Hypoglycaemia.
- Hyperglycaemia.
- Diabetic ketoacidosis.
- Dehydration and thrombosis.

A pre-Ramadan medical assessment is helpful where advice can be given about management of diabetes and fasting (see Box 13.11). Those with problems with hypoglycaemia, insulin treatment, or complications of diabetes may be at particularly high risk. Management strategies can be suggested for those who do elect to fast. Ramadan-focused structured education may helpful. The American Diabetes Association (ADA) has published useful guidance for assessing the risks of fasting and appropriate management of diabetes medication (📖 see Further reading, p. 731).

Box 13.11 Managing diabetes during Ramadan
- Blood glucose should be monitored more frequently.
- Insulin doses may need to be ↓.
- Type of insulin may need to be changed. Pre-mixed insulin is not recommended during fasting.
- Consume more low glycaemic index (GI) food before the fast. Fruit, vegetables, and salad should be included.
- Limit high GI and fatty foods when breaking the fast.
- Avoid dehydration—increase fluid intake during non-fasting hours.
- Break the fast in the event of hypoglycaemia (blood glucose <3.9mmol/L) and significant hyperglycaemia (blood glucose >16.7mmol/L).
- Avoid fasting on 'sick days'.

Weight management with insulin treatment

Treatment with insulin is often linked with ↑ weight. As ↑ weight often results in ↑ insulin requirements, this can become a vicious cycle. It is helpful to warn patients of this, and the following strategies may be helpful in its management:

• Control portion size, and monitor CHO intake.
• Do not miss meals—eat smaller ones.
• Keep physically active (see recommendations earlier in this chapter).
• Consider medications which may promote weight loss.
• Do not ↓ insulin doses to promote weight loss.

Annual review for patients with diabetes

All patients with diabetes should have an annual medical check-up. Diabetes UK defines '15 healthcare essentials' which patients are entitled to (℘ http://www.diabetes.org.uk).

These include:

- Assessment of glucose control: HbA1c, review of blood glucose records, and adjustment of doses.
- Documentation of insulin doses and other medications.
- Assessment of complications, including:
  - Diabetes retinal screening.
  - Urine albumin/creatinine ratio.
  - Foot examination (pedal pulses, monofilament sensation, vibration sense, temperature sense).
  - Biochemistry, including liver and renal function.
- Risk factor management:
  - Blood pressure—target 130/80mmHg.
  - Total cholesterol <4; LDL <2mmol/L.
  - Weight loss to achieve normal BMI.
- Evaluation of hypoglycaemia: history of the number, severity, and frequency of mild and severe hypoglycaemia. Evaluation of hypoglycaemia awareness.
- Support to stop smoking.
- Pre-conception care.
- Emotional and psychological support.
- Access to specialist diabetes healthcare professionals, if required.

Further reading

The Diabetes UK website has useful information about all topics on diabetes and life. Available at: ℘ http://www.diabetes.org.uk.

Al-Arouj M, Assaad-Khalil S, Buse J, et al. (2010). Recommendations for management of diabetes during Ramadan: update 2010. *Diabetes Care* **33**, 1895–902.

Lee P, Greenfield JR, Campbell LV (2009). Managing young people with Type 1 diabetes in a 'rave' new world: metabolic complications of substance abuse in Type 1 diabetes. *Diabet Med* **26**, 328–33.

Lumb AN, Gallen IW (2009). Diabetes management for intense exercise. *Curr Opin Endocrinol Diabetes Obes* **16**, 150–5.

Hospital inpatient diabetes management and diabetic emergencies

Data from the National Diabetes Inpatient Audit suggest that the number of hospital inpatients with diabetes ranges from ~10 to 30%. This does not mean that up to 1 in 3 inpatients are in hospital *because* of their diabetes but happen to have diabetes, in addition to whatever other condition has necessitated their admission. Whatever the reason for admission, patients with diabetes often have longer lengths of hospital stay, and the presence of diabetes remains an important comorbidity that must be dealt with by staff who are competent and confident in its management.

Over the last few years, the Joint British Diabetes Societies Inpatient Care Group has published several national guidelines on the management of several aspects of inpatient diabetes care. The following guidelines are largely derived from those, and full versions can be found on the internet (ℜ http://www.diabetologists-abcd.org.uk/JBDS/JBDS.htm).

Diabetic hyperglycaemic emergencies

Diabetic ketoacidosis

The diagnosis of diabetic ketoacidosis (DKA) is dependent on the combined presence of three biochemical abnormalities:

- Ketonaemia ≥3mmol/L or significant ketonuria (>2+).
- Blood glucose >11mmol/L or known diabetes mellitus.
- Bicarbonate (HCO_3^-) <15mmol/L and/or venous pH <7.3.

The presence of any of the following should prompt consideration of admission to a level 2/HDU environment:

- Blood ketones >6mmol/L, bicarbonate level <5mmol/L, pH <7.1.
- Hypokalaemia (<3.5mmol/L).
- Abnormal GCS or AVPU score.
- Oxygen saturation <92% on air.
- Systolic BP <90mmHg, pulse >100 or <60bpm.
- Anion gap >16 (anion gap = $(Na^+ + K^+) - (Cl^- + HCO_3^-)$).

The management of DKA

The resolution of DKA depends upon the suppression of ketonaemia, and measurement of blood ketones now represents best practice in monitoring the response to treatment. Bedside ketone monitors should be used to measure the plasma ketone concentrations (in particular, 3β-hydroxybutyrate) because this is the direct marker of disease severity.

Where available, the specialist diabetes team should ideally be involved as early as is practical after admission.

Monitor using venous blood gases (the differences in arterial and venous pH, bicarbonate, and K^+ are not great enough to alter management). Plasma ketones, venous pH, and bicarbonate measurements should be used as treatment markers (see Box 13.12).

Use a weight-based, fixed-rate intravenous insulin infusion (FRIII) at 0.1 units/kg/h, i.e. 7 units per hour for a 70kg individual. This enables rapid blood ketone clearance. The fixed rate may be adjusted in insulin-resistant states if the response is not fast enough. There is no need for a bolus dose of insulin if the IV insulin infusion (IVII) is set up promptly.

Continue SC basal insulin analogues. They provide background insulin when the IVII is discontinued. Short-acting insulin should be given before discontinuing the IVII.

Bicarbonate should not be given because it may worsen intracellular acidosis and it may precipitate cerebral oedema, particularly in children.

Box 13.12 Metabolic treatment targets in DKA

- Reduction in blood ketones by 0.5mmol/L/h.
- Increase in venous bicarbonate by 3mmol/L/h.
- Reduction in capillary blood glucose by 3mmol/L/h.
- Potassium maintained at 4.5–5.5mmol/L.

If these rates are not achieved, then the FRIII needs adjusting.

Initial actions (first hour of treatment)
- Rapid assessment and resuscitation of patient; commence IV fluids.
- Full clinical examination, with assessment of:
  - Respiratory rate; temperature; blood pressure; pulse; O_2 saturation.
  - Assess GCS. Consider NG tube if GCS is <12.
- Initial investigations should include:
  - Bedside capillary ketones and capillary glucose.
  - Venous gases for glucose, U&Es, pH, HCO_3^-.
  - FBC, blood cultures.
  - ECG, CXR, MSU.
- Continuous cardiac monitoring and pulse oximetry.
- Low molecular weight heparin.
- Consider any precipitating causes, and treat appropriately.

Fluid resuscitation
If the systolic blood pressure is <90mmHg, consider causes other than fluid depletion, such as heart failure, sepsis, etc. Give 500mL of 0.9% sodium chloride (NaCl) solution over 10–15min, and repeat if necessary. If there is no improvement in BP, consider the need for circulatory support.

If systolic BP is >90mmHg, use the rate of fluid replacement in Table 13.6.

Potassium replacement
Hypo- and hyperkalaemia are common in DKA. See Table 13.7.

Table 13.6 Fluid replacement rates

Fluid	Volume
0.9% NaCl 1L	1000mL over first hour
0.9% NaCl 1L with KCl	1000mL 2-hourly × 3
0.9% NaCl 1L with KCl	1000mL 4-hourly × 2

Reassessment of cardiovascular status at 12h is mandatory; further fluid may be required.

Table 13.7 Potassium replacement for different levels

Potassium level in first 24h (mmol/L)	Potassium replacement in mmol/L of infusion solution
Over 5.5	Nil
3.5–5.5	40mmol/L
Below 3.5	Additional potassium needed: either through increased infusion rate or use of concentrated potassium infusion (check local guidelines—may require transfer to HDU)

Insulin infusion
- Start a continuous FRIII via an infusion pump. 50 units human soluble insulin (Actrapid®, Humulin S®), made up to 50mL with 0.9% NaCl solution.
- Infuse at a fixed rate of 0.1 unit/kg/h (i.e. 7mL/h if weight is 70kg).

Ongoing management of DKA after the first 60min is covered in detail in the National Guidelines, available at: ℘ http://www.diabetologists-abcd.org.uk/JBDS/JBDS_IP_DKA_Adults.pdf.

This involves continual monitoring and reassessment of the patient to ensure that metabolic targets are being achieved (see Box 13.12), stabilization and treatment of precipitating factors, and that other medical interventions or monitoring (e.g NG tube, catheter) are not required.

Practice points
Infusion of large volumes of normal saline may lead to hyperchloraemic acidosis; however, this is not a cause of significant morbidity or prolongation of inpatient stay.

Convert back to SC insulin when biochemically stable (blood ketones <0.3, pH >7.3) and the patient is ready to eat and drink.

Involve the specialist diabetes team at an early stage. It is commonly said that DKA is usually a failure of self-management, so assessing the reasons behind admission and re-education to prevent recurrence are vital.

Hyperosmolar hyperglycaemic state

Whilst there is no formal definition of hyperosmolar hyperglycaemic state (HHS; previous name HONK), the following criteria have been adopted nationally across the UK:

- Hypovolaemia.
- Marked hyperglycaemia (30mmol/L or more).
- No significant ketonaemia (<3mmol/L) or acidosis (pH >7.3, bicarbonate >15mmo/L).
- Osmolality usually ≥320mmol/kg.

(Calculated osmolality = 2 Na$^+$ + glucose + urea)

NB A mixed picture of HHS and DKA may occur.

HHS typically occurs in the elderly, but, as type 2 diabetes is diagnosed in younger adults and teenagers, it is likely that HHS will present at younger ages as well. Unlike DKA, which usually comes on over a matter of hours, HHS comes on over many days, and consequently the dehydration and metabolic disturbances are more extreme.

Management of HHS

See ℘ http://www.diabetologists-abcd.org.uk/JBDS/JBDS_IP_HHS_Adults.pdf.

Initial assessment

Hyperglycaemia results in an osmotic diuresis and renal losses of water in excess of sodium and potassium. Fluid losses are estimated to be between 100 and 220mL/kg. Despite these severe electrolyte losses and total body volume depletion, the typical patient with HHS may not look as dehydrated as they are because the hypertonicity leads to preservation of intravascular volume.

The goals of treatment of HHS are to gradually and safely:

- Normalize the osmolality.
- Replace fluid and electrolyte losses.
- Normalize blood glucose.
- Treat the underlying cause.
- Prevent arterial or venous thrombosis.
- Prevent other potential complications, e.g. cerebral oedema/central pontine myelinolysis.
- Prevent foot ulceration.

As with DKA, venous blood can be used to assess pH, bicarbonate, U&Es, glucose, etc. in a blood gas analyser.

The presence of any of the following should prompt consideration of admission to a level 2/HDU environment:

- Osmolality >350mOsm/kg, sodium >160mmol/L.
- Venous/arterial pH <7.1.
- Hypokalaemia (<3.5mm/L) or hyperkalaemia (>6mmol/L).
- Glasgow Coma Scale (GCS) <12 or abnormal AVPU score.
- Oxygen saturation <92% on air.
- Systolic blood pressure <90mmHg, pulse >100 or <60bpm.
- Hypothermia.
- Acute or serious comorbidity, e.g. MI, CCF, or CVA.
- Urine output <0.5mL/kg/h or other evidence of acute kidney injury.

Fluid replacement and changes in osmolality

The goal of the initial therapy is expansion of the intra- and extravascular volume and to restore peripheral perfusion. Replace fluid with 0.9% sodium chloride. Measurement or calculation of osmolality should be undertaken every hour initially and the rate of fluid replacement adjusted to ensure a positive fluid balance sufficient to promote a gradual decline in osmolality. Fluid replacement alone (without insulin) will lower BG which will reduce osmolality, causing a shift of water into the intracellular space. This inevitably results in a rise in serum sodium.

The aim of treatment should be to replace approximately 50% of estimated fluid loss within the first 12h and the remainder in the following 12h, although this will be determined by the initial severity, degree of renal impairment, and associated comorbidities, which may limit the speed of correction.

A BG target of between 10 and 15mmol/L is a reasonable goal. Complete normalization of electrolytes and osmolality may take up to 72h.

The role of insulin in HHS

If significant ketonaemia is present (3β-hydroxybutyrate is >1mmol/L), this indicates relative hypoinsulinaemia, and insulin should be started at time zero.

If significant ketonaemia is not present (3β-hydroxybutyrate <1mmol/L), there is an argument for not starting insulin treatment immediately, as fluid replacement alone will result in a falling blood glucose, and reducing this too quickly may lead to lowering the osmolality precipitously. Insulin treatment, prior to adequate fluid replacement, may result in cardiovascular collapse, as water moves out of the intravascular space, with a resulting decline in intravascular volume.

The recommended insulin dose is a fixed rate intravenous insulin infusion (FRIII) given at 0.05 units/kg/h (e.g. 4 units/h in an 80kg person). A fall of glucose at a rate of up to 5mmol/L/h is ideal, and once the blood glucose has ceased to fall following initial fluid resuscitation, reassess fluid intake and renal function. Insulin may be started at this point or, if already in place, the infusion rate increased by 1 unit/h.

Potassium replacement

This is the same as DKA.

Anticoagulation

Because of the increased risk of arterial and venous thromboembolism, all patients should receive prophylactic low molecular weight heparin for the full duration of admission unless contraindicated. Full treatment dose anticoagulation should only be considered in patients with suspected thrombosis or acute coronary syndrome.

Other electrolytes

Hypophosphataemia and hypomagnesaemia are common in HHS; however, as with DKA, routine replacement is not recommended.

Foot protection

These patients are at high risk of pressure ulceration. An initial foot assessment should be undertaken and heel protectors applied in those with neuropathy, peripheral vascular disease, or lower limb deformity. The feet should be re-examined daily.

Intravenous insulin infusions used in hyperglycaemia

These can be either fixed-rate intravenous insulin infusions (FRIII) or variable rate (VRIII).

Fixed-rate intravenous insulin infusions

These are used in the initial stages of DKA until ketones are <0.3mmol/L *and* pH >7.3 *and* venous bicarbonate >18mmol/L, or in patients with HHS once their blood glucose has stopped dropping at 5mmol/L/h with the initial use of 0.9% sodium chloride. The starting doses are 0.1 unit/kg/h for DKA, and 0.05 unit/kg/h for HHS.

Intravenous crystalloid solution must always be given with an FRIII. In DKA, if the blood glucose levels are >14mmol/L, then this should be 0.9% sodium chloride; if blood glucose levels are <14mmol/L, then 10% dextrose solution should be run *alongside* the saline infusion.

Variable-rate intravenous insulin infusions

The aim of the VRIII is to achieve and maintain normoglycaemia. It should be made up in 50mL syringe with 0.9% sodium chloride—making a concentration of 1 unit per mL. See Table 13.8 for an example of how to prescribe a VRIII.

Use of intravenous insulin infusion

- If the patient is already on a long-acting insulin analogue, these should be continued.
- Monitor blood glucose hourly.
- If the blood glucose remains >12mmol/L for three consecutive readings and is not dropping by 3mmol/L/h or more, the rate of insulin infusion should be increased.
- If the blood glucose is <4.0mmol/L, the insulin infusion should be reduced to 0.5 units per hour, and the low blood glucose should be treated, irrespective of whether the patient has symptoms. If the patient has continued on their basal insulin, then their VRII can be switched off, but the regular blood glucose measurements need to continue. Ensure basal insulin has been given before stopping VRII.

Table 13.8 Prescribing a VRIII

Bedside capillary blood glucose (mmol/L)	Initial rate of insulin infusion (units per hour)
<4.0	0.5 (0 if basal insulin has been continued)
4.1–7.0	1
7.1–9.0	2
9.1–11.0	3
11.1–14.0	4
14.1–17.0	5
17.1–20	6
>20	Seek diabetes team or medical advice

Perioperative management of diabetes

Poor perioperative glycaemic control leads to poor outcomes in a variety of surgical specialities. There is detailed guidance available in the Joint British Diabetes Societies guideline on the perioperative management of adult patients with diabetes undergoing surgery or procedures ($\varnothing$ http://www.diabetologists-abcd.org.uk/JBDS/JBDS_IP_Surgery_Adults_Full.pdf).

There are several reasons why patients experience problems:
- Failure to identify patients with diabetes.
- Lack of institutional guidelines for management of diabetes.
- Poor knowledge of diabetes amongst staff delivering care.
- Complex polypharmacy and insulin-prescribing errors.

It is advocated that, whenever possible, the HbA1c should be below 69mmol/mol (8.5%) prior to surgery.

For most procedures where only one meal will be missed, hypoglycaemic therapy can be adjusted, as outlined in Table 13.9 (OHA) and Table 13.10 (insulin). The use of the VRIII (Table 13.8) should be limited to those who will miss more than one consecutive meal, those who require emergency surgery, and those for whom there was no time to optimize their glycaemic control prior to surgery. The rate of insulin infusion is as described in Table 13.8.

Table 13.9 Guideline for perioperative adjustment of non-insulin medication (short starvation period—no more than ONE missed meal)

Tablet	Day prior to admission	Day of surgery	
		AM surgery	PM surgery
Acarbose	Take as normal	Omit AM dose if NBM	Give AM dose if eating
Meglitinide (repaglinide or nateglinide)	Take as normal	Omit AM dose if NBM	Give AM dose if eating
Metformin (procedure not requiring use of contrast media)*	Take as normal	Take as normal	Take as normal
Sulfonylurea	Take as normal	Once daily—AM omit Twice daily—AM omit	Once daily—AM omit Twice daily—omit AM and PM
Pioglitazone	Take as normal	Take as normal	Take as normal
DPP-IV inhibitor	Take as normal	Omit on day of surgery	Omit on day of surgery
GLP-1 analogue	Take as normal	Omit on day of surgery	Omit on day of surgery

NBM, nil by mouth; AM, morning; PM, afternoon.

* If contrast medium is to be used and eGFR less than 50mL/min/1.73m², metformin should be omitted on the day of the procedure and for the following 48h.

Table 13.10 Guideline for perioperative adjustment of insulin (short starvation period—no more than ONE missed meal; in all cases, check blood glucose on admission)

Insulins	Day prior to admission	Day of surgery	
		AM surgery	PM surgery
Once daily basal (evening)	No dose change*	No dose change	No dose change
Once daily basal (morning)	No dose change	No dose change*	No dose change*
Twice daily pre-mixed insulin or basal insulin	No dose change	Half AM dose PM—no change if eating	Half AM dose PM—no change if eating
Twice daily free-mixing	No dose change	Give half total AM dose as intermediate-acting PM dose—no change if eating	Give half total AM dose as intermediate-acting PM dose—no change if eating
Basal bolus	No dose change	Omit AM and lunchtime short-acting insulins Basal—no change	Take usual AM insulin dose(s) Omit lunchtime dose

AM, morning; PM, afternoon.

* Some units would advocate reduction of usual dose of long-acting analogue by one-third. This reduction should be considered for any patient who 'grazes' during the day. Warn the patient that their blood glucose control may be erratic for a few days after the procedure.

Management of hypoglycaemia

(📖 see also Type 1 diabetes, p. 702.)

Hypoglycaemia is the commonest side effect of insulin and sulfonylurea treatment. Hypoglycaemia should be excluded in any person with diabetes who is acutely unwell, drowsy, unconscious, unable to cooperate, or presenting with aggressive behaviour or seizures. The hospital environment presents additional obstacles to the maintenance of good glycaemic control and the avoidance of hypoglycaemia.

Management of hypoglycaemia

Algorithm A: adults who are conscious, orientated, and able to swallow

Give 15–20g quick-acting carbohydrate of the patient's choice:
- 5–7 Dextrosol® tablets (or 4–5 Glucotabs®).
- 90–120mL of *original* Lucozade® (preferable in renal patients).
- 150mL non-diet cola (a small can).
- 5 Jelly babies or fruit pastilles or 10 Jelly beans.
- 3–4 heaped teaspoons of sugar dissolved in water*.
- 150–200 mL pure fruit juice*.

*Some centres advocate ONLY glucose for the treatment of hypos. Repeat capillary blood glucose measurement 10–15min later. If blood glucose is less than 4.0mmol/L, repeat step 1 up to three times.

If blood glucose remains less than 4.0mmol/L after 45min or three cycles, consider 1mg of glucagon IM (remembering that this may be less effective in patients prescribed sulfonylurea therapy) or IV 10% glucose infusion at 100mL/h.

Once the blood glucose is above 4.0mmol/L and the patient has recovered, give 15g long-acting carbohydrate:
- Two biscuits.
- One slice of bread.
- 200–300mL glass of milk (not soya).
- Normal meal if due (must contain carbohydrate).

DO NOT omit insulin injection if due (a dose review may be required).

Relative hypoglycaemia

Adults who have poor glycaemic control may start to experience symptoms of hypoglycaemia above 4.0mmol/L. Adults who are experiencing symptoms, but have a blood glucose level greater than 4.0mmol/L, should consume a small carbohydrate snack only (e.g. one medium banana or a slice of bread). All adults with a blood glucose level less than 4.0mmol/L, with or without symptoms of hypoglycaemia, should be treated as outlined in Management of hypoglycaemia in the section above.

Algorithm B: adults who are conscious but confused, disorientated, unable to cooperate, or aggressive but are able to swallow

- If patient is unable to follow algorithm A but is able to swallow, give *either* 1.5–2 tubes GlucoGel®/Dextrogel®, squeezed into the mouth between the teeth and gums, *or* (if ineffective) give glucagon 1mg IM.

- Monitor blood glucose levels after 15min. If still less than 4.0mmol/L, repeat steps 1 and 2 up to three times.
- If blood glucose level remains less than 4.0mmol/L after 45min, give IV 10% glucose infusion at 100mL/h.
- Once blood glucose is above 4.0mmol/L and the patient has recovered, give a long-acting carbohydrate, as outlined in Management of hypoglycaemia, see 📖 p. 746.
- DO NOT omit insulin injection if due (a dose review may be required).
- NB Patients given glucagon require a larger portion of long-acting carbohydrate to replenish glycogen stores (double the suggested amount above).

Algorithm C: adults who are unconscious and/or having seizures and/or are very aggressive OR patients who are nil by mouth

- Assess patient.
- If the patient has an insulin infusion *in situ*, stop it immediately.
- The following two options are both appropriate:
  - Glucagon 1mg IM (remembering that this may be less effective in patients prescribed sulfonylurea therapy and may take up to 15min to work).
  - If IV access available, give 75mL of 20% glucose or 150mL of 10% glucose over 12–15min. Repeat capillary blood glucose measurement 10min later. If blood glucose less than 4.0mmol/L, repeat.
- Once blood glucose is greater than 4.0mmol/L and the patient has recovered, give a long-acting carbohydrate, as outlined in Management of hypoglycaemia, see 📖 p. 746.
- DO NOT omit insulin injection if due (dose review may be required).
- If the patient was on IV insulin, continue to check blood glucose every 30min until it is above 3.5mmol/L, then restart IV insulin after review of dose regimen.

The management of stroke patients with diabetes

See ✎ http://www.diabetologists-abcd.org.uk/JBDS/JBDS_IP_Enteral_Feeding_Stroke.pdf. Also see Fig. 13.3.

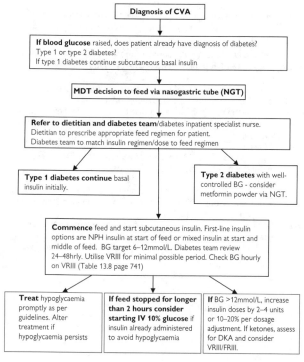

Fig. 13.3 Algorithm for managing diabetes in patient with a stroke and swallowing difficulties.

The critically ill patient

There is controversy regarding the best way to treat hyperglycaemia in critically ill patients. There have been a number of studies done in this population, although the vast majority have been done on patients in intensive care or cardiac surgical patients. The results have not been consistent, with some studies showing benefit and others showing potential harm. In addition, there is currently little consensus on the best way to treat hyperglycaemia-associated poor outcomes following an episode of acute coronary syndrome; however, studies to assess this are ongoing. If one accepts the premise that high blood glucose levels are associated with harm, then a pragmatic approach is to keep the blood glucose between 6 and 10mmol/L using whatever means necessary—oral medication, where appropriate, or a VRIII (Table 13.8 📖 p. 741). Local guidelines should be followed and guidance sought from diabetes specialist teams.

Further reading

Dhatariya K, Flanagan D, Hilton L, et al. (2011). Management of adults with diabetes undergoing surgery and elective procedures: improving standards. London. Joint British Diabetes Societies Inpatient Care Group for NHS Diabetes. Available at: ℘ http://www.diabetologists-abcd.org.uk/JBDS/JBDS_IP_Surgery_Adults_Full.pdf

Furnary AP, Zerr KJ, Grunkemeier GL, Starr A (1999). Continuous intravenous insulin infusion reduces the incidence of deep sternal wound infection in diabetic patients after cardiac surgical procedures. *Ann Thorac Surg* **67**, 352–62.

Gandhi GY, Nuttall GA, Abel MD, et al. (2007). Intensive intraoperative insulin therapy versus conventional glucose management during cardiac surgery: a randomized trial. *Ann Intern Med* **146**, 233–43.

Savage MW, Dhatariya KK, Kilvert A, et al. (2011). Joint British Diabetes Societies guideline for the management of diabetic ketoacidosis. *Diabet Med* **28**, 508–15.

Stanisstreet D, Walden E, Jones C, et al. (2010). The hospital management of hypoglycaemia in adults with diabetes mellitus. London, Joint British Diabetes Societies Inpatient Care Group for NHS Diabetes. Available at: ℘ http://www.diabetologists-abcd.org.uk/JBDS/JBDS_IP_Hypo_Adults.pdf

The NICE-SUGAR Study Investigators (2009). Intensive versus conventional glucose control in critically ill patients. *N Engl J Med* **360**, 1283–97.

Van den Berghe G, Wouters P, Weekers F, et al. (2001). Intensive insulin therapy in the surgical intensive care unit. *N Engl J Med* **345**, 1359–67.

Diabetes and pregnancy

Background
Diabetes is the most common medical complication of pregnancy, affecting approximately 1 in 250 pregnancies. Of the 650,000 women giving birth in England and Wales each year, 2–5% will involve women with diabetes. Approximately 87.5% of pregnancies complicated by diabetes are due to gestational diabetes (which may, or may not, resolve after pregnancy), with 7.5% being due to type 1 diabetes and the remaining 5% being due to type 2 diabetes. In both cases, there are risks both to the mother and the fetus, with a congenital malformation rate of up to 10% or 4–5 times that of the background population in women with very poor glycaemic control (periconception HbA1c >86mmol/mol or 10%). The risk can be reduced, but not entirely eliminated, by optimal pre-conception glycaemic control (HbA1c <53mmol/mol or 7% or lower if achieved without hypoglycaemia.) and 5mg folic acid supplementation (see Box 13.13).

Risks
Fetal
- Macrosomia (birthweight above the 90th percentile) remains the commonest complication of diabetic pregnancy, affecting 40–50% of offspring born to mothers with type 1 and type 2 diabetes. As well as causing birth trauma and delivery complications, macrosomic infants have increased longer-term risks of insulin resistance, obesity, and type 2 diabetes. Fetal hyperinsulinaemia causes growth of insulin-sensitive tissues, with increased abdominal circumference, due to hypertrophy of the fetal pancreatic cells, liver, and heart.
- Preterm delivery (before 37 weeks' gestation) occurs in approximately 37% of pregnancies, with resulting complications of hypoglycaemia (30–50% preterm infants), jaundice, and polycythaemia.
- Neonatal care admission: approximately 40% infants born to mothers with diabetes require additional neonatal care, most typically for complications of prematurity or macrosomia.
- Congenital malformation: cardiac, renal, and neural tube defects occur during the first 5–6 embryonic weeks, stressing the importance of optimizing glycaemic control before conception. The risk of having an infant with a major congenital malformation is comparable for women with type 1 and type 2 diabetes (2–4%) and twice that of the background population (1–2%). The contributions of hyperglycaemia and maternal obesity to the pathogenesis of congenital malformation are well recognized. Alterations in oxygen free radicals, myoinositol, arachidonic acid, and zinc metabolism have also been implicated.
- Fetal mortality (up to 2.2% of births in mothers with type 1 and type 2 diabetes).
- Stillbirth (increased risk if poor glycaemic control and after 38 weeks' gestation).

Box 13.13 Pre-conception management

- Pre-conception glycaemic control optimized, aiming for HbA1c <43mmol/mol (6.1%) if safely achievable without severe hypoglycaemia.
- High-dose folic acid supplements (5mg/day).
- Reviewing potentially teratogenic drugs, including ACE inhibitors, statins.
- Advice on losing weight for all women with BMI >27kg/m².
- Advice on stopping smoking, reducing alcohol intake, avoiding unpasteurized dairy products.
- Screening for retinopathy and nephropathy.
- Metformin may be used as an adjunct or alternative to insulin. All other oral hypoglycaemic agents should be discontinued and replaced with insulin. In HNF1A/4A-MODY already well controlled on low-dose SU glibenclamide can be substituted—see p. 692).

Maternal

- Increased risk of severe hypoglycaemia (SH), particularly during early pregnancy. Historically, the prevalence of SH was as high as 30–40% in type 1 diabetes but may now be declining with increased use of insulin analogues and pump therapy.
- Increased risk of pre-eclampsia, which is related to glycaemic control and complicates approximately 15% diabetic pregnancies.
- Worsening of diabetic nephropathy and progression of retinopathy: renal and retinal screening is recommended before pregnancy and during each trimester.
- Increased risk of diabetic ketoacidosis (DKA). Although rare, affecting <1% of pregnancies, DKA is associated with fetal loss in up to 20% of episodes. Women with suspected DKA should be admitted to level 2 critical care for immediate medical and obstetric care.
- Increased delivery by Caesarean section (66% in type 1 diabetes).
- Thromboembolic disease, while rare, is responsible for a third of all maternal deaths. All women with risk factors (age >35, BMI >30kg/m², proteinuria >5g/day) and/or other comorbidities should receive prophylactic low molecular weight heparin throughout pregnancy.
- Thyroid dysfunction is three times more common in type 1 diabetes pregnancy and should be assessed during pregnancy and post-partum.

Type 1 and type 2 diabetes

- Most women (95%) deliver normal healthy babies. The congenital malformation and spontaneous abortion rates are higher when the HbA1c is elevated (>6.1%; 43mmol/mol).
- Pregnancy is not recommended in women with HbA1c >86mmol/mol (10%).

Management during pregnancy

All pregnant women should be managed in a multidisciplinary clinic and reviewed every 1–2 weeks. A checklist for the clinic visit is listed in Box 13.14.

Maintain good glycaemic control

Good glycaemic control reduces the risk of DKA, fetal macrosomia, fetal loss, and congenital malformation. However, even with near perfect control, there is a small, but significant, risk of major congenital malformations and an unexplained risk of late stillbirths.

A basal bolus regimen is used to achieve the tight postprandial glucose targets. Fast-acting insulin analogues (aspart and lispro) are preferred and safe for use in pregnancy. Levemir® (not yet Lantus®) is licensed by the FDA for pregnancy while basal insulin analogues are not licensed in Europe at the time of writing. However, both Lantus® and Levemir® are increasingly used in type 1 diabetes in pregnancy to reduce the risk of hypoglycaemia.

Insulin pump therapy (CSII) is indicated for women with type 1 diabetes who cannot achieve optimal glycaemic control on multiple daily injections without disabling hypoglycaemia.

Insulin therapy

In type 1 diabetes, insulin requirements often fall in the first trimester, increase slightly in the second, and then continue to rise until about 36 weeks, falling back to pre-pregnancy levels after delivery.

Women with type 1 diabetes should be advised about the increased risk of severe hypoglycaemia and that hypoglycaemia awareness may decrease. Advice regarding care with driving (do not drive below 5mmol/L) is essential. Partners should be instructed how and when to administer glucagon.

In type 2 diabetes, insulin requirements vary considerably; approximately 1.0 units/kg per day initially and up to 2.0 units/kg per day later in the pregnancy.

Monitoring of diabetic complications during pregnancy

Screening for nephropathy and retinopathy is advised at the first antenatal appointment and repeated at 28 weeks. Diabetic retinopathy should not be considered a contraindication to rapid optimization of glucose control. If serum creatinine is abnormal (120micromol/L or more) or the estimated glomerular filtration rate (eGFR) is <45mL/min/1.73m^2, referral to a nephrologist is indicated.

Fetal monitoring

- Scanning of the fetus at 10–12 weeks to confirm dates, looking for congenital abnormalities.
- Screening for congenital malformations at 18–20 weeks.
- Fetal growth assessments at 28, 32, and 36 weeks.

Management of delivery and after delivery

- Women should be offered elective birth through induction of labour or by elective Caesarean section after 38 completed weeks.

Box 13.14 Checklist for type 1/type 2 diabetes in pregnancy during clinic visit

- Capillary blood glucose monitoring before and 1h after meals and before bed, i.e. 7–8 tests per day.
  - Fasting glucose of <5.9mmol/L.
  - 1h postprandial glucose of <7.8mmol/L.
- HbA1c <43mmol/mol (6.1%).
- Insulin therapy—basal bolus or insulin pump therapy. Metformin and/ or glibenclamide may be continued.
  - Reinforce risk of hypoglycaemia during first trimester (e.g. education on driving, glucagon injection) and DKA (e.g. ketone testing during illness).
- Monitoring of maternal weight, BP, and urinalysis.
  - Reinforce dietary advice throughout pregnancy.
  - Physical activity (at least 30min daily), with advice on monitoring BGs and adjusting diet and/or insulin.
  - Assessment for nephropathy and retinopathy at first antenatal visit and at 28 weeks.
- Screening for thyroid disorders.
- Fetal monitoring.
  - Scanning at 18–20 weeks for congenital abnormalities.
  - Growth scanning at 28, 32, and 36 weeks.
  - Review 1–2-weekly.
- At 36 weeks' clinic visit, discuss and document.
  - Mode and timing of delivery.
  - BG management and insulin infusion rate for delivery.
  - Benefits of breastfeeding (mother and baby).
  - Options for safe, effective post-partum contraception.
- Induction of labour or elective Caesarean section is usually advised at or around 38 completed weeks.

- During labour, capillary blood glucose should be monitored on an hourly basis and maintained between 4 and 7mmol/L.
- Intravenous dextrose and insulin infusion is recommended during labour and birth for women if blood glucose is not 4–7mmol/L.
- Blood glucose testing should be carried out routinely in babies of women with diabetes at 2–4h after birth.
- Women should commence pre-conception insulin doses or reduce late pregnancy doses by at least 50% as soon as possible after birth.

The potential for hypoglycaemia in mothers who are breastfeeding should be discussed. Extra carbohydrate snacks for the mother are often needed (10–15g CHO per feed), along with further reductions in pre-conception insulin requirements. One day's worth of breast milk contains about 50g of carbohydrate.

Gestational diabetes

Epidemiology

Pregnancy induces a state of insulin resistance, with increases in the levels of growth hormone, progesterone, placental lactogen, and cortisol, resulting in impaired glucose disposal. Hyperglycaemia during pregnancy occurs in up to 2–5% of women and is associated with increased risk of subsequent type 2 diabetes in up to 50% women over the next 5–10 years. The risk of subsequent type 2 diabetes is significantly reduced by diet and lifestyle and by metformin.

There is a clear association with increasing hyperglycaemia and poorer maternal and fetal outcomes. Intensive treatment with diet, metformin, and insulin (required in 10–20% women) reduces the risk of serious perinatal morbidity (death, macrosomia with associated complications of shoulder dystocia, bone fracture, and nerve palsy), Caesarean delivery, and maternal hypertensive disorders.

Diagnostic criteria for GDM are listed in Table 13.11.

High-risk groups

Most women with gestational diabetes are detected on routine screening at 24–28 weeks, but certain high-risk groups should be screened earlier. These risk factors include:

- Previous gestational diabetes.
- A large baby in their last pregnancy, e.g. >4.5kg.
- A previous unexplained stillbirth/perinatal death.
- Maternal obesity (BMI above 30kg/m^2).
- Family history of diabetes (first-degree relatives).
- Family origin with a high prevalence of type 2 diabetes:
  - South Asian.
  - Black Caribbean.
  - Middle Eastern.
- Polyhydramnios.

Screening

Screening is recommended at 16 weeks if previous gestational diabetes and, if normal, should be repeated at 24–28 weeks in high-risk groups. Box 13.15 details methods of screening.

Table 13.11 Diagnosis of gestational diabetes, according to the current WHO and proposed IADPSG diagnostic criteria

	Plasma glucose (mmol/L)	
WHO	Fasting >7.0mmol/L	Postprandial level ≥7.8mmol/L at 2h
IADPSG	≥5.1mmol/L	≥10.1mmol/L at 1h or ≥8.5mmol/L at 2h

NICE guidelines currently recommend WHO diagnostic criteria. Use of the IADPSG (International Association of Diabetes and Pregnancy Study Group) criteria is an attempt to standardize the diagnosis, based on the Hyperglycaemia and Adverse Pregnancy Outcome (HAPO) study.

Box 13.15 Methods of screening
- The NICE guidelines for GDM screening are currently under review. At present, screening is recommended only in high-risk groups.
- The 2h 75g oral glucose tolerance test (OGTT) should be used at 24–28 weeks, with earlier testing (16–18 weeks) and/or capillary glucose testing indicated in women with previous GDM.
- Fasting plasma glucose, random blood glucose, glucose challenge test, and urinalysis should not be undertaken.

Treatment
- Initial treatment is with dietary advice and exercise. There is an emphasis on watching the quantity of carbohydrate (especially at breakfast) and choosing carbohydrates from low glycaemic index sources, lean proteins, including oily fish, and a balance of polyunsaturated fats and monounsaturated fats.
- 30min of daily physical activity is recommended.
- Women with pre-pregnancy BMI ≥27kg/m² should also be advised to restrict calorie intake (to 25kcal/kg/day or less).

Oral hypoglycaemic therapy
Oral hypoglycaemic treatment is recommended if diet and exercise fail to maintain blood glucose levels in the target range (3.5–7.8mmol/L) and/or the growth scans suggest incipient macrosomia (abdominal circumference >70th percentile).

Metformin and/or glibenclamide are not licensed for use in pregnancy but are commonly used. Informed consent should be obtained.

Insulin therapy
- Required in 10–20% gestational diabetes pregnancies to maintain fasting blood glucose 3.5–5.9mmol/L and 1h postprandial <7.8mmol/L.
- Used in conjunction with diet and exercise or in addition to metformin.
- Regimen should be tailored to glycaemic profile and patient acceptability: boluses alone, basal alone, mixed or basal bolus.
- Most (but not all) women can stop insulin and/or oral hypoglycaemic treatments immediately after birth.

Post-partum follow-up
- Women with gestational diabetes should be offered lifestyle advice (including weight control, diet, and exercise) and a fasting plasma glucose measurement at the 6-week post-natal check and annually thereafter.
- NICE do not recommend a post-partum OGTT, but this is often used in high-risk multiethnic groups at increased risk of type 2 diabetes.

See Box 13.16 for a checklist for GDM during clinic visit.

Box 13.16 Checklist for gestational diabetes during clinic visit

- Monitoring BG, aim:
  - Fasting BG <5.9mmol/L.
  - 1h postprandial BG <7.8mmol/L (some advocate lower BG targets for obese women, e.g. <5.1 fasting and <7.0 after meals).
- Monitor maternal weight, BP, and urinalysis.
- Monitor fetal size (abdominal circumference)—increase treatment if abdominal circumference ≥70th percentile.
- Treatment:
  - Diet and lifestyle advice.
  - Oral hypoglycaemic agents if diet and exercise inadequate or incipient macrosomia: metformin/glibenclamide; insulin therapy— NPH and/or rapid-acting insulin analogues (aspart and lispro).
- Reinforce dietary advice throughout pregnancy.
- Advice on physical activity (at least 30min daily).
- At 36 weeks' clinic visit, discuss and document:
  - Mode and timing of delivery.
  - BG management and insulin infusion rate for delivery.
  - Increased risk of type 2 diabetes and evidence for delaying and prevention (diet and lifestyle or metformin).
  - Benefits of breastfeeding (mother and baby).
  - Options for safe, effective post-partum contraception.
  - Post-partum follow-up—fasting glucose or OGTT 6 weeks post-delivery.

Further reading

Crowther CA, et al. (2005). Effect of treatment of gestational diabetes mellitus on pregnancy outcomes. *N Engl J Med* **352**, 2477–86.

International Association of Diabetes and Pregnancy Study Groups Consensus Panel (2010). International Association of Diabetes and Pregnancy Study Groups recommendations on the diagnosis and classification of hyperglycemia in pregnancy. *Diabetes Care* **33**, 676–82.

Landon MB, et al. (2009). A multicenter, randomized trial of treatment for mild gestational diabetes. *N Engl J Med* **361**, 1339–48.

Macintosh MC, et al. (2006). Perinatal mortality and congenital anomalies in babies of women with type 1 or type 2 diabetes in England, Wales, and Northern Ireland: population based study. *BMJ* **333**, 177.

Metzger BE, et al. (2008). Hyperglycemia and adverse pregnancy outcomes. *N Engl J Med* **358**, 1991–2002.

National Institute for Health and Clinical Excellence (2008). NICE guideline 63: Diabetes in Pregnancy: Management of diabetes and its complications in pregnancy from the pre-conception to the post-natal period. Available at: ◦⃝ http://publications.nice.org.uk/diabetes-in-pregnancy-cg63/guidance.

Ratner RE, et al. (2008). Prevention of diabetes in women with a history of gestational diabetes: effects of metformin and lifestyle interventions. *J Clin Endocrinol Metab* **93**, 4774–9.

Rowan JA, et al. (2008). Metformin versus insulin for the treatment of gestational diabetes. *N Engl J Med* **358**, 2003–15.

Contraception and diabetes

Oral contraceptives

Standard advice regarding the pill should be given, with extra caution in at-risk groups, such as overweight smokers with a family history of thromboembolism and coronary heart disease. It is important to balance the risks and benefits of safe effective contraception with the consequences of unplanned pregnancy.

In those with microvascular disease or coronary risk factors, the progesterone-only 'mini-pill' (POP) is safer than the combined OCP, as it has no significant adverse effects on lipid metabolism, clotting, platelet aggregation, or fibrinolytic activity. It has been suggested that levonorgestrel- and norethisterone-containing POPs may reduce HDL2 cholesterol subfractions.

Barrier methods

These are less effective forms of contraception, with failure rate of 0.7–3.6/100 couple years, compared to nearly 0.2/100 with the combined OCP. As unplanned pregnancy carries significant risks, safer forms of contraception are recommended.

Intrauterine contraceptive devices (IUD)

There were historical concerns that diabetes might make a pelvic infection associated with an IUD more severe, but these are unconfirmed.

Implantable contraceptive

Etonogestrel (Nexplanon®) is a matchstick-sized progestin-only contraceptive, inserted under the skin of the inner upper arm, that offers safe, effective contraception for up to 3 years. It is a popular option for women who cannot, or do not want to, use the combined OCP.

Paediatric and transition diabetes

Diabetes is the third commonest chronic condition in childhood.

- Prevalence—there are 23,000 children and young people under 18 with diabetes in England; 97% type 1, 1.5% type 2, and 1.5% other types. The others are made up of secondary diabetes, e.g. cystic fibrosis, as well as single gene abnormalities.
- Incidence is currently around 26:100,000 children per year. This is rising at around 4% per year in most developed countries, and even faster in some developing nations.

Type 1 diabetes

Epidemiology

- Age of onset can be anything from 6 months onwards.
- There are typically two peaks of onset—at around ages 5–6 and 12–13 years. It is thought that this suggests viral infections as a cause.
- The environmental trigger is, however, unknown in most cases, and various pancreatic antibodies can be present months or years before the diagnosis is made.

Diagnosis

- Onset generally with polyuria and polydipsia in older children.
- 50–90% have new-onset bedwetting, having been dry previously.
- Younger children, including babies and toddlers, may have less easily recognized symptoms—constipation, lethargy, thrush, poor feeding.
- 30–40% under age 5 are in DKA at diagnosis, compared with 20–25% of older children.
- Symptoms of DKA in children can be abdominal pain, breathing difficulties, vomiting, dehydration, and shock.

The diagnosis should be made at the first presentation by doing a capillary BG measurement, rather than waiting for a urine sample or fasting BG sample. Management in children is highly specialized and is only done in secondary care centres with an appropriate MDT with training in diabetes in children. If BG greater than 11mmol/L, the child should be referred that same day to such a centre.

Type 2 diabetes

Increasing in Europe but not to the same extent as in the USA where half of children diagnosed with diabetes now have type 2. Associated with obesity but also in particular ethnic groups with a high genetic susceptibility. Children often have a family history and may have acanthosis nigricans, indicative of insulin resistance. At present, in the UK, only 1.5% of all children with diabetes have type 2. Therefore, only a few centres have a lot of experience, and adult diabetologists may be asked to assist with the management.

Other types of diabetes

Neonatal diabetes

Diabetes presenting before the age of 6 months is very rare and unlikely to be autoimmune in aetiology. This can be transient or permanent and is usually due to single gene abnormalities. Many of these babies require tiny doses of insulin, particularly if also of low birthweight, and this is best given using an insulin infusion pump. This should only be done in specialist centres.

Monogenic diabetes

Various single gene disorders can present in childhood.

Making a correct genetic diagnosis of neonatal diabetes or MODY is important, as insulin treatment may not be required (see p. 691).

Secondary forms of diabetes

- Most common is cystic fibrosis (CF-related diabetes; CFRD).
- Weight loss and frequent infections are signs of possible CFRD.
- CGM may be the best way of diagnosing subtle changes in glucose tolerance.
- All teenagers with CF should be screened.
- Management is with insulin.

Management of children with diabetes

In the UK, standards for best practice in caring for children with diabetes have been linked to payment of a 'best practice tariff'—a set amount of money paid for each young person cared for (up to their 19th birthday). To qualify for this, the following must apply:

- Every child or young person with diabetes will be cared for by a specialist team of healthcare professionals (consisting of a doctor, a nurse, and a dietician as a minimum) who have specific training in paediatric diabetes. DSN caseload 70–100 patients.
- For new diagnoses: the case must be discussed with the specialist team within 24h of the diagnosis and seen on the next working day.
- An age-appropriate structured education programme offered at diagnosis and with updates, as needed.
- Four clinic appointments with HbA1c check.
- Annual dietician contact.
- At least eight additional contacts per year from members of the specialist team (not all face-to-face) are recommended.
- Annual review with BP and retinopathy/renal screening from age 12.
- Annual psychology assessment and access to psychology services.
- 24h emergency phone advice for families/other health professionals.
- Involvement in the National Paediatric Diabetes Audit and Paediatric Diabetes Network.
- Policy for transition to adult services.
- Policy on managing high HbA1c and infrequent clinic attendance.

Type 1 diabetes in children

Insulin

Insulin is started at a total daily dose of 0.5 units/kg body weight in children. In puberty, the starting dose is 0.7 units/kg body weight.

Insulin regimens are the same as in adults, varying from centre to centre, with very little evidence base for one being superior. In toddlers, basal insulin tends to be given in the morning, moving to the evening in children aged >5 years. It is often used twice daily in puberty. Prandial insulin doses for food can be anything from 0.5 units for 40g of CHO in babies to 3–4 units for 10g in pubertal boys.

Continuous subcutaneous insulin infusion (CSII) pumps (📖 p. 704)
NICE guidelines allow for pumps to be funded in children under the age of 12 in whom multiple insulin injections are considered to be impractical or inappropriate. Over 12s have the same funding restrictions as adults.

Education

As in adults, this is the mainstay of management to allow parents and then children to self-manage their own condition.

- *Carbohydrate counting.* This may be taught at any stage but is better if done soon after diagnosis so that it becomes routine for the family.
- *Multiple carers.* One of the main differences between children and adults with diabetes is the need to teach many family members about the condition, including grandparents and childminders.

- *Blood testing.* Before every meal and at other times to work out whether mealtime doses are correct, as well as at other times for troubleshooting. Many children require 6–8 blood tests per day, and so there is much interest currently in continuous subcutaneous glucose sensing.
- *Exercise.* Children's exercise levels vary enormously from one day to the next. Therefore, advice about how to cope with the BG variability is essential and built into most structured education programmes.
- *Management at school and nursery:*
  - Children spend around a third to half of waking hours at school.
  - Schools need to support intensive management of diabetes.
  - This works best when volunteers at primary school are taught diabetes management. This includes either supervising or doing the BG testing, insulin injections, or pump boluses, and, in some places, the use of algorithms to calculate insulin doses for food and BG correction. This involves a lot of education, usually by the DSN.
  - All school staff (primary and secondary) should be aware of the symptoms of hypoglycaemia in a particular child and should know how to treat hypoglycaemia.

Acute complications are mainly treated as in adults (📖 see Expert management of type 1 diabetes, p. 694; Diabetes and life, p. 722; Hospital inpatient diabetes management and diabetic emergencies, p. 732). Specific points relevant to children are described in the following sections.

Hypoglycaemia
- Parents and carers should look out for symptoms, as children may not recognize them reliably until around 10 years old.
- Dose of glucagon for severe lows with fits or unconsciousness: 0.5mg if under 8 years old and 1.0mg if older.

Diabetic ketoacidosis
Management in those <18 years should be according to the British Society of Paediatric Endocrinology and Diabetes guidelines (🖰 http://www.bsped.org.uk/clinical/clinical_endorsedguidelines.html). Key features which are different from the new adult guidelines are:
- Lower volumes of fluid than in adults because of the risk of cerebral oedema.
- Fixed-rate insulin infusion at 0.1 units/kg/h.
- Delay in insulin administration until after 1h of fluids for the same reason.

Complications and associated conditions
Annual review should include:
- Blood pressure at all ages.
- Microalbuminuria and retinopathy screening: annually when >12 years.
- Examine feet to instil good practices.
- 3-yearly screening for coeliac disease (6–8% patients have condition).
- Annual thyroid function tests.
- Addison's disease—no screening, but consider if recurrent hypoglycaemia and lethargy.

Puberty and diabetes

- Insulin requirements rise from ~0.7 units/kg/day to up to 2.0 units/kg/day in early puberty in girls and late puberty in boys (timed with the growth spurt) because of the insulin resistance of puberty.
- Puberty can make the management of a chronic condition difficult as the teenager wishes, most of all, to be accepted into a peer group, and feeling different in any way makes this hard.
- Therefore, some young people will stop doing BG testing or miss insulin doses, particularly when out with friends.
- Supportive management with short-term goal-setting and counselling is important.
- Young people often need to be seen more frequently, rather than less, during this time.

Transition from paediatric to adult services

During the teenage years, there is a gradual change from parental management of the diabetes to the young person themselves being responsible for their own diabetes. Many parents think that as soon as the child reaches the age of 14–15, they can take care of their own diabetes and should be left to get on with it. This is NOT true. HbA1c levels continue to increase until the age of around 20, and it is only when young people settle down in their early 20s that diabetes becomes more stable.

Good research evidence shows that the longer the parents remain involved, the better the outcomes in terms of HbA1c and quality of life. Therefore, young people should be seen with their parents as long as they wish to, even in an adult clinic. Seeing them alone at the start of the consultation may help to uncover their own management style, but parental involvement should still be encouraged.

How a transition service should work

- The service should have a transition protocol, which should include agreeing the timing of transfer with the young person, discussed well in advance.
- Transfer should be to a service with a young adult clinic, rather than to general practitioners, as they do not generally have the expertise to manage young people with type 1 diabetes.
- Some evidence suggests that transition is more successful if there is a joint clinic between the paediatric MDT and the adult MDT.
- A dedicated transition service DSN should keep in contact with young people in the community when they default from clinics.
- There is evidence that defaulters have higher HbA1c levels, and so they do need to be followed up in specialist care.

Educational aspects of transition

It is helpful to have leaflets on all of the following issues available at each contact with young people. Advice should be non-judgemental, be offered from early teenage years, and take place with parents absent.

- Alcohol.
- Driving: a doctor is required to sign the provisional driving licence application form. The usual DVLA rules apply.

- Smoking.
- Recreational drugs.
- Contraception and pre-conception care.
- Sick day rules—to take account of living alone for the first time.
- Eating disorders:
  - Mild forms are common, especially, but not exclusively, in girls. Discussion should be towards helping the young person recognize the link between thoughts, feelings, and behaviour and to try to find alternative behaviours. Missed insulin injections are often a way of controlling weight.
- Higher education:
  - Often secondary specialist care is kept at home for appointments during the holidays, with local GP registration with the university/college student health system. Young people on insulin need a fridge to be provided in their University accommodation and to let people on their corridor know about diabetes. A discussion about how they will manage 'fresher's week', especially with alcohol, and other issues is helpful.
- Separation from parents:
  - The paediatric team will usually have spent many years communicating more with the parents than the children. However, now the young person may need to be helped to understand their diabetes for themselves, often requiring a new process of education from basics onwards.

Diabetic eye disease

Epidemiology

Diabetic retinopathy (DR) is a complication of diabetes, resulting from damage to the small blood vessels, generally occurring 10 years after diabetes onset (which may be some years before the diagnosis of type 2 diabetes). DR is the leading cause of blindness in the working age population. Cataracts are also more common in people with diabetes.

DR is extremely common with long durations of diabetes. A recent study of global prevalence of DR showed a prevalence of 35% for any DR, 7% had proliferative diabetic retinopathy (PDR), 7% had macular oedema, and 10% had sight-threatening diabetic eye disease (STED).

Recent studies have shown that, since 1985, people with diabetes have experienced lower rates of progression to proliferative DR and severe visual loss, probably reflecting improvements in diabetes care.

Some studies have suggested that non-White ethnic groups have higher prevalences of DR. However, this has been difficult to separate from confounding risk factors, such as age, duration of diagnosed diabetes, HbA1c, and blood pressure.

See Box 13.17 for classification of DR.

Box 13.17 Classification and features of diabetic retinopathy

- Background retinopathy (graded as R1 by the National Screening Committee—NSC):
  - Microaneurysms.
  - Haemorrhages—dot and flame-shaped.
  - Hard exudates.
  - Soft exudates/cotton wool spots.
- Pre-proliferative retinopathy (graded as R2):
  - Multiple blot haemorrhages.
  - Intraretinal microvascular abnormalities (IRMAs).
  - Venous beading.
  - Venous reduplication.
- Proliferative retinopathy (graded as R3):
  - New vessels on the disc (NVD) or within 1 disc diameter of it.
  - New vessels elsewhere (NVE).
  - Fibrovascular proliferation ± tractional retinal detachment.
  - Pre-retinal or vitreous haemorrhage.
  - Rubeosis iridis (± neovascular glaucoma).
- Maculopathy (graded as M0 if none and M1 if present):
  - Exudate within 1 disc diameter (DD) of the centre of the fovea.
  - Group of exudates within the macula.
  - Any microaneurysm or haemorrhage within 1 DD of the centre of the fovea only if associated with a best VA of ≤6/12 (if no stereo).
  - Retinal thickening within 1 DD of the centre of the fovea (if stereo available).

Other NSC grades
- R0—no retinopathy.
- O—other non-diabetic lesions seen (e.g. drusen and macular degeneration).
- P—evidence of previous laser therapy/retinal photocoagulation.
- U—unclassifiable, often due to cataracts.

Clinical and histological features of diabetic eye disease

The classification of diabetic retinopathy is based on clinical examination or on grading of retinal photographs, but changes in the pathophysiology may explain some of the clinical findings.

One of the first histological changes seen is thickening of the basement membrane and loss of pericytes embedded within it, forming acellular capillaries. Breakdown in endothelial cell tight junctions leads to increased capillary permeability. The microaneurysm is the hallmark of retinal microvascular disease in diabetes. Microaneurysms may be asymmetrical dilatations of the capillary wall where it is weakened or damaged, following the loss of the supporting pericytes and localized increases in hydrostatic pressure. Smooth muscle cell death, capillary weakening and closure, with the occurrence of intraretinal microvascular abnormalities (IRMA), and impaired autoregulation are all features of diabetic retinopathy.

The natural progression, with increasing retinal ischaemia, is from background to pre-proliferative to proliferative DR and ultimately to sight-threatening DR. Maculopathy can occur at any of these stages but does occur more frequently with more advanced disease.

Background retinopathy

Capillary microaneurysms are the earliest feature seen clinically as red 'dots'. Dot haemorrhages also occur, and these can be difficult to distinguish from microaneurysms and are collectively, referred to as HMA. Small intraretinal haemorrhages or 'blots' also occur, as can haemorrhage into the nerve fibre layer, which are often more flame-shaped. With ↑ capillary leakage, hard exudates, which are lipid deposits, can also be seen.

A *cotton wool spot* is a delay in transmission along the axoplasm of the nerve fibre layer of the retina, caused by ischaemia. It used to be considered a pre-proliferative feature, but, because it is not a good indicator of progression to proliferative retinopathy, it is now included in the background R1 category in the English national DR screening programme.

Pre-proliferative retinopathy

With increasing ischaemia, the retina shows signs of increasing numbers of blot haemorrhages, which are usually in a deeper layer of the retina than dot or flame-shaped haemorrhages.

Intraretinal microvascular abnormalities (IRMA) are tortuous intraretinal vascular segments varying in calibre. They derive from remodelling of the retinal capillaries and small collateral vessels in areas of microvascular occlusion.

Venous beading is a localized increase in calibre of the vein, and the severity is dependent on the increase in calibre and the length of vein involved.

Venous reduplication is dilation of a pre-existing channel or proliferation of a new channel adjacent to, and approximately the same calibre as, the original vein.

The Early Treatment of Diabetic Retinopathy Study (ETDRS) provided evidence that certain features were more indicative of progression to proliferative DR and suggested a '4–2–1' rule:

- 4 quadrants of severe haemorrhages or microaneurysms.
- 2 quadrants of IRMAs.
- 1 quadrant with venous beading.

If you have one of these features, there is a 15% risk of developing proliferative diabetic retinopathy within the next year; if two are present, the risk rises to 45%.

Proliferative retinopathy

(See Fig. 13.4.)

New vessels developing in diabetic retinopathy are characterized according to whether they develop at or near the optic disc (NVD) or elsewhere in the retina (NVE). They usually develop from the venous circulation and grow forwards in the vitreous gel, but they can also develop from the arterial circulation.

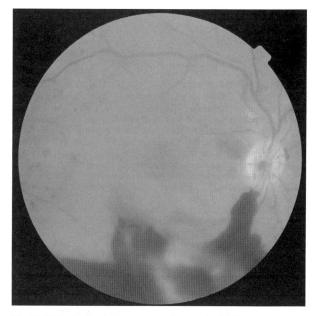

Fig. 13.4 This photograph shows new vessels at the disc (NVD) and haemorrhage from these new vessels in front of the inferior temporal arcade.

New vessels on the disc (NVD) are defined as any new vessel developing at the optic disc or within 1 disc diameter of the edge of the optic disc.

New vessels elsewhere (NVE) are defined as any new vessel developing more than 1 disc diameter away from the edge of the optic disc.

Both give no symptoms but cause the problems of advanced retinopathy, such as haemorrhage, scar tissue formation, traction on the retina, and retinal detachment which actually results in loss of vision.

The Diabetic Retinopathy Study (DRS) recommended prompt treatment with panretinal photocoagulation in the presence of DRS high-risk characteristics, which reduced the 2-year risk of severe visual loss by 50% or more and were defined by:

- The presence of pre-retinal or vitreous haemorrhage.
- Eyes with NVD equalling or exceeding 1/4 to 1/3 disc area in extent with no haemorrhage.
- NVE equalling >1/2 disc area with haemorrhage (from the NVE).

Untreated, eyes with high-risk characteristics had between 25.6% and 36.9% chance of severe visual loss within 2 years.

Proliferative eyes without high-risk characteristics had the following risks of severe visual loss:

- Untreated—2 years 7.0%, 4 years 20.9%.
- Treated—2 years 3.2% 4 years 7.4%.

Because the side effects of modern laser treatment are considerably less than the early lasers, most ophthalmologists treat eyes that develop new vessels of either the high- or low-risk categories.

Diabetic macular oedema

Diabetic macular oedema or maculopathy may be classified into focal, diffuse, and ischaemic types.

In focal maculopathy, focal leakage tends to occur from microaneurysms, often with a circinate pattern of exudates around the focal leakage.

In the diffuse variety, there is a generalized breakdown of the blood–retina barrier and profuse early leakage from the entire capillary bed of the posterior pole, sometimes accompanied by cystoid macular changes.

In ischaemic maculopathy, enlargement of the foveal avascular zone (FAZ) due to capillary closure is found with variable degrees of visual loss.

The Early Treatment Diabetic Retinopathy Study (ETDRS) reported that focal photocoagulation of 'clinically significant' diabetic macular oedema (CSMO) substantially reduced the risk of visual loss, CSMO being defined as:

- Thickening of the retina at or within 500 microns of the centre of the macula.
- Hard exudates at or within 500 microns of the centre of the fovea, if associated with thickening of the adjacent retina (no residual hard exudates remaining after disappearance of retinal thickening).
- A zone or zones of retinal thickening 1 disc area or larger, any part of which is within 1 disc diameter of the centre of the macula.

Eye screening

National screening programmes

The development of screening in Europe was first encouraged by the St. Vincent Declaration which, in 1989, set a target for the reduction of new blindness by one-third in the following 5 years.

National screening programmes, with consensus grading protocols, were introduced in the UK in 2002–2004. The National Institute for Health and Clinical Excellence (NICE) recommends that those with type 1 and type 2 diabetes have their eyes screened at the time of diagnosis and at least annually thereafter. There are differences in the protocols used globally in screening programmes. In England, the method used is two-field mydriatic digital photography, with screening performed by technician screeners or optometrists. Fixed locations and mobile units are both used. Monitoring of programme performance is via Quality Assurance Standards and Key Performance Indicators against which individual screening programmes are assessed.

Ad hoc eye examinations

It is important to remember that the patients who are most at risk of developing sight-threatening diabetic retinopathy and visual loss are the regular non-attenders for screening. Hence, it is important to examine the eyes of patients who have not attended for routine screening using the following method:

Visual acuity

Use a standard Snellen chart for distance, and check each eye separately. Let the patient wear their glasses for the test, and if vision is worse than 6/9, also check with a pinhole, as this will correct for any refractive (glasses) error. If it does not correct to 6/9 or better, consider more careful review; some maculopathy changes cannot be seen easily with a handheld ophthalmoscope, and an ophthalmology review may be needed. Cataracts are a more likely cause, so look carefully at the red reflex.

High blood glucose readings can lead to myopia and low blood glucose to hypermetropia. In both these circumstances, one would expect the vision to improve with a pinhole.

Eye examination

- Dilate the pupil before looking into the eye.
  - Use *tropicamide* 1%—dilates the pupil adequately in 15–20min and lasts only 2–3h.
  - In those with a dark iris, you may also need *phenylephrine* (2.5%), added soon after the tropicamide, to give adequate views.
  - The main reasons not to dilate are closed angle glaucoma and recent eye surgery, but as such patients are usually under an eye clinic already, most people are suitable for dilatation.
- Once the pupil is dilated, look at the red reflex to check for lens opacities. Examine the anterior chamber, as, although rare, rubeosis iridis is important to pick up. The vitreous is examined before

examining the retina. When examining the retina, use the optic disc as a landmark; follow all four arcades of vessels out from it; examine the periphery, and at the end, examine the macula, as this can be uncomfortably bright through a dilated pupil, and if done at the start, it makes it difficult for anyone to keep their eye still enough to complete the examination adequately. It is usually much easier for the patient to look directly at the light if a smaller spot size or a target on a green background are chosen for this aspect of the examination.

When to refer

Referral will depend on local preferences but are based on NSC management guidelines, as outlined in Box 13.18.

Box 13.18 Reasons for and timing of referral to ophthalmologist

- Immediate referral:
  - Rubeosis iridis/neovascular glaucoma.
  - Vitreous haemorrhage.
  - Advanced retinopathy with retinal detachment.
- Urgent referral (<2 weeks):
  - R3/proliferative retinopathy, as untreated NVD carries a 40% risk of blindness in <2 years and laser treatment reduces this.
- Routine referral (<13 weeks):
  - R2/pre-proliferative changes.
  - M1/maculopathy.
- Routine non-DR referral:
  - Cataracts.
- Other categories:
  - R0/no retinopathy—annual screening.
  - R1/background retinopathy—annual screening and inform diabetes care team.

Medical treatment for diabetic eye disease

Box 13.19 shows the risk factors for worsening retinopathy.

Glycaemic control

The DCCT and UKPDS confirmed the link between glycaemic control and the onset and progression of diabetic eye disease.

Worsening of DR can occur when glycaemic control improves rapidly, so careful monitoring of diabetic retinopathy is needed during this period (e.g. pregnancy). However, the long-term benefits of improved glycaemic control greatly outweigh the risks of early worsening.

Blood pressure control/therapy

UKPDS also showed that good blood pressure control is vital to reduce the onset and progression of DR.

Lipid control/therapy

Evidence that elevated serum lipids are associated with macular exudates and moderate visual loss and that partial regression of hard exudates may be possible by reducing elevated lipid levels comes from several studies. The FIELD study suggested that the use of fenofibrate in type 2 diabetes might reduce the need for laser treatment of diabetic retinopathy over a 5-year period. However, caution is needed with this interpretation, as the numbers of events were small.

Antiplatelet therapy

These agents have been tried in patients with diabetes, but the results are variable.

Lifestyle advice

Stopping smoking may reduce the risk of DR in type 1 diabetes. Changes to alcohol consumption or physical activity show no consistent effect.

Box 13.19 Risk factors for developing/worsening of diabetic retinopathy

Modifiable risk factors for DR:
- Glucose control.
- Systemic hypertension.
- Blood lipids.
- Smoking in type 1 diabetes.

Non-modifiable risk factors for DR:
- Duration of diabetes.
- Age.
- Genetic predisposition.
- Ethnicity.
- Pregnancy.

Surgical treatment for diabetic eye disease

Laser treatment

- The ETDRS protocol for panretinal photocoagulation recommends 1,200–1,600 argon laser burns of 500 micron spot size, with the treatment performed in two or more episodes, no more than 2 weeks apart, and that no more than 900 burns should be applied in one session.
- Laser therapy is usually performed as two sessions of outpatient treatment on conscious patients. Topical local anaesthetic drops allow a contact lens to be placed on the cornea for application of the laser through the contact lens. Modern multispot laser machines with reduced duration of the burn and the ability to apply predetermined pattern types, which can administer up to 25 spots at a time, have reduced the time taken and the discomfort of panretinal laser treatment. Hence, panretinal photocoagulation can usually be applied with local anaesthetic drops.
- The laser energy is absorbed by the choroid and the pigment epithelium.
- Laser treatment for clinically significant macular oedema reduces visual loss by >50%.
- Laser treatment aims to prevent further visual loss, especially in maculopathy, not to restore vision, and the distinction must be emphasized to all patients requiring treatment. The benefits from laser therapy currently outweigh the risks, which include accidental burns to the fovea if the eye moves during therapy, a reduction in night vision, and, in a small number, interference with visual field severe enough to affect the ability to drive. Most patients, however, retain the minimum field for driving.

Vitrectomy

The surgical techniques of vitrectomy for advanced diabetic retinopathy have improved over the last 30 years, which has been demonstrated by the improved surgical results during this period. Most modern systems employ three small (20–25 gauge) entry 'ports' into the eye, and a cutting/suction device, an intraocular light source, and an infusion cannula are inserted through these trans-scleral incisions.

The reasons why vitrectomy may be required are:

- Non-clearing vitreous haemorrhage.
- A large subhyaloid macular haemorrhage.
- Tractional retinal detachment.
- Combined rhegmatogenous (due to retinal tear)/tractional retinal detachment.
- Progressive severe fibrovascular proliferation.
- Taut posterior hyaloid in diabetic macular oedema.

Alternative surgical treatment—the use of intravitreal VEGF inhibitors

Ocular neovascularization (angiogenesis) and increased vascular permeability have been associated with Vascular Endothelial Growth Factor (VEGF), which does also have a neuroprotective effect.

There are three potential VEGF inhibitors: pegaptanib, ranibizumab, and bevacizumab. Ranibizumab is an antibody fragment derived from bevacizumab, which is a full-length humanized monoclonal antibody against human VEGF.

The Diabetic Retinopathy Clinical Research Network reported the results of a multicentre, randomized clinical trial of 854 eyes in 691 participants that evaluated ranibizumab plus prompt or deferred laser or triamcinolone plus prompt laser for diabetic macular oedema. Intravitreal ranibizumab with prompt or deferred laser was more effective through at least 1 year, compared with prompt laser alone for the treatment of DME involving the central macula. The expense of these agents has led to some limitation in their use in diabetic eye disease, but a NICE appraisal in 2013 has now recommended the use of ranibizumab in certain cases of diabetic macular oedema.

Favourable results have been reported with some regression of neovascularization and reduction in fluorescein leakage in some studies using bevacizumab and pegaptanib, but the effect is only transient (2–11 weeks).

Intravitreal injection is an effective means of delivering anti-VEGF drugs to the retina but has the potential complications of endophthalmitis and retinal detachment. Randomized controlled trials utilizing varying doses of the VEGF inhibitors are required to assess the long-term efficacy and safety and to define optimum treatment regimens. Cost effectiveness studies are also needed.

Cataract extraction

This is a common procedure, with a slightly higher complication rate than in the non-diabetic population. Although diabetes is a risk factor for the development of cataracts and studies have shown an increased risk of ocular complications in people with diabetes after cataract surgery, modern surgical techniques and appropriate preoperative laser treatment have led to an overall good visual outcome in the majority of patients.

Further reading

Elman MJ, Aiello LP, Beck RW, *et al.* (2010). Randomized trial evaluating ranibizumab plus prompt or deferred laser or triamcinolone plus prompt laser for diabetic macular edema. *Ophthalmology* **117**, 1064–77.

Keech AC, Mitchell P, Summanen PA, *et al.* (2007). Effect of fenofibrate on the need for laser treatment for diabetic retinopathy (FIELD study): a randomised controlled trial. *Lancet* **370**, 1687–97.

Klein R, Knudtson MD, Lee KE, Gangnon R, Klein BE (2008). The Wisconsin Epidemiologic Study of Diabetic Retinopathy: XXII the twenty-five-year progression of retinopathy in persons with type 1 diabetes. *Ophthalmology* **115**, 1859–68.

National Institute for Health and Clinical Excellence (2013). NICE appraisal: Ranibizumab for the treatment of diabetic macular oedema. Available at: ℜ http://www.nice.org.uk/nicemedia/live/14082/62873/62873.pdf.

No authors listed (1985). Photocoagulation for diabetic macular edema. Early Treatment Diabetic Retinopathy Study report number 1. Early Treatment Diabetic Retinopathy Study research group. *Arch Ophthalmol* **103**, 1796–806.

No authors listed (1987). Indications for photocoagulation treatment of diabetic retinopathy: Diabetic Retinopathy Study Report no. 14. The Diabetic Retinopathy Study Research Group. *Int Ophthalmol Clin* **27**, 239–53.

No authors listed (1991). Grading diabetic retinopathy from stereoscopic color fundus photographs--an extension of the modified Airlie House classification. ETDRS report number 10. Early Treatment Diabetic Retinopathy Study Research Group. *Ophthalmology* **98**(5 Suppl), 786–806.

Raymond NT, Varadhan L, Reynold DR, *et al.* (2009). Higher prevalence of retinopathy in diabetic patients of South Asian ethnicity compared with white Europeans in the community: a cross-sectional study. *Diabetes Care* **32**, 410–15.

Wong TY, Mwamburi M, Klein R, *et al.* (2009). Rates of progression in diabetic retinopathy during different time periods: a systematic review and meta-analysis. *Diabetes Care* **32**, 2307–13.

Yau JW, Rogers SL, Kawasaki R, *et al.* (2012). Global prevalence and major risk factors of diabetic retinopathy. *Diabetes Care* **35**, 556–64.

Diabetic renal disease

Background
Diabetic nephropathy is now the major cause of end-stage renal disease (ESRD) worldwide, representing over 50% of patients on renal replacement therapy in many Middle and Far Eastern countries (>20% in the UK), the majority having type 2 diabetes. Cardiovascular morbidity and mortality is much greater in diabetic patients with nephropathy, and many will die before reaching ESRD.

Definition
Diabetic nephropathy is defined by the presence of dipstick +ve proteinuria in a person with diabetes. This equates to an albumin concentration of 300mg/L (total protein 0.5g/L). Most patients will also have hypertension and retinopathy, and many will have renal impairment. Research studies use timed urine collections, with a diagnostic level of >300mg/day (about 200 micrograms/min). This level of albuminuria is termed overt or clinical nephropathy. Excretion rates between 20 and 200 micrograms/min are called microalbuminuria or incipient nephropathy and indicate a high risk for future ESRD, although as many as 30% may spontaneously revert to normal (see Table 13.12).

Chronic kidney disease (CKD) has been classified into stages, according to an estimated glomerular filtration rate (eGFR) derived from serum creatinine concentrations. Stages 1 and 2 (eGFR >90 and 60–89mL/min/1.73m^2, respectively) also require the presence of albuminuria or renal structural abnormality, but stages 3–5 (eGFR 30–59, 15–29, and <15mL/min/1.73m^2, respectively) do not (see Table 13.13). The problem is that this classification does not map easily to the classical definition of incipient and overt nephropathy. Moreover, not all CKD is due to diabetic glomerulosclerosis, particularly in the older person with type 2 diabetes, although the presence of retinopathy makes the likelihood of diabetic glomerulosclerosis >80%. Table 13.13 attempts to reconcile these diagnostic difficulties.

Epidemiology
The duration of diabetes is a major risk for the development of nephropathy, so point prevalence studies are hard to interpret. In addition, the incidence appears to be declining, at least in type 1 diabetes, so historical prevalence rates may be misleading. In an inception cohort of 277 type 1 patients from Denmark studied from 1979 to 2004, the cumulative incidence of microalbuminuria was 34% and for clinical nephropathy 15% after 20 years. For ESRD, rates of 2.2% and 7.8% have recently been reported from Finland after 20 and 30 years' duration, respectively.

Because the true date of onset of type 2 diabetes is hard to determine, cumulative incidence data are less reliable. However, the annual incidence of microalbuminuria was around 2% in the United Kingdom Prospective Diabetes Study (UKPDS), which is slightly more than that seen in type 1, and 3% per annum for clinical nephropathy in those with established microalbuminuria. Rates of ESRD are very dependent upon background ethnicity. In the UKPDS population of mainly white Europid patients, ESRD occurred in 0.6% after 10 years. Prevalence is equal in men and women. The rates are at least double for those of South Asian background.

Table 13.12 Definitions of nephropathy, based upon albuminuria

Urine specimen	Microalbuminuria	Clinical nephropathy
Overnight collection	20–199 micrograms/min	>200 micrograms/min
24h collection	30–299mg/day	≥300mg/day
Albumin concentration	20–300mg/L	>300mg/L
Albumin:creatinine ratio (ACR, Europe)	♂ 2.5–30mg/mmol ♀ 3.5–30mg/mmol	♂ >30mg/mmol ♀ >30mg/mmol
ACR (USA)	Both 30–300mg/g	>300mg/g

Table 13.13 Relative likelihood of diabetic kidney disease (DKD) by CKD stage and albuminuria

Stage	GFR (mL/min)	Diabetes		
		Normoalbuminuria	Microalbuminuria	Clinical nephropathy
1	>90	At risk for DKD	Probable DKD (T1DM) Possible DKD (T2DM)	DKD
2	60–89	At risk for DKD	Probable DKD (T1DM) Possible DKD (T2DM)	DKD
3	30–59	Probable DKD (T1DM) Possible DKD (T2DM)	DKD (T1DM) Probable DKD (T2DM)	DKD
4	15–29	Probable DKD	DKD	DKD
5	<15	Probable DKD	DKD	DKD

NB Likelihood >80% if concomitant retinopathy.

Making the diagnosis of diabetic renal disease

Timed urine collections are too cumbersome for routine clinical care, so spot samples (preferably first morning void specimens) are used, and, in order to allow for urine concentration, the albumin content is corrected for creatinine, giving an albumin:creatinine ratio or ACR. A +ve dipstick test or ACR on two or more occasions over 6 months is usually enough to confirm the diagnosis. Remember to exclude potential confounding causes of a +ve test (see Box 13.20).

An increased ACR in a person with type 1 diabetes is almost always due to diabetic kidney disease, but up to 15% of type 2 patients with microalbuminuria have atypical appearances on renal biopsy. The presence of retinopathy makes diabetic glomerulosclerosis much more likely. Nephrosclerosis and tubulointerstitial changes are the most commonly seen non-diabetic changes.

Rapidly developing nephrotic-range proteinuria, an accelerated loss of GFR (>5mL/min/year), the presence of features of other systemic disease (such as connective tissue disorders or myeloma), or accelerated hypertension should prompt investigation, as these features may suggest alternative, potentially treatable conditions. An increase in serum creatinine of >30% after initiation of ACE inhibitor therapy suggests possible renal artery stenosis.

Pathology

The earliest pathological feature in type 1 patients is kidney enlargement, mostly due to tubular hypertrophy and hyperplasia in response to glycosuria. These changes are not completely reversible with glycaemic correction in man, and their link to later nephropathy is uncertain. GFR is also increased in newly diagnosed patients (termed hyperfiltration), but this usually returns to normal with glycaemic correction.

Within 5 years of type 1 diabetes, small, but significant, increases in glomerular capillary basement membrane (GBM) thickness are seen due to an accumulation of matrix material, and recent studies have linked this to hyperfiltration. As nephropathy progresses, GBM width continues to increase, and matrix accumulation occurs in the glomerular mesangium (diffuse glomerulosclerosis). In advanced nephropathy, these accumulations can form large acellular (Kimmelstiel–Wilson) nodules (nodular glomerulosclerosis). Ultimately, the glomerular capillaries are obliterated by matrix material and become sclerosed and non-functioning. The increase in GBM width leads to increased passage of albumin into the filtrate. At the same time, there is a detachment and loss of podocytes on the epithelial side of the GBM, reducing the integrity of the filtration barrier to circulating proteins, thus leading to increasing proteinuria. These changes are also seen in type 2 diabetes, although this has been less well studied, and pathological appearances are often confounded by coexisting hypertension and ischaemia.

Tubulointerstitial changes are also seen, particularly in advanced nephropathy and in type 2 diabetes, and are due to a combination of

> **Box 13.20 Causes of a false positive test for albuminuria**
> - Vigorous exercise.
> - Urinary tract infection.
> - Presence of blood, e.g. menses.
> - Concentrated urine (less likely using ACR).
>
> *Causes of a false negative test for albuminuria*
> - Dilute urine (less likely using ACR).

nephron loss secondary to global glomerulosclerosis and direct disease, perhaps secondary to increasing proteinuria. The combination of glomerular capillary loss and tubulointerstitial disease results in a progressive loss of GFR toward ESRD.

Pathogenesis

Hyperglycaemia

Experimental studies suggest that an interaction between metabolic and haemodynamic changes secondary to hyperglycaemia are the drivers for nephropathy. Hyperglycaemia results in glycation of structural proteins (such as collagen), making them less easy to metabolize and altering their function. Increased levels of circulating and tissue advanced glycation end-products (AGEs) have been linked to microvascular and macrovascular complications.

Hyperglycaemia also induces the polyol (sorbitol) and hexosamine pathways and also results in the activation of protein kinase C which increases flux through glycolysis. In experimental studies, these changes can cause increased oxidative stress, increased thrombosis, and alterations in blood flow which can result in microvascular damage.

In human diabetes, epidemiological studies have shown that both duration and severity of hyperglycaemia are strong determinants of nephropathy risk. Moreover, cross-sectional studies have largely supported a role for these mechanisms.

Haemodynamic alterations

The raised GFR in people with newly diagnosed type 1 (and to a lesser extent type 2) diabetes has been shown in experimental studies to be due to dilatation of the afferent glomerular arteriole. This leads to an increase in glomerular capillary pressure which drives increased filtration (hyperfiltration). The increased pressure results in mechanical stress in the GBM which, in turn, is thought to stimulate matrix production and thickening via production of pro-fibrotic cytokines, such as transforming growth factor-β (TGF-β). Angiotensin II is thought to be a key mediator of these changes. Hyperfiltration has been associated with later nephropathy development in type 1 diabetes, but the link was no longer significant when corrected for hyperglycaemia. Its role in type 2 is much less certain.

Systemic hypertension is known to accelerate nephropathy development and loss of GFR, probably through similar mechanisms and mediators.

Genetic predisposition and ethnicity

Studies in families with multiple siblings with type 1 diabetes have shown concordance for nephropathy development, but it is not possible to completely exclude confounding factors. Over 20 different genetic polymorphisms have been linked to nephropathy; those linked to the ACE gene appear to be the strongest. No major gene effect has yet been identified.

Nephropathy rates are much higher in certain ethnic subgroups, notably the Pima and other Native American communities, Pacific Islanders, Australian Aborigines, and non-Ashkenazi Jews. Rates are also higher in those from Afro-Caribbean and Asian populations, compared to White Europid age- and duration-matched cohorts in the UK. The reasons are unclear but may be related to greater insulin resistance in the Asian population.

Smoking and other factors

A consistent link between cigarette smoking and nephropathy has been known for some time, but an aetiological mechanism is not yet known. Dietary protein (particularly animal) intake has also been linked to nephropathy in some epidemiological studies.

Natural history

This can be best described in terms of changes to the main clinical features of nephropathy—GFR, albuminuria, blood pressure, and cardiovascular disease.

GFR

The hyperglycaemia-driven GFR increases in early diabetes mostly resolve with glycaemic correction. Thereafter, GFR remains stable until other features of nephropathy are present, notably albuminuria and hypertension. Historically, GFR declined at a rate of 10mL/min/year once patients developed overt nephropathy, but this rate is now 2–4mL/min/year with effective blood pressure control. Rates of decline greater than this should prompt clinical review. The MDRD GFR equation (estimates GFR based on creatinine, age, sex and race) www.renal.org/egfrcalc is not very precise at GFR levels >90mL/min/1.73m^2, so it is hard to detect changes in early diabetes prior to the development of albuminuria.

Older people with type 2 diabetes may have CKD due to other non-diabetic causes, such as hypertension or renovascular disease. They often have a more benign course and stable renal function for many years.

Albuminuria

The development of albuminuria is usually the first clinical sign of nephropathy and is associated with a gradual loss of GFR. The rate of increase of albuminuria is heavily influenced by systemic blood pressure and dietary protein but is around 2% per year. Albuminuria fluctuates greatly on a daily basis as a result of glycaemic variation, diet and exercise, and antihypertensive therapy. Around 30% of patients with microalbuminuria can regress to normal; some of these will revert, but others will be normoalbuminuric for many years. It is unclear whether these patients with intermittent albuminuria will have progressive nephropathy. Once albuminuria exceeds an ACR of 10mg/mmol (~100mg/g), it is usually persistent and represents established nephropathy.

Blood pressure

Blood pressure is normal, or even low, at the onset of type 1 diabetes. It increases with albuminuria such that over 50% of patients are on anti-hypertensive therapy or have values >130/80mmHg by the time they develop persistent microalbuminuria. In contrast, over 35% of newly diag-nosed patients with type 2 diabetes in the UKPDS had a blood pressure >160/90mmHg or were on treatment. More than 80% of patients with overt nephropathy will be on antihypertensive therapy, irrespective of their type of diabetes. Thus, blood pressure increases are a concomitant factor of nephropathy in type 1 patients but may be more of a causa-tive factor in type 2 diabetes. What is certain is that high blood pressure drives nephropathy progression (increases in albuminuria and rate of loss of GFR), and its management is critical in the prevention of ESRD.

Cardiovascular disease

Patients with nephropathy have a greatly increased risk of cardiovascular disease partly because of increases in blood pressure, but also partly due to increased insulin resistance and serum lipid abnormalities. Mortality is increased at least 2-fold for patients with microalbuminuria. Recent data in people with type 1 diabetes from Finland suggest that mortality is increased only in those with increased albuminuria. The UKPDS cohort had an annual mortality of 2–4% for those with microalbuminuria, but this increased to nearly 20% in those with a serum creatinine >175micromol/L and/or renal replacement therapy (RRT). This explains why many patients fail to survive to RRT. Intensive management of modifiable cardiovascular risk factors has been shown to improve both morbidity and survival in people with type 2 diabetes and microalbuminuria, and the SHARP trial has established the effectiveness of lipid-lowering therapy in preventing cardiovascular events in patients with CKD stage 3 or worse.

Treatment for diabetic renal disease

Treatments can usefully be considered under the headings of glycaemia (and other metabolic corrections), blood pressure, cardiovascular risk factors, and diet.

Glycaemia

Both the DCCT/EDIC and the UKPDS studies confirmed that good glycaemic control can prevent the development of microalbuminuria. There are conflicting data on the role of glycaemic control in the progression of established nephropathy, although, as a rule, patients with worse control do less well and have a greater incidence of concomitant complications, such as retinopathy and neuropathy.

As GFR declines, insulin clearance by the kidneys is reduced, so doses may need adjustment. In addition, as most patients with overt nephropathy will also have a long duration of diabetes, they will be at greater risk of hypoglycaemic unawareness. These two factors make hypoglycaemia a real risk, so target HbA1c may need to be higher than for those without nephropathy.

A small study of pancreas transplantation in type 1 patients with established nephropathy and glomerulosclerosis showed that prolonged normoglycaemia for >10 years resulted in a reversal of matrix accumulation and GBM thickening. This demonstrates that the pathology may take as long to reverse as it does to develop and that nothing short of normoglycaemia may suffice for the resolution of established disease.

Blood pressure

There are no data supporting a role of antihypertensive therapies (specifically agents which block the renin–angiotensin system RAS) in the prevention of nephropathy in normoalbuminuric, normotensive people with type 1 or type 2 diabetes. Once blood pressure rises above 140/90mmHg in type 1 and 160/90mmHg in type 2, there are trial data showing that RAS-blocking agents can prevent the development of microalbuminuria and overt nephropathy. These studies have not been of a sufficient duration to demonstrate any impact on ESRD rates. Once overt nephropathy has developed, ACE inhibitors in type 1 and angiotensin II receptor blockers (ARBs) in type 2 diabetes have been shown to reduce the numbers developing ESRD, more so than other antihypertensive therapies. These drugs remain the cornerstone of treatment of blood pressure in nephropathy. Diabetes and renal guidelines suggest a target blood pressure of <130/80mmHg in patients with nephropathy.

Cardiovascular risk factors

The high rates of CV disease and the unfavourable lipid profiles seen in people with nephropathy make these attractive targets. In the Heart Protection Study (mainly type 2 patients), there was a reduction in CV events by around 25%, but few had nephropathy. Recently, the SHARP trial reported a significant reduction in risk for CV events of 17% in over 6,000 people with pre-dialysis CKD randomized to simvastatin/ezetimibe vs placebo. Lipid-lowering to a target LDL cholesterol of <2mmol/L should be undertaken in all people with diabetes and CKD. No consistent effect of lipid-lowering has been shown on the rate of loss of GFR or albuminuria.

Smoking rates are higher in those with nephropathy, compared to those without, and there are some data that cessation can help preserve renal function as well as CV risk.

Multifactorial intervention (including glycaemic control, ACE inhibitors, aspirin, lipid-lowering, smoking cessation, weight reduction, exercise, and antioxidant therapy—the Steno 2 trial) has been shown to reduce CV morbidity and mortality in 80 people with type 2 diabetes and micro-albuminuria. Thus, a broad clinical approach to management should be undertaken in all with diabetes and CKD.

Diet

High dietary protein has been shown to damage the kidney in experimental diabetes. In type 1 diabetes, protein restriction can reduce rate of loss of GFR, albuminuria, and mortality in people with established nephropathy. The data are less strong in type 2 diabetes. A dietary protein content <0.8g/kg is suggested, but patients find long-term adherence to be difficult.

As with all patients with CKD, people with diabetes may develop anaemia, hyperphosphataemia, vitamin D deficiency, and hyperkalaemia, particularly in stage 4. All of these may require expert dietary and nephrology input and should prompt referral.

When to refer to nephrology

Current CKD guidance from NICE suggests referral of all patients with CKD stage 4 or worse (GFR <30mL/min/1.73m²). All those with a rate of progression that suggests that they will develop ESRD within 2 years should be referred for preparation for RRT, as there is good evidence that survival is better with careful planning. Those with stable CKD, no significant albuminuria, and well-controlled blood pressure and glycaemia may not need referral.

Complications of CKD, such as anaemia and secondary hyperparathyroidism, or unusual features suggestive of non-diabetic CKD, such as nephrotic-range proteinuria, the presence of signs of non-diabetic systemic disease, or a rapidly declining GFR, should also prompt referral.

Survival in those requiring RRT is best for those who receive a renal transplant although remains less good than for those with non-diabetic renal disease. Simultaneous pancreas transplantation has not been shown to improve survival, although there are some data suggesting an improved quality of life in those achieving normoglycaemia. See Box 13.21.

Box 13.21 Criteria for referral for specialist review (take into account patient's wishes, serious comorbidities, and age)

- CKD stage 4 or 5 (eGFR <30mL/min/1.73m^2).
- Rapid decline of GFR (eGFR decline >5mL/min/1.73m^2/year or >10mL/min/1.73m^2/5 years).
- Microscopic or macroscopic haematuria and/or active urinary sediment.
- Signs of other systemic disease, such as SLE or systemic sclerosis.
- Blood pressure outside target despite four or more drugs at optimum titration.
- Heavy proteinuria (>1g/day or protein:creatinine ratio >100mg/ mmol or ACR >70mg/mmol).
- Family history of genetic causes of kidney disease (e.g. polycystic kidneys).
- Suspected renal artery stenosis.

For further details, see ℘ http://www.renal.org.

Further reading

Bilous R (2008). Microvascular disease: what does the UKPDS tell us about diabetic nephropathy? *Diabet Med* Suppl 2, 25–9.

Bilous R, Chaturvedi N, Sjolie AK, *et al.* (2009). Effect of candesartan on microalbuminuria and albumin excretion rate in diabetes: 3 randomised trials. *Ann Intern Med* **151**, 11–20.

DCCT/EDIC Research Group (2003). Sustained effect of intensive treatment of type 1 diabetes mellitus on development and progression of diabetic nephropathy. *JAMA* **290**, 2159–67.

De Boer I, Rue T C, Cleary PA, *et al.* (2011). Long-term outcomes of patients with type 1 diabetes mellitus and microalbuminuria. *Arch Int Med* **171**, 412–20.

Forbes JM, Coughlan MT, Cooper ME (2008). Oxidative stress as a major culprit in kidney disease in diabetes. *Diabetes* **57**, 1446–54.

Gaede P, Lund-Andersen H, Parving H-H, Pedersen O (2008). Effect of multifactorial interventions on mortality in type 2 diabetes. *N Engl J Med* **358**, 580–91.

Joint Specialty Committee on Renal Medicine of the Royal College of Physicians and the Renal Association, and the Royal College of General Practitioners (2006). Chronic Kidney Disease in Adults: UK Guidelines for identification, management and referral. London: Royal College of Physicians.

KDOQI (2007). KDOQI Clinical Practice Guidelines in Clinical Practice Recommendations for Diabetes and Chronic Kidney Disease. *Am J Kidney Dis* **49**(Suppl 2), S1–180.

Levey AS, Coresh J (2012). Chronic kidney disease. *Lancet* **379**, 165–80.

National Collaborating Centre for Chronic Conditions (2008). Clinical guidance 73. Chronic Kidney Disease. Early identification and management of chronic kidney disease in adults in primary and secondary care. Available at: ℘ http://guidance.nice.org.uk/CG73/QuickRefGuide/pdf/English.

Prigent A (2008). Monitoring renal function and limitation of renal function tests. *Semin Nucl Med* **38**, 32–46.

Diabetic neuropathy

Definition

Involvement of cranial, peripheral, and autonomic nerves may be found in patients with diabetes and termed diabetic neuropathy; this usually suggests a diffuse, predominantly sensory peripheral neuropathy. The effects on nerve function can be both acute or chronic as well as being transient or permanent. The commonest clinical consequences of neuropathy are:

- Altered sensation (both pain and ↑ sensitivity to normal sensation).
- Neuropathic ulcers, usually on the feet.
- Erectile dysfunction (with autonomic neuropathy).
- Charcot arthropathy.

See Box 13.22 for classification.

Pathology

Diabetic neuropathy is one of the microvascular complications of diabetes. Pathologically, distal axonal loss occurs with focal demyelination and attempts at nerve regeneration. The vasa nervorum often shows basement membrane thickening, endothelial cell changes, and some occlusion of its lumen. This results in slowing of nerve conduction velocities or a complete loss of nerve function. Both metabolic and vascular changes have been implicated in its aetiology.

Pathogenesis

Hyperglycaemia is probably the major underlying cause of the histological and functional changes, although vascular risk factors, such as hypertension and hyperlipidaemia, may also have a role. Several possible mechanisms have been suggested:

- Overloading of the normal pathways for glucose metabolism, resulting in ↑ use of the polyol pathway which leads to ↑ levels of sorbitol and fructose and ↓ levels of myoinositol and glutathione. This may result in more free radical damage and also lowers nitric oxide levels, thus altering nerve blood flow. Experimental models, using aldose reductase inhibitors which can improve aspects of diabetic neuropathy, support this theory.
- Accumulation of AGE (via non-enzymatic glycation) may contribute.
- In the more acute neuropathies, acute ischaemia of the nerves due to vascular abnormalities has been suggested as the cause. The underlying reason for this is still unclear. Insulin-induced 'neuritis' may occur when insulin therapy is started and blood glucose levels fall.
- Other potential aetiological factors include changes in local growth factor production and oxidative stress.

Further work is needed to clarify the exact role of each of the above mechanisms. In the meantime, studies showing improvements in neuropathy associated with good diabetic control strengthen the argument for the role of hyperglycaemia and offer us a treatment option.

Box 13.22 Classification of diabetic neuropathies

- Sensory neuropathy:
  - Acute.
  - Chronic.
- Autonomic neuropathy:
  - Erectile dysfunction.
  - Gastroparesis.
  - Postural hypotension.
- Mononeuropathy:
  - Entrapment neuropathy.
  - External pressure palsies.
  - Spontaneous mononeuropathy.
- Proximal motor neuropathy (diabetic amyotrophy).

Peripheral sensorimotor neuropathy

(See Box 13.23.)

Although hyperglycaemia can alter nerve function and often gives some sensory symptoms at diagnosis, correcting the hyperglycaemia can often resolve these. Chronic sensorimotor neuropathy is the most common feature of peripheral nerve involvement seen in patients with diabetes. The exact prevalence of diabetic neuropathy varies in most studies because of the different definitions and examination techniques used. For example, sensitive nerve conduction studies can show up to 80% of patients have abnormal results. In more normal practice, however, around 30% of patients have either symptomatic neuropathy or abnormalities on examination which are clinically significant. But at least 50% of these patients are asymptomatic. Prevalence increases with increasing duration of diabetes, so although 7–8% of type 2 patients have abnormalities at diagnosis, 50% can be expected to have them 25 years later.

Box 13.23 Features of peripheral sensorimotor neuropathy

- Usually insidious onset with numbness or paraesthesiae, often found on screening rather than as a presenting problem.
- Starts in the toes and on the soles of the feet, then spreads up to midshin level in a symmetrical fashion. Less often, in more severe cases, it also involves the fingers and hands.
- Affects all sensory modalities and results in reduced vibration perception thresholds, pinprick, fine touch, and temperature sensations.
- ↓ vibration sensation and absent ankle reflexes are often the first features found. Another risk factor for ulceration is the inability to feel a 10g monofilament.
- Less often, the skin is tender/sensitive to touch (allodynia) or frank pain can occur.
- Painful neuropathy affects up to 20% of a general clinic population. This pain may be sharp, stabbing, or burning in nature and at times very severe. This is also associated with sleep disturbance, mood disorders, and loss of quality of life.
- There may also be some wasting of the intrinsic muscles of the foot with clawing of the toes.

Mononeuropathies

Peripheral mononeuropathies and cranial mononeuropathies are not uncommon. These may be spontaneous or may be due to entrapment or external pressure. Of the peripheral mononeuropathies, median nerve involvement and carpal tunnel syndrome may be found in up to 10% of patients and require nerve conduction studies and then surgical decompression. Entrapment of the lateral cutaneous nerve of the thigh is also seen more commonly in those with diabetes, giving pain over the lateral aspect of the thigh. Common peroneal nerve involvement, causing foot drop and tarsal tunnel syndrome, is also recognized but less common.

Cranial mononeuropathies usually occur suddenly and have a good prognosis. Palsies of cranial nerves III and VI are most commonly seen (but still infrequent). In the IIIrd nerve palsy, sparing of the pupillary responses is usual. Spontaneous recovery is slow over several months, and no treatment, apart from symptomatic help such as an eye patch, is needed. Unlike entrapment neuropathies where decompression may help, no effective treatment is currently available in most cases of spontaneous mononeuropathy.

Proximal motor neuropathy (diabetic amyotrophy)

This is an uncommon, but disturbing, condition to have, mostly affecting ♂ in their 50s with type 2 diabetes. It presents with severe pain and paraesthesiae in the upper legs and is felt as a deep aching pain which may be burning in nature and can keep patients awake at night and cause anorexia, resulting in marked cachexia. This, with proximal muscle weakness and wasting of the quadriceps, in particular, can be very debilitating. The lumbar sacral plexus lower motor neurons are affected, and improvement is usually spontaneous over 3–4 months. Before making this diagnosis, however, consider other causes, such as malignancies and lumbar disc disease. An MRI scan of the lumbar sacral spine is advisable.

Oral antidiabetic agents may play a part in the aetiology of this problem, and conversion to insulin therapy is advised, although the anorexia experienced when the pain is severe can make this difficult. Although recovery happens over many months, only 50% recover fully, but no other treatment is currently known to improve on this.

Foot examination for diabetic neuropathy

- Mandatory at diagnosis and at least yearly in all asymptomatic patients.
- Test vibration, fine touch (with a 10g monofilament), and reflexes as a minimum. Using a neurothesiometer or biosthesiometer gives a more quantitative measure of vibration than a 128Hz tuning fork. Inability to feel the vibrating head at >25V in the toes is associated with a significant risk of neuropathic ulceration and should be considered a sign of 'at-risk' feet.

Differential diagnoses of peripheral neuropathy

- Uraemia.
- Vitamin B12 deficiency.
- Infections (e.g. HIV and leprosy).
- Toxins (e.g. alcohol, lead, mercury).
- Drugs (chemotherapeutic agents).
- Malignancy.

Treatment

(See Box 13.24.)

For all patients

Review by a podiatrist and, if indicated, an orthotist to give education on foot care and suitable footwear. If followed by regular podiatry review, this can help to prevent some problems developing.

Asymptomatic patients

Apart from good glycaemic control, no drugs are yet available.

Painful diabetic neuropathy (painful DN)

Pharmacological treatment of painful DN is not entirely satisfactory, as currently available drugs are often ineffective and complicated by side effects.

- Tricyclic compounds (TCAs) have been used as first-line agents for many years, but many patients fail to respond to them and side effects are frequent. Amitriptyline or imipramine 10mg taken at night may be started. Depending on side effects, the dose can be gradually increased up to 75mg/day.
- Duloxetine, a selective serotonin noradrenaline reuptake inhibitor (SNRI), is a first-line treatment for painful DN. It relieves pain by increasing synaptic availability of 5-HT and noradrenaline in the descending pathways that inhibit pain impulses. Duloxetine for painful DN has been investigated in three identical trials, and pooled data from these shows that 60–120mg/day doses are effective in relieving symptoms, starting within a week and lasting the full treatment period of 12 weeks. The main side effect is nausea, but this is often self-limiting. It is advisable to start at 30mg/day taken with food for a few days.
- The anticonvulsant gabapentin, gradually titrated from 100mg bd to 1,800mg/day, is also effective. Doses up to 3,600mg/day can be used.

Box 13.24 Pharmacological treatment of painful DN

Only two (duloxetine and pregabalin) have been formally approved by the EMA and FDA for the treatment of painful DN.

- Tricyclic antidepressants (TCAs):
  - Amitriptyline 25–75mg/day.
  - Imipramine 25–75mg/day.
- Serotonin noradrenaline reuptake inhibitors (SNRIs):
  - Duloxetine 60–120mg/day.
- Anticonvulsants:
  - Gabapentin 300–3,600mg/day.
  - Pregabalin 300–600mg/day.
- Opiates:
  - Tramadol 200–400mg/day.
  - Oxycodone 20–80mg/day.
  - Morphine sulphate SR 20–80mg/day.
- Capsaicin cream (0.075%)—applied sparingly 3–4 times per day.
- IV lidocaine (for refractory painful neuropathy)—5mg/kg, given IV over 1h with ECG monitoring.

- Pregabalin has been shown in seven clinical trials to be effective in the management of painful DN. Starting dose is 75mg bd, increased to a 150mg bd maintainance dose, with a maximum dose of 600mg/day.
- Other drugs include other anticonvulsants, in particular carbamazepine, opiates, such as tramadol and oxycodone, and, for refractory cases, intravenous lidocaine. The antioxidant alpha-lipoic acid is also an effective treatment and is widely used in Germany, Eastern Europe, and China. Topical capsaicin, a substance P depleter, is also used; local discomfort at the site of application initially means many patients do not persevere with treatment to see a favourable outcome.

Despite these treatments, however, many sufferers have suboptimal pain relief. Non-pharmacological treatments, such as acupuncture, TENS, and, for severe resistant cases, electrical spinal cord stimulation, may be used. A recent consensus panel evaluated all published clinical trial data and recommended that first-line therapies for painful DN to be a TCA, the SNRI duloxetine or the anticonvulsants pregabalin or gabapentin, taking into account patient comorbidities and cost.

General treatments

Specific treatments for each form of neuropathy have already been discussed, but there is some evidence for more general therapies.

- Poor diabetic control appears to be associated with worsening neuropathy, and improving glycaemic control is advocated in any patient, especially if neuropathy is present.
- Cardiovascular risk factors, such as hypertension, smoking, obesity, and hyperlipidaemia (especially hypertryglyceridaemia), are risk factors for peripheral neuropathy. Clinical trials are now required to test whether CV risk reduction improves neuropathy outcomes.

Autonomic neuropathy

The commonest effect of autonomic neuropathy is erectile dysfunction which affects 40% of ♂ with diabetes (although this is multifactorial). The recent interest in *sildenafil* has highlighted this. Only a small number develop severe GI, cardiac, or bladder dysfunction. Abnormal autonomic function tests can be expected in 20–40% of a general diabetic clinic population. The ↑ problems during surgery from cardiac involvement should be remembered.

Clinical features

• Erectile dysfunction.
• Postural hypotension—giving dizziness and syncope in up to 12%.
• Resting tachycardia or fixed heart rate/loss of sinus arrhythmia—in up to 20%.
• Gustatory sweating—sweating after tasting food.
• Delayed gastric emptying, nausea/vomiting, abdominal fullness.
• Constipation/diarrhoea.
• Urinary retention/overflow incontinence.
• Anhidrosis—absent sweating on the feet is especially problematic, as it increases the risk of ulceration.
• Abnormal pupillary reflexes.

Assessment

If AN is suspected, check:
• Lying and standing BP (measure systolic BP after 2min standing; normal is <10mmHg drop; >30mmHg is abnormal).
• Pupillary responses to light.

Other less commonly performed tests to consider if the diagnosis is uncertain or in high-risk patients include:
• *Loss of sinus arrhythmia.* Measure inspiratory and expiratory heart rates after 5s of each (<10 beats/min difference is abnormal; >15 is normal).
• *Loss of heart rate response to Valsalva manoeuvre.* Look at the ratio of the shortest R–R interval during forced expiration against a closed glottis, compared to the longest R–R interval after it (<1.2 is abnormal).
• *BP response to sustained hand grip.* Diastolic BP prior to the test is compared to diastolic BP after 5min of sustaining a grip equivalent to 30% of maximal grip. A diastolic BP rise >16mmHg is normal; <10mmHg is abnormal. A rolled-up BP cuff to achieve the required hand grip may be used.
• For gastroparesis, consider a radioisotope test meal to look for delayed gastric emptying. Blood glucose should be <10mmol/L, as hyperglycaemia exacerbates delayed gastric emptying.

Treatment

This is based on the specific symptom and is usually symptomatic only.

In all patients, improvement in diabetic control is advocated in case any of it is reversible, but this is not usually very helpful or effective.

Postural hypotension

Stopping drugs that may result in, or exacerbate, postural hypotension, including diuretics, β-blockers, anti-anginal agents, tricyclic agents, etc.

- Advising patients to get up from the sitting or lying position slowly and crossing the legs.
- Increasing sodium intake up to 10g (185mmol) per day and fluid intake to 2.0–2.5L per day (caution in elderly patients with heart failure).
- Raising the head of the bed by 10–20°, as this stimulates the renin–angiotensin–aldosterone system and results in a decrease in the nocturnal diuresis.
- Drinking approximately 500mL of water, which stimulates a significant pressor response and improves symptoms of postural hypotension.
- Using custom-fitted elastic stockings extending to the waist.
- Pharmacological treatment with fludrocortisone, starting at 100 micrograms per day, whilst carefully monitoring for supine hypertension, ankle oedema, and hypokalaemia. Potassium supplementation may be required when higher doses are used, and it is important to monitor urea and electrolytes.
- In severe cases, the following drugs: alpha-1 adrenal receptor agonist midodrine (2.5–10.0mg tds), sympathomimetic ephedrine (25mg tds), and occasionally octreotide and erythropoietin (25–75U per kg three times a week until a haematocrit level approaching normal is achieved), may be tried.

Erectile dysfunction

Libido is not normally affected and pain is also unusual, so look for hypogonadism and Peyronie's if they are present. Autonomic neuropathy is the likely cause, but many drugs, especially thiazides and β-blockers, can also cause it, as can alcohol, tobacco, cannabis, and stress. These should be assessed by direct questioning. Examination should include:

- Genitalia and 2° sexual characteristics.
- Peripheral pulses—as vascular insufficiency may play a part.
- Lower limb reflexes and vibration thresholds—to confirm that neuropathy is present.

Biochemical screening should at least include:

- Prolactin.
- Testosterone.
- Gonadotrophins (LH/FSH).

Exacerbating factors, such as alcohol and antihypertensive drugs, should be modified. The main therapies are:

- Oral therapies include: sildenafil (start at 25–50mg, ↑ to 100mg if needed, and taken 1h prior to sexual intercourse), vardenafil (start at 10mg, ↑ to 20mg if needed, and taken 25–60min prior to sexual intercourse), tadalafil (start at 10mg, ↑ to 20mg if needed, and taken 30min to 12h prior to sexual intercourse).
- Intraurethral *alprostadil* (start at 125 micrograms, ↑ to 250 or 500 micrograms if needed).
- Intracavernosal *alprostadil* (trial dose is 2.5 micrograms; treatment is 5–40 micrograms).
- Vacuum devices.

None of these is ideal. Sildenafil, although an oral therapy, is effective in only 60% of those with diabetes and is contraindicated with severe heart disease and those on nitrates, which rules many out.

Gastroparesis

Management of diabetic gastroparesis includes:

- Optimization of glycaemic control, as hyperglycaemia can delay gastric emptying. Insulin pump therapy is commonly used.
- Stopping drugs that can delay gastric emptying, such as calcium channel blockers, GLP-1 analogues, and anticholinergic agents, such as antidepressants, etc.
- Antiemetics (metoclopramide and domperidone).
- Erythromycin which may enhance activity of the gut peptide motilin.
- Gastric electrical stimulation ('pacing') is a treatment option in patients with drug-refractory gastroparesis and can increase the quality of life and decrease hospital admissions by alleviating nausea and vomiting.

Severe gastroparesis, causing recurrent vomiting, is associated with dehydration, swings in blood sugar, and weight loss and is, therefore, an indication for hospital admission. The patient should be adequately hydrated with intravenous fluids, and blood sugar should be stabilized by intravenous insulin; antiemetics could be given intravenously, and if the course of the gastroparesis is prolonged, total parenteral nutrition or feeding through a gastrostomy tube may be required.

Autonomic diarrhoea

The patient may present with diarrhoea which tends to be worse at night, or alternatively some may present with constipation. Both the diarrhoea and constipation respond to conventional treatment.

- Diarrhoea associated with bacterial overgrowth may respond to treatment with a broad-spectrum antibiotic, such as erythromycin 250mg qds for 7 days or tetracycline 250mg bd for 7 days.
- Bile acid malabsorption may be treated with colestyramine.
- The antidiarrhoeal synthetic opioids (e.g. loperamide 2mg qds) and codeine phosphate (30mg qds) can improve symptoms by decreasing peristalsis and increasing rectal sphincter tone.
- Refractory diarrhoea may be treated with the α2-adrenergic receptor agonist clonidine and the somatostatin analogue octreotide. Octreotide suppresses gastrointestinal motility and inhibits the release of motilin, serotonin, and gastrin but may result in recurrent hypoglycaemia due to impaired counter-regulation.

Neuropathic bladder

- Bladder dysfunction is a rare complication of autonomic neuropathy, involving the sacral nerves. The patient presents with hesitancy of micturition, increased frequency of micturition, and, in serious cases, with urinary retention associated with overflow incontinence.
- Patients are prone to urinary tract infections. Ultrasound scan of the urinary tract, intravenous urography, and urodynamic studies may be required.

- Treatment manoeuvres include mechanical methods of bladder emptying by applying suprapubic pressure or the use of intermittent self-catheterization.
- Anti-cholinesterase drugs, such as neostigmine or pyridostigmine, may be useful.
- Long-term indwelling catheterization may be required in some, but this unfortunately predisposes the patient to urinary tract infections and long-term antibiotic prophylaxis may be required.

Anhidrosis

Dry feet can cause cracks in the skin and act as a site for infection. Emollient creams may help prevent this.

Gustatory sweating

Increased sweating, usually affecting the face and often brought about by eating (gustatory sweating), can be very embarrassing to patients and difficult to treat.

- Oral anticholinergic agents, including oxybutynin, propantheline, and glycopyrronium bromide, may improve symptoms; however, adverse reactions, including dry mouth, constipation, potential worsening of gastroparesis, and confusion, limit their use.
- Clonidine has been used with some success but is also limited by side effects, including hypotension and dry mouth.
- Systemic side effects have led to the investigation of non-systemic approaches. Topical glycopyrronium bromide, a quaternary ammonium antimuscarinic compound, has been shown to significantly decrease the incidence, severity, and frequency of sweating with eating and is tolerated well.
- Botulinum toxin has been used for gustatory sweating, though, in most literature, it is limited to use in unilateral, surgically related cases.

Further reading

Tesfaye S, Boulton AJ (eds) (2009). *Diabetic neuropathy*. Oxford: Oxford University Press.

Tesfaye S, *et al.* on behalf of the Toronto Expert Panel on Diabetic Neuropathy (2011). Painful Diabetic Peripheral Neuropathy: Consensus Recommendations on Diagnosis, Assessment and Management. *Diabetes Metab Res Rev* [Epub ahead of print].

Vinik AI, Ziegler D (2007). Diabetic cardiovascular autonomic neuropathy. *Circulation* **115**, 387–97.

The diabetic foot

Diabetic foot problems are a leading cause of morbidity. Box 13.25 illustrates the burden of diabetic foot ulceration in the UK.

See Box 13.26 for clinical features and Box 13.27 for Wagner's classification of diabetic foot lesions.

Risk factors for foot ulcer development

Several factors predispose to ulcer formation, and awareness of these should highlight 'at-risk' patients for education and other preventive strategies. Ulcers can occur anywhere on the foot, but the tips of claw/hammer toes and over the metatarsal heads are the most frequent sites. Risk factors include:

- *Peripheral neuropathy* (seen in up to 80% of diabetic patients with foot ulcers) reduces awareness of pain and trauma caused by footwear and foreign bodies in shoes. Look for reduced sensation on 10g monofilament and reduced vibration perception thresholds (e.g. reduced sensation to a 128Hz tuning fork for <10s or >25V with a biothesiometer).
- *Autonomic neuropathy*, leading to anhidrosis, can dry out the skin and cause it to crack, so allowing a portal of entry for infection. These feet are often warm and dry, with distended veins.
- *Motor neuropathy* can result in altered foot muscle tone, wasting of small muscles, raising of the medial longitudinal arch, and clawing of the toes. This puts more pressure through the metatarsal heads and heels, predisposing to callus and ulcer formation. Electrophysiology can help examine this but is not in widespread routine use.
- *Peripheral vascular disease* (seen in up to 10% of patients) and *microvascular circulatory disease* lead to local ischaemia, ↑ the potential for ulcer formation and delaying wound healing. Always examine peripheral pulses, and consider Doppler studies if abnormal. An ankle:brachial artery ratio of >1.1 suggests arterial disease (the ratio of the BP in the ankle and the arm measured while at rest).
- *Duration of diabetes* is an independent risk factor, as is ↑ age. Remember type 2 diabetes may be present and undiagnosed for some time.
- The presence of *other microvascular complications*, such as nephropathy and retinopathy, is also a risk factor for foot ulcer development.
- *Previous ulceration* is an important risk factor, and anyone with previous problems needs very careful monitoring/follow-up.
- *Lack of diabetes monitoring* and lack of previous examinations of the feet are also recognized risk factors.
- *Mechanical, chemical, or thermal trauma/injury* is often the predisposing factor, and any profession or pastime that increases the risk of these is a risk factor.

Box 13.25 Epidemiology of foot ulceration in the UK

Prevalence of foot ulceration	5–10%
Number of people with diabetes with foot ulcers	61,000
Proportion of people with diabetes undergoing lower limb amputation each year	0.2%
Number of people with diabetes undergoing lower limb amputation per year	6,000
Annual NHS expenditure on diabetes foot-related care	~£650 million

Box 13.26 Clinical features of diabetic feet

Neuropathic feet	Ischaemic feet
• Warm.	• Cold/cool.
• Dry skin.	• Atrophic/often hairless.
• Palpable foot pulses.	• No palpable foot pulses
• No discomfort with ulcer.	• More often tender/painful.
• Callus present.	• Claudication/rest pain.
	• Skin blanches on elevation and reddens on dependency.

Box 13.27 Wagner's classification of diabetic foot lesions

- Grade 0—high-risk foot, no ulcer present.
- Grade 1—superficial ulcer, not infected.
- Grade 2—deep ulcer, with or without cellulitis, but no abscess or bone involvement.
- Grade 3—deep ulcer with bone involvement or abscess formation.
- Grade 4—localized gangrene (toe, forefoot, heel).
- Grade 5—gangrene of the whole foot.

Treatment of the diabetic foot

This is a multidisciplinary problem, requiring collaboration between diabetologists, diabetes nurse specialists, podiatrists, orthotists, vascular surgeons, plastic surgeons, and orthopaedic surgeons. Treatment is aimed at several distinct areas, namely:

- At-risk feet with no current ulceration.
- Treating existing ulcers.
- Treating infected ulcers.
- Treating osteomyelitis.
- Treating vascular insufficiency.

The typical clinical features of diabetic feet are listed in Box 13.26.

At-risk feet with no current ulceration

When at-risk feet are identified in any patient with diabetes, standard advice should be given, and this will need to be repeated/reinforced regularly. This advice would usually include:

- General advice on nail care, hygiene, and care with footwear—often best from the podiatrist.
- Reinforce the need for regular daily examination of the feet by the patient or carer.
- Consider regular podiatry review as well as self-monitoring. Also reinforce the need for urgent review if the patient discovers problems.
- Consider the need for modification of footwear or special footwear if there are abnormalities with foot posture or problems with pressure loading on certain parts of the foot. Padded socks can also reduce trauma. Advise the patient to examine shoes before putting them on, wear lace-ups or shoes with lots of room for the toes, and avoid ill-fitting fashion shoes. In some people, protective toecaps can be useful.
- Avoid walking barefoot.

At the moment, no other therapy is advocated in this group of patients, but, as discussed in the neuropathy section, good diabetic control is important and other agents may be useful in the future, such as aldose reductase inhibitors, inhibitors of non-enzymatic glycation, and various growth factors.

Existing ulcers

All ulcers should be considered deep/involving bone until proved otherwise.
Box 13.27 shows one classification of diabetic foot lesions.

Management

- Optimize diabetic control.
- Reduction of oedema is important to aid healing.
- Regular debridement of callus and dead tissue/skin is important for both neuropathic and ischaemic ulcers. Debridement is usually best with a scalpel and forceps, although chemical agents can occasionally help. But, as these agents can also damage healthy tissue, use under careful supervision. More recently, the use of sterile maggots has

been shown to be effective. After debridement, apply dressings, but change these regularly. Be careful that dressings do not impair a poor circulation or cause further skin trauma or pressure effects.

- *Infection control.* Infection may be localized, but any evidence of deeper infection or sinus formation raises the possibility of osteomyelitis. Systemic symptoms of an infection may be minimal as may pain/tenderness in the foot itself, so be suspicious of more severe infection than you can see. The organisms may be ordinary skin commensals given a port of entry, but send swabs for culture and think of *Staphylococcus aureus* or streptococci as likely organisms.
  - If a sinus is present, probe it, and, if down to bone, assume there is osteomyelitis. Culture anything you get out. Plain radiographs may show bone erosion or destruction with osteomyelitis; radioisotope scans using technetium can show ↑ uptake in both infection and Charcot arthropathy. The use of MRI scanning can be useful to differentiate in this situation.
  - If infection is present, use antibiotics according to local microbiology guidelines and culture results. Commonly: 'triple therapy' with *flucloxacillin* (500mg qds), *ampicillin/amoxicillin* (500mg tds), and *metronidazole* (200mg tds); or co-amoxiclav (*amoxicillin/clavulanic acid*, 250/125mg tds) or *ciprofloxacin* (500–750mg bd) and *clindamycin* (300–450mg bd). IV treatment initially if the infection is severe, and, for the deeper infections, several months of therapy may be needed. For osteomyelitis, again follow local guidelines, but agents, such as *ciprofloxacin* or *sodium fusidate* which have better bone penetration, can be used, again for several months. Linezolid is also a useful therapy as a second- or third-line agent, but care with hepatic and renal impairment, and the need to monitor for potential thrombocytopenia, anaemia, or pancytopenia may limit its use.
  - In some patients, this approach fails to control osteomyelitis adequately, and resection/amputation is required, so regular surgical liaison is imperative.
- *Reducing trauma* and *pressure relief* in neuropathic ulcers. Padded socks can reduce shear stress and trauma. Suitable shoes and insoles can help to relieve pressure to allow healing to occur as long as unnecessary walking is minimized. If this is not enough, a pneumatic boot/Aircast boot or a total contact cast may be needed. These allow the patient to be mobile but take the weight away from the ulcerated area or foot and put through to the calf instead. The involvement of both podiatrists and orthotists is essential.
- *Revascularization.* Always consider coexistent vascular disease. Vascular bypass grafting/reconstruction or angioplasty can give excellent results, with a 70–95% limb salvage rate often quoted. The improved blood supply will also help healing of existing ulcers and may negate the need for amputation or allow the area requiring resection to be minimized. If vascular intervention is unsuccessful or not possible, then amputation is required, preferably as a below-knee procedure to give a better mobilization potential post-operatively.

The Charcot foot

Epidemiology

This is a relatively rare complication of diabetes: an average district general hospital clinic will have 3–10 patients with this problem.

Pathogenesis

It is suggested that blood flow increases due to sympathetic nerve loss. This causes osteoclast activity and bone turnover to increase, so making the bones of the foot more susceptible to damage. Even minor trauma can, therefore, result in destructive changes in this susceptible bone.

Clinical features

The most likely site is the tarsal–metatarsal region or the metatar-sophalangeal joints. Initially, it gives a warm/hot, swollen, and often uncomfortable foot, which may be indistinguishable from cellulitis and gout. Peripheral pulses are invariably present, and peripheral neuropathy is evident clinically.

Plain radiographs will be normal initially and later show fractures with osteolysis and joint reorganization with subluxation of the metatar-sophalangeal joints and dislocation of the large joints of the foot. Isotope scans with technetium are abnormal from early on, but differentiation from infective or other inflammatory causes can be difficult. MRI scanning may prove more useful for this in the future, as may [111]indium-labelled white cell studies if infection is suspected.

Eventually, in the untreated patient, two classic deformities are seen:
• A 'rocker bottom' deformity due to displacement and subluxation of the tarsus downwards.
• Medial convexity due to displacement of the talonavicular joint or tarsometatarsal dislocation.

Management

If diagnosed early, immobilization may help to prevent joint destruction. Exactly how best to do this is not agreed, but using a non-walking plaster cast or an Aircast type of boot is needed for at least 2–3 months while bone repair/remodelling is going on. Some advocate immobilization for anything up to a year.

The use of bisphosphonates does not seem to alter outcomes.

Further reading

National Institute for Health and Clinical Excellence (2004). Type 2 diabetes—footcare. Available at: ◌ http://www.nice.org.uk/CG10.
National Institute for Health and Clinical Excellence (2011). Diabetic foot problems—inpatient management. Available at: ◌ http://www.nice.org.uk/guidance/CG119.
Rogers LC, et al. (2011). The Charcot foot in diabetes. *Diabetes Care* **34**, 2123–9.

Macrovascular disease

People with diabetes have a significantly greater risk of macrovascular complications (coronary heart disease, cerebrovascular disease, and peripheral vascular disease) than the non-diabetic population. Around three-quarters of people with diabetes will die as a result of macrovascular disease, and a diagnosis of type 2 diabetes equates to a cardiovascular risk equivalent of ageing 10–15 years.

Epidemiology

The exact prevalence and incidence of macrovascular disease and its outcomes will vary, depending on the age, gender, and ethnic mix of the patients being assessed. The previous belief that cardiovascular disease is less common in type 1 diabetes has been proven wrong, and, in general, vascular complications account for around three-quarters of deaths in both type 1 and type 2 diabetes. Although the atheroma seen is histologically the same as in a non-diabetic population, it tends to be more diffuse and progresses more rapidly. It also occurs at an earlier age, and women with diabetes lose the cardiovascular protection seen in the non-diabetic population.

- Overall, peripheral vascular disease occurs in up to 10% of patients, and they have up to 15-fold greater risk of needing a non-traumatic amputation than the non-diabetic population.
- Thromboembolic cerebrovascular events increase in individuals with diabetes, compared to the non-diabetic population.
- The risk of having a myocardial infarction is also increased 2–4 times in individuals with diabetes.

Secondary prevention

- Stop smoking.
- Strict control of blood pressure.
- Lipid-lowering drugs.
- Early control of blood glucose.
- Aspirin: this is *no longer* recommended for primary cardiovascular protection in subjects with diabetes.

Pathogenesis

The risk factors for atherosclerosis, such as smoking and family history, still apply in a diabetic population. Some factors, however, are more common in those with diabetes and may also confer a greater risk to the diabetic population. These include:

- *Glycaemic control*. Short-term studies, such as ACCORD, VADT, and ADVANCE, investigating the effects of tight glycaemic control on the development of macrovascular disease have been disappointing. These showed that optimizing glucose control has no value in preventing vascular ischaemic events. However, longer-term studies, such as DCCT-EDIC in type 1 diabetes and UKPDS in type 2 diabetes, have clearly demonstrated that early glycaemic control is key for the prevention of cardiovascular disease later in life. However, strict glycaemic control should not occur at the expense of increased hypoglycaemia, which can be life-threatening.

- *Hypertension.* More common in both type 1 and type 2 patients and results in vascular endothelial injury, so predisposing to atheroma formation. The UKPDS suggests BP control is a more important individual risk factor for CVD than glycaemic control. Therefore, there are strict criteria to control BP in patients with diabetes, particularly in the presence of microvascular complications.
- *Hyperlipidaemia.* Common, e.g. hyperinsulinaemia in insulin-resistant type 2 patients causes reduced HDL cholesterol, elevated triglycerides (and VLDL), and smaller denser, and therefore, more atherogenic LDL cholesterol. Results from the FIELD study, investigating the effects of lowering triglyceride levels with fibrate treatment in diabetes, failed to show a beneficial effect on vascular complications, which may have been partially related to study design. On the other hand, the use of statins in diabetes has been shown to reduce cardiovascular events in a number of studies, and this is now routine practice for both primary and secondary cardiovascular protection in diabetes.
- *Obesity.* An independent risk factor, more common in type 2 patients. Central obesity, in particular, is more atherogenic.
- *Insulin resistance* or elevated circulating insulin/proinsulin-like molecule levels are known to increase the risk of atherosclerosis in both diabetic and non-diabetic populations. This may be linked to impaired endothelial function.
- *Altered coagulability.* Circulating fibrinogen, plasminogen activator inhibitor (PAI)-1, and von Willebrand factor levels are altered in diabetes, whereas platelet activity is enhanced. Antiplatelet agents, mainly aspirin, were previously recommended for primary cardiovascular protection, but recent evidence (e.g. POPADAD study) does not support such practice. ASCEND, running till 2017, is a large study that will address the role of asprin in primary prevention in diabetes further. However, aspirin continues to be used for secondary cardiovascular protection in diabetes. No specific treatment exists at present to address changes in level/activity of coagulation factors.

The UKPDS has shown the major risk factors for coronary heart disease in type 2 patients to be elevated LDL cholesterol, decreased HDL cholesterol, hypertension, hyperglycaemia, and smoking.

See Box 13.28 for the management of myocardial infarction in those with diabetes.

Box 13.28 Management of acute myocardial infarction

Patients with diabetes are more likely to have a myocardial infarction and more likely to die from it than the non-diabetic population. This may be due to a greater likelihood of myocardial pump failure. Several studies highlight this (see Table 13.14).

Up to 20–40% of patients admitted to hospital with a myocardial infarction will have hyperglycaemia, many of whom will not have been previously diagnosed with diabetes.

As in the non-diabetic population, streptokinase, aspirin, and acute angioplasty have proven benefits. The previous contraindication for thrombolysis in those with proliferative diabetic retinopathy has been questioned by many, although this is less an issue these days as primary angioplasty is used, rather than thrombolytic therapy, in most centres. Tight glycaemic control (blood glucose 7–10mmol/L) using IV glucose and insulin for at least 24h followed by SC insulin, as used in the DIGAMI study, also has benefits. In this study, patients with an admission blood glucose >11.0mmol/L who were treated with this regimen had a 7.5% absolute risk reduction in mortality at 1 year and an 11% risk reduction at 3.5 years, compared to the control group (i.e. 33% mortality with treatment vs 44% in controls at 3.5 years). This equates to one life saved for every nine treated with this regimen. The exact reason for this is unclear. However, DIGAMI 2 study failed to show a benefit for insulin therapy post-MI, but the various groups had similar glycaemic control, making results interpretation from this trial problematic.

- It is suggested that all patients with a blood glucose >11mmol/L benefit from glucose-lowering therapy, whether previously known to have diabetes or not. Using an admission HbA1c to detect those with undiagnosed or stress-related hyperglycaemia can be useful but should not result in withholding the acute treatment of this hyperglycaemia in such patients. It may, however, help to identify those who may be troubled by hypoglycaemia and may not, therefore, be suitable for SC insulin or sulfonylureas in the intermediate or long term.
- Using ACEIs early after myocardial infarction gives a 0.5% absolute risk reduction in 30-day mortality and a 4–8% risk reduction over 15–50 months in a general population. Analysis of the diabetic subgroup in the GISSI-3 study showed a 30% relative risk reduction in 6-week mortality for the diabetic subgroup (8.7% vs 12.4%), compared to a 5% reduction for non-diabetics. In view of the greater proportion of diabetics with poor left ventricular function after myocardial infarction compared to the non-diabetic population, this difference is very important.

Table 13.14 Studies of patients with myocardial infarction

Trial and outcome examined	Non-diabetic subgroup (%)	Diabetic subgroup (%)
ISSI-2: non-streptokinase 4-year mortality	27	41
GUSTO: in-hospital mortality	6.2	10.6
GISSI-2: re-infarction rates	14	30

Lipid abnormalities found in patients with diabetes

Hyperlipidaemia in a patient with diabetes, at any level of cholesterol, is associated with a greater risk of macrovascular disease than in a non-diabetic individual. Patients with diabetes may have altered activity of insulin-dependent enzymes, such as lipoprotein lipase, which results in delayed systemic clearance of certain lipids. This, combined with altered hepatic production of apoprotein B-containing lipoproteins, gives a more atherogenic profile.

Usual findings are of increased triglyceride-containing lipoproteins, chylomicrons, and VLDL. Although more common in the insulin-resistant type 2 patients, this can also be seen in type 1 patients, particularly in those with poor glycaemic control. Another abnormality is low HDL cholesterol (HDL2 especially), commonly seen in type 2 diabetes patients and individuals with insulin resistance. Other atherogenic changes include a tendency to develop small dense LDL cholesterol particles and a greater tendency to oxidative damage which renders them even more atherogenic. Lipoprotein a (Lpa) levels, which are thought to contribute to the atherothrombotic process, are also often raised.

Other causes of lipid abnormalities should be kept in mind when assessing individuals with diabetes, such as familial hypercholesterolaemia or familial combined hyperlipidaemia (🕮 see Chapter 14, p. 828). Screening for secondary causes of hyperlipidaemia, such as hypothyroidism, obstructive liver disease, nephrotic syndrome, and alcohol abuse, should also be performed.

Evidence from trials

The diabetic subgroups from the major lipid-lowering trials (see Table 13.15), such as the 4S study (Scandinavian Simvastatin Survival Study), CARE (Cholesterol and Recurrent Events Trial), LIPID (Long-term Intervention with Pravastatin in Ischaemic Disease), and WOSCOPS (West of Scotland Coronary Prevention Study), show impressive reductions in mortality, re-infarction, and stroke, although the numbers in each were relatively small (see Table 13.15). In 4S, for example, the simvastatin-treated diabetic subgroup had a 23% rate of major coronary events, compared to 45% in the diabetic placebo group, while the non-diabetic simvastatin group had 19% major coronary events and the placebo non-diabetic group had 27%. On the basis of this, it is suggested that if 100 patients with diabetes who have angina or are post-MI are treated with simvastatin for 6 years, 24 of the 46 expected coronary deaths and non-fatal myocardial infarctions can be prevented.

More recent lipid-lowering trials in individuals with diabetes, such as CARDS (Collaborative Atorvastatin Diabetes Study), showed significant benefit of statin treatment in this population. However, ASPEN (Atorvastatin Study for the Prevention of Endpoints in Non-insulin dependent diabetes) demonstrated no effects, but this may have been due to study design and protocol changes during the study.

Table 13.15 Important lipid-lowering studies

Study	4S	WOSCOP	CARE	LIPID
Type of study	2° prevention of CHD	1° prevention of CHD	2° prevention of CHD	2° prevention of CHD
Duration of study (years)	6	5	5	6
Number studied	4,444	6,595	4,159	9,014
Mean total cholesterol (mmol/L) (cholesterol at inclusion)	6.8 (5.5–8.0)	7.0 (>6.5)	5.4 (<6.2)	5.6 (4.0–7.0)
Age range (years)	35–70	45–64	21–75	31–75
% men	81	100	86	83
% with diabetes	4.5	1	17	8.6
Treatment	Simvastatin 20–40mg daily	Pravastatin 40mg daily	Pravastatin 40mg daily	Pravastatin 40mg daily
Event reduction for	34% for non-diabetics 55% for diabetics	31% overall	23% for non-diabetics 25% for diabetics	23% overall

Management

Patients with diabetes are given dietary advice to help control blood glucose, which also contributes to improving lipid profile. In a patient who is already following a good 'diabetic diet', however, there is often not much room for improvement.

Other standard advice should also be given:
- Stop smoking—reduces risk of death by about 50% over a 15-year period.
- Reduce weight if overweight/obese.
- Increase physical activity.

Lipid-lowering therapy

The use of general cardiovascular risk stratification tables is not recommended for individuals with diabetes. NICE guidelines recommend for those with type 1 diabetes, statin treatment is used in those with raised albumin excretion rate or ≥2 features of metabolic syndrome or other risk factors (e.g. age >35 years or high-risk ethnic group). For those with type 2 diabetes, statin treatment is recommended in all those >40 years old, unless their CV risk is low (<20% over 10 years, using the UKPDS risk engine), and in those under 40 years with multiple CV risk factors.

Treatment aims for lipids

- Total cholesterol <4.0mmol/L.
- LDL cholesterol <2.0mmol/L.
- HDL >1.0 mmol/L.
- Triglycerides <2.3mmol/L.

Pharmacological interventions to increase HDL levels have not been shown to improve clinical outcome. HDL can be raised non-pharmacologically using lifestyle measures (weight loss, exercise, and stopping smoking).

Remember that a fit patient with diabetes has a similar risk when compared to a non-diabetic of the same age and gender who has also had a coronary event. More strict lipid targets are advocated by many, especially for those patients who are post-coronary artery bypass grafting or post-angioplasty.

In those with mixed hyperlipidaemia, consider a fibrate or a statin licensed for this indication. A fibrate will reduce triglycerides by 30–40% and LDL cholesterol by 20% while a statin would reduce triglycerides slightly less (10–15%) and LDL cholesterol slightly more (25–35%). Fibrates also alter the LDL cholesterol to its less atherogenic form. The choice of agent must be tailored to the individual patient. For hypercholesterolaemia alone, a statin is first-choice, as in the non-diabetic patient, and, in severely resistant patients, combination therapy with statins and ezetimibe or statin and fibrates may be required. Combination of statin and ezetimibe may reduce LDL more effectively than increasing the statin dose alone, although there is no evidence that such combination therapy is translated into better clinical outcome, compared to monotherapy with higher-dose statin.

Hypertension

Epidemiology

Hypertension is twice as common in the diabetic population as in the non-diabetic population, and standard ethnic differences in the prevalence of hypertension still hold true. It is known that hypertension worsens the severity and increases the risk of developing both microvascular and macrovascular disease. Using a cut-off of >160/90mmHg, hypertension occurs in:

- 10–30% of patients with type 1 diabetes.
- 20–30% of microalbuminuric type 1 patients.
- 80–90% of macroalbuminuric type 1 patients.
- 30–50% of Caucasians with type 2 diabetes.

Using the UKPDS suggested target of 140/80, hypertension is even more common.

Pathogenesis

- *Type 1 patients.* Hypertension is strongly associated with diabetic nephropathy and microalbuminuria and occurs at an earlier stage than that seen in many other causes of renal disease.
- *Type 2 patients.* Hypertension is associated with insulin resistance and hyperinsulinaemia. Hyperinsulinaemia can directly cause hypertension by increased sympathetic nervous system activity, enhanced proximal tubule sodium reabsorption, and stimulation of vascular smooth muscle cell proliferation.

Management of hypertension

Treatment aim

NICE guidelines recommend all patients with diabetes should have a blood pressure <140/80mmHg or 130/80 in the presence of diabetic complications.

The hypertension study in the UKPDS highlights the benefits for type 2 patients of such a treatment level on mortality, diabetes-related endpoints, and microvascular endpoints. In this study, a 10/5mmHg difference in BP was associated with a 34% risk reduction in macrovascular endpoints, a 37% risk reduction in microvascular endpoints, and a 44% risk reduction in stroke. The Hypertension Optimal Treatment (HOT) study supports these targets.

Predisposing conditions

Other conditions causing both hypertension and hyperglycaemia should be considered, e.g. Cushing's syndrome, acromegaly, and phaeochromocytoma.

End-organ damage

Assess evidence of end-organ damage (eyes, heart, kidneys, and peripheral vascular tree, in particular).

Assessment of cardiac risk factors

Treat associated risk factors for coronary heart disease.

Treatment

General

Modify other risk factors, such as glycaemic control, smoking, and dyslipidaemia. Then consider:
- Weight reduction if obese.
- Reduced salt intake (<6g/day).
- Reduced alcohol intake (<21 units/week in ♂, <14 in ♀).
- Exercise (20–40min of moderate exertion 3–5 times/week).

Pharmacological

Most agents currently available will drop systolic BP by no more than 20mmHg at most. In the UKPDS BP study, one-third of those achieving the current BP targets required three or more drugs. Recently, the NICE guidelines for BP treatment were updated and now advocate an 'A/CD' approach. That is starting with 'A', an ACEI (or an angiotensin II receptor blocker/antagonist if the ACEI is not tolerated), and then adding in either a 'C'/calcium channel blocker or a 'D'/thiazide-type diuretic, with an α-blocker, a β-blocker, or further diuretic therapy then added if this fails to reduce BP adequately.
- In the presence of microalbuminuria or frank proteinuria, an ACEI is first-line, or an angiotensin II receptor antagonist if not tolerated.
- In Afro-Caribbean patients, ACEI and β-blockers are less effective than calcium channel blockers and diuretics. A diuretic may be needed to improve the efficacy of the ACEI in these patients.
- Several agents, such as high-dose thiazides and β-blockers, can worsen diabetic control and exacerbate dyslipidaemia, so tailor the drugs

chosen to each patient. Interestingly, a recent review of data from the Nurses Health Study and the Health Professionals Follow-up study (HPFS) suggested that, while these agents may increase the risk of developing diabetes, it may not be associated with an increased risk of cardiovascular or total mortality.

- In those with angina, a β-blocker has added benefits.
- In those with PVD, consider vasodilators, e.g. calcium channel blockers.

In summary, to reduce the risk of macrovascular complications in diabetes, we should ensure:

- Early glycaemic control: strict glycaemic control to achieve HbA1c of 6.5% or less, with avoidance of hypoglycaemia. In individuals with long-standing diabetes and advanced arterial disease, strict glucose control is probably less effective at reducing cardiovascular events.
- Strict blood pressure control: aiming for BP <140/80mmHg or <130/80mmHg for those with micro- or macrovascular complications.
- Treatment of dyslipidaemia, aiming for total cholesterol of <4.0mmol/L, LDL <2.0mmol/L, HDL >1.0mmol/L, and triglyceride <2.3mmol/L.
- Patient should be encouraged to lose weight through healthy diet and regular exercise.
- Aspirin therapy has currently no role in primary cardiovascular protection but continues to be used for secondary prevention.

Further reading

Ajjan RA, Grant PJ (2011). The role of antiplatelets in hypertension and diabetes mellitus. *J Clin Hypertens* **13**, 305–13.

Betteridge DJ (2011). Lipid control in patients with diabetes mellitus. *Nat Rev Cardiol* **8**, 278—90.

Chrysant SG, Chrysant GS (2011). Current status of aggressive blood glucose and blood pressure control in diabetic hypertensive subjects. *Am J Cardiol* **107**, 1856–61.

Hill D, Fisher M (2010). The effect of intensive glycaemic control on cardiovascular outcomes. *Diabetes Obes Metab* **12**, 641–7.

Malmberg K for the DIGAMI (DM, Insulin Glucose Infusion in Acute Myocardial) study group (1997). Prospective randomized study of intensive insulin treatment on long term survival after acute myocardial infarction in patients with DM. *BMJ* **314**, 1512–15.

National Institute for Health and Clinical Excellence (2006). Hypertension: management of hypertension in adults in primary care. NICE clinical guidelines 34 (partial update of NICE clinical guideline 18), June 2006. NICE: London. Available at: ℘ http://www.nice.org.uk/nicemedia/pdf/cg034niceguideline.pdf

National Institute for Health and Clinical Excellence (2008). Type 2 diabetes: the management of type 2 diabetes. Management of blood pressure and lipids. NICE Clinical Guideline CG 66 (May, 2008). Available at: ℘ http://www.nice.org.uk/nicemedia/live/11983/40803/40803.pdf.

UKPDS Group (1998). Tight blood pressure control and risk of macrovascular and microvascular complications in type 2 diabetes: UKPDS 38. *BMJ* **317**, 703–13.

Zuanetti G, Latini R, Maggioni AP, et al. (1997). Effect of the ACE inhibitor lisinopril in diabetic patients with acute myocardial infarction. Data from GISSI-3 Study. *Circulation* **96**, 4239–45.

Lipids and hyperlipidaemia

Lipids and coronary heart disease

Physiology

The two main circulating lipids triglycerides and cholesterol are bound with phospholipid and apolipoproteins to make them more water-soluble for transportation throughout the body. The apolipoproteins on the surface of these soluble complexes have functional characteristics and are specific for each lipoprotein:

- *Chylomicrons.* Contain 85% triglycerides and 4% cholesterol and can be up to 0.001mm in diameter (light-scattering and presence, therefore, gives a milky appearance to plasma). Main transport vehicle of fat (50–150g/day) from intestine, and assembled and secreted by the mucosa of the small intestine and after fat ingestion. Their triglyceride content is broken down in peripheral tissues by lipoprotein lipase. Initially, they contain apoprotein B-48 (apo B-48) and acquire apo E and apo C-II from circulating HDL. Following the triglyceride removal in the capillary bed, the chylomicron remnants are removed by specific apo B and apo E receptors in the liver.

- *Very low density lipoproteins (VLDLs).* Contain 50% triglyceride, 15% cholesterol, and 18% phospholipid. They are the main carrier of triglycerides from the liver (approximately 50g/day). The VLDL contain apo B-100 and apo E. VLDL triglycerides are also broken down by lipoprotein lipase in peripheral tissue to generate IDLs or other remnants (LDL) which are removed by the liver.

- *Intermediate density lipoproteins (IDLs).* These VLDL remnants contain mostly cholesterol and phospholipid and are either removed by the liver or metabolized to form LDLs.

- *Low density lipoproteins (LDLs).* Contain 45% cholesterol, 10% triglycerides, and 20% phospholipid. LDL has apo B-100 on its surface and is the predominant cholesterol transport vehicle in the circulation. The liver has specific LDL receptors to extract it from the circulation. Half of the body's circulating LDL is removed from the plasma each day, mostly by the liver. Small, dense LDL (5–50% of the LDL pool) is easily oxidized. This is likely to occur whilst the LDL particle has been retained in the vascular wall. Modified LDL is taken by macrophages, and an extensive uptake will be the basis of foam cell formation in the atheromatous plaque.

- *High density lipoproteins (HDLs).* Made in the liver and gut; contain 17% cholesterol, 4% triglycerides, and 24% phospholipid. HDL transports 20–50% of circulating cholesterol. The main apoprotein is apo AI which attracts free cholesterol from peripheral tissues to form the first step of 'reverse cholesterol transport'.

In practice, patients are managed by their levels of cholesterol (total, LDL, HDL) and triglycerides. Elevated total or LDL cholesterol with normal triglycerides is hypercholesterolaemia. Isolated elevation of triglyceride is hypertriglyceridaemia, and both together is combined or mixed hyperlipidaemia.

There is an exponential relationship between hypercholesterolaemia and coronary heart disease (CHD). A man with a TC of 6.5mmol/L has double the risk of CHD of a man with a TC of 5.2mmol/L, and half the risk of a man with a cholesterol of 7.8mmol/L. Intervention studies show that reductions in total and LDL cholesterol reduce coronary and cerebrovascular events as well as mortality.

HDL cholesterol has an inverse relationship with CHD, i.e. increased levels appear protective. Low HDL cholesterol concentrations may be due to lack of physical exercise, obesity, or the presence of hypertriglyceridaemia and occurs in smokers.

A low HDL is very often seen in the presence of hypertriglyceridaemia.

Although much debated over the past decades, recent evidence suggests that hypertriglyceridaemia is directly related to CHD. Combined hyperlipidaemia carries a substantial excessive CHD risk.

The specific role of low HDL is less clear, as the monogenic 'low HDL syndromes' often do not carry an excessive CHD risk.

A novel and useful way of quantifying the presence of potentially atherogenic lipoprotein concentrations in plasma is to use apo B which is a marker of lipoprotein particle number.

Pathogenesis

Hyperlipidaemia is due to a combination of genetic and environmental factors. Obesity is one of the strongest 2° factors. It is a major risk factor for atherosclerosis.

- 1° *hyperlipidaemias*—usually genetically determined.
- 2° *hyperlipidaemias*—due to a combination of other conditions, drugs, and dietary anomalies.

Atherosclerosis

In atherosclerosis, subintimal plaques start in medium-sized blood vessel walls when cholesterol from LDL accumulates. A cholesterol-rich necrotic core, surrounded by smooth muscle cells and fibrous tissue, then develops. These plaques can calcify. If the surface of the plaques ulcerates, thrombosis occurs which can obliterate the lumen of a blood vessel.

Plaques may result from diffusion of elevated LDL cholesterol, a qualitative abnormality of LDL cholesterol, endothelial cell damage, or a combination of these. Endothelial cell damage may be due to:

- Physical trauma, e.g. with hypertension.
- Toxins, e.g. tobacco or alcohol.
- Low-grade infection or inflammation, e.g. Chlamydia.
- Immune complex damage.

CHD/atherosclerosis risk factors

♂ gender, ↑ age, and a +ve family history are all linked with a greater risk for atherosclerosis. There are also several modifiable risk factors:

- *Cigarette smoking.* >10 cigarettes/day increase the CHD odds ratio by 6.7-fold while stopping smoking reduces risk of myocardial infarct (MI) by 50–70% within 5 years.
- *Hypertension.* Increases the CHD odds ratio by 2.7-fold. Each 1mmHg drop in diastolic blood pressure reduces the MI risk by 2–3%. But remember, aspirin reduces MI risk by 33%.
- *Diabetes mellitus.*
- *Hyperlipidaemia.* A 10% fall in total cholesterol (TC) results in a 25% decrease in CHD risk, and plaque regression with reducing lipids is well documented.
- *Other.* Less strongly associated factors include type A personality and hyperuricaemia.

Assessment of CVD risk

Risk assessment tables/calculators for CVD or CHD are now available, such as the Sheffield tables, the New Zealand tables, the Joint British Societies Coronary Risk Prediction Chart, and QRISK. These calculate the likelihood of the patient's absolute risk of CVD over a period of years and/or the individual's relative risk, assuming CVD is not present at this time. The data used for assessment include sex, age, blood pressure, presence of left ventricular hypertrophy, smoking, diabetes mellitus, and the measured values of total cholesterol (TC), HDL cholesterol, or the ratio of TC:HDL cholesterol. The tables give a prediction which is useful for estimating the need for treatment.

Risk assessment tables/calculators can be accessed online or downloaded to clinic room computers.

Joint British Society Coronary Risk Prevention Score

Available at: ℘ http://www.bhsoc.org/index.php?cID=269.

This chart was updated in 2009 to include older patients aged >70 years and to show risk thresholds of <10%, 10–20%, and >20% over 10 years (in line with NICE guidance for statin use).

QRISK

Available at: ℘ http://www.qrisk.org/.

QRISK, which uses data from British subjects, appears to be better at predicting outcome. The other risk assessment tables are calculated, based on data from the Framingham study which appears to overestimate the risk in the UK. QRISK also takes ethnicity into account and allows UK postcode entry to calculate the effects of deprivation.

UKPDS risk engine

Available at: ℘ http://www.dtu.ox.ac.uk/riskengine/index.php.

The UKPDS risk engine provides risk calculation in patients with type 2 diabetes.

General cautions when interpreting calculated risk

- CVD risk may be higher than indicated in the charts for:
  - Those with a family history of premature CVD (♂ <55 years and ♀ <65 years). This is accounted for in QRISK.
  - Those with raised triglyceride levels.
  - Those who are not diabetic but have impaired glucose tolerance.
  - Women with premature menopause.
  - As the person approaches the next age category. As risk increases exponentially with age, the risk will be closer to the higher decennium for the last 4 years of each decade.
- The estimates of CVD risk from the chart are based on groups of people, and in managing an *individual*, the physician also has to use clinical judgement in deciding how intensively to intervene on lifestyle and whether or not to use drug therapies.

- An individual can be shown on the chart (or by using the calculator in QIntervention ℘ http://qintervention.org/) the direction in which the risk of CVD can be reduced by changing smoking status, BP, or cholesterol.

Individuals at risk of hyperlipidaemia

- Those with premature CHD (<55 years in ♂, <65 years in ♀).
- Those with signs of other atherosclerotic disease (e.g. PVD, ischaemic cerebrovascular disease).
- Those with diabetes mellitus.
- Those with signs of insulin resistance, such as acanthosis nigricans.
- Post-menopausal ♀ not on HRT.
- Those with a high alcohol intake (♀ >14 units/week, ♂ >21).
- Those with a family history of hyperlipidaemia.
- Those with a family history of early CHD or other atherosclerotic disease.
- Those with known 2° causes of hyperlipidaemia (📖 see p. 836).

Lipid measurements

Measurements should not be taken during an acute illness or during periods of rapid weight loss, as these artificially lower the results. This is particularly important from 24h after an MI for up to 6 weeks (less if thrombolysed), as during this time, the levels of TC and LDL cholesterol may be falsely reduced.

Pregnancy or recent weight gain will increase lipid levels. Following rapid weight gain or weight loss, leave at least 1 month before reassessing lipid levels.

Full lipid profile

Measures TC, HDL cholesterol, LDL cholesterol, and triglycerides.

This needs to be a fasting sample. If non-fasting, only TC and HDL cholesterol measurements are accurate. Triglycerides rise postprandially, and LDL is usually calculated with the formula below so is inaccurate if not fasting. It is also invalid if triglycerides are >4.5mmol/L:

$$LDL \text{ (in mmol/L)} = TC - HDL - 0.45 \text{ (triglycerides)}$$

The use of TC alone can be misleading, as isolated HDL elevation can increase the value. Use of a TC:HDL or an LDL:HDL ratio is preferred, especially in ♀ and people with diabetes mellitus. Most risk calculation tables now use these ratios, rather than total values alone.

Variations between assay method and different samples should not lead to >3% variation, but more than one measurement should be used to decide on initial pharmacological intervention.

ApoB

ApoB is the carrier protein of LDL and VLDL. As there is one molecule of apoB per lipoprotein particle, measuring apoB in plasma gives insight to the total number of potentially atherogenic lipoprotein particles. Some studies suggest that apoB is a more accurate CVD risk indicator than LDL cholesterol or non-HDL cholesterol and may, therefore, serve as a useful CVD risk indicator. ApoB concentration is largely independent of fasting.

Primary hyperlipidaemias

Background

A primary hyperlipidaemia is defined by a knowledge of a monogenic or polygenic cause. Although the clinical features of 1° hyperlipidaemia are driven by a specific defect, the phenotype is also susceptible to environmental pressure. Some of the primary hyperlipidaemias are very aggressive and need strict clinical attention. At present, the family history and the phenotypic findings in other family members are used as a surrogate for a genetic diagnosis. DNA-based diagnosis is established for type III hyperlipidaemia and is being implemented for familial hypercholesterolaemia. The latter can be useful not just for initial diagnosis, but also for family screening.

Severe isolated hypertriglyceridaemias are classically recessive, and genetic diagnosis is of little help or unavailable in clinical routine.

Polygenic hypercholesterolaemia

This is the most common cause of isolated hypercholesterolaemia. LDL clearance appears to be reduced by a variety of mechanisms, and the E4 allele of apo E is a common association. Patients do not have the characteristic xanthelasmata or extensor tendon deposits (xanthomata) seen in familial hyperlipidaemia, and occasionally it can be difficult to distinguish from familial hypercholesterolaemia. If young offspring of cases with polygenic hypercholesterolaemia are tested, it would be unsurprising if they have normal cholesterol concentrations, which is in contrast to children of those with familial hypercholesterolaemia.

Familial hypercholesterolaemia (FH)

FH is an autosomal dominant disorder. Its gene frequency is thought to be 1 in 500 in Western Europe and North America. In FH, hypercholesterolaemia is mainly (>95%) due to an increase in LDL cholesterol, caused by LDL receptor mutations (on the short arm of chromosome 19) reducing the number of high-affinity LDL receptors by up to 50%, so reducing LDL clearance and thus prolonging the circulating time before catabolism from the normal 2.5 days to >4.5 days. More than 1,000 different mutations have, so far, been described. Less commonly, FH is due to familial defective apolipoprotein B-100 (3–4%) and proprotein convertase subtilisin/kexin 9 gene (*PCSK9*) mutation (<1%). These can lead to several situations, causing elevation of circulating LDL cholesterol by:

- Not producing any LDL receptors.
- Failure of LDL receptors to move to the cell surface.
- Abnormal binding of the receptor to LDL.
- Inability to adequately internalize LDL for metabolism.

Patients with untreated FH have a very high risk of premature CHD.

See Box 14.1 for clinical features.

Pharmacological treatment of FH

Treatment is with high-dose statins and ezetimibe, with bile acid sequestrants, fibrates, and nicotinic acid as next-line treatments. Aim to reduce LDL-C by >50%. Children should be treated by age 10. Homozygote FH should be treated in a specialist lipid clinic.

It is estimated that >50% of heterozygous FH patients will die from CHD before 60 years of age if left untreated. One in 20 patients under 60 years old surviving an MI are FH heterozygotes. Homozygous FH may need non-pharmacological therapies, such as plasmapheresis, or surgical procedures, such as ileal bypass, portocaval shunts, or liver transplantation. These treatments are not readily available and, along with pharmacological treatments, may be superseded by gene therapy in the future.

Clinical diagnosis is made by measurement of blood lipids, searching for clinical stigmata, and noting the family history. DNA sequencing can sometimes be used for specific diagnosis. Once an index case is detected, further testing should involve immediate family members and can be done at any age, using so-called 'cascade screening'. In neonates, LDL can be measured in cord blood, although this screening method may be unreliable in heterozygote FH. Screening children is best carried out before 10 years of age (at this age, a total cholesterol of above 5.5mmol/L is highly indicative of FH) and then again at adolescence and early adulthood. Typically, between the ages of 1 and 16 years, heterozygotes will have a 2-fold higher cholesterol level than unaffected siblings, so standard lipid profiles can be used. Over 16 years of age, use a full fasting lipid profile and clinical examination.

Box 14.1 Clinical features of FH
- TC >7.8mmol/L (>12.5mmol/L in homozygotes), LDL high from birth.
- Normal triglycerides.
- Clinical stigmata: xanthelasmic deposits around the eyes and on the tendons (i.e. fingers, hands, elbow, knee, and the Achilles tendon). Tendon xanthoma is more specific for FH than corneal arcus or xanthelasma. 7% of heterozygote FH (aged >19 years) and 75% of homozygotes have tendon xanthomas (but may not be present until age >40 years).
- Onset of a corneal arcus aged 30–40 years.
- Achilles tendonitis in childhood.
- Homozygotes can have CHD presenting in childhood and certainly before the age of 30.
- Heterozygotes usually present after 30 years of age.
- FH may occur without clinical stigmata but with strong family history of early-onset CHD, e.g. <50 years.

Familial combined hyperlipidaemia (FCHL)

- FCHL is a high-risk syndrome for CHD.
- Population frequency has been estimated to 1/200.
- The aetiology is not yet known. Despite its seemingly dominant appearance, the risk is clearly conveyed by a number of different unknown genes.
- It is the most common type of inherited dyslipidaemia, estimated to cause 10% of cases of premature CHD.
- It has no unique clinical manifestations, and the diagnosis is based on raised lipids (>95th centile for age) and a family history of premature CHD in first-degree relatives. In contrast to FH, tendon xanthomata should not be present.
- The lipid phenotype can vary within individuals and family members such that combined hyperlipidaemia, isolated hypercholesterolaemia, and isolated hypertriglyceridaemia can be seen within the same individual at different times and in different family members.
- Very likely to have raised Apo B concentrations.
- Should be treated aggressively and very often needs the combination of several different pharmacological agents.

Familial hypertriglyceridaemia

- Is defined as a subentity of FCHL, but clearly less common, perhaps with a frequency of 1/1,000, often as an autosomal dominant trait with elevated VLDL levels, and is frequently accompanied by a moderate hypercholesterolaemia. Triglyceride concentrations are rarely higher than 10mmol/L.
- Suspect this condition where there is a subtle hypertriglyceridaemia without any obvious causes (obesity, type 2 diabetes, etc.), together with a positive CHD or stroke family history.
- The condition can sometimes be surprisingly responsive to statins.

Rare genetic hypertriglyceridaemias

Two rare, but important, familial causes of severe hypertriglyceridaemia are *lipoprotein lipase deficiency* and *apolipoprotein C-II deficiency*. Both are autosomal recessive conditions which present in childhood and are characterized by the presence of hyperchylomicronaemia.

- *Lipoprotein lipase (LPL)* is the enzyme needed to metabolize chylomicron triglycerides; complete absence of this enzyme or production of an inactive form are both recognized defects. Some cases of apo C-II (the apolipoprotein-activating LPL) deficiency have been described. Heterozygous LPL deficiency has a mild phenotype. Recently, additional causes have been described in cases with mutations in the protein-binding LPL to the endothelium (GP1-HDLBP) and also with mutations in Apo AV. The overwhelming clinical concern is pancreatitis. At present, the only useful treatment is an extremely low fat diet.
- *Pseudohypertriglyceridaemia* should be suspected when a very stable hypertriglyceridaemia (typically around 5mmol/L) is seen in someone without any obvious secondary causes (obesity, type 2 diabetes, etc.). The condition is X-linked (essentially restricted to ♂) and caused by glycerol kinase (GK) deficiency. Typically, upon inspection of a fasting plasma sample, it is clear (hypertriglyceridaemia in the range of 5mmol/L always show some opalescence). Test for free glycerol. This is a harmless condition that should be left untreated.

Familial dysbetalipoproteinaemia

- Also known as *type III hyperlipidaemia* or *broad beta disease*.
- It is associated with early-onset CHD.
- It is an uncommon disorder affecting 1/10, or less, of people with the Apo E2/E2 genetic background (which is 1/100 in most populations).
- The condition leads to specific elevation of IDL and chylomicron remnants which are both cholesterol- and triglyceride-rich. Typically, the rise of cholesterol and triglycerides is equimolar, and very high concentrations can be seen (15mmol/L of TG and 15mmol/L of cholesterol).
- Diagnosis is confirmed by genetic testing.
- A characteristic clinical feature is the presence of palmar striae xanthoma; tubero-eruptive xanthomata, found over the tuberosities of the elbows and knees, may also be present.
- Due to the recessive nature of the apo E2 genotype and the required additional environmental pressure, family history is rarely revealing.
- Apo E2/E2 genetic background is not enough to precipitate the syndrome; an additional factor is needed. This is typically obesity, type 2 diabetes, hypothyroidism, β-blocker, or thiazide diuretic medication. The oral contraceptive pill can also elicit type III hyperlipidaemia.

Elevation of Lp(a)

- Lp(a) is an LDL-like lipoprotein particle, but it is not cleared via the LDL receptors. Less than 5% of the population have raised Lp(a), and the distribution is very skewed. Synthesis appears to be highly genetically driven. Recent evidence suggests this is a highly atherogenic lipoprotein particle. Raised Lp(a) should be suspected in someone with early presentation of CHD, stroke, or peripheral vascular disease, with moderately elevated cholesterol that is seemingly resistant to statin therapy. At present, the only available pharmacological means by which lowering of Lp(a) can be achieved is with niacin. However, there is no formal evidence to suggest that niacin reduces cardiovascular events in people with raised Lp(a).

Rare familial mixed dyslipidaemias

These should be considered in any patient with unexplained neurology, organomegaly, or corneal opacities.

- *Familial lecithin:cholesterol acyltransferase (LCAT) deficiency.* In this recessively inherited disorder, an enzyme necessary for intravascular lipoprotein metabolism is deficient, resulting in elevated cholesterol and triglycerides. Clinically, corneal lipid deposits result in visual disturbances and renal deposits in glomerular damage, proteinuria, and often renal failure. Red blood cell morphology.

- *Tangier disease (analphalipoproteinaemia* or *familial alphalipoprotein deficiency).* In this autosomal recessive condition, apo A-I, which is found on HDL, is deficient. HDL level is low, as is TC while triglycerides are normal or high. Cholesterol accumulation gives enlarged orange-coloured tonsils, hepatosplenomegaly, polyneuropathy, and corneal opacities.

- *Fish eye disease.* A rare disorder from northern Sweden, with high VLDL levels, low HDL, and a triglyceride-rich LDL. As well as hypertriglyceridaemia, dense corneal opacities occur, giving visual impairment.

- *Abetalipoproteinaemia.* Results in intestinal fat accumulation due to failure of secreting chylomicrons. Cholesterol levels are low, with no LDL and VLDL in many cases, which results in fat accumulation in the gut and nerves. Vitamin E injections may prevent some of the neurological abnormalities observed (ataxia, nystagmus, dysarthria, and motor plus sensory neuropathies) but usually not the retinitis pigmentosa and acanthocytes which also feature.

- *Hypobetalipoproteinaemia.* This autosomal dominantly inherited condition gives a TC of 1–4mmol/L and can be associated with organomegaly and neurological changes in middle age due to fat deposition and abnormal red cell morphology. The homozygous state is similar to abetalipoproteinaemia.

- *Hyperalphalipoproteinaemia* or *HDL hyperlipoproteinaemia.* Results in mildly elevated HDL and TC and may be beneficial. If very high HDL is seen together with a type III-like pattern, hepatic lipase deficiency could be suspected. Raised HDL can also occur with exercise, exogenous oestrogen, phenytoin and phenobarbital use, or from alcohol. Very high consumption of alcohol is one of the few circumstances when high HDL is seen together with raised triglycerides.

Secondary hyperlipidaemias

Background

Secondary hyperlipidaemias are common, and the predominant precipitating factors are obesity and type 2 diabetes They may consist of isolated elevations of cholesterol or triglycerides or be combined. Treatment is based upon managing the primary disorder disease before making a further decision on the raised lipids. Not infrequently, more than one cause is apparent in secondary hyperlipidaemias.

Causes

(Summarized in Table 14.1.)

- *Obesity* (📖 see Consequences of obesity, p. 857).
- *Diabetes mellitus* (📖 see Lipid abnormalities found in patients with diabetes, p. 814).
- *Fatty liver disease.* Almost invariably associated with elevated TG.
- *Diet.* Excessive consumption of saturated fats, carbohydrate, sugary drinks, and alcohol. Raised triglycerides by alcohol are normally only seen after excessive consumption. Occasionally, the unusual combination of elevated HDL cholesterol with raised triglycerides is seen.
- *Hypothyroidism.* Estimated to occur in 4% of those with hyperlipidaemia, and compensated (subclinical) hypothyroidism in a further 10%. Usually resulting in hypercholesterolaemia with a TC of 7–12mmol/L. It also worsens primary hypercholesterolaemias due to ↓ synthesis of hepatic LDL receptors.
- *Chronic renal disease.* ↓ creatinine clearance is accompanied by hypertriglyceridaemia and ↓ HDL cholesterol. Proteinuria, in the nephrotic syndrome, is associated with hypercholesterolaemia. It also raises Lp(a). After kidney transplantation, ciclosporin may increase LDL.
- *Liver disease.* Especially with cholestasis, resulting in abnormal LDL cholesterol. Primary biliary cirrhosis often results in TC >12mmol/L, which is close to treatment resistance. The accumulating cholesterol is contained in a fraction called LpX, absent in healthy humans. These are large aggregates of phospholipids and free cholesterol and do not resemble conventional lipoproteins. However, severe hepatocellular damage may also lower LDL cholesterol by ↓ production of its component parts and the enzymes which metabolize it.
- *Cushing's syndrome.* Glucocorticoids increase VLDL production, thus hypertriglyceridaemia. The associated weight gain and glucose intolerance can make this effect more pronounced.
- *Lipodystrophies.* A very rare group of disorders, hallmark of which is regional, partial, or generalized fat loss, associated with hyperlipidaemia, especially unusually raised triglycerides. Also associated with glucose intolerance. See 📖 Genetic causes of severe insulin resistance, p. 693.

- *Drugs*. Medications commonly implicated are:
  - β-blockers, especially the non-cardioselective ones.
  - Thiazide diuretics.
  - Exogenous oestrogens.
  - Anabolic steroids.
  - Glucocorticoids.
  - Isotretinoin.
  - Protease inhibitors (said to cause hyperlipidaemia in 50% after 10 months of treatment).
- *Pregnancy*. Cholesterol rises throughout pregnancy, mostly in the second trimester. Triglycerides also rise but in the final trimester and mostly in those with underlying genetic abnormalities. Both return to normal by 6 weeks post-partum.

Table 14.1 Secondary causes of dyslipidaemia

Elevated LDL cholesterol	Elevated triglycerides	Reduced HDL cholesterol
Diet (high saturated fats, high calories)	Diet (weight gain + excess of sugary drinks and alcohol)	Diet (some low-fat diets)
Drugs (glucocorticoids, thiazide + loop diuretics, ciclosporin)	Drugs (glucocorticoids, β-blockers, oestrogens, isotretinoin)	Drugs (anabolic steroids, tobacco, β-adrenergic blockers)
Hypothyroidism	Hypothyroidism	Type 2 diabetes
Nephrotic syndrome	Type 2 diabetes	Insulin resistance syndromes/obesity
Chronic liver disease	Insulin resistance syndromes	Chronic renal failure
Cholestasis + biliary obstruction	Cushing's syndrome	
Pregnancy	Chronic renal failure	
	Peritoneal dialysis	
	Pregnancy	

Management of dyslipidaemia

Background

Hyperlipidaemias are common, and a decision to use pharmacological means to lower hyperlipidaemias should depend on estimated cardiovascular risk. For this purpose, useful risk scoring systems have been developed, but it is important to use these wisely. Importantly, they should not be used for certain primary and familial conditions with very high cardiovascular risk.

It can be a challenge to the physician to describe benefits of the medication or the necessary change in lifestyle to the patient, as treatment rarely comes with an obvious 'reward' and the true effect may only be described as a certain CHD risk reduction noticeable a decade or more ahead.

Overall, the use of statins has an extremely good evidence base, whereas most alternative or complementary options have less solid evidence.

Primary and secondary prevention

It is universally accepted that lowering hypercholesterolaemia using statins in secondary prevention reduces future cardiovascular events and overall mortality. It is estimated that a 10% fall in TC results in a 25% decrease in CHD risk. Regression and remodelling of atheromatous lesions have also been clearly demonstrated. The presence of type 2 diabetes mellitus puts the patient in the category for secondary prevention. Acute coronary syndrome should be treated aggressively (high-dose atorvastatin 80mg), which shows early benefit with statin treatment. In post-MI patients, omega-3 fatty acids are recommended, as it reduces the incidence of sudden death due to arrhythmias.

A decision to reduce cholesterol primary prevention is much dependent on the overall cardiovascular risk (🕮 see p. 826). The reduction in absolute risk is marginal in patients with few other risk factors and should be evaluated critically. An estimated risk of CHD >2% per annum has unquestionable support for initiation of pharmacological treatment. However, even young patients with primary and familial conditions should be treated aggressively without applying risk scoring systems.

Specific interventions

Dietary advice

Current recommendations are that fats should constitute <30% of energy consumed and saturated fats must be <30% of the total fat content. To achieve this, vegetable and marine mono- and polyunsaturated fats should be high in the diet, whereas animal and dairy fat should be low. Total dietary cholesterol should not exceed 300mg per day. Foods advocated include fresh fruit and vegetables, which are also important sources of antioxidants. A high fibre content is cholesterol-lowering. Four months should be given to see if dietary manipulation will work in patients with low-to-moderate risk. It is unusual to see more than a 15% fall in cholesterol from dietary measures, but certain individuals can respond better. Alcohol should be <14 units/week for a ♀ and <21 units/week for a ♂.

Plant sterols and stanols, 2–3g daily, can reduce blood cholesterol by 10–15%. They are available commercially in enriched margarine spreads, yoghurt, and milky drinks.

Weight control
All overweight patients must be encouraged to lose weight. Weight reduction is closely attuned to dietary advice and physical exercise. Most weight is lost in the first 4 months of a regimen. A 10kg weight loss in an obese subject can reduce LDL cholesterol by 7% and increases HDL cholesterol by 13%. The effect on raised triglycerides can be much greater and clinically very useful.

Physical activity
Physical activity, especially aerobic exercise, is recommended. This should be realistic and adapted to the individual's capacity. Although exercise levels in the range of 70% of VO$_2$max for 30–40min at least 3–5 times per week is extremely useful, it is often unrealistic, and very good effects are seen by walking, etc. Acute exercise will transiently change lipoprotein levels and increase lipoprotein lipase activity. These effects become more permanent with regular training. Triglyceride levels fall, HDL cholesterol levels rise, especially the HDL2 subfraction with more vigorous exercise, and the LDL cholesterol is of the less dense variety which is not so atherogenic. The changes are dose-dependent with ↑ exercise, and a 20% alteration in each variable is achievable after 6 weeks. Particularly good effects are seen in type 2 diabetes mellitus.

Modification of other risk factors
Other risk factors, such as hypertension, smoking, and diabetes mellitus, must be addressed.

Drug therapy

Numerous agents can be used for both 1° and 2° prevention in patients in whom non-pharmacological approaches have either been unsuccessful or deemed insufficient.

HMG CoA reductase inhibitors (statins)

Table 14.2 shows the comparative potency of common statins.

Indications

Raised LDL, heterozygous + homozygous FH, mixed hyperlipidaemia. Not all these medications are licensed for use in children and should be used with caution in ♀ of childbearing age because of potential teratogenicity. The medication should be stopped for at least 3 months before pregnancy is planned. Women of childbearing age must ensure effective contraception when on these drugs.

Mechanism of action

Inhibition of 3-hydroxy-3-methylglutaryl coenzyme A (HMG CoA) which is the rate-limiting enzyme in cholesterol synthesis. Its activation increases hepatocyte LDL receptor numbers which leads to increased clearance of LDL and VLDL remnants. See Table 14.2 for comparative lipid-lowering profile and Table 14.3 for dosage.

Side effects

Statins are usually very well tolerated. The most common side effect is muscle ache which, in extremely rare cases, also develops into myositis. Hepatotoxicity is not common but does exist. LFTs and creatine kinase should be measured before they are prescribed and used with caution in those with an excessive alcohol intake. It is recommended that the medications should be discontinued if the liver enzymes aspartate transaminase (AST) and/or alanine transaminase (ALT) show more than a 2–3-fold elevation above the upper limit of normal. LFTs should, therefore, be checked within 3–4 months of treatment and, at most, annually in the long term if the patient is without symptoms. Myositis is rare, but the frequency increases with concomitant medications, e.g. ciclosporin, fibrates, or when renal impairment or untreated hypothyroidism are present. Clinically, there is a picture of swollen tender muscles and creatine kinase being >10× the upper limit of normal. Rhabdomyolysis is even rarer.

Interactions

Several statins are metabolized through CYP3A4. Grapefruit juice should be avoided. Statins can interact with *ciclosporin*. There is an interaction with *warfarin* for atorvastatin, simvastatin, and rosuvastatin, but it is often not clinically significant and would only lead to small adjustments of the warfarin dose. *Erythromycin* interacts with all statins. *Digoxin* interacts with atorvastatin and simvastatin. *Rifampicin* interacts with fluvastatin and pravastatin. Atorvastatin and rosuvastatin may also interact with the *oral contraceptive pill*, *antacids*, and some *antifungals*.

Table 14.2 Comparative lipid-lowering profile of statins

Statin	% fall in LDL-C	% fall in triglycerides	% rise in HDL-C
Atorvastatin	38–54	13–32	3–7
Fluvastatin	17–34	8–12	3–6
Pravastatin	18–34	5–13	5–8
Rosuvastatin	50–63	10–28	3–14
Simvastatin	26–48	12–38	8–12

Management of statin intolerance

Muscle problems after start of statin treatment is common. Although it has been demonstrated that Q10 is reduced in muscle samples after statin treatment, there is no evidence from randomized controlled trials that supplementation of Q10 is of any benefit. The two main strategies are to change statin or to reduce the dose. The first option normally involves switching from simvastatin or atorvastatin to a low dose of pravastatin (10 or 20mg). The second option involves a very low dose of a second-generation statin, e.g. rosuvastatin 5mg every second day. Non-statin agents are possible but should be used with caution, as the evidence base for cardiovascular benefits is low (i.e. fibrate alone, ezetimibe alone, etc.).

Fibrates

Indications

Raised plasma triglycerides or IDL, i.e. mixed hyperlipidaemias which have not responded adequately to diet or other therapies. Fibrates should normally be seen as add-on therapy beyond statins. However, fibrates constitute first-line therapy in type III hyperlipidaemia. These medications are less effective than statins at lowering cholesterol but better at ↑ HDL cholesterol and more effective in lowering triglycerides. Reduce triglycerides by 20–60%, increase HDL by 5–20%, and reduce LDL by 5–25%.

Mechanism of action

Increases VLDL triglyceride clearance by ↑ lipoprotein lipase activity and LDL receptor-mediated LDL clearance while ↑ HDL synthesis. The effect on LDL cholesterol may vary in isolated hypertriglyceridaemia, and an increase in LDL cholesterol can be seen in type IV hyperlipidaemia. See Table 14.3 for dosages.

Side effects

Occasionally cause nausea, anorexia, or diarrhoea and precipitate gallstones. They should not be used in patients with severe liver disease (AST/ALT >2–3× upper limit of normal) and renal dysfunction (creatinine >150micromol/L), as they are conjugated in the liver prior to excretion by the kidney. Myopathy, although rare, is the main concern, and the risk of this increases if used with statins.

Interactions

Use with caution in combination with *statins*. Can enhance the effects of *warfarin* and *antidiabetic agents* and is contraindicated in those on *orlistat*.

Anion exchange resins (bile acid sequestrants)

Indications

High LDL, i.e. hypercholesterolaemia. Largely superseded by statins, these are now best used as adjuncts when LDL has not fallen enough with a statin alone. They are also the only drug licensed for use during pregnancy.

Mechanism of action

Bind to bile acids in the gut, so reducing their enterohepatic circulation and ↑ bile acid excretion. This increases hepatocyte cholesterol requirements which increases LDL receptor production, so reducing circulating LDL levels. Under optimum conditions, LDL cholesterol can be reduced by 20–30%; triglycerides rise by 10–17%, and HDL increases by 3–5%.

Side effects

These agents remain in the gut, so constipation, bloating, nausea, and abdominal discomfort are not uncommon. Constipation, found in 35–40% of those on these agents, can be helped with bulking laxatives. Less often, a bleeding tendency due to vitamin K malabsorption can be seen. These agents can also exacerbate hypertriglyceridaemia, but HDL cholesterol is often ↑ slightly. To reduce the side effects, start with low doses and build up gradually over the next 3–4 weeks while maintaining a good fluid intake.

Interactions

These agents can reduce the absorption of *warfarin*, *digoxin*, β-*blockers*, *pravastatin*, *fluvastatin*, and *hydrochlorothiazide*. Many other agents, such as *simvastatin*, have not been checked, so to avoid any potential interaction, advise patients to take all other drugs 1–3h *before* or 4–6h *after* the resin.

Nicotinic acid and acipimox

Indication

High LDL, VLDL, IDL, or triglycerides. Nicotinic acid is the most effective medication for ↑ HDL cholesterol. In practice, however, their use is limited by the side effect profile, especially flushing.

Mechanism of action

Work by inhibiting lipolysis in adipocytes, so altering fatty acid flux and reducing VLDL synthesis and HDL clearance, or by inhibiting VLDL triglyceride synthesis. Plasma triglycerides fall by 20–50%, and LDL by 5–25% while HDL levels rise (by 10–50%).

Side effects

Common, with 30% unable to tolerate these agents. Vasodilatation, giving cutaneous/facial flushing, occurs in most patients but tends to improve after 2–3 weeks of therapy. Pruritus and dry, burning sensation in the skin can be seen. High doses of aspirin were previously given to reduce this effect, but this is now rarely practised due to the side effects of high-dose aspirin. Patients should also be instructed to avoid hot drinks and spicy food. Gastritis is also a common side effect, whereas liver side effects are rare. Raises uric acid almost invariably, and exacerbation of gout can be seen. Rarely, precipitation of acanthosis nigricans and retinal oedema are also recognized side effects. *Nicotinic acid* can adversely affect glucose control in prediabetic states and in diabetes mellitus. *Acipimox*, a nicotinic acid analogue, seems to be less problematic but is also less potent. In 2013 following the results of the HPS2-THRIVE study, the European Medicines Agency suspended licences for nicotinic acid preparations on the grounds that they were ineffective and associated with adverse effects. Acipimox remains available.

Omega-3 fatty acids (Omacor®, Maxepa®)

Indications
Hypertriglyceridaemia.

Mechanism of action
Inhibit the secretion of VLDL due to ↑ intracellular apo B-100 destruction. Normal patients see both a fall in VLDL and LDL, but LDL may rise in the hypertriglyceridaemic individual. Should be seen as add-on therapy to statins. Lower doses (1g per day) have demonstrated positive effects on cardiovascular prevention, but the mechanism of action is likely to be through an antiplatelet effect.

Side effects
As high doses are needed, this is a high calorie load and may increase obesity. More commonly, gives nausea and belching. Omacor® produces fewer unwanted effects and is less calorific, as it is used in a smaller dose.

Interactions
None significant.

Cholesterol absorption blocker
Ezetimibe is the only available compound. Should be used as second-line treatment after a statin.

Indications
LDL cholesterol-lowering in patients who are intolerant of statins or in combination with a statin in those that are not adequately controlled with a statin alone. Also in the very rare condition of sitosterolaemia where there is an ↑ absorption of plant sterols.

Mechanism of action
Dietary and biliary cholesterol absorption is selectively inhibited. Ezetimibe (10mg) monotherapy produces an 18% fall in LDL cholesterol and an increase in HDL cholesterol of 1–3%, and triglycerides are not affected. In combination therapy with a statin, ezetimibe reduces levels by an additional 22% to that obtained by statin alone.

Interactions
None significant.

Which drug to use when (for diet-resistant dyslipidaemias)

Elevated LDL cholesterol only
- First choice:
  - Statins.
- Second choice:
  - Cholesterol absorption blocker.
- Then:
  - Fibrates.
  - Nicotinic acid (not available in Europe).
  - Bile acid sequestrants.

Elevated triglycerides only
- First choice:
  - Fibrates.
- Second choice:
  - Omega-3 fatty acids or nicotinic acid.

All three groups can occasionally be used together if one or two of the above groups are insufficient.

Mixed hyperlipidaemia
- First choice:
  - Statin.
- Second choice:
  - Statin + fibrate (but needs close monitoring).
  - Statin + fibrate + nicotinic acid (but needs close monitoring).

As with elevated LDL alone, combination therapy may sometimes be useful, with emphasis on avoiding side effects and interactions as above.

The relative doses of lipid-lowering drugs are shown in Table 14.3.

Aims of treatment

Primary prevention:
- TC <5.2mmol/L.
- LDL cholesterol <4mmol/L.
- HDL cholesterol >1mmol/L in ♂; >1.2 in ♀ (TC:HDL ratio <6).
- Triglycerides <1.7mmol/L.

Secondary prevention. For patients with CHD or post-MI (2° prevention) and diabetes mellitus, the target should be:
- TC <4mmol/L.
- LDL cholesterol <2mmol/L.
- HDL cholesterol >1.0mmol/L in ♂; >1.2mmol/L in ♀.
- Triglycerides <1.5mmol/L.
- Apo B <1g/L.

If these optimal levels are not achievable, at least a 25% fall from pretreatment serum TC concentration or 30% reduction in LDL cholesterol is acceptable, whichever gets to the lowest.

Table 14.3 Dosage of lipid-lowering drugs

Drug	Dose/day
Statins	
Atorvastatin	10–80mg
Fluvastatin	20–80mg
Pravastatin	10–40mg
Rosuvastatin	10–40mg (5–20mg in patient of Asian origin)
Simvastatin	10–40mg
Fibrates	
Bezafibrate	400–600mg
Ciprofibrate	100mg
Fenofibrate	67–267mg
Gemfibrozil	0.9–1.2g
Anion exchange resins	
Colestyramine	12–36g (in single dose or up to 4×/day)
Colestipol hydrochloride	5g 1–2×/day (max 30g/day)
Colesevelam	1–2g 2×/day
Nicotinic acid group	
Acipimox	500–750mg in divided doses
Nicotinic acid MR	375–2,000mg
Nicotinic acid	300mg–6g in divided doses
Nicotinic acid with laropriprant	1,000–2,000mg
Omega-3 fatty acids	
Omacor®	1–4g
Cholesterol absorption blocker	
Ezetimibe	10mg

Further reading

Bhatnagar D, Soran H, Durrington PN (2008). Hypercholesterolaemia and its management. *BMJ* **337**, a993.

Chapman MJ, Ginsberg HN, Amarenco P (2011). European Atherosclerosis Society Consensus Panel. Triglyceride-rich lipoproteins and high-density lipoprotein cholesterol in patients at high risk of cardiovascular disease: evidence and guidance for management. *Eur Heart J* **32**, 1345–61.

Graham I, Atar D, Borch-Johnsen K, et al. (2007). European guidelines on cardiovascular disease prevention in clinical practice: full text. Fourth Joint Task Force of the European Society of Cardiology and other societies on cardiovascular disease prevention in clinical practice (constituted by representatives of nine societies and by invited experts). *Eur J Cardiovasc Prev Rehabil* **14** Suppl 2, S1–113.

Watts GF, Karpe F (2011). Triglycerides and atherogenic dyslipidaemia: extending treatment beyond statins in the high-risk cardiovascular patient. *Heart* **97**, 350–6.

Hippisley-Cox J, Coupland C, Vinogradova Y, et al. (2008). Predicting cardiovascular risk in England and Wales: prospective derivation and validation of QRISK2. *BMJ* **336**, 1475–82.

The National Institute for Clinical Excellence guidelines on lipid modification. Available at: ℝ http://guidance.nice.org.uk/CG67.

The National Institute for Clinical Excellence guidelines: identification and management of familial hypercholesterolaemia. Available at: ℝ http://www.nice.org.uk/CG71.

The online access to metabolic and molecular basis of inherited disease. Available at: ℝ http://www.ommbid.com/OMMBID/the online metabolic and molecular bases of inherited disease/b/parttoc/part 12.

Obesity

Definition of obesity

Obesity is defined as an excess of body fat sufficient to adversely affect health. Body mass index (BMI) and waist circumference, as a measure of fat distribution, are the most commonly used measures, but a clinical staging system is increasingly used to determine risk and management (see Box 15.1). BMI is an imprecise measure of adiposity and does not account for fat distribution, which may better determine metabolic and cardiovascular risk at lower BMI.

Lower cut-off values for BMI and waist circumference are applicable to non-Caucasian ethnic groups: cut-off points for increased risk varies from $22kg/m^2$ to $25kg/m^2$ in different Asian populations, and for high risk from $26kg/m^2$ to $31kg/m^2$.

Central obesity may reflect increased visceral (intra-abdominal fat) stores and/or 'ectopic' fat (fat stored in liver, muscle, pancreas, and epicardium) more directly linked to pathophysiology, such as insulin resistance.

Assess overall clinical status, using BMI, waist circumference, and stage (see Box 15.1).

Obesity is associated with increased secretion of adipose tissue products, including hormones, cytokines (adipocytokines), and growth factors such that it is now regarded as a disease of chronic low-grade systemic inflammation. Many of its adverse sequelae relate to this pathology.

Box 15.1 Edmonton Obesity Staging System (EOSS)

Stage 0
- No apparent obesity-related risk factors, physical symptoms, psychopathology, functional limitations, and/or impairment of well-being.

Stage 1
- Obesity-related subclinical risk factor(s) (borderline hypertension, impaired fasting glucose, elevated liver enzymes, etc.), *mild* physical symptoms (e.g. dyspnoea on moderate exertion), psychopathology, functional limitations, and/or impairment of well-being.

Stage 2
- Established obesity-related chronic disease(s) (hypertension, type 2 diabetes, sleep apnoea, osteoarthritis, reflux disease, polycystic ovary syndrome, anxiety disorder), moderate limitations in activities of daily living, and/or well-being.

Stage 3
- Established end-organ damage (myocardial infarction, heart failure, diabetes complications, incapacitating osteoarthritis), significant psychopathology, functional limitation(s), and/or impairment of well-being.

Stage 4
- Severe (potentially end-stage) disability/ies from obesity-related chronic diseases, disabling psychopathology, functional limitation(s), and/or impairment of well-being.

Epidemiology of obesity

Overweight and obesity are rapidly increasing globally; the highest rates of obesity (>30%) are seen in the USA, Mexico, and the Middle East. One billion adults are currently overweight (BMI 25–29.9kg/m^2), and a further 475 million are obese. When Asian-specific cut-off points for the definition of obesity are taken into account, the number of adults considered obese globally is over 600 million.

In the UK, prevalence has doubled in 25 years: 26.1% of adults (aged 16 years and over) were obese in 2010, and 55% of the population is either overweight or obese.

Global estimates of childhood obesity suggest 200 million school-aged children are either overweight or obese, of whom 40 million are obese.

In the UK, 10.1% of boys and 8.8% of girls aged 4–5 years and 20.6% of boys and 17.4% of girls aged 10–11 years are obese

Prevalence of obesity varies with age (peak prevalence at 50–70 years), socio-economic class (15% women and 21% men in social class I; 34% and 30% in social class V) and social deprivation in women (22% least to 31% most deprived).

Aetiology of obesity

Overweight and obesity results from a complex interaction between environmental pressures and risks and genetic susceptibility. Heritability of obesity is about 60%, but the rapid increase in obesity prevalence over the past 30 years argues in favour of predominantly environmental drivers. However, there is increasing interest in the possibility of epigenetic influences on obesity related to maternal obesity, diet, gestational diabetes, and even possibly environmental pollutants, such as polyfluorinated compounds and polycyclic aromatic hydrocarbons.

Genetic factors

Monogenic obesity

Mutations in genes (usually related to appetite control within the hypothalamus) are associated with obesity of early childhood onset, usually with hyperphagia. However, only about 5% of all severe childhood and 2% of adult obesity are associated with identified genetic causes. Of these, mutations in the melanocortin 4 receptor (MC4R) are the most frequent and are associated with increased linear growth, fat and lean mass, hyperphagia (moderate) and severe hyperinsulinaemia, but normal puberty and fertility.

An increasing number of genes associated with the development of obesity have been identified through genome-wide association studies. The FTO 'fat mass and obesity associated' gene was originally linked to type 2 diabetes; the association was actually found to be due to the higher BMI of diabetic cases in comparison to non-diabetic controls; common variants in the first intron result in a $+0.4\text{kg/m}^2$ elevation in BMI per risk allele. Similar to the situation with type 2 diabetes, possession of 'risk' single nucleotide polymorphisms (SNPs) only accounts for a small increase in susceptibility to obesity or adult BMI.

Environmental factors

The drivers of obesity can be considered under two main headings: increased energy (food) intake or decreased energy expenditure due to physical inactivity, as the major determinants of obesity in genetically susceptible individuals. Societal changes, e.g. increased availability of high caloric density foods and sedentary lifestyle, have been one of the main causes of changes in this balance.

Secondary causes

These are uncommon because, even when linked to weight gain, the disease usually manifests itself from its particular pathophysiology.

- Hypothyroidism: an important cause to exclude in children but rarely presents simply with weight gain in adults.
- Cushing's disease/syndrome: rare, but an important cause to exclude in obese patients presenting with 'overlap' signs and symptoms which can include striae, depression, and hypertension.

- Hypothalamic lesions: gonadal failure, visual disturbances, headache, or raised intracranial pressure often predominate as presenting signs, rather than weight gain and hyperphagia.
- Polycystic ovary syndrome (PCOS): strongly linked to overweight and obesity but mechanism unclear. Features of hyperandrogenism and oligomenorrhoea may result from obesity itself.
- Iatrogenic: drugs, e.g. antipsychotic medication, hypoglycaemics (including insulin) glucocorticoids. Also recreational drugs, e.g. cannabis.

Pathophysiology of obesity

Energy balance and body weight are regulated, but the main drive of this allostatic physiology is towards energy acquisition (and thus fat deposition) and defence against weight loss. Although physiology can be 'overridden' by cognitive and behavioural control (e.g. diet, exercise) long-term, these mechanisms (within our obesogenic environment) usually prove insufficient in the long-term either to protect against or reverse weight gain.

Long-term signals associated with body fat stores are provided by leptin and insulin. In human obesity, leptin levels are high, rather than low, correlating with fat mass, suggesting either that leptin 'resistance' is present or that leptin is a starvation, rather than obesity, signal (see Box 15.2 and Table 15.1).

Gut peptide hormones released after food intake provide acute signals of hunger, satiety, and fullness (see Box 15.3). Although originally thought to be short-term signals, the importance of the gut–brain axis as a regulator of body weight in humans has become increasingly apparent from the effects of bariatric surgery. Ghrelin, a hunger hormone, rises before, and probably is involved with, initiation of food intake. Satiety hormones released after food include glucagon-like peptide-1 (GLP-1), an incretin hormone secreted by ileal L-cells in the distal intestine that stimulates insulin secretion, and peptide YY secreted from the ileum and colon. Oxyntomodulin (also derived from preproglucagon) reduces food intake and increases energy expenditure after systemic administration.

Weight is gained or lost usually in the proportion of 70% fat and 30% lean tissue, implying that approximately 30MJ (7,000kcal) surplus or deficit is needed to gain or lose 1 kg in body mass. During the first days of a very low energy or ketogenic diet, liver glycogen may be the primary source of stored energy to meet metabolic needs; since it provides about 8MJ/kg, initial weight loss is more rapid than with less severe energy restriction.

Box 15.2 Leptin

- Synthesized in, and secreted by, adipose tissue (subcut > visceral).
- Encoded by *LEP* gene (chromosome 7q31.3).
- Hypothalamic receptors, activated through entry via arcuate nucleus (exposed to peripheral circulation), decrease food intake and increase energy expenditure (by sympathetic activation).
- Stimulated by glucocorticoids.
- Human obesity persists, despite high circulating levels of leptin (proportional to fat mass), suggesting resistance to effects or that, in human physiology, leptin signals low body fat stores, such as in starvation.
- Mutations in *LEP* lead to a rare syndrome of hyperphagia, obesity, hypogonadism, and impaired immunity. Features are reversed by recombinant leptin replacement.
- In conditions of selective decrease in adipose tissue mass (lipodystrophy, HIV or HIV therapy-associated lipoatrophy, severe anorexia nervosa), leptin replacement therapy reverses insulin resistance.
- In response to fasting, leptin levels fall rapidly before, and out of proportion to, changes in fat mass, triggering the neuroendocrine response to acute energy deprivation.
- Trials of leptin augmentation in common obesity do not lead to weight loss or maintenance of weight loss.

Table 15.1 Leptin deficiency

Type	Frequency	Features
Complete congenital	Rare	hyperphagia hypogonadotrophic advanced bone age hyperinsulinaemic immune dysfunction
Heterozygous	5–6 %	
Leptin resistant gene mutations	Rare	hypogonadotrophic abnormal GH and TSH secretion
POMC mutation	Rare	ACTH ↓ red hair, pale skin
MCR 4 mutation	Rare	↑ growth ↑ bone mineral density

Box 15.3 Gut peptide hormones linked to weight regulation

Ghrelin
- The only known 'hunger' hormone.
- Derived from preproghrelin secreted in the stomach, cleaved to active form acyl ghrelin (28 amino acid peptide) and obestatin.
- Acts on hypothalamic GH secretagogue receptors (GHSR1a) to increase the release of GH from the pituitary.
- Peripherally injected ghrelin increases food intake through the stimulation of ghrelin receptors on hypothalamic neuropeptide Y-expressing neurons and agouti-related protein-expressing neurons.
- Levels in obesity not consistently elevated but are markedly reduced by bariatric surgery (sleeve gastrectomy and gastric bypass).
- Circulating ghrelin increases preprandially and decreases postprandially and is thought to regulate premeal hunger and meal initiation.
- GHSR1a is also expressed in other brain areas, linking to the mesolimbic reward neuropathway and to central pathways of energy balance.
- Ghrelin is also involved in modulating reward and motivation in enhancing the hedonic and incentive response to food-related cues.

Glucagon-like peptide-1 (GLP-1)
- Secreted by L-cells in the distal intestine.
- Stimulates insulin secretion and (in animals) islet cell differentiation and proliferation.
- Inhibits glucagon secretion; inhibits gastric emptying.
- Unlike GIP, levels of GLP-1 are reduced in patients with diabetes.
- Levels raised preferentially by protein, accounting, in part, of protein's higher satiating effects compared to other macronutrients.
- GLP-1 analogues (exenatide and liraglutide) are associated with ~5% weight loss.
- Liraglutide (see 🕮 p. 716), in higher doses than used for diabetes treatment, produces sustained weight loss >10% in non-diabetic subjects.
- Levels markedly elevated after bariatric surgery.

Peptide YY
- 36 amino acid peptide synthesized and released in L-cells in distal GI tract.
- Conversion of PYY1-36 to active PYY3-36 by dipeptidyl peptidase IV (DPP-IV).
- PYY3-36 shows affinity for hypothalamic neuropeptide Y neurones.
- PYY levels are low in the fasting state, rapidly increase in response to food intake, peak at 1–2h after a meal, and remain elevated for several hours.
- In addition to regulating food intake, PYY3-36 has additional metabolic beneficial effects on energy expenditure and fuel partitioning.

Consequences of obesity

Most metabolic, physiological, and organ systems are affected by obesity and can be considered under the '4 M' headings: mental, metabolic, mechanical, and monetary (see Box 15.4).

- Mortality rates rise steadily at BMI >5kg/m^2. Obesity and physical inactivity have both independent and dependent effects on all-cause mortality.
- Loss of life expectancy: BMI >35kg/m^2—5–7 years at age 45.
- Type 2 diabetes: elevation in BMI, the dominant risk factor for development of diabetes. Relative risk (RR) in overweight men 2.4, women 12.4; at BMI 30kg/m^2 >10; increased to 50–90-fold at BMI >35.
- Hypertension: RR for overweight men 1.8, women 2.4.
- Dyslipidaemia: moderate relationship with total cholesterol, closer relationship with triglycerides, HDL cholesterol.
- Stroke: RR 1.2 for overweight and 1.5 for obese men and women.
- Asthma: obese 2 ×, overweight 1.4 × more likely to develop asthma.

Box 15.4 Obesity associations and consequences

'Mental'	'Mechanical'	'Metabolic'	'Monetary'
Depression	Sleep apnoea	Type 2 diabetes	Lower educational achievement
Low self-esteem	Hypoventilation	Dyslipidaemia	Employment discrimination
Attention deficit disorder	Osteoarthritis	Hypertension	Lower income
Eating disorder	Chronic pain	IHD	Chronic disability
Cognitive impairment	Gastro-oesophageal reflux	Gout	Increased healthcare costs
	Incontinence	NAFLD and NASH	
	Thrombosis	Cancer	
	Intertrigo		

Management of an obese patient

The use of a structured approach, modified from management of other chronic diseases, consists of *Ask*, *Assess*, *Advise*, *Agree*, and *Assist* (5 As).

Ask permission to discuss weight

A non-judgemental approach, using motivational interviewing techniques, that also explores the patient's readiness to change is recommended.

Assess 'root causes' of obesity and obesity-related risk

History

- Weight history from birth onwards (early onset may suggest genetic syndromes).
- Previous treatment/management strategies and their success.
- Current eating habits and triggers for eating/activity levels.
- Family history of obesity and obesity-related disease.
- Symptoms or previous diagnosis of obesity-related diseases, including CVD, diabetes, psychological issues (eating disorder, depression, low self-esteem), OA, obstructive sleep apnoea, PCOS.
- Symptoms of reflux.
- Other risks, such as smoking and alcohol intake.
- Drugs that might exacerbate weight gain.
- Patient's beliefs and expectations.
- Optimal management of other diseases, obesity-related or not.

Examination

- Height, weight, fat distribution.
- General: evidence for syndrome (e.g. small hands and facies in Prader–Willi syndrome), mood.
- Skin: acanthosis nigricans and skin tags (insulin resistance), intertrigo, fat distribution (partial lipodystrophy).
- Cardiovascular: hypertension, heart failure, and other causes for breathlessness.
- Respiratory: airway, obstructive sleep apnoea (somnolence), pulmonary hypertension, cardiopulmonary fitness (consider 6-minute walk test).
- GI: hepatomegaly, herniae (may influence bariatric surgery).
- Musculoskeletal: mobility.
- Consider other diagnoses: hypothyroidism, Cushing's syndrome, haemochromatosis.

Investigations

- Blood count and iron studies (iron deficiency anaemia from reflux or GI bleeding; polycythaemia from hypoventilation).
- Renal function.
- Liver function (non-alcoholic steatohepatitis).
- Glucose, HbA1c, and possibly insulin (prediabetes, diabetes).
- Fasting lipid profile (raised triglycerides, total and LDL cholesterol, lowered HDL cholesterol).
- Vitamin D (often deficient in the obese).
- Thyroid function (hypothyroidism).
- ECG (atrial fibrillation, left ventricular hypertrophy).

Additional tests
- Liver ultrasound if abnormal liver function to confirm NAFLD.
- Echocardiogram if heart failure suspected.
- Pharmacological stress testing if ischaemic heart disease suspected (subject may be unable to undertake exercise test).
- Endoscopy if anaemia—gastroscopy if reflux disease, colonoscopy if colon cancer suspected.
- Gynaecological referral if post-menopausal bleeding (high incidence of endometrial cancer in obese women).
- Dexamethasone suppression (overnight or low-dose) if Cushing's disease suspected.
- Transferrin, then genetic testing for haemochromatosis in patients with type 2 diabetes and abnormal liver function.

Advise on risks of obesity, benefits of weight loss and treatment options, and the need for a long-term strategy. Treatment options include:
- Stress management and self-assertiveness training.
- Dietary intervention.
- Physical activity.
- Psychological counselling.
- Anti-obesity medication.
- Bariatric surgery.

Agree on:
- Weight loss goals.
- Behavioural goals and health outcomes.
- Management plan.

Assist in addressing drivers and barriers to weight management; offer referral to appropriate provider (primary care for diet and lifestyle programmes, psychology services if binge eating disorder or severe depression, secondary care if obesity severe or complex).

General principles

Dietary energy restriction produces greater weight loss than exercise. Increased physical activity and exercise predicts weight loss maintenance.

Patients' expectations frequently exceed realistic goals or need.

A weight loss of 5–10% of the initial body weight reduces many of the health risks associated with obesity and reduces cancer and diabetes-related mortality; a 5kg loss in adults with prediabetes reduces progression to diabetes by 60%, maintained even if weight regain occurs. In patients with a BMI >35kg/m^2, greater weight loss (>10kg or 15%) is likely to be needed to produce a sustained improvement in comorbid diseases; 10–15% may be needed.

Diet, physical activity, and behavioural therapy
- Dietary advice should aim to reduce energy intake to produce a 2.5MJ (600kcal)/day deficit (calculated from standard equations of resting energy expenditure and assuming a physical activity level (PAL) of 1.3). Both low carbohydrate (<30g/day) and low fat (<30% total daily energy) produce equivalent weight loss (4–5kg) at 1 year. High-protein diets may be more satiating.

- Commercial providers (e.g. Weight Watchers, Rosemary Conley) can achieve equivalent, or better, results than GPs or pharmacists.
- Low (3.4–5MJ; 800–1,200kcal/day) and very low (<3.5MJ, 800kcal/day) diets produce more rapid initial weight loss and, in combination with behaviour therapy and pharmacotherapy, produce sustained weight loss greater than that achieved with conventional diets.
- Regular exercise induces cardiorespiratory fitness and leads to a beneficial effect on other risk factors, with a reduction in blood pressure and improvement in lipid profile.
- The PAR-Q physical activity readiness questionnaire provides a quick and validated screening tool to risk-assess patients before they start an exercise programme.
- 225–300min/week of moderate intensity exercise (equivalent to 7.5–10.5MJ, 1,800–2,500kcal) is recommended for weight loss maintenance.
- Behavioural interventions may include self-monitoring of behaviour and progress, stimulus control, goal-setting, problem-solving and assertiveness training, relapse prevention and management but has only been shown to provide modest benefit in terms of weight outcomes

Anti-obesity drugs

In Europe, only orlistat is licensed; elsewhere, phentermine is widely prescribed. Several new drugs (lorcaserin, a 5HT2c agonist; Qnexa®, a combination of phentermine and topiramate; Contrave®, a combination of naltrexone and bupropion) are currently under review by the US licensing authorities. The GLP-1 agonist liraglutide is in phase 3 trials, at higher doses than used for treating diabetes, as a weight loss drug in non-diabetic patients. Off-label use of drugs is not recommended: the history of anti-obesity pharmacotherapy has seen many adverse effects emerge, even with well-investigated and developed drugs, such as sibutramine (withdrawn in 2010 due to adverse cardiovascular outcomes) and rimonabant (withdrawn in 2009 due to depression and suicide risk).

Orlistat

- Intestinal pancreatic lipase inhibitor; reduces fat absorption.
- Increases dietary fat loss to 30% (compared to <5% on placebo).
- Best used in those at medical risk from obesity: BMI >30kg/m² or BMI >27 with established comorbidities (e.g. diabetes, heart disease, dyslipidaemia).
- May have modest insulin-sensitizing effects over and above weight loss (reduced portal triglyceride levels).
- Only use in patients who achieve at least 2.5kg weight loss in 4 weeks using a dietary programme alone (NICE guidelines). This ensures adequate dietary compliance with a low-fat diet (ideally <50g/day) and minimizes GI side effects.
- Average weight loss of 8% at 1 year.
- NICE guidelines:
  - At 3 months, stop if <5% weight loss.
  - At 6 months, stop if <10% weight loss (of initial weight).

- Contraindications: cholestasis, hepatic dysfunction, malabsorption, pregnancy, breastfeeding, concomitant use of fibrate, acarbose, renal impairment (creatinine >150micromol/L), anticoagulation (possible ↓ vitamin K absorption with orlistat).
- Consider vitamin supplementation (especially vitamin D) if used beyond 1 year.
- Side effects (must warn patient): flatus (24%), oily rectal discharge, fatty stool (20%), faecal urgency (22%), fat-soluble vitamin deficiency, incontinence (8%). Limited by dietary fat reduction (to <35% of energy).

Bariatric surgery

Three types of surgery are commonly performed—all usually done laparoscopically. The most compelling data for the success of bariatric surgery at producing weight loss and improving the clinical outcomes for obese patients come from the 20-year follow-up data of the Swedish Obese Subjects study (a case control study started at a time when surgical techniques were not as advanced as nowadays). The persistent weight loss in the surgical groups was associated with a much reduced mortality: the unadjusted overall hazard ratio was 0.76 in the surgery group (P = 0.04), compared with the control group, and the hazard ratio adjusted for sex, age, and risk factors was 0.71 (P = 0.01). Other studies have confirmed that bariatric surgery is associated with reduced all-cause mortality, including deaths from CVD, diabetes, and cancer.

In patients with type 2 diabetes, benefit extends beyond weight loss. Up to 80% of people with type 2 diabetes may experience remission of their diabetes (normoglycaemia without the need for hypoglycaemic medication), the exact remission rate being determined by the type of surgery and the duration of diabetes prior to surgery.

Gastric bypass (see Fig. 15.1)

Patients will lose approximately 50–75% of their excess weight (30–40% absolute weight loss) within 12–18 months of surgery. The large majority (>80%) of patients will have a significant improvement or resolution of their weight-related illnesses, and most patients report dramatic changes to their quality of life. Routine supplementation of vitamins, minerals, and vitamin B12 is required.

The gastric bypass works in the following way:
- There is a restriction in food intake, as the stomach is reduced to the size of a large egg.
- Food bypasses digestive secretions, causing some malabsorption.
- Profound changes are seen in gut hormones that control hunger, satiety, and glucose metabolism (reduced ghrelin, increased and earlier release of GLP-1 and PYY).
- Other mechanisms, involving changes in gut flora and bile salt metabolism that affect appetite and CV risk, are also postulated.

Sleeve gastrectomy (see Fig. 15.2)

Patients will lose approximately 50–75% (30–40% absolute weight loss) of their excess weight within 12–18 months of surgery. Again, >80% have a significant improvement in weight-related illnesses and improved QoL. Routine supplementation of vitamins is required for the first year.

The sleeve gastrectomy works in the following way:
- 75% of the stomach is removed, restricting the volume of food patients are able to eat in one sitting.
- Gastric emptying is faster which alters gut hormone profiles, resulting in satiety (reduced ghrelin, increased and earlier release of GLP-1 and PYY).

Gastric Bypass

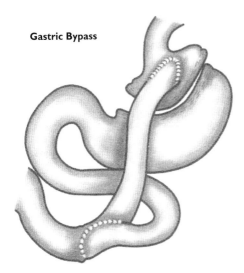

Fig. 15.1 Gastric bypass.

Sleeve Gastrectomy

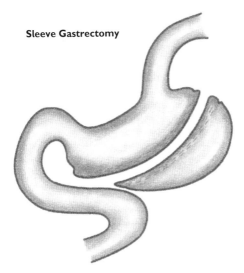

Fig. 15.2 Sleeve gastrectomy.

Adjustable gastric banding (see Fig. 15.3)

Patients will lose approximately 50% of their excess weight (30% absolute weight loss) within 2–3 years of surgery. Routine supplementation of vitamins, minerals, and vitamin B12 is not usually needed beyond the first year.
The gastric band works in the following way:

- Gastric restriction is achieved by placing an adjustable silastic band around the upper gastric cardia that can be tightened or loosened by injecting saline into a tube that connects to a port under the skin. The restriction slows the speed of eating.
- Patients are required to attend clinic for band consultations every 2–3 months until the right degree of band adjustment is achieved.

Pre- and post-operative care needs to be provided by specialist multidisciplinary teams.

Bariatric surgery and diabetes

In 2011, the International Diabetes Federation recommended that bariatric surgery:

- Constitutes a powerful option to ameliorate diabetes in severely obese patients, often normalizing blood glucose levels, reducing or avoiding the need for medications, and providing a potentially cost-effective approach to treating the disease.
- Is an appropriate treatment for people with type 2 diabetes and obesity not achieving recommended treatment targets with medical therapies.

Adjustable Gastric Band

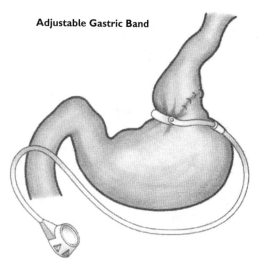

Fig. 15.3 Adjustable gastric banding.

- Should be an accepted option in people who have type 2 diabetes and a BMI >35 and even an alternative treatment option in patients with a BMI between 30 and 35 when diabetes cannot be adequately controlled by optimal medical regimen, especially in the presence of other major cardiovascular disease risk factors.

Further reading

Chandarana K, Gelegen C, Karra E, et al. (2011). Diet and gastrointestinal bypass–induced weight loss. The roles of ghrelin and peptide YY. *Diabetes* **60**, 810–18.

Hinney A, Vogel CIG, Hebebrand J (2010). From monogenic to polygenic obesity: recent advances. *Eur Child Adolesc Psychiatry* **19**, 297–310.

Kelesedis T, Kelesidis I, Chou S, et al. (2010). Narrative review: the role of leptin in human physiology: emerging clinical applications. *Ann Intern Med* **152**, 93–100.

National Institute for Health and Clinical Excellence (NICE) Clinical guideline 43: obesity guidance on the prevention, identification, assessment, and management of overweight and obesity in adults and children. Available at: ℘ http://www.nice.org.uk/nicemedia/live/11000/30365/30365.pdf.

Ramachandran S, Farooqi IS (2011). Genetic approaches to understanding human obesity. *J Clin Invest* **121**, 2080–6.

Rucher D, Padwal R, Li SK, et al. (2007). Long term pharmacotherapy for obesity and overweight: updated meta-analysis. *BMJ* **335**, 1194–9.

Scottish Intercollegiate Guidelines Network (2010). Management of obesity: a national clinical guideline. Edinburgh. Available at: ℘ http://www.sign.ac.uk.

Sharma AM, Kushner AF (2009). A proposed clinical staging system for obesity. *Int J Obes (Lond)* **33**, 289–95.

Sjöström L, Peltonen M, Jacobsen P, et al. (2012). Bariatric surgery and long-term cardiovascular events. *JAMA* **307**, 56–65.

Tsigos C, Hainer V, Basdevant A, et al. (2008). Management of obesity in adults: European clinical practice guidelines. *Obesity facts* **1**, 106–16.

Pitfalls in laboratory endocrinology

Introduction

As with all biochemical investigations, their usefulness lies in careful and appropriate selection, combined with discerning interpretation. Where neither is possible nor simple, the chemical pathologist, or other members of the analysing laboratory, would always be happy to help.

The results obtained by the wide variety of analytical techniques can be altered by many factors, some associated with an underlying pathology and others not. A brief consideration of potential confounding factors seems relevant here.

Box A1.1 Factors influencing laboratory investigations

- Pre-analytical factors:
  - Sample timing—in relation to dose, stimulation, suppression, diurnal variation, etc.
  - Which tube, preservative, order of blood collection into a variety of different tubes?
  - Rapidity and temperature of transport required to maintain sample stability, or when to centrifuge and separate.
  - Biological variation—within-person variation (see Box A1.2).
  - Which stimulation/suppression test?
- Analytical factors:
  - Assay specificity, sensitivity, and overall performance.
  - Assay standardization—quality control, quality assurance.
  - Analytical performance—precision, accuracy, robustness, etc.
  - Hook effects (e.g. prolactin) in very high concentrations, requiring dilution and re-measurement to exclude as a confounding factor.
  - Sample interference—haemolysis, lipaemia, or icteric/elevated bilirubin levels. Most analysers have automatic detection levels of each interference.
  - Antibody interference—heterophilic antibodies can increase assayed, but not biologically active, measurements.
  - Particularly problematic assays—very low concentrations, poorly specific antibodies, commonly occurring interferences, etc.
- Post-analytical factors:
  - Reference interval.
  - Units of standardization.
  - Interpretation in the specific clinical setting and dynamic function test—complicated results are often best addressed by joint endocrinologist's and chemical pathologist's input in MDT meetings.

Box A1.2 Examples of within-person (biological) variation

- Aldosterone, 29%
- Androstenedione, 16%
- CA125, 36%
- CA153, 5.7%
- CEA, 10.6%
- DHAS, 3.4%
- Prolactin, 24%
- SHBG, 9%
- Testosterone (♂), 10%
- TSH, 20%

Variation expressed as cv (%) (Coefficient of variation = (standard deviation/mean) × 100).

Analytical factors

Most endocrine assays are immunoassays which rely on binding of an analyte by a diagnostic antibody. The binding specificity will depend on the care and attention with which the manufacturer has chosen the reagents. Typical interferences in small molecules are due to slightly different molecular forms and typically occur with steroid and digoxin assays. Peptide hormones are more complex because so many differently glycosylated forms of those peptides exist.

Standards for pituitary hormones are generally derived from purified pituitary extracts which contain a mixture of peptides. This leads to different assays having quite marked biases between each other due to different binding affinities of the antibodies to the different isoforms. A similar situation exists with hCG for which many multiple molecular forms co-exist. Attempts to find international consensus for standards which can be used in diagnostic systems are being made, particularly for growth hormone and glycated haemoglobin at the present time.

Analytical performance or assay reproducibility is important in determining the critical differences between patient samples. A significant difference between consecutive samples at 95% confidence will require a difference of 1.96 x the method standard deviation at the appropriate concentration.

The hook effect occurs when very high analyte concentrations flood the available antibody *in vitro* and this leads to artefactually low results. It is less common nowadays as assays have large dynamic ranges but new cases continue to be reported, and there are published case reports for all hormones and tumour markers.

Antibody interference is a widespread problem that affects approximately 1% of immunoassays. It is insidious and is due to endogenous antibodies which interfere with analyte binding *in vitro*. Most importantly, they cannot be detected by usual quality control mechanisms. There are a number of laboratory techniques that can be used to clarify whether such interference is present but it is inherent on the clinician to alert the laboratory to a potential clinical mismatch.

Some assays can only be classified as problem assays. These include thyroglobulin and low concentrations of oestradiol (<300pmol/L) and testosterone (<5nmol/L). The former is due to the high prevalence of endogenous anti-thyroglobulin antibodies which are particularly prevalent in patients with thyroid disease. The latter are due to antibody specificity; however, it is hoped that this will be resolved with the introduction of mass spectrometry into routine clinical practice.

Post-analytical factors

Interpretation of assay results is made in relation to reference ranges provided by the laboratory. These usually represent the 95th centiles of a population of healthy individuals. However, the definition of normality is subjective and reference ranges are affected by such factors as age, gender, and in some cases by ethnicity. Moreover, for hormones, time of day, month, and season will be important. For some analytes, it is diffi cult to obtain appropriate samples to construct ranges such as in children and circumstances that are difficult to obtain in health e.g. following pharmacological stimulation or samples of CSF.

If the central 95th centile reference ranges are used, there is a 5% chance that a result will be out-of-range due to chance. As the number of tests taken are ↑, so will the risk of a chance abnormality. The increase will be x% (where $x = 1 – 0.95^a$ and a is the number of tests performed).

Literature from the USA and European journals may use different units—beware! SI units use molar or mass (g) and volumes reported in litres.

Most assays are standardized with international preparations. These are usually the molecular forms that are most prevalent when basal samples are taken. However, following stimulation non-standard molecules are released into the circulation which have different clearance rates and different binding characteristics to the diagnostic antibodies *in vitro*. This can lead to marked differences between methods. For example, following stimulation by ACTH corticosteroid precursors are released which will compete with cortisol for binding in the assay; similarly following stimulation of GH release different isoforms of GH are secreted and the most abundant 20 and 22kDa isoforms clear at different rates leading to variations in recognition by the diagnostic antibodies at different times during the test.

Box A1.3 Disastrous outcomes

- *Assay interference*: a series of patients has been described in whom aggressive therapy for choriocarcinoma was instituted for diagnoses that were based on assays affected by *in vitro* artefacts.
- *Antibody specificity*: a patient has been described who had prolactin measured by 3 different assays giving 3 different answers. The solution awaited a clinical answer when the hyperprolactinaemia resolved after stopping the offending medication.
- *Interference by insulin auto-antibodies*: a patient has been described with recurrent hypoglycaemia due to insulin auto antibodies caused by myeloma. This patient demonstrated *in vivo* interference by endogenous antibodies as well as *in vitro* interference.
- *Hook effect*: a patient presents with a large pituitary tumour that appears to be non-functioning as the prolactin is normal and the patient is treated surgically. The following day the blood sample is reassayed after dilution and the high prolactin is uncovered when the antibody is no longer flooded by excess prolactin.

Appendix 2
Reference intervals

Introduction

All values are for serum unless specified otherwise.

Box A2.1 Definitions
- Serum. A serum sample is collected in a plain tube, left to permit clotting, then centrifuged and separated.
- Plasma. A plasma specimen is collected in a tube containing EDTA or lithium heparin, centrifuged immediately, and separated.

Box A2.2 Table notes

[a] EDTA tube cold spun immediately and frozen on separation.

[b] Serum, cold spun, flash frozen.

[c] Fasting sample collected into 2 × EDTA tubes, cold spun, and flash frozen.

[d] Acid-containing container (20mL 6M HCl).

Table A2.1 Thyroid function

Analyte	SI units	Traditional units	Conversion factor
TSH	0.35–5.50mU/L	0.35–5.50mU/L	1
Free T_4	10.5–20pmol/L	0.8–1.6ng/dL	12.9
Total T_3	0.9–2.8nmol/L	60–190ng/dL	0.015
Free T_3	3.5–6.5pmol/L	2.3–4.3pg/mL	1.54
Thyroid-binding globulin		13–28ng/L	
Thyroid-stimulating hormone receptor antibodies		<7U/L	
Antithyroid peroxidase antibodies		<50IU/mL	

Table A2.2 Adrenal and gonadal function

Analyte		SI units	Traditional units	Conversion factor
Cortisol (9 a.m.)		180–620nmol/L	6.5–22.5ng/dL	27.6
Aldosterone (Charing Cross)	Random	100–800pmol/L	3.6–28.9ng/dL	27.7
	Supine	100–450pmol/L	3.6–16.2ng/dL	27.7
Plasma renin activity (Charing Cross)	Random	0.5–3.1pmol/mL/h	N/A*	
	Supine	1.1–2.7pmol/mL/h	N/A	
	Ambulant (30min)	2.8–4.5pmol/mL/h	N/A	
Serum 11-deoxycortisol		24–46nmol/L		
DHEAS	♀	1.9–9.4micromol/L	5.1–25.4pg/mL	0.0027
	♂	2.8–12micromol/L	7.6–32.4pg/mL	0.0027
Androstenedione	♀	3.0–8.0nmol/L	10.5–27.5 micrograms/L	3.49
	♂	3.0–8.0nmol/L	10.5–27.5 micrograms/L	3.49
17-hydroxy-progesterone (Barts)	♀			
	Follicular	1–8.7nmol/L	3.3–28.7 micrograms/L	3.3
	Luteal	<18nmol/L	<59.4 micrograms/L	
	♂	1–8.7nmol/L	3.3–28.7 micrograms/L	3.3
	Neonatal	20nmol/L	<66 micrograms/L	
Oestradiol	♀ Follicular	69–905pmol/L	248–325pg/mL	3.6
	Midcycle	130–2095pmol/L	468–7542pg/mL	3.6
	Luteal	82–940pmol/L	295–3384pg/mL	3.6
	♂	43–151pmol/L	155–544pg/mL	3.6
Progesterone	♀	0–90nmol/L	0–288ng/mL	3.2
	♂	0–10nmol/L	0–32ng/mL	3.2
Testosterone	♀	0.5–2.6nmol/L	1.7–9ng/mL	3.5
	♂	8.4–28.7nmol/L	29–100ng/mL	3.5
DHT (Barts)	♀	0.1–0.8nmol/L	2.9–23ng/dL	0.034
	♂	1–2.9nmol/L	29–85ng/dL	0.034
SHBG	♀	18–114nmol/L	18–114nmol/L	1
	♂	13–71nmol/L	13–71nmol/L	1
Adrenaline (after 30min resting)		0.03–1.31nmol/L		
Noradrenaline (after 30min resting)		0.47–4.14nmol/L		

* A variety of different units are used by non-UN labs.

Table A2.3 Pituitary hormones

Analyte		SI units	Traditional units	Conversion factor
FSH	♀ Follicular	2.5–10.2U/L	2.5–10.2mU/mL	1
	Midcycle	3.4–33.4U/L	3.4–33.4mU/mL	1
	Luteal	1.5–9.1U/L	1.5–9.1mU/mL	1
	Post-menopausal	23–116U/L	23–116mU/mL	1
	♂	1.4–18.1U/L	1.4–18.1mU/mL	1
LH	♀ Follicular	1.9–12.5U/L	1.9–12.5mU/mL	1
	Midcycle	8.7–76.3U/L	8.7–76.3mU/mL	1
	Luteal	0.5–16.9U/L	0.5–16.9mU/mL	1
	Post-menopausal	15.9–54U/L	15.9–54mU/mL	1
	♂	1.5–9.3U/L	1.5–9.3mU/mL	1
Prolactin	♀	60–620mU/L	3–31ng/mL	20
	♂	45–375mU/L	2.2–19ng/mL	20
IGF-1	20 years	16–118nmol/L	120–885ng/mL	7.5
	40 years	14–47nmol/L	105–353ng/mL	
	60 years	10.5–35nmol/L	79–263ng/mL	
	>60 years	7.0–28nmol/L	52–210ng/mL	
IGF-1:IGF-2 ratio		>10		
ACTH[a]		2.2–17.6pmol/L	10–80ng/L	0.22
Inhibin B (Charing Cross)		80–150pg/mL		

[a] EDTA tube cold spun immediately and frozen on separation.

Table A2.4 Bone biochemistry

Analyte	SI units	Traditional units	Conversion factor
Parathyroid hormone[b]	1.3–7.6pmol/L	13–73pg/mL	0.1
Total 25-hydroxy-colecalciferol[b]	25–125nmol/L	10–50ng/mL	2.5
25-hydroxycalcitriol			2.4
Deficiency	<30nmol/L	<12.5ng/mL	
Insufficiency	30–79nmol/L	12.5–33ng/mL	
Sufficiency	80–150nmol/L	33–63ng/mL	
1,25-dihydroxy-colecalciferol[b] (Liverpool)	43–144pmol/L	18–60pg/mL	2.4
Calcitonin[a]	<0.10ng/L		
P1NP[b] procollagen extension peptide	20–60 micrograms/L		

[a] EDTA tube cold spun immediately and frozen on separation.

[b] Serum, cold spun, flash frozen.

Table A2.5 Plasma gastrointestinal and pancreatic hormones

Analyte	SI units	Traditional units	Conversion factor
Insulin (fasting)	18–77pmol/L	2.6–11.1mU/L	6.9
C-peptide (fasting)	0.27–1.28nmol/L	0.8–3.88ng/mL	0.33
Gastrin[c]	0–40pmol/L	0–89pg/mL	0.45
Glucagon[c]	0–50 pmol/L	0–179pg/mL	0.28
Vasoactive intestinal polypeptide (VIP)[c]	0–30pmol/L	0–71pg/mL	0.42
Pancreatic polypeptide[c]	0–300pmol/L	0–1250pg/mL	0.24
Somatostatin[c]	0–150pmol/L		
Chromogranin A[c]	0–60pmol/L		
Chromogranin B[c]	0–150pmol/L		
Neurotensin[c]	0–100pmol/L		

[c] 2× EDTA tubes cold spun and flash frozen.

Table A2.6 Tumour markers

Analyte	SI units
β-hCG	0–4U/L
Carcinoembryonic antigen (CEA)	0–3U/L
Prostate-specific antigen (PSA)	0–4 micrograms/L
Alpha fetoprotein	0–7IU/mL

Table A2.7 Urinary collections (1)

Analyte	♀ SI units (micromol/24h)	♂ SI units (micromol/24h)
Normetadrenaline[d]		
20–40 years	3.0	3.6
40–60 years	3.45	4.25
60–80 years	3.65	4.5
Metadrenaline[d]		
20–40 years	1.4	1.9
40–60 years	1.4	1.9
60–80 years	1.4	1.9
3-methoxytyramine[d]		
20–40 years	2.75	3.3
40–60 years	2.55	3.1
60–80 years	2.3	2.8

[d] Acid-containing container (20mL 6M HCl).

Table A2.8 Urinary collections (2)

Urinary analyte	SI units (mmol/L)	Traditional units	SI units (mmol/24h)	Conversion factor
Cortisol			0–560	
Calcium	1.25–3.75	50–150mg/L	2.5–7.5	0.025
Phosphate	7.5–25	0.2–0.8mg/L	12.9–42	32.3
Potassium	20–60	20–60mmol/L	♀: 34–103 ♂: 37–139	1.0
Sodium	50–125	50–125mmol/L	♀: 61–214 ♂: 83–287	1.0
5-hydroxyin-doleacetic acid[d]		1.9–7.7mg/24h	10–40Umol/L/24h	5.2
Aldosterone			14–53nmol/L	

[d] Acid-containing container (20mL 6M HCl).

Table A2.9 Table of analyses

Analyte	SI Units	Other Units		Conversion factor
Fasting Glucose[1]				
Normal	≤6.0 mmol/l	≤108mg/dl		
Impaired fasting glycaemia	≥6.1<7.0 mmol/l	≥11<126mg/dl		
Diabetes	≥7.0 mmol/l	≥126mg/dl		
2-hour glucose in 75g OGTT:				18
Normal	<7.8 mmol/l	<140 mg/dl		
Impaired glucose tolerance	≥7.8 <11.1 mmol/l	≥140<200mg/dl		
Diabetes	≥11.1 mmol/	≥200mg/dl		
HbA1c (non-diabetic range)	< 48 mmol/ mol	<6.5		mmol/mol value = (% value × 10.93) − 23.5 % value=(0.0915 × mmol/mol value) + 2.15[2]
Total Cholesterol[3]	≤ 6.5 mmol/l	195 mg/dl		
HDL-Cholesterol[3]	>1.5 mmol/	>60 mg/dl		38.6
LDL-Cholesterol[3]	≤4	115 mg/dl		
Fasting triglycerides	0.55–1.9 mmol/l	49–168 mg/dl		88.5
Adiponectin Inversely correlated with body % fat	N/A	Males µg/ml 5–25	Females µg/ml 5–35	N/A
Leptin Correlated with % body fat	N/A	Males ng/ml 1–10	Females ng/ml 4–25	N/A

[1] Figures quoted are World Health Organisation definitions. The American Diabetes Association have a lower cut off for normal fasting glucose of 5.6 mmol/l or 100mg/dl

[2] Not straightforward, best to download a converter to your smartphone or print out a chart for the clinic wall.

[3] The appropriate cholesterol level for an individual depends on cardiovascular risk, presence of diabetes and whether primary or secondary prevention. The figures quoted would be appropriate for primary prevention. See also 📖 pp. 810, 824.

Patient support groups and other endocrine organizations

Addison's Disease Self-Help Group
Conditions: Addison's disease
Web: http://www.adshg.org.uk/

ALDLIFE
Conditions: Adrenoleukodystrophy and adrenomyeloneuropathy
Phone: 0208 473 7493
Email: info@aldlife.org
Web: http://aldlife.org/

Androgen Insensitivity Syndrome Support Group
Conditions: Complete and partial androgen insensitivity syndrome and related conditions (e.g. Swyer's syndrome, 5 alpha-reductase deficiency, Mayer-Rokitansky-Kuster-Hauser (MRKH) syndrome)
Web: http://www.aissg.org/

Anorchidism Support Group
Conditions: Anorchidism
Helpline: 01708 372597
Email: asguk@asg4u.org
Web: http://www.asg4u.org/

Association for Multiple Endocrine Neoplasia Disorders
Conditions: Multiple endocrine neoplasia disorders and associated endocrine growths.
Phone: 01892 516076
Email: info@amend.org.uk
Web: http://www.amend.org.uk/

British Thyroid Foundation
Conditions: Disorders of the thyroid gland
Phone: 01423 709707
Email: Via form on website
Web: http://www.btf-thyroid.org/

British Thyroid Association
Web: www.british-thyroid-association.org

Butterfly Thyroid Cancer Trust
Conditions: Thyroid cancer
Phone: 01207 545469
Email: enquiries@butterfly.org.uk
Web: http://www.butterfly.org.uk/

Child Growth Foundation
Conditions: Growth related conditions including Turner syndrome, growth hormone deficiency and premature sexual maturity
Phone: 0208 995 0257
Email: info@childgrowthfoundation.org
Web: http://www.childgrowthfoundation.org/

CLIMB (Children Living with Inherited Metabolic Conditions)
Conditions: Inherited metabolic diseases
Phone: 0800 652 3181
Email: enquiries@climb.org.uk
Web: http://www.climb.org.uk/

Living with CAH – Congenital Adrenal Hyperplasia Support Group
Conditions: Congenital Adrenal Hyperplasia
Phone: 01525 717536
Email: Via form on website
Web: http://www.livingwithcah.com/

Daisy Network
Conditions: Premature menopause
Email: daisy@daisynetwork.org.uk
Web: http//www.daisynetwork.org.uk/

Diabetes UK
Conditions: Diabetes mellitus
Phone: 0845 120 2960
Email: careline@diabetes.org.uk
Web: http://www.diabetes.org.uk/

dsdfamilies
Conditions: Disorders of sex development
Web: http://www.dsdfamilies.org/

FIPA Patients
Conditions: Familial isolated pituitary adenoma
Email: info@fipapatients.org
Web: http://www.geneticalliance.org.uk/

The Gender Trust
Web: www.gendertrust.org.uk

Genetic Alliance UK
Conditions: All genetic disorders
Web: http://www.geneticalliance.org.uk/

Hypoparathyroidism UK
Conditions: Hypoparathyroidism and other parathyroid conditions
Email: liz@hpth.org.uk
Web: http://www.hypoparathyroidism.orn.uk/

Infertility Network UK
Conditions: All conditions related to male and female fertility
Phone: 0800 008 7464
Email: admin@infertilitynetworkuk.com
Web: http://www.infertilitynetworkuk.com/

Kallman Syndrome Organisation
Conditions: Kallman's syndrome
Email: Via form on website
Web: http://www.kallmanns.org

Klinefelter's Organisation
Email: ask@klinefelter.org.uk
Web: http://www.klinefelter.org.uk/

Klinefelte's Syndrome Association
Conditions: Klinefelter's syndrome
Phone: 0845 230 0047
Email: coordinator@ksa-uk.co.uk
Web: http://www.ksa-uk.co.uk/

Men's Health Forum's
Conditions: General information on male health
Web: http://www.menshealthforum.org.uk/

National Association for Premenstrual Syndrome (NAPS)
Conditions: Premenstrual syndrome
Phone: 0844 815 7311
Email: contact@pms.org.uk
Web: http://www.pms.org.uk/

National Osteoporosis Society
Conditions: Osteoporosis
Phone: 0845 450 0230
Email: nurses@nos.org.uk
Web: http://www.nos.org.uk/

NET Patient Foundation
Conditions: Neuroendocrine tumours
Phone: 0800 434 6476
Email: Via form on website
Web: http://www.netpatientfoundation.com/

Paget's Association
Conditions: Paget's syndrome
Phone:
Email:
Web: http://www.pagets.org.uk/

Pituitary Foundation
Conditions: Disorders of the pituitary gland
Phone: 0845 450 0375
Email: helpline@pituitary.org.uk
Web: http://www.pituitary.org.uk/

Prader-Willi Syndrome Association UK
Conditions: Prader-Willi syndrome
Phone: 01332 365 676
Email: admin@pwsa.co.uk
Web: http://pwsa.co.uk

Restricted Growth Association
Conditions: Conditions which cause restricted growth
Phone: 0300 111 1970
Email: office@restrictedgrowth.co.uk
Web: http://www.restrictedgrowth.co.uk/

Sexual Advice Association
Conditions: Male and female sexual disorders
Phone: 020 7486 7262
Email: info@sexualadviceassociation.co.uk
Web: http://www.sda.uk.net/

The Gender Trust
Conditions: Gender identity
Email: info@gendertrust.org.uk
Web: http://www.gendertrust.org.uk/

Thyroid Eye Disease Charitable Trust
Conditions: Thyroid eye disease
Phone: 0844 800 8133
Email: ted@tedct.co.uk
Web: http://www.tedct.co.uk/

Turner Syndrome Support Society
Conditions: Turner syndrome
Phone: 0300 111 7520
Email: Via form on website
Web: http://www.tss.org.uk/

Unique
Conditions: Conditions caused by rare chromosome disorders
Phone: 01883 330766
Email: info@rarechromo.org
Web: http://www.rarechromo.org/

Verity (PCOS)
Conditions: Polycystic ovary syndrome
Web: http://www.verity-pcos.org.uk/

Weight Concern
Conditions: Obesity
Web: http://www.weightconcern.org.uk/

Women's Health Concern
Conditions: General information on female health
Web: http://www.womens-health-concern.org/

You & Your Hormones
Conditions: General information on endocrine conditions
Web: http://www.yourhormones.info

Index

Approximate weight conversions

kg	st	lb	kg	st	lb	kg	st	lb
0.5		1	40	6	3	75	11	11
1		2	41	6	7	76	12	0
1.5		3	42	6	8	77	12	1
2		4	43	6	11	78	12	5
2.5		6	44	6	13	79	12	6
3		7	45	7	1	80	12	8
3.5		8	46	7	3	81	12	10
4		9	47	7	6	82	12	13
4.5		10	48	7	8	83	13	1
5		11	49	7	10	84	13	3
5.5		12	50	7	13	85	13	6
6		13	51	8	0	86	13	7
			52	8	3	87	13	10
10	1	8	53	8	4	88	13	11
15	2	6	54	8	7	89	14	0
20	3	1	55	8	10	90	14	3
21	3	4	56	8	11	91	14	4
22	3	7	57	9	0	92	14	7
23	3	8	58	9	1	93	14	8
24	3	11	59	9	4	94	14	11
25	3	13	60	9	6	95	14	13
26	4	1	61	9	8	96	15	1
27	4	3	62	9	11	97	15	4
28	4	6	63	9	13	98	15	6
29	4	8	64	10	1	99	15	8
30	4	10	65	10	3	100	15	10
31	4	13	66	10	6	101	15	13
32	5	0	67	10	7	102	16	1
33	5	3	68	10	10	103	16	3
34	5	6	69	10	13	104	16	6
35	5	7	70	11	0	105	16	7
36	5	10	71	11	3	106	16	10
37	5	11	72	11	4	107	16	11
38	6	0	73	11	7	108	17	0
39	6	1	74	11	8	109	17	3

Adapted with permission from Webster-Gandy J, Madden A, and Holdsworth M (2006). Oxford Handbook of Nutrition. Oxford University Press: Oxford